The Essential Guide to Religious Traditions and Spirituality for Health Care Providers

Edited by

STEVEN L. JEFFERS, PhD

MICHAEL E. NELSON, MD

VERN BARNET, DMin

MICHAEL C. BRANNIGAN, PhD

Forewords by

PERRY A. PUGNO, MD, MPH, FAAFP, FACPE
American Academy of Family Physicians

CARL E. LUNDSTROM, MD
Mayo Clinic, Rochester, MN

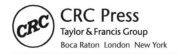

CRC Press
Taylor & Francis Group
Boca Raton London New York

CRC Press is an imprint of the
Taylor & Francis Group, an **informa** business

First published 2013 by Radcliffe Publishing Ltd

Published 2019 by CRC Press
Taylor & Francis Group
6000 Broken Sound Parkway NW, Suite 300
Boca Raton, FL 33487-2742

First issued in papaerback 2020

ISBN 13 : 978-0-367-57659-2 (pbk)
ISBN 13 : 978-1-84619-560-0 (hbk)

Visit the Taylor & Francis Web site at
http://www.taylorandfrancis.com

and the CRC Press Web site at
http://www.crcpress.com

British Library Cataloguing in Publication Data

A catalogue record for this book is available from the British Library.

Typeset by Darkriver Design, Auckland, New Zealand

Dedication

This book is dedicated to the memory of Steven L. Jeffers. He is the individual who had the idea that eventually grew into this book and without his tireless energy it would have never been completed. It was Steve who recruited the authors for almost every chapter and spent hours editing the chapters as each was received. Unfortunately, he died in an accident prior to the completion of the book and so never got to see the text in its final form. However, his spirit will continue to live on in this work.

Michael E. Nelson, MD
Vern Barnet, DMin
Michael C. Brannigan, PhD

Prologue

I would be remiss in my duty as an editor if I did not provide additional insight into how this book was "born." Steve Jeffers was a fixture in the hallways and care areas of Shawnee Mission Medical Center, always looking to provide spiritual support to the health care workers, from patient transporters to nurses to physicians to the hospital's chief executive officer. He found me one morning in the intensive care unit and, as was my wont, I was complaining about a young lady who had low blood pressure. She also had low blood counts, but would not consent to a transfusion because of her religious beliefs. I asked her if her spiritual tradition would allow for transfusion of products that did not include cells, but she did not know the answer to this. I noted to Steve that it would certainly be helpful to clinicians if there were a resource one might use that explained the restrictions of the various spiritual traditions. Steve returned a few days later and suggested that we write a "Spiritual PDR" that would be similar to the PDR (Physician's Desk Reference) for medication. I suggested that this would be a good project for *him* and that I would not have the time to participate. Those who knew Steve are aware that a "no" to him didn't really mean no. It just meant that he would ask again at a later time.

A number of weeks later I received an email asking me to review a manuscript (I don't recall which spiritual tradition), which was the initial chapter of the book. I thought I had made it clear that I couldn't participate, but I read it and made a few suggestions, thinking my work was now done. How wrong I was! In relatively rapid succession I received additional manuscripts, which I dutifully checked for "medical readability" and sent back to Steve with suggestions as to what might be of additional interest to health care personnel. This process later morphed into 5:30 a.m. or 6 a.m. meetings to review the chapters and make changes to the structure of the book. I still thought I had made it clear that I did not have time to participate. Steve would enthusiastically incorporate my suggestions and, should I recommend that an additional tradition be included (as I did with the Afro-Atlantic religions), he would find an author for that chapter, somehow convincing an individual with expertise to write it.

In the fall of 2007 it was clear that the book was well on its way to completion, and Steve requested that I provide him with a short bio as he was adding me as an editor. I explained to him that I did not want to be listed as an editor and reiterated that I did not have time to participate. In the spring of 2008, we had received initial positive responses from a publisher and Steve again requested that I send him a bio as it was important to have an editor who was a physician. Procrastination is the best weapon against persistence and I employed this as skillfully as a fencer uses his épée. Quite unexpectedly and unfortunately, Steve died in the late summer of 2008. It was agreed by all involved in the project that this book would be a fitting tribute to an individual who had invested so much time in the care of others.

I had a copy of the book on a thumb drive, which I had used during our morning editing sessions and during the evening when I made the changes we would subsequently discuss. Of course, I thought that I would be able to access all of the authors' contact information on his computer in his office in the hospital, as I did not have any of this. As there were still some chapters that had not been completed, it would be necessary to contact the authors for final revisions and addition. However, I subsequently found out that all of his communications had been deleted after his death, leaving me only with the names of the authors on the headers of their chapters. I received help from the kind people in the Spiritual Wellness section of Shawnee Mission Medical Center in getting additional contact information for many of these individuals. Some of the individuals were easily located because Steve knew them from his contacts in this area. Others were much more difficult to find, or even to identify.

One anecdote bears repeating. I was trying to contact the individual who had authored an incomplete chapter on Sufism. I was unable to find him in the local phone book and finally "googled" his contact information. Excited that I would finally get to speak with this author, I made a call, which was answered by a pleasant man whose name was on the chapter heading. I explained that I was attempting to complete the book for which he had authored a chapter and asked if he was still interested in finishing the chapter on Sufism. This was met by a protracted silence ended by a query, "What?" I repeated my introduction and again asked if he were interested in participating to which he replied, "What the hell are you talking about and what is Sufism?" I verified that his name was the same as the author's but came to find out that he was a plumber from Des Moines, Iowa, and he had never even heard of Sufism. A new author was subsequently identified. Unfortunately, similar episodes occurred with other chapters as well, resulting in a time to completion that was much longer then I had anticipated.

However, I must personally thank all of the authors who have graciously shared their knowledge and who have done so much to help bring this work to completion. In all of my communications, whether by email (now numbering over 1000), phone calls (well into the hundreds), or even snail mail (two or three folks), there has been nothing but friendly and helpful responses. While this book is dedicated to the memory of Steve Jeffers, it is important for readers to know that this project would never have existed without the gracious assistance of these many fine authors.

I would also like to thank Gillian Nineham and Jamie Etherington from Radcliffe Publishing, who have helped to move this project to completion. In addition, I would like to thank Camille Lowe of Undercover for all of her assistance, especially in keeping me on schedule. Finally, I need to thank Lore, Brad and Graham for their patience through this process.

Mike Nelson
September 2012

Table of Contents

Table of Contents

Preface

The *vision* of Shawnee Mission Medical Center's Institute for Spirituality in Health is to help create an atmosphere wherein delivery of health care occurs within an environment that values medical skills complemented by spirituality, which is often expressed in the language of faith.

The *mission* of the Institute is to facilitate collaboration among various groups to improve the physical, emotional, and spiritual health of patients and their families, while respecting every individual's faith.

In this world of ethnic, cultural, and religious pluralism, we believe people have the right to expect that their spiritual and religious traditions should be acknowledged and respected in social and professional settings. That same expectation holds true for patients in a clinical setting, who often experience "crises of faith" caused by the onset of adverse physical conditions.

In the fall of 2007, the institute initiated a new educational program for physicians, entitled "Spirituality and Faith Traditions of the World in the Healthcare Setting," at Shawnee Mission Medical Center. At the first meeting, the facilitator asked the physicians what they wanted to obtain from this series. The consensus was to learn about other faith traditions in order to be more respectful of their colleagues and supportive of their patients with spiritual traditions different from their own.

Those physicians' desire to become more knowledgeable of various spiritual and religious traditions leads us to conclude that we could all learn a great lesson from crayons for living in this world. Collectively, crayons are a vast array of different colors, but they all live harmoniously in the same box. When different-colored crayons are used in creating a piece of art, it is the combination of those colors that turns the resultant work into a beautiful masterpiece. We think it is fair to say that the world in which we live is analogous to an artist's creation. A resplendent piece of handiwork is created when various cultures, ethnic groups, and spiritual and religious traditions are woven together into a tapestry, rich with different hues, reflecting society's diversity.

It is our belief that knowledge of other cultural, ethnic, and faith traditions can enable us to be better citizens of the world in which we live and work. It can also aid in highlighting the common elements our own backgrounds share with differing traditions, and may prove to be one way of enriching our own personal culture, ethnicity, faith, and spirituality.

We also want to point out how important it is for clinicians to establish good working relationships with chaplains and other spiritual care providers in order to offer the broadest possible range of care to patients and their families.

Even though this book is lengthy and contains much information, it is impossible to provide an exhaustive resource on such a broad topic. Thus, there are religious and spiritual traditions that were not included.

We hope that future editions of the book will contain even more religions and spiritual traditions and will have a more global impact on health care.

This book would not have been possible without the commitment and hard work of many people throughout the United States and abroad who wrote the chapters on the various spiritual and religious traditions. These individuals have provided an invaluable service for the health care community. The authors of the many faith traditions contained in this volume were honored to be asked to contribute to this resource. They sincerely hope that their efforts have helped all who use this book enhance the overall care of patients.

We greatly appreciate all of you who purchased our book to use in your care of the sick and dying. All of the royalties from our publisher go to the Foundation for Shawnee Mission Medical Center for use in funding other initiatives of the Institute for Spirituality in Health.

Steven L. Jeffers, PhD
Michael E. Nelson, MD
Vern Barnet, DMin
Michael C. Brannigan, PhD
September 2012

Foreword by Perry A. Pugno, MD

For the busy health care professional of today, there are few publications that can justify a place on the office shelf, let alone be the sort of reference that would be found on every ward and in every department of a modern hospital. Yet, that is precisely the book you have picked up and are reading now.

This publication directly addresses one of the most significant unmet needs of our time. To my knowledge, this is the only resource available that can provide an unbiased, directly pertinent, and comprehensive (but still brief) summary of the core beliefs related to health, life, and death of every major spiritual belief system in the world today.

It is a well-documented reality that when people are sick or injured (and frightened), they will turn their thoughts to the spiritual side of their lives. Health care providers who can "connect" with patients and their spiritual needs during these most challenging times of their lives can not only bring added comfort to patients but also have a positive and healing impact on patients' illnesses or injuries. What health care provider wouldn't want that for patients?

In this resource, Dr. Steven Jeffers and his colleagues have compiled a comprehensive reference that should see daily use in hospitals and clinics. Using the conceptual framework of "being fully present," Dr. Jeffers has included important and useful information on every spiritual tradition from American Indian Spirituality to

Zoroastrianism. The early sections provide approach models to assist health care providers in addressing patients' spiritual needs at the most appropriate level for that individual's comfort. For each spiritual tradition or religion, the authors provide information including pertinent historical facts; basic teachings and practices; clinically useful concepts of life, illness, and death; and helpful perspectives on challenging topics such as organ donation, gender issues, and end-of-life care. Each section also includes inspirational and comforting readings and prayers from the particular religion or spiritual belief system.

I can see this book being used in a whole host of different ways. It will undoubtedly be a great resource for anyone wanting to learn more about different religious traditions or wanting to understand how best to support individual patient needs. It will be a time-saver to busy clinicians who want to quickly understand the core belief systems of their patients without having to invest in long, often stressful, conversations with the sick and scared people under their care. I can see, too, that health care facility in-service training personnel will find this a gold mine of helpful information as they plan educational programs about the patient populations their institutions serve, and risk managers will find helpful perspectives in it to assist in establishing procedures and initiatives to avoid unnecessary communication problems with patients and their families. What a great resource!

It is my sincere belief that, properly used, this book will help any health care worker, from nursing assistant to subspecialty surgeon, provide a unique kind of supportive care to their patients based in a rich understanding of that individual's particular spiritual beliefs and needs. In this era of super high-tech medicine and molecular-level therapy, how wonderful it is to finally have a resource that can help all thoughtful health care providers comfort and heal our fellow humans at this most intimate and personal level.

Perry A. Pugno, MD, MPH, FAAFP, FACPE
**Director, Division of Medical
Education
American Academy of Family
Physicians
Leawood, KS**
September 2012

Foreword by Carl E. Lundstrom, MD

As a general internist in clinical practice, I was first amazed and then enthusiastic about the potential of this volume. I have been working in the arena of the intersection of spirituality and health care for some years, first as a clinician in a religious-based hospital and more recently in a major academic medical center involved in issues of spirituality as it might apply to both the practice and the professional. The utility of this resource will be a major benefit to anyone trying to connect with and understand patients. To be involved in health care in our world now means to be holistic in approach. This book will advance many of our interactions in a complex health care system.

Just as Dr. Jeffers was led into dealing with this subject by a survey at his institution, we also have noted similar findings in researching the feelings and desires of both our patients and our staff. In our case, after obtaining 336 responses from physicians, we were impressed with the data that 85% believed that spirituality is a factor in the healing process, while 96% believed that patient's spirituality would influence medical care. In addition, 74% of physicians surveyed thought that spirituality and religion were integral parts of their own lives. Other recent studies continue to confirm this type of response. We also observe that in spite of this information, many practitioners have trouble knowing how to approach this area of care. Here in this book are many practical suggestions

about application as well as information on which to base the application.

This book is helpfully divided into two major sections. The first might appear as a prelude to the major portion of the volume conveying specific information about a very comprehensive number of faith traditions. This impression would be misleading, however. The first section may actually be more helpful to health care professionals in the way that it gives basic, well-documented information about the relevance of the rest of this book. It also helps us all in knowing how to apply all of this information. The two concepts that I found highlighted in the first section were the ideas about healing versus curing, and the concept that "Spirituality is like a river flowing through every person." Taken seriously, these ideas certainly impress us with the vital nature of this holism.

Another focus is defining spirituality and then contrasting it with religiosity. One of the immediate reactions of many of my clinical colleagues to dealing with this arena is to want to avoid it or to give it solely to the clergy for handling. The first part of this book lays a great foundation for helping us in the medical profession achieve our best relationship with patients who look to us for words that might validate some of these powers for healing that we all have within us. Some view discussing religion as divisive, but understanding not only the definition and importance of spirituality but also the approach to the patient removes some of the controversy and allows us to proceed therapeutically. Here again the first section of this book becomes extremely valuable!

The second and larger section of this book contains material that is needed to approach individuals of very diverse backgrounds. We have seen many instances of medical problems related to an incomplete understanding of a patient's milieu. A classic example would be the patient who refuses certain treatments because of the perception or the reality that the treatment violates a religious or spiritual precept. For the busy clinician, knowing something about where the patient is coming from will help to avoid such situations. Having this material organized in a manner that speeds the comprehension is even better! I was most appreciative of the fact that the material in the second section is produced by experts in the various faiths/cultures. These comments thereby have more authority and relevance than otherwise. Dr. Jeffers, however, cautions the reader about application, knowing that individuals may well have their own outlook slightly at variance with authorities even in their own tradition.

Thanks to the production of this book, we will all be much more able to connect with our patients and assist in the healing process. I am anticipating the daily usefulness of this material on my desk! I laud Dr. Jeffers and all his collaborators in their efforts to help us all!

Carl E. Lundstrom, MD
Consultant, Division of General
Internal Medicine
Chair, Spirituality in Healthcare
Committee
Mayo Clinic
Rochester, MN
September 2012

Reasons For and How to Use This Book

It is the patient's religious or spiritual beliefs that are to be supported or encouraged, not the beliefs of the doctor or other health professional.[1]

This resource is intended as a guide for health care professionals to enable them to provide optimal care of patients. However, the reader should not assume that specific spiritual care interventions listed in the Seventh-Day Adventist, Hinduism, or Bahá'í sections, for example, would be appropriate to utilize in the care of every patient of those respective traditions. To assume that would be *standardizing* care based on a certain model. The goal of providing spiritual care is that it be *individualized* to a particular patient. This book can prove invaluable in accomplishing individualized care if used correctly. For instance, if you have a patient who is a Scientologist, you might say something like, "I know that some Scientologists have been comforted by touch assists; would that be helpful for you?" By adopting this approach, you have utilized the material in the text, but did not presume all Scientologists would benefit from the same intervention, thereby individualizing the plan of care by involving the patient. Many patients and their families will be favorably impressed that you are knowledgeable of their particular faith tradition.

Reasons for this Book

Why is a book on how to provide spiritual care for people in a clinical setting important? An overarching reason relates to the World Health Organization's (WHO) definition of health cited in the preamble to its constitution adopted in 1946: "Health is a state of complete physical, mental and social wellbeing and not merely the absence of disease or infirmity."[2] Even though spirituality is not in this definition, it indicates that health is more encompassing than its relationship to the physical. Furthermore, the role of spirituality in health did not experience its "revival" in the medical community until the latter half of the twentieth century. However, the role of spirituality in health became part of an ongoing discussion among WHO members in the 1970s culminating in a proposal from a special group of the WHO Executive Board that the preamble to the 1946 constitution be amended to read: "Health is a dynamic state of complete physical, mental, spiritual and social well-being and not merely

---

[2] Citation from the Preamble to the Constitution of the World Health Organization, July 22, 1946. (The Avalon Project at Yale Law School, available at: www.yale.edu/lawweb/avalon/decade/decad051.htm).

---

[1] Koenig, H. (2002). *Spirituality in Patient Care*. Philadelphia, PA: Templeton Foundation Press, 57.

the absence of disease or infirmity."[3] The preamble was not changed, but the discussion of spirituality as it relates to health continues in medical communities around the globe. Other reasons for the value of such a book are outlined in the following paragraphs.

One reason relates to the facility itself – the hospital.

- A hospital is a **place of celebration**: Healthy babies are born; broken bones are mended; symptoms that generate fear are diagnosed as benign; pains are stilled. Hope abounds. God's goodness is apparent, or so it seems.
- A hospital is a **place of sorrow**: Babies are born dead or deformed; feared symptoms are confirmed. Hope is dashed. God is distant, or so it seems.
- A hospital is a **place of precision**: "As we suspected, you have an infected gall bladder. I can schedule you for surgery tomorrow, and you should be out of here by the end of the week."
- A hospital is a **place of disappointing imprecision**: "We're just not sure what's causing all this."

In sum, a hospital is a place of joy and sadness, of life and death. People are born in a hospital; people are cured in a hospital; people die in a hospital. The beautiful and ugly seem to occur in hospitals. For many people, the very thought of being in a hospital for even "routine, non-life-threatening procedures" produces anxiety and fear which can result in a "crisis of faith."

A second reason this book is important relates to the people served by a hospital – the patients – and how they are perceived and/or treated by clinicians. Many physicians were trained in the "biotechnical model" of medicine, which views the patient as a single-dimensional entity. Thus, healing is perceived as correcting a biological dysfunction. Unfortunately, in the modern health care environment, people can get lost in the sophistication of technology and the focus on physical healing. However, patients are far more complex. They are people comprised of body, mind, spirit, and stories/memories who have some form of illness that affects all aspects of the multidimensional whole. The various aspects of a patient are interdependent, interrelated links that are weakened with the onset of illness. Illness, then, can be understood as brokenness with loss of integration in various aspects of wholeness:

- **Physical**: symptoms, signs, dysfunction
- **Mental**: deficient understanding of cause and effect
- **Emotional**: suffering, fear, anger, hurt, loss, grief
- **Social**: relationships – expectations, practices, roles
- **Spiritual**: meaning and purpose of life, future, hope, guilt, God.

Based on this perspective of the makeup of a patient, an appropriate plan of care must include an in-depth diagnosis of the whole person. Who was the patient before the illness – physically, mentally, emotionally, socially, spiritually? Who is the patient now in these same areas? How does the patient see self? What are the perceived changes? How does the patient respond to these changes? What does the patient anticipate with "healing?" Who will the patient then be? Is that future self-picture realistic?[4]

---

3   World Health Organization. (1997). Review of the Constitution http://apps.who.int/gb/archive/pdf_ files/EB101/pdfangl/angr2.pdf (accessed 4 Sept 2012).

---

4   Jeffers, S. (2001). *Finding a Sacred Oasis in Illness.*

A third reason for the importance of this book is to help health care institutions excel in spiritual care of patients and, thus, comply with policies for accreditation. The Joint Commission on Accreditation of Health Care Organizations (JCAHO) has "Standards" and "Elements of Performance" within those standards that reference spiritual care. "Each patient has a right to have his or her cultural, psychosocial, spiritual and personal values, beliefs and preferences respected." Because of this, "The hospital accommodates the right to pastoral and other spiritual services for patients."[5]

A fourth reason for the importance of this book is that research supports the view that patient spirituality enhances patient well-being and this view is also supported by health care providers. A growing body of literature that highlights the results of many of those studies suggested that a healthy spirituality prevents illness, helps in coping with illness and improves treatment outcomes.[6]

A fifth reason for the importance of this book is that patients and their families have the right to expect that their faith traditions and spirituality will be acknowledged, respected and nurtured. Not that many years ago, fulfilling those expectations was much easier than it is today because there was greater religious homogeneity than is present in the twenty-first century. The religious and spiritual pluralism in modern US society makes the practice of providing spiritual care and support much more difficult. The vast majority of health care providers, including chaplains, are not conversant with a wide array of religions and spiritual practices, and yet people embracing this diversity of faith traditions present themselves daily for services in hospitals.

A sixth reason for the importance of this book is to emphasize the "bridge between faith and medicine" concept concerning one of the most emotionally charged issues in modern health care – honoring patient requests in withholding/withdrawing life support in medically futile situations. The American Medical Association issued a statement regarding this matter to the United States Supreme Court in 1996.

The right to control one's medical treatment is among the most important rights that the law affords each person. [We] strongly support the recognition and enforcement of that right. Health care professionals are committed to their ethical and legal obligations to honor patient requests to withhold or withdraw unwanted life-prolonging treatment and to provide patients with all medication necessary to alleviate physical pain, even in such circumstances where such medication might hasten death. Through these means, patients can avoid entrapment in a prolonged, painful, or overly medicalized dying process.[7]

Overland Park, KS: Leathers Publishing, 1.

5   Joint Commission on Accreditation of Health Care Organizations. (2007). *Comprehensive Accreditation Manual for Hospitals: The Official Handbook (CAMH)*. Oakbrook Terrace, IL: Joint Commission Resources. Standard RI.2.10 and Element of Performance for RI.2.10 (2,4); Standard PC 2.20 (4); Standard PC.3.120 (2); Standard PC.8.70 and Element of Performance PC.8.70 (1,2).

6   Mueller, P. S., D. J. Plevak, and T. A. Rummans. (2001). Religious involvement, spirituality and medicine: implications for clinical practice. *Mayo Clinic Proceedings*, 76(12), 1225–1235. Mueller and his colleagues conducted a literature search and found that the overwhelming majority of over 1200 studies on spirituality in health indicated a positive relationship between spiritualty and better health outcomes.

7   *Washington v. Glucksburg*, No. 96–110, Supreme Court of the United States, Brief of the American Medical Association, et al. as Amici Curiae (November 12, 1996), 1. Quote excerpted

Furthermore, according to the Society of Critical Care Medicine, attention to patient spirituality is essential for optimal end-of-life care. In a March, 2008 article in *Critical Care Medicine*, Robert D. Truog, MD, et al. state:

> Spirituality plays an important role in how critically ill patients and clinicians cope with illness and death ... Each person's understanding of spirituality should be explored. Assessment of spiritual needs is not the exclusive domain of the chaplain but is part of the role of critical care clinicians, who should possess fundamental skills in spiritual assessment and referral.[8]

Daniel Sulmasy, MD, broadens the scope to include physicians in general: "If physicians value their patients as persons, they have an obligation of being respectful of what is important to them. To ignore the religious beliefs of a religious patient is to ignore the patient."[9]

Throughout the pages of this book in virtually every faith tradition discussed, there is a constant refrain: "withholding/withdrawing life support does not violate the teachings of the faith; it is an individual decision." The actual wording contained in the "Specific Medical Issues" sections of each of the various religious traditions in this volume might differ from these, but the message is consistent.

Thus, medicine and religion agree that death is a natural part of the human experience and "extraordinary" measures should not be used to "prolong" the dying process.

How to Use this Book

This resource is a user-friendly, comprehensive reference book containing specific and detailed information about multiple faith traditions that is important for health care personnel to be aware of in order to provide optimal spiritual care in a clinical setting.

The book begins with several introductory chapters. The Introduction sets the stage with a story of a physician/patient encounter, historical overview of spirituality in medicine and rationale for the book based on data from research. That is followed by chapters on Spirituality and Religion: An Overview of Three Families of Faith; Spirituality, Religion, and Culture; Spirituality and Religion: Relevance in the Clinical Setting?; Spirituality and Religion in the Clinical Setting: Pros and Cons; and Spiritual Care in the Clinical Setting: Assessment and Application. The overarching principles contained in these chapters are important for clinicians to keep in mind when utilizing the material contained in the faith-specific sections.

The majority of the book's contents is a compilation of articles, authored by people throughout the United States: from American Indian Spirituality to Zoroastrianism – a literal A–Z compendium. Many chapters conclude with a section on special days of the particular religious and/or spiritual tradition and a glossary of terms. The writers and reviewers of each essay are experts in the respective subject matter; this is evident in the annotated biographical information

---

from Colby, W. (2006). *Unplugged*. New York: AMACOM, 195.

8   Truog, R., M. L. Campbell, J. R. Curtis, et al.; for American Academy of Critical Care Medicine. (2008). Recommendations for end-of-life care in the intensive care unit: a consensus statement by the American Academy of Critical Care Medicine. *Critical Care Medicine*, 36(3), 955.

9   Sulmasy, D. (1997). *The Healer's Calling*. Mahwah, NJ: Paulist Press, 60.

contained in the "About the Contributors" section.

All of the belief-specific sections conform to the same format for purposes of standardization and user-friendliness. The outline of the content of each document is as follows:
- History and Facts
- Basic Teachings
- Basic Practices
- Principles for Clinical Care
  - Dietary Issues
  - General Medical Beliefs
  - Specific Medical Issues
  - Gender and Personal Issues.
- Principles for Spiritual Care through the Cycles of Life
  - Concepts of Living and Dying for Spiritual Support
  - During Birth
  - During Illness
  - During End of Life
  - Care of the Body
  - Organ and Tissue Donation
  - Scriptures, Inspirational Readings, and Prayers.

The first three sections – History and Facts, Basic Teachings, and Basic Practices – are intended to provide some general information about the particular belief and/or give the clinician some background of the faith that may facilitate understanding of information in subsequent sections. With respect to the user-friendliness aspect, if a clinician needs information about a specific religious tradition's teachings on the use of blood products or life support in medically futile scenarios, he or she can consult "Specific Medical Issues" in the "Principles for Clinical Care" portion of that faith-specific section. The same would be true of the need for information about

dietary or gender issues. If there is a need for information about spiritual care issues at birth, during illness, at end of life, care of the body and/or organ or tissue donation, the health care provider would consult the "Principles for Spiritual Care through the Cycles of Life" section.

Throughout the text, we have sought "lay friendly" explanations for non-English terms and concepts. We asked each of the faith-specific section authors to presuppose no knowledge of the particular faith on the part of the intended audience. Our purpose in making that request was to produce an easily understandable and useful resource. In keeping with that goal, we have tried to avoid including scholarly debates and nuances in what we intend as a practical reference work for health care providers. Our summaries of the various faiths have been written with that purpose in mind and should not be regarded as statements with which all authorities or members of any particular faith will agree. We recognize that regional and global variations exist within all spiritual traditions and that all of these are not addressed within this work. However, we hope that this book will motivate the user to research additional resources if discrepancies are identified. Also, we recognize that some traditions may have been excluded and we apologize, but this was not done willfully.

The principal reason for the writing of this book is that attention to people's spiritual well-being (or distress) is an important component of whole person care, especially during difficult times of illness and the approach of death. We believe that this type of support can best happen when a multidisciplinary approach (chaplains, physicians, nurses, social workers, and other members of the health care team) is applied.

Finally, we sincerely hope that the utilization of this resource will, at least in some small way, contribute to the actualization of that goal.

About the Editors

Steven L. Jeffers, PhD, was the founder and director of the Institute for Spirituality in Health at Shawnee Mission Medical Center, a regional medical center in the suburbs of Kansas City. He received a Bachelor of Arts in religion from Palm Beach Atlantic College, a Master of Divinity from Midwestern Baptist Theological Seminary with a concentration in Greek and New Testament and a Doctor of Philosophy in the Program in the Humanities from Florida State University, where he studied the Greco-Roman Classics, Bible and world religions.

Prior to his current work, Dr. Jeffers was a seminary professor with extensive experience in faith congregational ministry. In his role with the Institute, he worked with physicians, other health care providers, and civic, business, and religious leaders of various faith traditions to advocate for the effective, compassionate care of patients and families and the integration of spirituality into the practice of medicine. He gave leadership for the implementation of the institute's initiatives to provide lay and professional education, publications and research on the relationship of spirituality and health care. He was an author of several books along with the publication of articles in peer-reviewed journals.

Dr. Jeffers was a frequent lecturer in medical and nursing schools, hospitals, businesses, graduate seminaries and faith communities of various traditions. He organized conferences for health care professionals and clergy on spirituality in health care topics and spoke at end-of-life care coalitions throughout the United States. He was also active in interfaith dialogue and spoke about how to provide spiritual care for patients of various faith traditions in a clinical setting to physicians, other health care providers and students. Finally, Dr. Jeffers developed and implemented a program at Shawnee Mission Medical Center of bringing physicians and clergy together for monthly meetings of informal dialogue related to enhancing the well-being of patients, families, health care providers, and faith communities. Tragically, he died in a motor vehicle accident in August 2008.

Michael E. Nelson, MD, is a physician practicing at Shawnee Mission Medical Center in Merriam, Kansas. He received his undergraduate training in chemistry and molecular biology at the University of Colorado. He attended medical school at the University of Kansas where he also completed his residency in internal medicine. This was followed by a fellowship in pulmonary and critical care medicine at the same institution. He has his board certification in internal medicine, pulmonary diseases, critical care medicine, and sleep medicine. Dr. Nelson served as the inaugural chairman of the Institute for Spirituality in Health and lectured with Dr. Jeffers on end-of-life care. He is the author of several book chapters as well as journal articles and abstracts pertaining to his areas of medical expertise, but this is his first foray into literature involving spirituality.

The Reverend Vern Barnet, DMin, completed his doctoral work at the University of Chicago and Meadville-Lombard Theological School in 1970. Honored by Buddhist, Christian, Jewish, Hindu, Muslim, Sikh, and other groups, he has taught world religions at several universities and seminaries. Since 1994, he has been a religion columnist for the *Kansas City Star*, and his articles and reviews have appeared in many national publications.

After international interfaith work, he organized the Kansas City Interfaith Council in 1989, with 13 faiths, from American Indian to Zoroastrian. Following 9/11 he led the region's unprecedented "Gifts of Pluralism" conference, which fostered interfaith initiatives featured on a half-hour CBS-TV special. Among his many civic activities, he chaired the Jackson County government's Diversity Task Force that studied the effects of 9/11 on people of faith in the five-county Kansas City area.

His interfaith work led to Kansas City being chosen as the site for the nation's first "Interfaith Academies," sponsored by Harvard University's Pluralism Project, Religions for Peace-USA, and other groups. Ellie Pierce, principal researcher for the Pluralism Project, said: "At the Pluralism Project, we consider Kansas City to be truly at the forefront of interfaith relations. This is – in no small part – due to the tireless efforts of Vern Barnet, whose work and writings have been an inspiration to all of us at the Pluralism Project."

With great affection, he remembers the originator of this book, the Reverend Steven L. Jeffers, PhD, who attracted him and others of many faiths in developing the Institute for Spirituality in Health at Shawnee Mission Medical Center.

Michael C. Brannigan, PhD (Philosophy), MA (Religious Studies, University of Leuven, Belgium) is the George and Jane Pfaff Endowed Chair in Ethics and Moral Values at The College of Saint Rose in Albany, New York. He holds the first endowed chair in the college's history. He is also part of the Alden March Bioethics Institutes' Core Teaching Faculty at Albany Medical College. His specialties lie in ethics, intercultural ethics, medical ethics, and Asian philosophy. Along with numerous articles, his books include: *Everywhere and Nowhere*; *The Pulse of Wisdom: The Philosophies of India, China, and Japan*; *Healthcare Ethics in a Diverse Society* (co-authored); *Ethical Issues in Human Cloning* (ed.); *Cross-Cultural Biotechnology*; and *Ethics Across Cultures*. His most recent books are his revised edition of *Striking a Balance: A Primer on Traditional Asian Values*, and the newly published *Cultural Fault Lines in Healthcare: Reflections on Cultural Competency*. Prior to coming to Albany, he was Vice President for Clinical and Organizational Ethics at the Center for Practical Bioethics in Kansas City, Missouri. Before that, he was Executive Director and founder of the Institute for Cross-Cultural Ethics at La Roche College, Pittsburgh, Pennsylvania, where he was also Professor of Philosophy and department Chair. He chairs the Association for Practical and Professional Ethics Diversity Committee, and serves on the editorial boards of *Health Care Analysis: An International Journal of Health Care Philosophy and Policy* and *Communication and Medicine*. He writes a monthly column on ethics for the Albany, New York, *Times Union* newspaper; see www.timesunion.com/brannigan/. For fun, he plays piano, ocean kayaks, and practices martial arts.

About the Contributors

African American Baptist/Protestantism

Pastor L. Henderson Bell has served the Mt. Pleasant Missionary Baptist Church of Kansas City, Missouri, for the past 26 years. During his tenure of ministry at Mt. Pleasant Baptist Church, he has served in multiple community roles, one of which was President of the Kansas City Baptist Ministers Union. He also served as Vice President to the Missouri State organization of Baptist Ministers. He was the transitional president of the Progressive National Baptist Convention Mid-West Region. He also served as a Vice-President at large with the Progressive National Baptist Convention, performing ministerial task to the several constituent churches of the Progressive National Baptist Convention, Inc. on a national level. Pastor Bell served for 17 years as the homiletics instructor at Western Baptist Bible College. He is a regular on the teaching circuit of the Progressive National Baptist convention and has traveled to London, England, Nassau Bahamas, and many other areas for the promotion of the Progressive National Baptist Convention's philosophy of unified religion.

African Methodist Episcopal Church (AME)

Rev. Natalie Mitchem is an ordained Itinerant Elder in the African Methodist Episcopal Church. She has a Master of Divinity degree from Lutheran Theological Seminary in Philadelphia, Pennsylvania, and a Bachelor of Science Degree from North Carolina Central University in Durham, North Carolina. She is the First Episcopal District Health Commission Coordinator appointed by Bishop Richard F. Norris. The First Episcopal District Health Commission coordinates a comprehensive wellness and health program for pastors and churches located in New Jersey, Pennsylvania, Delaware, New York, and Bermuda. The churches in the First Episcopal District partner with local health resources and provide health information and health screenings on an annual basis within the AME churches. The Health Commission is dedicated to ministering to mind, body, and spirit.

American Indian Spirituality

Kara Hawkins is Secretary of the Greater Kansas City Interfaith Council and the American Indian Spirituality faith member. She is a board member of the Institute for Spirituality in Health at Shawnee Mission Medical Center in Shawnee Mission, Kansas, and participates in its monthly physician/clergy dialogues. Ministerial trainer (1995) and faculty member (2003) of the Alliance of Divine Love, Inc., she writes a monthly column for its international newsletter, *Dayspring: Kara's Korner – American Indian Spirituality.*

Jimm G. GoodTracks is author of numerous manuscripts and books relating to the language, culture, and spirituality of the Ioway-Otoe-Missouria people, including the

Iowa-Otoe-Missouria Language Dictionary (University of Colorado, Center for the Study of the Languages of the Plains and Southwest, Boulder, 1992), a comprehensive glossary-style dictionary providing over 9000 words, phrases, and sentences as rendered by elders who spoke it as their first language. An enhanced encyclopedic edition is available in an onsite edition at the Kansas State Historical Society Library archives. He has been the recipient of various grants to expand the language projects, including a 2007–2009 grant from the National Science Foundation, DEL (Documenting Endangered Languages), Washington, DC. He is now retired as a professional MSW licensed social worker. He holds a Master of Social Welfare degree from the University of Kansas, Lawrence, Kansas.

Amish

Linda L. Graham has passed since this writing. She was an Associate Professor of Nursing at Indiana University–Purdue University Fort Wayne. She received a master's degree in community health nursing from Indiana University–Indianapolis, and was a doctoral candidate in Education through Purdue University. Linda worked in various nursing roles with the Old Order Amish beginning in 1985, and she published and presented on both cultural and nursing issues with this population.

James A. Cates is a board-certified clinical psychologist in practice in northeast Indiana. He is Coordinator of Special Projects for the Amish Youth Vision Project, a program that teams with Amish parents, clergy, and lay leaders to address alcohol and drug use among Amish teens. James also publishes and presents on both

cultural and psychological issues with this population.

Any merit this work possesses is primarily the product of a number of members of the Amish community who consistently provide their support and encouragement. Because of their humility, they prefer not to be named, and we reluctantly comply.

Note on Amish, Brethren in Christ, Church of the Brethren, Hutterite, and Mennonite documents: Donald B. Kraybill, who received his Doctor of Philosophy in sociology from Temple University, has reviewed these sections. Kraybill served as chair of the sociology and social work department at Elizabethtown College from 1979 to 1985 and directed the Young Center from 1989 to 1996. He was provost of Messiah College (PA) from 1996 to 2002, and then returned to Elizabethtown College in 2003. Nationally recognized for his scholarship on Anabaptist groups, Kraybill is the author or editor of more than 18 books and dozens of professional articles. His books have been translated into six different languages. Kraybill's research on Anabaptist groups has been featured in magazines, newspapers, and on radio and television programs across the United States and in many foreign countries. He has served as a consultant for various projects related to Amish and other Anabaptist groups. The National Endowment for the Humanities and various private foundations have supported his research projects. Kraybill is the editor of the Johns Hopkins University Press's series Young Center Books in Anabaptist and Pietist Studies.

Assemblies of God
Emanuel Williams retired in 2009 from serving as the Healthcare Chaplaincy

Representative for the General Council of the Assemblies of God (AG). In this role he provided oversight for the 130 AG health care chaplains serving in hospitals, nursing homes, and hospices throughout the United States. He was appointed to this position in 2002 following 17 years as hospital chaplain at Georgia Baptist Medical Center in Atlanta, Georgia. Rev. Williams attended the University of California. Following his graduation, he entered the army as an infantry second lieutenant and served for 28 years, which included two tours in Vietnam. Upon his retirement from the army as a lieutenant colonel, Rev. Williams sensed a call to ministry and completed a Master of Divinity degree at Emory University. Subsequently, he served as a chaplain at Georgia Baptist Medical Center and as associate pastor at three local AG churches. He is currently a member of Tabernacle AG, where he teaches the adult Sunday School class and serves as the church pianist.

Alvin F. Worthley has served as Director of Chaplaincy Ministries since August 2002. Chaplain Worthley oversees the ministries of over 446 chaplains in various settings throughout the world. Chaplain Worthley was born in Sherburn, Minnesota, and graduated from North Central Bible College. He received his Master of Divinity from Trinity Evangelical Divinity School and is presently working on his Doctorate of Ministry from Regent University. He is an ordained Assemblies of God minister with the Potomac District. Prior to his current position, Chaplain Worthley was Assistant Administrator of Chaplaincy Services for the Federal Bureau of Prisons in Washington, DC. He also served as chaplain at the Federal Bureau of Prisons in Springfield, Missouri, from 1981 to 1989 and pastored from 1965 to 1977. Chaplain Worthley has been an advisory board member of the Billy Graham Institute for Prison Ministry from 1991 to 1996 and Vice President of the American Protestant Correctional Chaplains Association.

Bahá'í Faith

Barb McAtee has been a member of the Bahá'í Faith for 40 years. For most of those years, she has served as a member of a local Bahá'í Spiritual Assembly in various locations. She also served at the National Bahá'í Center for 2 years. Since 1993, she has devoted much time and energy to interfaith activities. This began when she became inspired to found a campus organization, *KUMC Interfaith*, at the University of Kansas Medical Center in Kansas City, Kansas. For 10 years, weekly meetings were held at lunchtime, featuring speakers from a wide diversity of faiths. In 1995, she was invited to serve on the Greater Kansas City Interfaith Council, to which she still belongs. She also serves on the board of the Institute for Spirituality in Health of Shawnee Mission Medical Center in Merriam, Kansas.

David Edalati, MD, is a fourth-generation Bahá'í, who came to the United States in 1977, prior to the Iranian Islamic Revolution. He served as a member of Kansas City, Kansas Bahá'í Local Spiritual Assembly. He attended Lawrence High School, graduated from Kansas University, obtained his medical degree from the University of Kansas School of Medicine, and completed residency in Internal Medicine at University of Missouri at Kansas City. He is in practice in Internal Medicine, and he specializes in wound care and hyperbaric medicine. He is a wound care consultant at Shawnee Mission Medical Center and is on staff at St. Luke's South, Overland Park Regional Medicine, Providence Medical Center, Specialty Hospital of Mid America, Select Specialty Hospital, and Mid America Rehabilitation Hospital. He is the past medical director of Specialty Hospital and complex.

Baptists

C. Michael Fuhrman received his undergraduate degree from Southwest Baptist University and a Master of Divinity degree and PhD in New Testament from the Southern Baptist Theological Seminary in Louisville, Kentucky. He has served in the local church as a pastor for over 20 years, and since 1998 has served as Professor of Christian Studies at Southwest Baptist University in Bolivar, Missouri. He is a member of the Society of Biblical Literature and the Association of Ministry Guidance Professionals.

Brethren in Christ

Samuel M. Brubaker is a descendant of one of the founders of the Brethren in Christ. Born in 1939, he was raised in the Brethren in Christ culture of Lancaster County, Pennsylvania. His parents engaged in farming, and were active supporters and lay participants in the activities and ministries of the Brethren in Christ. After 3 years' study at the Brethren in Christ institution Messiah College, Brubaker completed his baccalaureate degree at Elizabethtown College. He then entered the University of Pennsylvania, School of Medicine, from which he graduated in 1964. Following 1 year of internship at Philadelphia General Hospital, he practiced general medicine for 4 years, including 3 years' missionary service at Navajo Brethren in Christ Hospital in New Mexico. Residency training in

General Surgery at Presbyterian Hospital, Philadelphia, was 1969–73. He practiced surgery full time in Ohio from 1973 to 2002. He is a Diplomate of the American Board of Surgery, and a Fellow of the American College of Surgeons. Brubaker has been active in the Brethren in Christ denomination. He has served as teacher, deacon, and congregational secretary; he was member of Regional Conference Board of Directors and Stewardship Commission, and served as regional representative to Great Lakes division of Mennonite Central Committee; he served the General Conference on its Board for Missions, Board of Administration, Commission on Stewardship, Board of Brotherhood Concerns and as denominational representative to the Social Action Commission of the National Association of Evangelicals. Semiretired from the practice of surgery, Brubaker now lives in Mechanicsburg, Pennsylvania.

Buddhism (Mahāyāna)

Guy McCloskey is a 40-year practitioner of Nichiren Buddhism within the Soka Gakkai tradition. He has fulfilled multiple organizational roles within the most diverse Buddhist community in the United States and is currently responsible for all Soka Gakkai International-USA publications, including the *Living Buddhism* bi-monthly study magazine, *World Tribune* weekly newspaper, and books such as the best-selling *The Buddha in Your Mirror* and *The Buddha Next Door: Ordinary People, Extraordinary Stories*. He is an active member of the Buddhism Section of the American Academy of Religion and the Society for Buddhist-Christian Studies.

Clark Strand is Contributing Editor to *Tricycle: The Buddhist Review*. He is a former

Zen Buddhist monk and the author of *Seeds from a Birch Tree: Writing Haiku and the Spiritual Journey* and *The Wooden Bowl: Simple Meditation for Everyday Life* (both from Hyperion). In 1996, he left his position as Senior Editor of *Tricycle: The Buddhist Review* to write and teach full-time. He now lives in Woodstock, NY, where he leads the Koans of the Bible Study Group.

Buddhism (Theravada)

Kongsak Tanphaichitr, MD, FACP, FRCP(C), FACR, FAAAAI, is Professor of Clinical Medicine, Washington University in St. Louis, Missouri. He is a practicing physician and is board certified in rheumatology, allergy and immunology, and internal medicine. Kongsak is Treasurer of Thai American-Physicians Foundation. He is also Chairman of the Buddhist Council of Greater St. Louis and Secretary, Wat Phrasriratanaram, Buddhist Temple of Greater St. Louis. Kongsak is the author of the books *Buddhism Answers Life* and *Essence of Life: Mindfulness and Self-Awareness*. In 2008, he was awarded the Dharma Wheel Pillar by H.R.H. Princess Sirindhorn of Thailand for propagating Buddhism to the World. Born in Thailand to a devout Buddhist family, Kongsak has had a life-long interest in Buddhism. He was once ordained as a Theravada Buddhist monk in 1967, with H.H. Somdej Phra Nyanasamvara, the Supreme Patriarch of Thailand, as his preceptor. He has been practicing the Four Foundations of Mindfulness for many years, with particular attention to the Self-Awareness technique through practicing the Dynamic Meditation of Luangpor Teean.

Buddhism (Background and Vajrayana)

Chuck Stanford is an ordained Lama within the Tibetan Buddhist tradition. His 20-year course of study has included multiple trips to Dharamsala, India where he received teachings from H.H. Dalai Lama and to Golok, Tibet. Lama Stanford is cofounder of the Rime Buddhist Center, where he serves as Executive Director. In his role as the Center's spiritual leader, he teaches classes on meditation and Buddhism and performs Buddhist ceremonies, including weddings and funerals. Lama Stanford is the Buddhist member for the Greater Kansas City Interfaith Council. In addition, he has written a monthly column on Buddhism for the religion section of the *Kansas City Star* newspaper since 1995. In 1998 after doing extensive research in Dharamsala, India, he wrote an article on Tibetan Medicine that was published in the *Kansas City Star*. He has also written other freelance articles on Buddhism and Tibetan culture. He has written a book entitled *Basics of Buddhism*, which is used as a study guide by the Rime and other Buddhist Centers. Lama Stanford serves on a number of boards, including Greater Kansas City Interfaith council; Harmony; Board of Bioethics for the Kansas City University of Medicine and Bioethics; Shawnee Mission Medical Center's Institute for Spirituality in Health board; Friends of the Department of Religious Studies at the University of Kansas; and Missouri Department of Corrections Religious Programming Advisory Council. In addition, he works as a part-time chaplain at the United States Disciplinary Barracks at Fr. Leavenworth.

Teri Brody, MD, is a board-certified physician in Family Practice after training at the University of Kansas Medical Center. As Associate Professor of Family Medicine at the University of Kansas Medical Center, she maintained active patient care practice as well as training medical students in clinical care of diverse patient population and problems. She later joined a five-physician, private family medicine practice based in Olathe, KS, with active privileges at four local hospitals. Her teaching and clinical practice emphasized the whole patient within context of family and community. Dr. Brody has been a Tibetan Buddhist rime practitioner for 30 years, studying with multiple lamas from all four schools of Tibetan Buddhism. She sponsored a Shambhala Dharma Center in home for a year before becoming a founding board member and regular participant at the Rime Buddhist Center. She is a 9-year senior Dharma teacher of all aspects of Tibetan Buddhism at the Rime Buddhist Center and periodic guest speaker at regular weekly services. She teaches basic Dharma principles for everyday life for practitioners of all faiths.

Catholic and Protestant General Introductions

Robert E. Johnson, PhD, is Professor of Church History at Central Baptist Theological Seminary in Shawnee, Kansas, and also teaches Christian Theology at Rockhurst Jesuit University in Kansas City, Missouri. He is a minister with the American Baptist Churches, USA, and previously taught at colleges in Brazil and Russia. He is also editor of the *American Baptist Quarterly*, a journal of history and theology published by the American Baptist Historical Society.

Catholic (Eastern Rite)

Paul Hura, MD, is a first-generation Ukrainian American who was born in South Dakota and then moved to Chicago as a young child. He is a cradle Eastern Rite Catholic. Hura earned a Bachelor of Arts degree in political science and a Doctor of Medicine in 1996. After marrying, he moved to Kansa City in 1999, where he practices medicine and raises a family. Hura and his family are members of St. Michael the Archangel Catholic Parish in Overland Park, Kansas.

Catholic (Roman Catholicism)

Rev. Jerry L. Spencer, MA, BCETS, BCECR, BCSM, BCBT, Diplomate in AAET, received his Bachelor of Arts and Master of Arts degrees from St. Thomas Seminary in Denver, Colorado. Father Spencer is the parish priest at Holy Name Catholic Church in Kansas City, Kansas. For 40 years, Father Spencer has been the Catholic Chaplain at the University of Kansas Medical Center/University of Kansas Hospital, a Level 1 Trauma Center, where he has ministered to hundreds of individuals and their families in times of crisis and trauma. He received his Clinical Pastoral Education at clinical sites affiliated with the Menninger Foundation in Topeka. He is also a member of the Mental Health Subcommittee of the Red Cross under the Department of Homeland Security.

Christian Church (Disciples of Christ)

Rev. Quentin B. Jones received a Bachelor of Arts degree from the University of Arizona in Tucson, Arizona, in 1971 and a Master of Divinity degree from Austin Presbyterian Theological Seminary in Austin, Texas, in 1974. Jones was ordained to ministry in the Christian Church (Disciples of Christ) at Central Christian Church, Corpus Christi, Texas, on November 16, 1975. He was also endorsed as a chaplain by the Christian Church (Disciples of Christ) in 1989 after completing an internship and four quarters of Clinical Pastoral Education at Memorial

Medical Center in Corpus Christi, Texas. Jones has served Disciples' churches in Associate Pastor and Senior Pastor positions from 1975 to 2001. During that time, he also served as a volunteer chaplain in hospitals and for fire and police departments. From 2001 to the present, Jones serves as chaplain and Ethics Committee chairman for Lakeview village, an adult retirement community with a skilled nursing facility, in Lenexa, Kansas.

Christian Science

Philip G. Davis, is the Manager of the Committee on Publication for The First Church of Christ, Scientist in Boston. In this role, he directs the work of a worldwide team of individuals who work with local media and their governments to provide accurate information about Christian Science and to make sure the public has continued access to the practice of Christian Science in law. Phil has been a professional Christian Science practitioner for over 20 years. He is also one of about 200 authorized Christian Science teachers in the world. Prior to his current position, Phil has held numerous other positions for his church, some of which are Committee on Publication (Church spokesperson) for Illinois from 1989 to 1993; manager of the church's federal office in Washington, DC, from 1993 to 1998 representing the church to Congress, the government, and the White House; manager of Christian Science Practitioners and Christian Science Nurse Activities at Church headquarters in Boston from 1998 to 2001, holding hundreds of interviews, meetings, and workshops with practitioners and nurses around the world.

Christianity General Introduction

Dr. Molly T. Marshall is an ordained minister in the American Baptist Churches denomination. She holds a Bachelor of Arts from Oklahoma Baptist University, and Master of Divinity and Doctor of Philosophy degrees from The Southern Baptist Theological Seminary in Louisville, Kentucky. Further graduate work was completed at Tantur Ecumenical Institute in Jerusalem, Israel, Cambridge University in Cambridge, England and Princeton Theological Seminary in Princeton, New Jersey. Marshall began her career in theological education in the early 1980s as a theology professor at The Southern Baptist Theological Seminary. She is currently President and Professor of Theology and Spiritual Formation at Central Baptist Theological Seminary in Shawnee, Kansas. In addition to a regular preaching schedule in churches, Marshall is a nationally recognized lecturer at colleges, universities, and other graduate seminaries as well as a widely published author of books, book chapters, journal articles, and Bible study curriculum.

Church of God Movement (Anderson, IN)

Barry L. Callen, EdD, DRel, is Distinguished Professor Emeritus of Christian Studies at Anderson University, Anderson, Indiana. An ordained minister of the Church of God (Anderson, IN), he holds academic degrees from Geneva College, Anderson University School of Theology, Asbury Theological Seminary, Chicago Theological Seminary, and Indiana University. He has authored or edited 35 books, served as dean of Anderson University and its School of Theology, directed the Center for Pastoral Studies on the Anderson campus, and currently serves as editor of Anderson University

Press, editor of the *Wesleyan Theological Journal*, corporate secretary of Horizon International, and is Special Assistant to the General Director of Church of God Ministries, Inc., Anderson, Indiana.

The Church of Jesus Christ of Latter-Day Saints (Mormon)

The chapter was researched and written by a team of individuals in the Public Affairs Department from the international headquarters of the Church of Jesus Christ of Latter-Day Saints in Salt Lake City, Utah.

Church of the Nazarene

Dr. Darius Salter was Professor of Christian Preaching and Pastoral Theology at Nazarene Theological Seminary in Kansas City until 2007 when he became Senior Pastor of a Nazarene Church in Texas. He also served as Chairman of the Pastoral Studies Department at Western Evangelical Seminary in Portland, Oregon. He was the Executive Director of the Christian Holiness Association, an interdenominational fellowship consisting of 17 denominations, 50 colleges and universities, and two missionary organizations, from 1979 to 1986. Dr. Salter directed the Doctor of Ministry program at Nazarene Theological Seminary from 1991 to 1996, and the Supervised Ministries program from 1991 to 2001. Dr. Salter's educational background includes the Master of Divinity from Asbury Theological Seminary and the Doctor of Philosophy from Drew University. He is the author of several books.

Dr. Judith A. Schwanz is an ordained minister in the Church of the Nazarene. She holds an Master of Science in psychology and the Doctor of Philosophy in systems science/psychology from Portland State University. She taught for 13 years at Western Evangelical Seminary (now George Fox Evangelical Seminary, part of George Fox University), and is currently Professor of Pastoral Care and Counseling at Nazarene Theological Seminary. She is the author of *Blessed Connections: Relationships That Sustain Vital Ministry*, published by the Alban Institute.

Church of Scientology

Nancy O'Meara, the daughter of an Army Colonel and his registered-nurse wife, has been a Scientologist for 35 years. She and her husband reside in Los Angeles where Nancy currently serves as a senior editor of the Church of Scientology International's *FREEDOM* magazine. In recent years, Nancy has traveled from Tokyo to Budapest, Seattle to London, and many cities in between, acting as an interfaith representative with the Church of Scientology, as well as serving on the Board of the Foundation for Religious Freedom. Nancy has coauthored a well-reviewed book on religious tolerance (*The "Cult" Around the Corner*) and a booklet on using supportive, noninvasive methods to help those suffering mental troubles (*Better Ways to Help the Troubled Soul*). She is in progress on another book, *Defeating Hate*, which addresses methods used to create arbitrary divisions between people and proposing tools to attack and neutralize those methods.

Church of the Brethren

Kathryn "Kathy" Goering Reid is the former Executive Director of the Association of Brethren Caregivers, an agency of the Church of the Brethren and Associate General Secretary of the Church of the Brethren. Currently, she is the Executive Director of the Family Abuse Center, a domestic violence service provider in Waco, Texas. She was ordained in the Church of the Brethren and in the Mennonite Church USA. Kathy had nearly 20 years of experience as a pastor of congregations in Texas and California. After graduating from Manchester College, Indiana (BA), Kathy completed a Master of Education degree from Georgia State University and a Master of Divinity degree from Pacific School of Religion. Kathy is also the author of two Christian Education Curriculums: *Preventing Child Sexual Abuse: Ages 5–8* and *Preventing Child Sexual Abuse: Ages 9–12*. She is also the coauthor of *Children Together: Teaching Girls and Boys to Value Themselves and Each Other*. Kathy and her husband Steve are coauthors of the book *Uncovering Racism*.

Community of Christ

Wallace B. Smith, MD, is currently President Emeritus of the Community of Christ Church, Chair of the World Hunger Committee of the Church, volunteer chaplain at Independence Regional Medical Center in Independence, Missouri, and frequent guest speaker in local congregations. Dr. Smith received an Associate of Arts degree from Graceland College in Lamoni, Iowa, a Bachelor of Arts degree from the University of Kansas in 1950, and a Doctor of Medicine from the University of Kansas Medical School in 1954. He served as a flight surgeon for the United States Navy from 1955 to 1958. He did residencies in internal medicine and ophthalmology from 1958 to 1962. Thereafter, Dr. Smith was in private practice as an ophthalmologist from 1962 to 1976. In 1976, he retired from medical practice to become President of the Reorganized Church of Latter Saints, now called the Community of Christ, at its world

headquarters in Independence, Missouri. Dr. Smith served in that position until his retirement in 1996. He remains active in church activities.

Confucianism

Edward R. Canda, PhD, is Professor and Director of the Office for Research on Spiritual Diversity in Social Work at the School of Social Welfare of the University of Kansas in Lawrence, Kansas. He has a Master of Arts in religious studies (University of Denver) specializing in East Asian religions and Master of Social Work and Doctor of Philosophy degrees in social work (The Ohio State University). His research focuses on issues of spiritual diversity in social work, especially from cross-cultural and international perspectives. He has studied Confucianism for about 33 years with mentoring from Dong-Jun Yi, PhD, who is Emeritus Professor of Korean Philosophy at Sungkyunkwan University in the Republic of Korea. Dr. Canda has more that 140 publications and more than 100 scholarly presentations around the world, most dealing with intersections between culture, spiritual diversity, and social work. For more information about Dr. Canda, and for extensive resources on spiritual diversity in health and social work, see his homepage and the online Spiritual Diversity and Social Work Resource Center at www.socwel. ku.edu/canda.

Episcopal Church (Episcopal Church in the United States of America)

Marshall S. Scott is Chaplain at Saint Luke's South Hospital in Overland Park, Kansas. He is a graduate of the University of Tennessee (Bachelor of Arts in religious studies) and the School of Theology of the University of the South (Master of

Divinity). He has had extensive clinical education in pastoral care. He is a board-certified chaplain of the Association of Professional Chaplains, and has served on the Association of Professional Chaplains Commission on Quality in Pastoral Care. He is an Episcopal priest and past president of the Assembly of Episcopal Healthcare Chaplains. He has served in chaplaincy full or part time since 1980. He has published articles in the *Journal of Pastoral Care*, the *Caregiver Journal*, and *Chaplaincy Today*. He is the author of the web log, "Episcopal Chaplain at the Bedside," where he reflects on issues in pastoral care, ethics, and the Episcopal Church.

Evangelical Covenant Church

Thomas B. Anderson is an ordained Covenant Pastor who has served Community Covenant Church in Lenexa, Kansas for 16 years. He has written a major booklet entitled *This We Believe*, which is a defining statement about the beliefs of the Covenant Church. In addition, he has served on the National Board of Ministry for 8 years and has served as Chairman of the Board of Education of Minnehaha Academy.

Hare Krishna

Kathleen Buckley was born and raised in California and joined the Hare Krishna movement in 1969. She took initiation in 1972 from her spiritual teacher, A.C. Bhaktivedanta Swami (Srila Prabhupada) and was given the Sanskrit name Nagapatni Devi Dasi. She is currently helping to raise her grandchildren and continues to be a practicing member of the International Society for Krishna Consciousness (ISKCON), better known as the "Hare Krishnas." Nagapatni writes:

Please forgive any mistakes or short-comings in the writing of this chapter. May my efforts help other Hare Krishna followers to be well cared for when facing the end of life and ultimately, return home, back to Lord Krishna.

I would like to thank Sangita Devi Dasi (Susan Pattinson, R.N., CHPN) for her guidance in writing this chapter. Her compassion for the dying could fill an ocean. She originated the hospice program in ISKCON and is the author of *The Final Journey-Complete Hospice Care for Departing Vaishnavas* (Torchlight Publishing). Her friendship is one of the greatest treasures in my life.

Great appreciation and gratitude to His Grace Hridayananda Goswami, PhD. Srila Prabhupada once commented, "His intelligence is as great as a demigod's." He generously edited and polished this work.

Hinduism

Anand Bhattacharyya served as the President of Hindu Temple and Cultural Center of Kansas City from 1982 to 1988. From 1988 to 2002, he was a member of the Kansas City Interfaith Council representing the Hindu faith tradition. Since 1990, he has been speaking to different faith and civic groups, schools and colleges about Hinduism, in general, and Hindu religious philosophy in particular. He is a regular contributor to the "Faith Section" of the *Kansas City Star*. He is a Board Member of the Institute for Spirituality in Health of Shawnee Mission Medical Center. He was the Vice President of the Friends' Board of the Department of Religious Studies in Kansas University before he retired in 2007. He is a retired professional engineer (electrical).

Arvind Khetia is a retired engineer from Black & Veatch after working for 22 years.

Since 1994, he has participated in the "Voices of Faith" column of the *Kansas City Star*, in which he answers questions from the Hindu perspective. He has also given presentations on Hinduism to various schools, universities, faith communities, and hospitals and actively participates in interfaith activities.

Kris Krishna was born in Taunggyi, Burma (now Myanmar). He moved to India, obtained a master's degree in mechanical engineering and worked there for about 10 years before immigrating to the United States in 1972. He and his pediatrician wife, Padma, lived in the Philadelphia area from 1972 to 1977 before coming to Kansas. Kris joined the Kansas City Interfaith Council in 2002. Occasionally, he writes a column in the "Faith Section" of the *Kansas City Star*. He also presents lectures on Hinduism to various groups of people in the community.

Hutterites

Rod Janzen is Distinguished Scholar and Professor of History at Fresno Pacific University, Fresno, California. He is the author of a number of books and articles on the Hutterites, including *Perceptions of the South Dakota Hutterites in the 1980s* (Freeman Publishing Company, 1984), *The Prairie People: Forgotten Anabaptists* (University Press of New England, 1999), *Paul Tschetter: The Story of a Hutterite Immigrant Leader, Pioneer, and Pastor* (Wipf & Stock, 2009), and *The Hutterites in North America* (Johns Hopkins University Press, 2010). He also authored *The Rise and Fall of Synanon: A California Utopia* (Johns Hopkins University Press, 2001). Born in Dinuba, California, Rod is an active member of the Mennonite Church.

Islam

A. Rauf Mir, MD, FACP, is a Consulting Nephrologist and emeritus Medical Director of Kansas City Dialysis and Transplant Center. He is serves as Clinical Professor of Medicine at the University of Missouri-Kansas City School of Medicine, and served as the Chief of Nephrology at Research Medical Center in Kansas City, Missouri. Dr. Mir is a board member of the Midwest Transplant Network and the Ethics Committee of the National Kidney Foundation. Dr. Mir is on the board of directors of the Greater Kansas City Interfaith Council, founding member of the Islamic Society of Greater Kansas City (established 1972), member of the Islamic Society of North America since 1972, member of the American Muslim Council in Washington, DC, member of the board of directors of the Kashmiri American Council in Washington, DC, and 2002–2003 President of the Islamic Medical Association of North America.

Mahnaz Shabbir is President of Shabbir Advisors, an integrated strategic management consulting company. She is a board member of the Greater Kansas City Interfaith Council, Crescent Peace Society, CRES (Center for Religious Educational Studies), and UMAA (Universal Muslim Association of America). She is also the past president of the Heartland Muslim Council. Her article, "I am an American Muslim Woman" appeared in the *Kansas City Star* and was syndicated throughout the United States. Since 2001, Shabbir has given over 200 lectures, locally, nationally, and internationally to organizations interested in knowing more about diversity issues. Shabbir was featured in the CBS special "Open Hearts, Open Minds" in October 2002 and interviewed in 2003 on *Voice of*

America. In February 2005, she presented an hour-long program on the radio show, *Voice of the Cape*, that aired in Cape Town, South Africa, to 150 000 listeners. In May and July 2008, Shabbir was interviewed on Channel Islam International broadcasting to 150 countries worldwide from Johannesburg, South Africa. Shabbir is also on the faculty at Baker University teaching strategic planning and marketing classes in the school of Professional and Graduate Studies, Park University teaching classes in health care administration and at Avila University teaching diversity classes. She is frequent lecturer at the Command and General Staff College at Fort Leavenworth and Fort Belvoir, Virginia.

Jainism

Christopher Key Chapple is the Navin and Pratima Doshi Professor of Indic and Comparative Theology at Loyola Marymount University. Dr. Chapple received his undergraduate degree in Comparative Literature and Religious Studies from the State University of New York at Stony Brook and his doctorate in the History of Religions through the Theology Department at Fordham University. He served as Assistant Director of the Institute for Advanced Studies of World Religions and taught Sanskrit, Hinduism, Jainism, and Buddhism for 5 years at the State University of New York at Stony Brook before joining the faculty at Loyola Marymount University. Dr. Chapple's research interests have focused on the renouncer religious traditions of India: Yoga, Jainism, and Buddhism. He has published several books, including *Karma and Creativity* (1986), *Nonviolence to Animals, Earth, and Self in Asian Traditions* (1993), *Hinduism and Ecology* (2000), a coedited volume, *Jainism and Ecology: Nonviolence in the Web of Life* (2002), *Reconciling Yogas* (2003), and *Yoga and the Luminous: Patanjali's Spiritual Path to Freedom* (2008).

Contributors to the Jain document include Gulab Kothari from Overland Park, Kansas along with a number of notable Jain authorities which include: Dilip V. Shah, President of the Jain Associations in North America (JAINA); Dr. Sulekh Jain, Texas, Former President of JAINA; Dr. Dilip Bobra, Arizona, a cardiologist who writes extensively on ethical issues in bioscience based on Jain principles; Naresh Jain, New Jersey, Chair, Interfaith Committee of JAINA; Anop Vora, New York, Former President of JAINA; Prakash Modi, Toronto, Member, Interfaith Committee of JAINA; and Dr. Pravin Shah, North Carolina, Chair, JAINA Education Committee.

Jehovah's Witnesses

James N. Pellechia is a third-generation Jehovah's Witnesses and is Associate Editor of Watch Tower publications at the international offices of the Watch Tower Society in New York City; he served as its Director of Public Affairs in 1996–2000. He is the producer of feature and documentary films, including the award-winning film *Jehovah's Witnesses Stand Firm Against Nazi Assault*, and a lecturer on modern history of Jehovah's Witnesses. Pellechia has presented at international academic conferences, university seminars, and research institutions, including the United States Holocaust Memorial Museum. His publications include *The Spirit and the Sword: Jehovah's Witnesses Expose the Third Reich*. He is a member of the Society of Professional Journalists President's Club, attended Union College and Columbia University, and served as board member and vice president of Jehovah's Witness Holocaust–Era Survivor's Fund, Inc.

Judaism

Rabbi Amy Wallk Katz, PhD, received her rabbinic ordination from the Jewish Theological Seminary of America. Rabbi Katz has devoted most of her rabbinate to education. Besides earning a doctorate in education, Rabbi Katz has worked in both formal and informal educational settings, working with both children and adults. Rabbi Katz served the Kansas City Jewish community for 10 years as the founding director of the Department of Adult Jewish Learning. In addition, Rabbi Katz was president of the Rabbinical Association of Greater Kansas City for 3 years, and served on the board of the Midwest Center for Holocaust Education and the Women's Division of the Jewish Federation of Greater Kansas City. She served as the associate rabbi of Congregation Beth Shalom in Overland Park, Kansas. Currently, she is the senior rabbi at Temple Beth El in Springfield, Massachusetts.

Lutheranism

Rev. John D. Kreidler is an ordained pastor of the Evangelical Lutheran Church in America. He is currently serving as the Bishop's Associate for Administration in the Central States Synod of the Evangelical Lutheran Church in America, a position he accepted in 2001. He is a 1977 graduate of Christ Seminary–Seminex, St. Louis, Missouri. He has had clinical pastoral education experiences at St. John's Hospital, Springfield, Illinois; Lutheran General Hospital, Park Ridge, Illinois; and Larned State Hospital, Larned, Kansas. Beginning in 1978, Rev. Kreidler served as a prison chaplain with the Illinois Department of Corrections. In 1980 he began 21 years of service with the Federal Bureau of Prisons, holding positions of increasing responsibility in various correctional institutions. His final position was as Regional Chaplaincy Administrator for the North Central Region of the Federal Bureau of Prisons.

Mennonites

Robert J. Carlson is an ordained Mennonite clergy, holding credentials in the Western District affiliated with the Mennonite Church USA. He has been a long-time member of the Mennonite Chaplains Association. He is Supervisor Emeritus of the Association for Clinical Pastoral Education, a retired Board Certified Chaplain of the Association of Professional Chaplains, and a Retired Fellow in the American Association of Pastoral Counselors. He holds a Master of Sacred Theology from Wesley Theological Seminary, and a Bachelor of Divinity and a Doctor of Ministry from San Francisco Theological Seminary. He holds a Licensed Clinical Marriage and Family Therapist license in the State of Kansas. He was a Director of Pastoral Services and Clinical Pastoral Education Supervisor at Prairie View, Inc. (Newton, Kansas), for 25 years. He was also Clinical Pastoral Education Supervisor at St. Luke's Hospital (Kansas City, Missouri) and the Veterans Affairs Medical Center (Kansas City, Missouri). He is an active member of the Rainbow Mennonite Church in Kansas City, Kansas.

Orthodox Christianity

V. Rev. Dr. Steven Voytovich is an ordained priest of the Orthodox Church in America. He holds a Bachelor of Science degree in business from the University of Minnesota; Master of Divinity, Master of Arts in liturgical music, and Doctor of Ministry degrees from St. Vladimir's Orthodox Theological Seminary in Crestwood, New York; and a Master of Arts degree in Community Counseling from Fairfield University, Fairfield, Connecticut. Fr. Steven was pastor of St. Alexis Orthodox Church in Clinton, Connecticut, from its roots as a mission parish in 1994 until 2010. He is the Director of the newly established Orthodox Church in America Department of Institutional Chaplains. He is a board-certified chaplain with the Association of Professional Chaplains, a certified Clinical Pastoral Education Supervisor with the Association for Clinical Pastoral Education and the College of Pastoral Supervision and Psychotherapy, and a Licensed Professional Counselor. He has been engaged in institutional ministry for over 15 years and is currently the Director of Clinical Pastoral Education at Episcopal Health Services, in Far Rockaway, NY. He has previously published an article "Pastoral Education and the Orthodox Slav" in the *Journal of Supervision and Training in Ministry* (2002). Rev. Voytovich has been active in the International Congress for Pastoral Care and Counseling, where he served on the Executive Committee, and presented a paper, "Relational Story of Joseph in Egypt: Implications for Cross-Cultural Training" during the Congress held in Poland (August 2007).

Paganism

Caroline Baughman has served as the Pagan member of the Greater Kansas City Interfaith Council since 2002 and is a long-time member of Gaia Community. She was a lay leader with Gaia Community for several years, served on their board, and also helped develop their ritualist training classes. Mrs. Baughman also taught "C.U.E.S. to Healing" on faculty for 4 years at the University of Missouri–Kansas City School of Medicine. Course curriculum covered both student personal development and medical interviewing, including "how to take a spiritual history." Baughman has been a featured speaker on National Public Radio; she has presented workshops from a Pagan perspective on rites of passage through the lifecycle, sacred sexuality, and death, dying, and the afterlife. Mrs. Baughman has received training from Enchantment's Grove in New York City, the Gaia Community in Kansas City, Missouri, and has studied at Diana's Grove in Salem, Missouri.

Mike Nichols is the celebrated author of *The Witches' Sabbats* (both book and website) – the ultimate resource on Pagan holidays and related writings – and a contributing author to *Creating Circles and Ceremonies*. He has been a featured speaker on National Public Radio, Spiral Dance Radio, and Eclectic Pagan Podcast (episodes 16 and 22) on iTunes. Nichols does extensive online teaching and writing, occasionally guest lectures at Pagan festivals, and performs in a Pagan band called Spellbound. A pioneer in the American neo-Pagan movement, Nichols taught classes in Witchcraft for 20 years continuously, from 1970 to 1989, in Columbia and Kansas City, Missouri, through the Communiversity and at his bookstore, The Magick Lantern. He was also the editor of *The Lantern's Light*, a semiquarterly journal. A founding member of the Coven of New Gwynedd, Nichols was the first Wiccan representative on the Greater Kansas City Interfaith Council.

Presbyterian Church (USA)

Robert H. Meneilly is a graduate of Monmouth College, Monmouth, Illinois, and Pittsburgh Theological Seminary. He also did additional studies at Theological Institutes in Scotland at St. Andrews University. Meneilly was founding minister of The Village Presbyterian (USA) Church in Prairie Village, Kansas, where he served as Senior Pastor for 47 years. He was also one of the founders of The Interfaith Alliance in Washington, DC, and the Mainstream Coalition in Johnson County, Kansas. Meneilly received the Harry S. Truman Good Neighbor Award and is the author of several books.

Quakers (Liberal)

Chel Avery, a former Registered Nurse and hospice volunteer, has a master's degree in Communications from Temple University. She served for 7 years as Director of the Quaker Information Center in Philadelphia, Pennsylvania (www.quakerinfo.org), responding to inquiries from within and without the Religious Society of Friends. Her work on this section benefited from the consultation of Pat Brown and Joan Broadfield of Philadelphia Yearly Meeting and Ben Richmond of Friends United Meeting, among others in the Friends community.

Quakers (Pastoral)

Brenda McKinney has been a Quaker for 25 years and has served in several leadership positions in the church. She is a graduate of North Carolina State University with a Bachelor of Science in science education. She also received a physician assistant degree from Wake Forest University in 1983 at, what was then, the Bowman Gray School of Medicine. She then worked as a physician assistant in emergency medicine, public health, and orthopedic surgery. At the present time, she is working in employee health at Wake Forest University Baptist Medical Center. Brenda is married to Brent McKinney, who also helped with creating the document. Brent McKinney has served two terms as Friends United Meeting clerk and serves on the board of advisors for Earlham School of Religion and the board of trustees for Guilford College, both Quaker schools. Viola Britt, wife of Billy Britt who was a former superintendent of the Quaker North Carolina Yearly Meeting edited the document.

Secularism

Michael Irwin, MD, MPH, who was born in 1931 in London, England, completed his medical education at St. Bartholomew's Hospital, London (1949–1955), and Columbia University, New York (1960). He worked for 32 years in the United Nations System. His main senior appointments were UNICEF Representative in Bangladesh (1977–1980); UNICEF Senior Adviser on Childhood Disabilities (1980–1982); Medical Director, United Nations (1982–1989); and Medical Director, World Bank and IMF (1989–1990). After retiring to England in 1993, Irwin was Chairman or Vice-Chairman of the Voluntary Euthanasia Society (1995–2003) and Chairman of the United Nations Association (1995–1998). He also served as President of the World Federation of Right-to-Die Societies (2002–2004). In 2006, he founded the Secular Medical Forum with the main objective of presenting a secular opinion on present-day medical and health care practices throughout the United Kingdom.

Seventh-Day Adventist Church

William G. Johnsson, PhD, is a minister of the Seventh-Day Adventist Church. A native of Australia, he has served as a missionary in India, seminary professor, writer, editor, and international public speaker. Previously editor of the *Adventist Review* and *Adventist World* (the global church paper for Seventh-Day Adventists) magazines, he currently is the assistant to the world church president for interfaith relations. Johnsson has authored 23 books and more than 1000 articles.

Shintoism

William R. Lindsey received his Doctor or Philosophy degree from the University of Pittsburgh. He teaches courses on religion in Japan, religion and the Japanese state, and religion in Korea. His research on early modern Japanese health and lifestyle guides has been published in both English and Japanese. His most recent work, *Fertility and Pleasure: Ritual and Sexual Values in Tokugawa Japan* (University of Hawai'i Press, 2007), studies the role of ritual and religious symbols in the composition of health and lifestyle discourses directed toward early modern Japanese women. Currently, he is an Associate Professor in the Department of Religious Studies at the University of Kansas.

Sikhism

Gurinder Singh, MD, MHA, was born at Patiala, Punjab, India. He had medical and ophthalmology training in India and worked for 3 years with a mission hospital providing ophthalmic care to the needy and poor in the countryside by organizing free eye camps; he performed operations on more than 4000 eye patients in remote places of four states. Dr. Singh received further medical training at Hamburg University in Germany for 3 years before moving to the United States. In the United States, he continued his medical training at the University

of California, Los Angeles followed by a fellowship at Harvard Medical School/Massachusetts Eye and Ear Infirmary in Boston. He is a scientific reviewer for several major United States ophthalmology journals, has lectured at major ophthalmology meetings, and taught courses in American Academy of Ophthalmology meetings. Dr. Singh has approximately 100 scientific publications, including five book chapters. Currently, he is in private practice and is Clinical Professor of Ophthalmology at the University of Kansas Medical Center for the last 14 years.

Karta Purkh Singh Khalsa has been a Sikh for 30 years. His mentor and guide, Harbhajan Singh Yogi (Yogi Bhajan), presented the teachings of Kundalini Yoga and Meditation as a resource for finding contentment within discontent, for finding healing within disease, and for finding light within darkness. Karta Purkh Singh has participated in interfaith work for almost as long as he has been a Sikh.

Spiritualism

Rev. Lelia E. Cutler was ordained as a minister by the National Spiritualist Association of Churches (NSAC) in August 1988. She has been in Spiritualism more than 30 years and has served in various leadership roles through many years; in addition to NSAC, she has served Spiritualist churches with the International General Assembly of Spiritualists, The Spiritual Churches of Science and Revelation, The Bridge of Light, The Universal Spiritualist Association and some independent organizations. Lelia has been President of the NSAC Board since October 2003. She was the National Financial Officer/Treasurer for the NSAC, serving on the National Board for fourteen years. She is also the National Treasurer for the Morris Pratt Institute and the Center for Spiritual Studies.

Sufism

Batina Hinds was born as Ruth Van Dam and these names are still part of her name. She was born while her father was learning to be a minister at a Baptist seminary in Philadelphia. Raised in a fairly conservative Christian Minister's home, she grew up loving God and Jesus as Divine Beings. She gradually figured out that the Divine is what she learned and so much more. Many of the mystical words of Jesus were not emphasized and she felt herself drawn to these while she developed a dream to be a missionary medical doctor. To do this, Batina attended a Baptist college and has received subsequent masters-level degrees in teaching Reading, teaching English as a second language (mostly linguistics and highly analytical), and mental health counseling. She has worked in all three capacities: Reading teacher from kindergarten through high school, teaching English as a second language on community college and university levels including doctoral students, and working as a psychotherapist in a psychiatric hospital, community health centers, and private practice for the past 18 years. She was thankful to discover Sufism, which fit with her path with the Divine, and she is now an ordained Sufi Minister or Cherag and a Healing Conductor and has found some Sufi practices to be most useful in helping people to heal their bodies, hearts, and souls.

Taoism

Peter F. Cunneen is a practitioner of Oriental medicine having earned a master's degree in acupuncture and traditional Chinese medicine from Yo San University in Los Angeles, California. He has taught Chinese medicine, philosophy, and medical history at several New York area colleges. A past president of the Integral Way Society and a professional member of the National Qi Gong Association, he has been a Taoist mentor with the College of Tao, studying and sharing of the knowledge gained from this ancient source since 1986. Currently, he is practicing medicine and teaching through Chi Rivers Constructive Life Learning Center in Geneva, Switzerland.

Donald D. Davis received a Doctor of Philosophy degree in psychology from Michigan State University. Currently he serves as a professor of psychology and Asian Studies at Old Dominion University in Norfolk, Virginia. He has studied, practiced, and taught Taoism, *tai chi*, and *qigong* for the past 25 years. He teaches them at Tidewater Tai Chi Center in Norfolk and Virginia Beach, Virginia.

Unitarian Universalism

Kathy Riegelman, MDiv, BCC, is affiliate minister at All Souls Unitarian Universalist Church, Kansas City, Missouri. Ordained as a Unitarian Universalist Community Minister, she serves as a chaplain at St. Joseph Medical Center in Kansas City, Missouri. Kathy is active in interfaith work in Kansas City and has served as the convener of the Greater Kansas City Interfaith Council.

United Church of Christ

Greg Heinsman, MDiv, BCC, received a Bachelor of Arts from Central Bible College in 1994 in Springfield, Missouri, and a Master of Divinity degree from Assemblies of God Theological Seminary in 1998 in

Springfield, Missouri. He completed eight units of Clinical Pastoral Education at St. Luke's/Shawnee Mission Health System from August 1998 to August 2000. Heinsman was ordained by the Southern District of the Assemblies of God on April 13, 2000, and became a board-certified chaplain through the Association of Professional Chaplains on March 3, 2001. He received Privilege of Call in November 2003 with the Missouri Mid-South United Church of Christ and Ecclesiastical Endorsement with the United Church of Christ in December 2003. He also served as Supply Interim Pastor at Evangelical United Church of Christ from September 2006 to February 2007. Heinsman has been a staff chaplain at Saint Francis Medical Center in Cape Girardeau, Missouri, from August 2000 to the present.

United Methodist Church

Jeanne Hoeft, PhD, is Associate Professor of Pastoral Theology and Pastoral Care at Saint Paul School of Theology, a United Methodist Seminary in Kansas City, Missouri. She received her Master of Divinity degree from Emory University and her Doctor of Philosophy in religious and psychological studies from the University of Denver and Iliff School of Theology. She is an ordained elder in the United Methodist Church and has been a pastor in Florida and Colorado congregations. For more than 20 years she has been involved in the work to resist violence, particularly violence against women, children, youth, and oppressed social groups. She continues to write and speak on this topic for both religious and nonreligious settings.

Amanda Caruso is a student at Saint Paul School of Theology preparing to be a Deaconess in the United Methodist Church.

Unity

Rev. Thomas W. Shepherd, MDiv, is chair of Theological and Historical Studies in the Ministry and Religious Studies Department of Unity Institute, located at Unity Village, Missouri. Although best known for his popular Q&A column "I've Always Wondered About ..." in *Unity Magazine*, Tom Shepherd is also the author of *Friends in High Places* (Unity Books, 1985), and *Glimpses of Truth* (UFBL Press, 2000). He also published two science fiction novels under the pen name Thomas Henry Quell. An ordained Unity minister, Tom's first career path took him soldiering, to include a tour in Vietnam as a decorated medical evacuation helicopter pilot. After Vietnam, Tom left the army to earn a Bachelor of Science in education (*cum laude*) at the University of Idaho and Master of Divinity (*magna cum laude*) from Lancaster Theological Seminary. He returned to active duty and completed 20 years service as an Army Chaplain. An ethnic German American who describes himself as "Pennsylvania Dutch," Shepherd has served as senior minister of Christ Church Unity of Augusta, Georgia; Assistant Executive Director and Theologian-in-Residence for Johnnie Colemon's Universal Foundation for Better Living; and senior minister of Sunrise Unity Church, Sacramento, California, before joining the seminary faculty at Unity School of Christianity.

Vodou and Afro-Atlantic Religions

Dowoti Désir is the founder of the Durban Declaration and Program of Action Watch Group (the DDPA Watch Group), a human rights organization focused on race, racial discrimination, and xenophobia in the global south. She was the first Executive Director of The Malcolm

X and Dr. Betty Shabazz Memorial and Educational Center, a not-for-profit focused on human, civil, and educational rights. The former Associate Publisher of the *AFRIcan Magazine*, Ms. Désir has served as an Adjunct Professor in the Africana Studies Department of Brooklyn College, City University of New York. A Federal Advisor to the African Burial Ground of New York City, her interests in cultural production include international development and the creative economy in Africa, where she has worked on national initiatives led by the governments of Zambia, Rwanda, and Uganda. As a journalist, Ms. Désir writes about the various issues that impact African descendants, contemporary art in the African Diaspora, and the Afro-Atlantic religions and sacred arts. A *Manbo Asogwe* in Haitian Vodou, she is both a priest and a scholar who has officiated various rites at the request of the Federal Government General Services Administration for the New York African Burial Ground and The Five Points Memorial; Museum of Natural History for the exhibition the *Sacred Art of Haitian Vodou*; and Cornell University Africana Studies Department. Ms. Désir lectures extensively on Haitian Vodou and the spiritual traditions of the Afro-Atlantic at a variety of institutions throughout the United States, including the Figge Museum in Quad City, Iowa, where she was commissioned to create a permanent altar to the Haitian *lwa* or Spirits, Harvard University School of Divination, Union Theological Seminary, Columbia University, New York University, several colleges of the City University of New York, and the Institute for the Advancement of Puerto Rican Studies in Carolina, Puerto Rico. Her writings on the *orisa*-based cultures can be found in the Wabash Center's *Teaching Theology and Religion*, and Vanderbilt University's *Afro-Hispanic Review*, among others.

Zoroastrianism

Maneck N. Bhujwala was born in Bombay (now called Mumbai), India, in 1940, studied at St. Xavier's High School, obtained his electrical engineering degree in Baroda, and worked at the Bombay Municipal Corporation, before coming to the United States to study for his master's degree in electrical engineering at the University of New Mexico, Albuquerque. He has worked as a design automation engineer and manager of software development and quality assurance at several computer engineering software and aerospace companies including NASA Ames Research Center over 32 years. While working, he also obtained his Master of Business Administration from San Jose State University, cofounded Zoroastrian associations in northern and southern California, obtained priesthood training, and serves the community as a junior priest and represents Zoroastrianism in interfaith organizations and at interfaith events. He is married to Mahrukh, who was born in India, and he has a daughter, Shehnaz, born in Pasadena, California.

Contributors to this chapter include Khojeste P. Mistree, one of the eminent teachers of Zoroastrianism who has lectured all over the world on various topics related to the religion, particularly the scriptures and historical practices. He is cofounder of the Center for Zoroastrian Studies, a research organization in Mumbai, India. James R. Russell, PhD, Mashtots Professor of Armenian Studies in the Department of Near Eastern Languages and Civilizations of Harvard University in Cambridge, Massachusetts, also contributed as a reviewer/editor. A final contributor is *Ervad*

About the Contributors

Jal N. Birdy, Vice President of Traditional
Mazdayasni Zoroastrian Anjuman (TMZA),
Corona, California.

Acknowledgments

We are truly grateful to each of the writers and reviewers of the various faith and belief system sections for providing the accuracy in representing the histories, basic teachings and basic practices of their respective traditions as well as supplying the relevant, practical material necessary for providing appropriate spiritual care in a clinical setting. Throughout the process of assembling the material for this book, we have learned much from so many people. This list of contributors (i.e. authors of individual sections), to whom we are deeply indebted for their masterful work, follows the order of the faith-specific sections found in the Table of Contents.

Rev. Kara Hawkins, DMin, American Indian Spirituality; Barb McAtee and David Edalati, MD, Bahá'í Faith; Guy McCloskey, Mahayana Buddhism; Kongsak Tanphaichitr, MD, Theravada Buddhism; Lama Chuck Stanford and Teri Brody, MD, Vajrayana Buddhism; Kathryn Goering Reed, Anabaptist Traditions: General Introduction; Linda Graham and James Cates, PhD, Amish; Samuel Brubaker, MD, Brethren in Christ; Kathryn Goering Reed, Church of the Brethren; Rod Janzen, PhD, Hutterites; Robert Carlson, DMin, Mennonites; Robert E. Johnson, PhD, Catholic and Protestant Traditions: General Introductions; Paul Hura, MD, Eastern Rite; Father Jerry Spencer, Roman Catholicism; Michael von Rosen and colleagues from the Public Affairs Department, The Church of Jesus Christ of Latter-Day Saints (Mormon); Wallace Smith, MD, Community of Christ; James Pellechia, Jehovah's Witnesses; Steven Voytovich, DMin, Orthodox Christianity; Rev. L. Henderson Bell, African American Baptist/Protestantism; Rev. Natalie Mitchem, African Methodist Episcopal Church (AME); Rev. Emmanuel Williams and Rev. Alvin Worthley, Assemblies of God; Michael Fuhrman, PhD, Baptists; Quentin Jones, MDiv, Christian Church (Disciples of Christ); Philip Davis and Debbi Lawrence, Christian Science; Barry Callen, EdD, Church of God Movement (Anderson, IN); Marshall Scott, MDiv, Episcopal Church (Episcopal Church in the United States of America); Rev. Tom Anderson, Evangelical Covenant Church; Rev. John D. Kreidler, Lutheranism; Judith Schwanz, PhD, and Darius Salter, PhD, Church of the Nazarene; Robert Meneilly, DD, Presbyterian Church (USA); William Johnsson, PhD, Seventh-Day Adventist Church; Greg Heinsman, MDiv, United Church of Christ; Jeanne Hoeft, PhD, United Methodist Church; Thomas W. Sherherd, MDiv, Unity; Chel Avery and Jim Kenney, Liberal Quakers (Friends); Brenda McKinney, Pastoral (Programmed) Quakers; Edward Canda, PhD, Confucianism; Nagapatni, Hare Krishna; Anand Bhattacharyya, Arvind Kheita, Kris Krishna, and Roy Hegde, Hinduism; A. Rauf Mir, MD, and Mahnaz Shabbir, Islam; Christopher Chapple, PhD, Jainism; Rabbi Amy Katz, PhD, Judaism; Caroline Baughman, Paganism; Nancy Omeara, Church of Scientology; Michael

Irwin, MD, Secularism; William R. Lindsey, PhD, Shinto; Gurinder Singh, MD, and Karta Purkh Singh Khalsa, Sikhism; Rev. Lelia E. Cutler, Spiritualism; Batina Hinds, Sufism; Peter Cunneen, Taoism; Kathy Riegelman, Unitarian Universalism; Dowoti Désir, Vodou; and Maneck Bhujwala, Zoroastrianism.

We are also thankful for the physicians who served as members of an editorial advisory council. David Hightower, MD, Gordon Kelley, MD, and Andrew Schwartz, MD, read various portions of the manuscript and offered many suggestions for improvement.

Finally, we are deeply appreciative of Vern Barnet, DMin, and Michael Brannigan, PhD, who authored several portions of the book and provided tremendous support in helping assemble the contributors for the various faith and belief system sections.

Steven L. Jeffers, PhD
Michael E. Nelson, MD

Setting the Stage

Story: A Surgeon's "Star of David" Necklace

One weekend day in the summer of 2005, I went to the Kansas City Jewish Arts Festival. During the day's enjoyment, I stopped at the booth of a vendor selling Judaic jewelry. Among the wares was a gold necklace with a Star of David pendant. While I am not usually one to adorn myself with jewelry, that necklace caught my attention, so I bought it.

The next day as I was preparing for work, I realized that my new Star of David was very prominent on my chest, just above the V-neck of my shirt. Immediately, an uncomfortable feeling came over me. Did I, a Jewish surgeon who practiced medicine in a Christian-sponsored hospital, want to be so bold in announcing my faith? Would wearing this necklace be offensive to patients and hinder my doctor-patient relationships? After some careful thought, I recalled seeing many people wearing necklaces that bore a person's name, a religious symbol, a relationship, or a country's flag. I concluded that wearing this necklace with a symbol of my religious faith was not something unique. People do it all the time. It did take some time, though, for my overactive self-consciousness about wearing the necklace to subside. However, little did I know, then, of the role that necklace would play in the care of one of my patients.

Several months later, I had a consult with a patient and her daughters to discuss open heart surgery. I discovered in the dialogue that the patient had experienced many surgeries as a child because of extensive burns. As a result, she was reluctant to have any other such procedures, especially heart surgery. During our discussion, and to my surprise, she suddenly looked with focused intent on my necklace and asked, "Is that a Star of David?" I said it was and asked her if she was Jewish. She replied that she was a "practicing" Christian. Then, she asked me to tell her about my faith. So, I proceeded to tell her about Judaism. She abruptly stopped me, almost in mid-sentence. "I don't mean Judaism. I want to know how *you* practice and observe your faith and how your faith influences the way you live your life." At that point, I began sharing with her and her daughters how my faith was (and will be in the future) the foundation upon which I made (and will make) various choices and decisions during life's journey.

After concluding our clinical and spiritual discussion with a request for any other questions or concerns, I left the room to await the decision about the proposed surgical procedure. An hour later, I was informed that the patient had decided to proceed with the surgery, which would be scheduled for the following day.

When the surgery was finished, I met with the patient's daughters and discussed the conduct of the operation, along with post-operative expectations and prognosis for recovery. As expected, they had a plethora of questions, all of which I answered. When

I arose from the chair to leave the family consultation room, one of the daughters said to me, "I want you to know that my mother decided to have her heart surgery after she saw your Star of David." She also related that the importance of faith in my personal and professional life gave her mom a great sense of comfort and security. After leaving the room and while walking down the hallway, I began chuckling to myself, "My Star of David, about which I was so concerned might be offensive to others, turned out to be a gift, a blessing to someone who was not even Jewish."

—Andrew M. Schwartz, MD,
cardiothoracic surgeon

This story serves to highlight one important element in providing spiritual care in a religiously pluralistic society – the distinction between spirituality and religion. The major thing that was significant for the patient was not that Dr. Schwartz was Jewish, but that he was a man of faith, a spiritual man. Furthermore, this scenario chronicling the interactions of a physician with a patient and her family is not typical in the medical community. However, the authors and the many contributors to this resource hope that stories such as this one will begin to proliferate and become commonplace in the health care setting.

Purpose Statement of the Book

The experience of illness is often a time when people draw on their faith and spirituality, as do their physicians (as the story about the surgeon's Star of David indicates), to find comfort, strength, and hope. Literature from the medical community has identified the value that both patients and physicians place on integrating spirituality and religion into the practice of medicine.[10,11,12] The benefits of a healthy spirituality or religious involvement have been correlated to improved coping mechanisms[13,14] and better health care outcomes. However, despite these positive findings, many practitioners continue to struggle with finding a comfortable approach for including religion and spirituality in their professional lives.[15,16,17]

Addressing the whole person – body, mind, and spirit – is a fundamental principle of quality patient care. Acknowledging the spiritual and religious dimensions of people is integral to that process. This book is a tool to better enable health care workers to be sensitive and responsive to the spiritual and religious needs and concerns of their patients.

In the following pages, the reader will find chapters that discuss the following:

10 Mansfield, C., J. Mitchell, and D. E. King. (2002). The doctor as God's mechanic? Beliefs in the southeastern United States. *Social Science and Medicine*, 54(3), 399–409.

11 Ehman, J. W., B. B. Ott, T. H. Short, et al. (1999). Do patients want physicians to inquire about their spiritual or religious beliefs if they become gravely ill? *Archives of Internal Medicine*, 159(15), 1803–1806.

12 Maugans, T. and Wadland, W. (1991). Religion and family medicine: a survey of physicians and patients. *Journal of Family Practice*, 32(2), 210–213.

13 Pargament, K., B. Cole, L. Vandecreek, et al. The vigil: religion and the search for control in the hospital waiting room. *Journal of Health Psychology*, 4(3), 327–341.

14 Koenig, H., K. I. Pargament, J. Nielsen, et al. (1998). Religious coping and health status in medically ill hospitalized older adults. *Journal of Nervous and Mental Disease*, 186(9), 513–521.

15 Sperry, L. (2000). Spirituality and psychiatry: incorporating the spiritual dimension into clinical practice. *Psychiatric Annals*, 30(8), 518–523.

16 Groopman, J. (2004). God at the bedside. *New England Journal of Medicine*, 350(12), 1176–1178.

17 Sloan, R., E. Bagiella, and T. Powell. (1999). Religion, spirituality, and medicine. *Lancet*, 353(9153), 664–667.

- Spirituality and religion: an overview of the three families of faith
- Spirituality, religion, and culture
- Spirituality and religion: relevance in the clinical setting?
- Spirituality and religion in the clinical setting: pros and cons
- Spiritual care in the clinical setting: assessment and application.

These sections are intended to provide a general overview of the various relationships among physical health, overall well-being, and spirituality and religion as these factors relate to and affect patient care. Most of the text, though, offers principles to provide spiritual care for patients of varying faith traditions and philosophies of life – a literal "A to Z" compendium, from American Indian Spirituality to Zoroastrianism.

Historical Overview of the Relationship between Spirituality and Medicine

The practice of medicine and its connection with spirituality and religion date back over 2 millennia.[18] Herophilus, a physician who lived in Alexandria, Egypt, in the third century BCE, stated: "When health is absent, wisdom cannot reveal itself, art cannot become manifest, strength cannot be exerted, wealth is useless and reason is powerless."[19] These words confirm the belief of many people that human well-being involves more than good physical health.

In addition to the physical dimension of health, there are also mental, emotional, spiritual, professional, financial, and relational dimensions.

As this book will point out, numerous cultures, early in their history, have thought of illness, disease, and health as matters of both body and spirit. Later, when "physicians" approached healing in distinct ways – some addressing the spiritual component and others dealing with the bodily features – their practices were not antithetical to each other. Illness and health were seen in ways that encompassed the spiritual and the physical needs of those who were ill. Medicine and spirituality were linked as complementary avenues to healing rather than as separate and opposing silos. This latter view (i.e., separate and opposing silos) became more prominent particularly in Western medicine, as medical practice professed to be more "scientific" and "rational." Nonetheless, cultures throughout the world continue to stress the connections among the spiritual, natural, and bodily when it comes to illness and health, so that illness and health remain an affair of both the spirit and the body.

One of the earliest records of this interplay of spirituality and medicine can be found in the ancient Near East. The polytheistic (belief in a plurality of deities) and animistic (belief in a sacredness toward nature) worldviews of the ancient Mesopotamian and Egyptian cultures (ca. 3100 BCE to the fourth century BCE) accompanied an understanding of illness and health as influenced by religious beliefs and spiritual forces. Even though its monotheistic (belief in one deity) worldview was radically different, the same could be said for ancient Israel (ca. 1300 BCE–70 CE). For example, the Hebrew term for "healer" is

---

18 Jeffers, S., M. McKenna, and A. Schwartz. (2006). A portion of the historical overview of medicine was extracted from the preface of the unpublished manuscript "Physicians and clergy in concert."
19 Von Staden, H. ed. (1989). *The Art of Medicine in Early Alexandria*. London: Cambridge University Press. Citation of Herophilus extracted from wall in Department of Public Health Building, Kansas City, Missouri.

derived from the verb *rapha*, meaning "to sew together" or "to repair." This "sewing together" acknowledged the unity of body and spirit in the enterprise of healing.[20] Whereas cooperation with the forces of gods and nature played a role in health for Mesopotamians and Egyptians, the degree to which Hebrews remained faithful to their covenant with Yahweh also influenced health and illness. Thus, healing for these ancient cultures involved the integration of spiritual, bodily, and moral dimensions. "Moral" refers to values underlying what we believe to be "right" and "wrong," "benevolent" and "malevolent," "justified" and "unjustified." Considerations of what is "moral" therefore naturally include physical and spiritual aspects.

Things began to change, though, when both early Greek dualistic philosophy (viewpoint of seeing the mind and body as separate) and dualistic Christian thought (as found in some of the writings of the apostles Paul and John) interacted in such a way as to enable a split between bodily and spiritual spheres. As this rift between matters of the spirit and those of the body became more apparent in Western intellectual history, the spiritual and physical domains became further distinguished, opposed, isolated, and mutually exclusive.

Despite this growing separation between body and spirit, at least in the early centuries CE, spirituality managed to sustain a harmony with medicine. We see this in the active role played by religious institutions in the practice of healing. For instance, in the fourth century, religious establishments built the first hospitals to care for society's population. Over the next 1000 years, religious groups continued to build hospitals as well as provide medical training and the licensing of physicians. Prior to the nineteenth century, many physicians were priests and monks. The practice of nursing also evolved from religious groups.[21]

The European Renaissance witnessed a "rebirth" of art and science, beginning in the early 1300s, and this, along with the scientific revolution in the sixteenth and seventeenth centuries, generated a dramatic change in the relationship between medicine and spirituality. We cannot underestimate the impact of the scientific revolution on views of illness, health, and the further separation of medicine and spirituality. Francis Bacon's (1561–1626) emphases upon "observation and experimentation" for the "advancement of learning" along strict rational grounds contributed to the development of a more empirically based scientific methodology. His *Novum Organum* (1620) and its rallying call of *scientia est potentia* (knowledge is power) extended its reach into medicine as "real knowledge" became further distinguished from matters of religion and the spiritual.[22]

Historians trace the philosophical underpinnings of western medicine to the French mathematician, scientist, and philosopher, René Descartes (1596–1650), who postulated that the universe operated according to mechanical laws without ref-

20 Amundsen, D. and G. Ferngren. (1995). History of medical ethics. In W. T. Reich, editor in chief. *Encyclopedia of Bioethics*, Vol. 3. New York, NY: Macmillan, 1443.

21 Koenig, H. (2001). Religion, spirituality, and medicine: how are they related and what does it mean? *Mayo Clinic Proceedings*, 76(12), 1189–1191.

22 The previous three and a half paragraphs, although slightly different, are cited in "Spiritual and Cultural Diversity: Innner Resources for Healing," (2008), chapter 5 in Steven L. Jeffers and Dennis Kenny's *Putting Patients First: Best Practices in Patient-Centered Care*. 2nd ed. San Francisco, CA: Jossey-Bass.

erence to meaning and purpose. The result of this new concept was the inauguration of the biomedical model, wherein physicians were trained first and foremost as scientists. Thus, medicine as an "art," where compassion and care for patients were paramount, at times became diminished by the "science" of medicine.[23]

As the Enlightenment (eighteenth century) in European thought followed in the wake of the scientific revolution, medicine acquired more credibility when based upon the scientific and the rational. In the century that followed, technological progress in medicine allied with scientific methodology and empowered medicine with heightened authority over matters of religion and spirituality, now increasingly viewed as abiding in the realm of "nonscience." At the same time, stricter accreditation requirements (further legitimating the power of knowledge) enabled laypersons to achieve their medical licenses so that laypersons as degreed professionals, not clergy or nuns, soon became the healers. This lead to the erection of a wall between faith and medicine, especially in Western medicine, that has existed for hundreds of years. However, during the last several decades of the twentieth century, that wall started to crumble.

As described throughout this book, though, this fissure between body and spirit was less prominent in numerous other cultures and traditions. For instance, Asian cultures and traditions managed to preserve a perspective of the human as a unity of body and spirit, so that they generally do not view illness and disease as the exclusive

preoccupation of scientific medicine. Asian societies continue to endorse the compatibility of both traditional approaches to healing, which assume the primacy of spirituality as a necessary ingredient in healing, and medicine, which tends to rely more on the physiological character of illness causation and healing. Whether it concerns the weight of karma (in Hindu and Buddhist traditions), *kami* (divine forces of nature in Japanese Shinto), or shaman as both priest and healer, Asian worldviews assume an integration of human, natural, and spiritual.

Despite US medical education's continued emphases on both the physiological character of illness and disease and "curing" as opposed to "healing" (curing entails restoring the body to some measure of "normalcy," whereas healing involves restoring balance to the whole person, not recovery in a strict physiological sense), a revival in recognizing the relationship between medicine and spirituality is now taking place. This compels us to ask: Are more physicians tending to be more aware of some unity of body and spirit? If so, how can physicians integrate spiritual care into medical practice? Are they willing to do so? Do they feel comfortable and even competent in addressing spiritual and religious issues? The answer to this last question may often be no, as the research presented in the Appendix will show.

Goal: Personalizing Spiritual Care

Despite the lack of training of physicians, other health care workers, and even clergy in the field of providing spiritual care in a clinical setting, there is a growing awareness of the positive effects that a person's spirituality has on health outcomes.

While the authors believe that this

---

23 Droege, T. (1991). *The Faith Factor in Healing.* Philadelphia, PA: Trinity Press. Droege was cited by Puchalski, C. M. (2001). Spirituality and health: the art of compassionate medicine. *Hospital Physician, 37*(3), 30–36.

book will be an invaluable resource for the health care community, there is one very important word of counsel. One should not assume that everything in the section on Hinduism, for example, would be appropriate for every Hindu patient. One must remember that every patient is unique. The personal spirituality and spiritual needs may well vary from one Hindu patient to another. Therefore, it is far better to ask how to be helpful in supporting spiritual and emotional concerns of the Hindu patient and then utilize the faith specific beliefs and practices that are appropriate in serving that patient's needs. This concept of providing individualized spiritual care is eloquently articulated by Rabbi Michael Zedek:

> Physicians and healthcare workers who know a patient's religious affiliation know nothing more than a label.[24]

Similarly, T. J. Mansen and S. W. Haak write:

> When it is assumed that satisfying the rites and rituals of a particular religion meets a patient's spiritual needs, interventions may become standardized rather than individualized to the patient's needs.[25]

The truth of the message about serving the needs and concerns of patients as individuals and not "lumping" people of a stated religious tradition, ethnic group, and so forth, into a single group cannot be overstated. Even so, having a general understanding of a particular patient's faith tradition or philosophy of life and some guiding spiritual care principles of that specific belief system can greatly enhance a care provider's ability in serving the patient by:

- providing the health care team with a shared background about the patient's beliefs
- alerting the health care providers of "what to look for" (i.e., signs and symptoms of spiritual and/or emotional distress)
- providing appropriate questions to ask the patient
- assisting in the development of the relationship between health care providers and patients.

The authors sincerely hope this resource will aid you in personalizing spiritual care to patients and that it will help you in "bridging faith and medicine" in your respective institutions.

---

24 Zedek, M., interview by Steven Jeffers, Center for Practical Bioethics' Compassion Sabbath February 4, 2000.
25 Mansen, T. and S. Haak. (1996). Evaluation of health assessment skills using a computer videodisk interactive program. *Journal of Nursing Education*, 35(8), 382–383.

Spirituality and Religion: An Overview of the Three Families of Faith

Introduction

The West produced the idea of "religion" as a separate sphere of culture. Art, government, and medicine, for example, now distinct enterprises, were formerly expressions of a pervasive spiritual impulse or energy. This universal energy, not to be parted and pieced, has become fragmented in modern, secularistic culture. This partly explains why an increasing number of people feel that today's religious institutions often fail to satisfy their deepest longings for connection, perspective, and health.

Medicine was a largely spiritual practice in Western culture until relatively recently. With the rise of science in the seventeenth century, the sense of divine order, *scala naturae*, the "great chain of being," was lost. The sense of unity in the culture was, to use the words of the English poet and clergyman John Donne, "all in pieces, all coherence gone." Scientific and technological advances, especially since the American Civil War, further parted medicine and spirituality.

Unquestionably, specialized study of human anatomy, physiology, and related fields freed from the control of certain religious constraints (such as the prohibition against autopsy) led to the continuing advancement of medicine as a science. However, that advance is sometimes challenged, as in this anonymous and widely circulated spoof:

A Short History of Medicine

"I have an earache."

2000 BCE	Here, eat this root.
1000 CE	That root is heathen. Here, say this prayer.
1850 CE	That prayer is superstition. Here drink this potion.
1940 CE	That potion is snake oil. Here, swallow this pill.
1985 CE	That pill is ineffective. Here take this antibiotic.
2000 CE	That antibiotic is artificial. Here, eat this root.

Yet, despite the vastly increased resources of medical knowledge, drugs, surgical and laboratory techniques, and highly trained physicians, nurses, and other health care professionals, the human need to understand the significance of one's medical condition remains important, and this need can be usefully understood as an enduring spiritual concern. Furthermore, in the best medical practice, attention to the *person* and not simply the *ailment* has never disappeared. In recent decades, the spiritual dimension of healing has been increasingly recognized as an essential component in health care. Because North America is increasingly populated by folks of many and varied faith traditions, it may be helpful to set forth a general pattern for understanding what is of ultimate importance to the different faiths and how this may affect health care.

First, we discuss *spirituality, religion, relationship between spirituality and religion*, and *sacred*. Then, we outline the three families of faith: primal, Asian, and monotheistic faiths.

Spirituality, Religion, and the Sacred

"Religion is an experience which no definition exhausts,"[26] so it is not surprising that hundreds of definitions of religion and related terms have been proposed. For example, religion is sometimes defined as "belief in a Supreme Being," but such a definition is inadequate for certain faiths like Buddhism in which there is no Creator God, and is misleading for other religions in which belief is not a critical element, as, for example, a normative definition of a Jew is someone with a Jewish mother.

In order to think comprehensively about caring for patients who come from the many traditions covered in this book, we explain how we use three words, *sacred, spirituality*, and *religion*. These explanations are not intended to replace the reader's own personal understanding of the terms but, rather, to clarify how they may be used in many contexts. Sensitively probing the patient may yield rewarding personal depths to these terms – as, indeed, the reader's own self-examination may prove beneficial.

Sacred

The word "sacred" may be used for isolated events, objects, or circumstances, such as Catholic Mass, the Muslim Qur'an, or the

Hindu wedding ceremony. While associating the divine with the sacred is helpful, we suggest an even more fundamental use for the term: the point or points from which the meanings of people's lives emerge, on which they ultimately depend. Such a use is sufficiently open that "nonbelievers," even if they do not embrace this term, may understand and respond to questions like the following:

- What gives meaning to my life?
- What do I most cherish?
- What is of ultimate worth to me?
- What is so important that my life depends on it, and what must I do to honor it?
- What provides comfort and encouragement in the face of adversity?

Experiences of awe and wonder, of profound connectedness to all things or to a transcendent source, or from sensing a pattern or purpose in one's life may illumine such questions. Such experiences are sometimes called "peak" or "mountain top" experiences that reveal a power or process in which a person finds one's way. Genuine answers to such questions usually do not arise simply just from thinking about them but, rather, from experiences in which the sacred is disclosed as supreme worth, fundamental significance, ultimate value, or utmost concern. Akin to "sacred" is the term "holy," which derives from Indo-European and Old English word forms that developed into modern words such as holistic, whole, wholesome, heal, and hale (healthy). Both "holy" and "sacred" are opposites of the profane, the secular, the fragmented, the partial, the instrumental, the means rather than the end. The cross, the menorah, the holy water, the stone, the Holy Book, incense, bells, gestures, and such, as well as personal items, may all be symbols imbued

26 Jones, R. M. (1922). *Spiritual Exercises in Daily Life*, New York: Macmillan, vii.

with sacred power, and thus in themselves considered sacred.

Spirituality: Breathing with a Sense of the Sacred

The newborn infant must breathe, and with that, a spiritual life ensues. The words that various tongues use for spirituality show that the spirit is not an exclusive field but, rather, is with us as we take every breath. In English, "spirit" is part of words like "respiration," "inspiration," and "aspiration." Similarly, Hebrew, Sanskrit, Greek, and Chinese languages (among others) employ terms similar to "breath" as a metaphor for spirituality. *Ruach*, an early Hebrew word for "soul," means wind or breath. Adam came to life when God breathed into his nostrils. The Sanskrit term for the soul, *atman*, means breath, related to the English word "atmosphere." The first lesson in yoga is how to breathe. The Greek word for soul, *psuche*, from which we derive "psychology," also means breath, life. Similarly, the word *pneuma*, meaning spirit or air, comes into English in words such as "pneumatic" and "pneumonia." In Chinese, this vital force is *ch'i*, the breath that informs the world, expanding and contracting, making every being spiritual, even stones.

Thus, one way of describing spirituality is "breathing with a sense of the sacred," living so that every breath we take reminds us of the ultimate mystery of our existence and our best responses to questions like those listed earlier in this chapter. Spirituality heals all fractures, remedies all ruptures, and brings balm to all wounds to the big picture we have of ourselves and the world. Spirituality can be understood as the source that energizes people with significance, the capacity to discern meaning in anything

they experience. Even if a person may not be able to walk physically, the metaphorical language of Edward Canda, PhD, points the way: "Spirituality is the way to walk in a sacred manner, to walk in harmony with the beauty all around us and within us."[27]

Since most people have developed some form of spirituality (whether they use this term or not), it is important to recognize that spirituality is a way of being that affects how people respond to what they experience in life. A caregiver can be more effective by attending to the patient's sense of spirituality expressed in personal values, beliefs, and practices, especially when difficult decisions are required.

From many interviews, Ian Mitroff, PhD, identifies several characteristics of spirituality:
- universal and timeless
- broadly inclusive
- ultimate source and provider of meaning and purpose to life
- sacredness of everything
- integrally connected to inner peace and calm
- expression of awe felt in the presence of the transcendent
- provision for inexhaustible source of faith.[28]

---

27 Canda, Edward. *Kansas City Star*, September 16, 1995, F4.

28 Mitroff, I. (1999). *A Spiritual Audit of Corporate America*. San Francisco, CA: Jossey-Bass. Dr. Mitroff related to the author in a personal communication in January 2007 that the characteristics of spirituality listed were a compilation from everyone he interviewed as to what spirituality meant to them. His interviews were preparation for writing his 1999 book on spirituality in corporate culture. This paragraph, although slightly altered, appears in "Spirituality and cultural diversity: inner resources for healing" (2008) by Steven L. Jeffers and Dennis Kenny, a chapter in *Putting Patients First: Best Practices in Patient-Centered Care*. 2nd ed. San Francisco, CA: Jossey-Bass.

Notice that these characteristics apply whether or not a person believes in God. Kenneth Pargament, PhD, says, "Spirituality is not necessarily about God, and yet spirituality is a search for the sacred."[29] He identifies the realms in which the search may take place: time/space, events, cultural products, roles in life, and physical attributes. Many hospital patients throughout the United States and the world profess no affiliation with any "formal" religion or are practicing none, yet they identify themselves as spiritual. Touch, aromas, crystals, meditation, and other devices, practices, and rituals unrelated to any particular religious tradition may give meaning and purpose to life for these persons and therefore can be considered spiritual. They may not use the word God but instead refer to their Higher Power. Walking in the park, gardening, playing with children, watching a sunrise or sunset, and so forth,[30] may be spiritual activities because of the beauty, relationships, or sense of the cosmos that are awakened or affirmed.

The "Spiritual Care in the Clinical Setting: Assessment and Application" chapter provides more practical guidelines within this understanding of spirituality. By utilizing this approach in attempting to provide spiritual care to patients, one practices "Individualized care." This is possible only when the patient's approach to spirituality can be united with the other components of a comprehensive plan for treating each patient.

Religion: Organized Spirituality

Today, the word "religion" commonly has organizational and institutional connotations: church, mosque, synagogue, temple, and so forth. However, a basic meaning of "religion" appears to originate in the Latin word *religio*, "to bind together in mutual obligation," as in one's duty to one's God, or more generally, one's ultimate commitment or the seeking and responding to the sacred. (This derivation can be recalled in the word "ligament," which apparently derives from a related Latin root.) In this sense, while secularistic culture entices people to many isolated, broken commitments, religion, on the other hand, puts them all in perspective by asking the ultimate questions about the sacred that integrate otherwise disconnected and fragmentary thoughts and feelings. The sense of religion as binding or aligning ourselves with the sacred may be especially useful when a patient is confronting a serious illness. Often those who experience a severe health crisis may reevaluate their priorities, their relationships, and the future directions for their lives as the changes involved in the crisis presents an opportunity to see things afresh.

As mentioned earlier, countless definitions of religion have been proposed, based on belief or content, based on the functions religion performs, and based on the forms in which religion is expressed. Scholars often consider religion as comprised of four interlocking components, the four Cs: Creed (belief), Community (such as church

---

29   Pargament, K. God help me: spirituality as a resource in self-care. Care for the Caregiver Bioethics Conference, Loma Linda University, Loma Linda, CA. interview by Steven Jeffers, 2001.

30   Klitzman, R. (2008). *When Doctors Become Patients*. New York, NY: Oxford University Press, 8. Klitzman cites a study by psychiatrist Robert Lifton on how people are able to connect with sources of meaning in difficult situations (his research was with survivors of the bombings of Hiroshima and Nagasaki in 1945); Lifton suggested that spirituality, along with work, family, and nature, was a way in which people could find some sense of hope and meaning in adversity.

or synagogue or *ummah*), Code (moral expectations), and Cultus (ritual practices). Religion includes conceptual, performatory, social, and other dimensions. In his widely used college textbook *Exploring Religion*, Roger Schmidt defines religion as "a human seeking and responding to what is experienced as holy."[31] While many of us might prefer this definition or describe religion as the earnest practice of spirituality, for the purposes of this book, we will use "religion" more narrowly to denote institutions, communities, and traditions that have arisen to nurture and promote spirituality.

The Relationship between Spirituality and Religion

As just suggested, the relationship between spirituality and religion is problematic today and deserves to be further explored. Spirituality is not a religion, and yet it pervades Baháʾí, Buddhist, Christian, Hindu, Islamic, Jewish, and all other religious traditions, in the sense that these are organized ways in which people have expressed their individual spirituality and the spiritual approach of their groups and cultures.

Every moment of life becomes an opportunity to see the world anew, so it may not be helpful to think of spirituality as an attainment. Mike Yaconelli stated, "spirituality is not a formula; it is not a test. It is a relationship. Spirituality is not about competency; it is about intimacy. Spirituality is not about perfection; it is about connection."[32] Thus, spirituality assists in the discovery of how to live in the world. Religions develop out of such discoveries. Using theistic language,

Elizabeth Taylor, PhD, RN, says, "Religion is a system of symbols, beliefs, myths, and rites experienced as profoundly significant, primarily because it provides individuals, groups, and societies with a means of drawing close to and in oneness with God."[33] Religion is a cultural form in which spirituality (its source) may be expressed.

Dale Matthews, MD, has contrasted religion and spirituality this way: Religion is more focused on establishing community, more objective and measurable to the external observer, more formal in worship, more based in behavior, and more focused on outward practices. Some people perceive religion as more authoritarian, with patterns of prescribed and proscribed behavior, more particularizing, distinguishing one group from another, and more orthodox and systematic in doctrine. In contrast, spirituality, as the term is commonly used nowadays, is typically more focused on individual growth, more subjective and less measurable to the external observer, less formal in worship, more emotion-based arising from inner experience. Spirituality may also be understood as less authoritarian, with few prescriptions or proscriptions; it may be more universalizing, discouraging separateness from others; it may be less orthodox and systematic in doctrine.[34]

As we have used the terms "spiritual" and "sacred," some people who consider themselves spiritual may also be very religious, but others may deny religious interest. Furthermore, some folks profess to be religious but do not show evidence of spiritual

31 Schmidt, R. (1988), *Exploring Religion* 2nd ed. Belmont, CA: Wadsworth Publishing.

32 Yaconelli, M. (2002). *Messy Spirituality*. Grand Rapids, MI: Zondervan, 5.

33 Taylor, E. Spiritual Dimensions of Health Care [course NURS 422], University of Southern California, Department of Nursing. interview with Steven Jeffers. 2000.

34 Matthews, D. (1998). *The Faith Factor*. New York, NY: Penguin Group, 183.

development. Because of this, it is helpful to distinguish spirituality and religion because many people separate them.

This distinction is important for spiritual care providers to keep in mind; all people are not religious per se, but a spiritual dimension is potential in everyone. Those who identify as spiritual but not religious may be saying they have experiences of the sacred or believe their life is part of a grand pattern, but they do not associate themselves with a particular religious group or tradition. The chapters on Paganism and Secularism, for example, illustrate why this point is essential. In performing spiritual assessments of patients to determine needs and concerns, it is often wise to use nonreligious terminology, at least until the patient discloses his or her spiritual and/or religious tradition. We recommend attention both to the patient's spirituality and to the patient's religion. This book provides information organized by religion because religion may provide critical clues for the spiritual care of the patient.

The Three Families of Faith

There are many ways of classifying the extraordinarily complex phenomena of religion. To understand the contexts in which most people develop their spiritual perspectives, it is helpful to know about various religious traditions, because religions differ greatly in how they approach the sacred. Many have found the following system to be a useful starting point for seeing differences and similarities. However, like any classification, it suffers from overgeneralization and exceptions. It should be regarded only as a place to begin one's study.

Here are three additional caveats. First, almost every faith has various forms. There is, for example, no single "American Indian" tradition; there are markedly different variations within some 500 tribes. Second, with each specific faith included in this book, an individual professing that faith may not fully understand the faith or may even depart from its usual characteristics in a particular situation. Third, while each of the three families of faith that we present here has an arena of typical emphasis (nature, personhood, covenanted community), this does not mean that these arenas cannot be found in every faith, even if they are not emphasized. With globalization and the increasing mutual influence and assimilation of faiths today, what is characteristic of one faith may be found in other faiths, even if the believer is unaware of its source. For example, while karma is a distinctly Asian religious notion, many Christians now employ the term when they are trying to understand the pattern or meaning of their lives – "It must have been bad karma."

Thus this overview of world religions should be used only as background from which specific questions may be developed. Furthermore, this particular synopsis of faiths and their cultures is based on the idea of the sacred as outlined earlier: that which points to ultimate concern or commitment or meaning, that on which people's lives depend.

Here are three families, each to be discussed in a little more detail later.

1. The primal religions generally find the sacred in the world of nature. These religions include those of American Indians, tribal Africans, and pagan traditions (such as Wicca).

2. The Asian religions generally locate the sacred in inner awareness. These religions include the faiths arising in China (Confucianism and Taoism as

well as Chinese folk religion) and the faiths beginning in India (Hinduism, Buddhism, and Jainism).

3. The Monotheistic religions generally find the sacred disclosed in the history of covenanted community. These religions include the three Abrahamic faiths of Judaism, Christianity, and Islam, as well as Sikhism, Unitarian Universalism, and Bahá'í. This is not to say that the sacred is nature, or is inner awareness, or is the history of covenanted community. Rather, in general, these families often locate the sacred in these realms. Of course, there are exceptions, variations, and subtleties. Shinto is an Asian religion that in this scheme belongs primarily with the primal faiths. Zoroastrianism is a special case since it greatly influenced the monotheistic faiths, while its origins are not Abrahamic.

Primal Faiths

Many primal religions behold the sacred in the world of nature. American Indian Spirituality serves as an example. Unlike creationists, who would dispute the notion that humans may be related to primates, the American Indian may celebrate one's bear, fox, or frog lineage, an ancestry that indicates intimacy with nature. This is why totem poles may portray one's forebears in animal form.

When most Americans need food, the sanitized supermarket is the source, not the wild. However, to recall the former days of the Plains Indians, when a hunter shoots a deer, he may have said:

I am sorry I had to kill you, Little Brother. My children were hungry. My family needs your meat. See, I hang your antlers in the tree. I decorate them with streamers. I smoke tobacco in your memory. Each time I cross this path, I shall honor your spirit.

Most people seldom talk to their groceries, but the American Indian perceives the sacred in the deer because his life literally depends upon it.

Even today, when an American Indian woman in the Southwest extracts clay from the ground to make a pot for storing food, she may offer a prayer to the earth. Stones themselves are considered "people." The streams, the air, the mountains – all are alive with sacred power, and deserve respect as one's relatives, not to be used as objects for selfish ends.

Health care providers will want to be alert to a sense that disease and accident occur by falling out of harmony with nature. Some patients may desire rituals to help to restore them to harmony with nature. The classic example is of the American Indian who, thrown by a horse, goes to the "regular" white doctor to have his bones set and to the traditional healer to find out why he was thrown by the horse.

Asian Faiths

Many Asian religions behold the sacred in a person's inner life. As an example of this, here is a Hindu story.

In the forest, 10 000 *rishis* (sages) worshipped the god Shiva in only one, static manifestation. Shiva decided to appear, to show them that his manifestations are multitudinous; that his personality is many, not one; that he is motion, movement, and dance.

But the *rishis*, whose preconceptions were challenged, rejected him. They called forth a great tiger that ferociously attacked Shiva at his throat. Shiva, with his little fingernail, skinned the tiger and wrapped the skin around him as a cloak. Then the *rishis* chanted a magic spell, and a great serpent emerged from the ground, wrapped himself around the body of Shiva, and began to writhe and twist and choke Shiva to death. But Shiva disabled the serpent, and cast its long body around his neck as a streamer of garlands. The *rishis'* incantations finally caused a demon dwarf to attack Shiva with a mace. But Shiva placed his little toe on the demon's back and began to dance.

All the gods came to see this dance, in which Shiva took every threat and made them props in his performance, showing people that whatever comes their way, however frightening, can be rendered harmless, even enriching, as they accept it into their dance – now moving forward, now retreating, now high, now low: the divine personality in many forms, always in process, moving in the eternal dance of the cosmos. This transforming power within is sacred; from it arises the meaning of individuals' lives.

A shallow way of translating this lesson is to say that while we cannot always control what happens to us, we are in command of our attitudes. In some forms of Hinduism, this is expressed by saying that Atman, the God within, is identical with Brahman, the Universal God.

The many dimensions of awareness are celebrated also by Buddhist *mandalas* (sacred designs for meditation). Even the ferocious-looking Buddhist temple guardian figures challenge people to observe their mental projections, to see that what they really fear may reside within. Through yoga, meditation, rites, and other techniques for observing the Self (or, in the case of Buddhism, the not-Self), Asian traditions provide paths for release from the perils of the ego.

Health care providers will want to be alert to a sense that misfortune may arise from a past life or from some inner process that needs to be cured or strengthened, and that practices such as meditation may be an important part of the path toward recovery.

Monotheistic Faiths

Because most users of this book may be immersed in one of the monotheistic religions (together, they comprise over half of the world's population, and the majority of the US population), it may be difficult to see the typical characteristics of this family, just as people don't usually notice the air they breathe because they are immersed in it. However, by comparing monotheism with the other families of faith, one can see that in the monotheistic faiths, the sacred is revealed in the realm of the history of covenanted community. This history and the accumulated wisdom is conveyed in scriptures, sometimes called the Word. This contrasts with the sacred in the world of nature for primal faiths, and it contrasts with the Asian faiths that discern the sacred in ineffable inner awareness. For the monotheistic traditions, nothing can be more sacred than God, who is One, ruling the universe and moving throughout history toward justice. Communities in covenant with God are instructed by prophets about how to live, and, in the case of Christianity, people are offered redemption through Christ as the Living Word. In some interpretations of these faiths, God is found in meeting other people, in the way people behave with one another, and in the allegiance people give to the expression of justice and peace.

Judaism serves as an example. Moses, though brought up an Egyptian, felt a strange kinship with the children of Israel, who had been pressed into bondage. He discovered who he really was by affirming his relationship with them, leading them out of the land of slavery, into the holiness of freedom. This story became a paradigm through which Jews have identified themselves. The Law revealed by Moses and his successors in written form provided the way in which Israel could be organized for holy living.

The succeeding Hebrew prophets analyzed the historical forces acting on their nation and proclaimed divine patterns as they commented on domestic economic issues and foreign affairs. Their prophecies were not so much prognostications and predictions as they were social commentaries and warnings. This Jewish tradition, that God is working out his will for justice, is expressed, for example, in what may be one of the most prized documents in US history, Lincoln's second inaugural address, which seeks to discern the meaning of the Civil War in the context of divine Providence with the freeing of the slaves and the preservation of the Union. As people relieve the suffering and oppression of their brothers and sisters, so, too, are their own spirits liberated into the vitality of the community, submitting to the commandments on which their lives and well-being as a society depend. For Jews, the holy community is the mystical Israel; for Christians, it is the Body of Christ, the church; for Muslims, it is the *ummah*; and for Sikhs, it is the *khalsa*.

Health care providers will want to be alert to some monotheists who may feel that their illness arises from lack of faith or disobedience to a divine command; for them, dealing with a sense of guilt, perhaps through ritual confession, may be important. As later chapters indicate, prayer, scripture reading, and the Eucharist or communion may provide spiritual comfort, reassurance, and restoration. On one hand, some patients may focus primarily on faith healing rather than medical attention, and on the other, some may completely separate their spirituality from medical conditions. Nonetheless, the inclusion of a sense of community may be especially important for spiritual support.

The Three Families of Faith and the World Today

The Abrahamic faiths (Judaism, Christianity, and Islam) have often drawn an important distinction between the Creator and the Creation. US culture has sometimes turned this distinction into a rupture, which makes it difficult to talk about a spirituality that encompasses everything of meaning. The realm of spirit has been confined to specific times, places, and activities (Sunday at church, for example) instead of being understood as a circle whose center is everywhere and whose circumference is nowhere.

Judaism ameliorates this split by emphasizing the world as God's creation. Christianity addresses the split by celebrating Jesus as both human and divine – the alpha and the omega, one without beginning or end. While utterly clear that nothing can be compared with God, Islam deliberately fosters the integration of all learning; even politics is seen as a religious activity insofar as justice and peace are pursued. In contrast to secularistic culture, the beliefs of these traditions are often made very explicit.

In Asian and primal traditions, faith is more likely to be implicit in all activities, rather than explicit or confined in expression to one particular arena (such as Sunday morning). Taoism, for example, teaches that the *Tao*, the Way, is present everywhere so that only the "ignorant" try to define it or specify its domain.

Today, the joining of East and West and primal traditions makes it possible to see spirituality not so much as an interest in an isolated or exclusive activity, but more like a pair of glasses through which one sees everything. Spirituality becomes not a fragment of existence but, rather, an experience of life in its fullness. It is not so much an arena as an orientation. It is not where people stand, but how people show up.

Because the many different religious traditions are now learning about one another as never before through interfaith dialogue, the modern age has an unprecedented opportunity – and health care workers have an increased responsibility.

Summary

While terms like spirituality, religion, and sacred have varied meanings, we have suggested some ways of understanding these terms so that the different orientations of persons of primal, Asian, and monotheistic faiths may be approached in the health care environment.

Furthermore, people with no professed faith and/or those only nominally religious may seek to recover earlier religious or spiritual teachings and practices to help them in making some sense of a critical illness or the experience of dying. This search for meaning or purpose within a medical situation may be expressed through self-hatred, anger at God, or a sense of loss of participation in community. For example, health care workers may hear patients ask, "God! Why are you doing this to me?" Folks may feel unmoored and ask, "What have I done to deserve this? Why is this happening to me?"

In many of these situations, helping patients understand or develop a sense of meaning from what they are facing can improve the results of their treatments and enable a sense of "peacefulness in the midst of the storm." The chapters on specific faith traditions expand upon this overview and provide specific strategies for providing spiritual care in the various faith traditions.

Spirituality, Religion, and Culture

In the previous chapter, spirituality and religion were discussed. In this chapter, we will look at the idea of culture, particularly its influence upon and relationship to spirituality and religion and views of health and illness. We begin the discussion with the Buddhist tale of *Kisagotami*, the mother whose infant son died from a disease. Grief-stricken, she carried his corpse in her arms wherever she went, seeking a cure. Then, *Kisagotami* met Gautama, the Buddha, who is sometimes called the Physician. Her son was not cured, but she was healed. As we shall see, this story nicely illustrates some key components of culture.

The Tale of Kisagotami

Kisagotami became in the family way, and when the 10 months were completed, gave birth to a son. When the boy was able to walk by himself, he died. The young girl, in her love for it, carried the dead child clasped to her bosom, and went about from house to house asking if anyone would give her some medicine for it. When the neighbors saw this, they said, "Is the young girl mad that she carries about on her breast the dead body of her son!" But a wise man thought to himself, "Alas! this Kisagotami does not understand the law of death, I must comfort her." The wise man said to Kisagotami, "My good girl, I cannot myself give medicine for it, but I know of a doctor who can attend to it." The young girl said, "If so, tell me who it is." The wise man continued, "Gautama can give medicine, you must go to him."

Kisagotami went to Gautama, and asked, "Lord and master, do you know any medicine that will be good for my boy?" Gautama replied, "I know of some." She asked, "What medicine do you require?" He said, "I want a handful of mustard seed." Gautama continued, "I require some mustard seed taken from a house where no son, husband, parent, or slave has died." The girl said, "Very good," and went to ask for some at the different houses, carrying the dead body of her son astride on her hip. She asked, "In my friend's home has there died a son, a husband, a parent, or a slave?" They replied, "Lady, what is this that you say! The living are few, but the dead are many." Then she went to other houses, but one said, "I have lost a son"; another, "I have lost my parents"; and another, "I have lost my slave." At last, not being able to find a single house where no one had died from which to procure the mustard seed, she began to think, "This is a heavy task that I am engaged in. I am not the only one whose son is dead. In the whole of the Savatthi country, everywhere children are dying, parents are dying." Thinking thus, she acquired the law of fear and putting away her affection for her child, she summoned up resolution, and left the dead body in a forest; then she went to Gautama and paid him homage. He said to her, "Have you procured the handful of mustard seed?" "I have not," she replied; "the people of the village told me, 'The living are few, but the dead are many.'" Gautama said to her, "You thought that you alone had lost a son; the law of death is that among all living creatures there is no permanence." When Gautama had finished preaching the law, Kisagotami was established in the reward of Sotapatti, and all the assembly who heard the law were also established in the reward of Sotapatti.

Thinking about Culture

There are many ways to think about culture, ranging from general views to those more narrow and specific. By "culture," people often mean geographical, regional, or national boundaries – for example, Scandinavian, Asian, Canadian, German, or Turkish cultures. They also think of culture as reflected through traditional belief systems, such as Jewish, Muslim, Hindu, or Christian cultures. Culture can also involve shared beliefs that pertain to age, gender, socioeconomic status, social status, occupation, sexual orientation, and so forth. However one thinks of culture, it represents that which distinguishes members of one group from members of another group. As Dutch organizational anthropologist Geert Hofstede claims, culture therefore constitutes "the collective programming of the mind which distinguishes the member of one group or category of people from another."[35]

Culture's Ubiquity

It is certain that people cannot escape culture. It is ubiquitous. It influences individuals without their even being aware of its power. To illustrate, there is in our US society a "consumer culture" that takes and exploits the benefits of a free-market economy. Indeed, consumerism may well be a new "religion" in culture if it provides people with a sense of vital meaning.[36] This is certainly consonant with our culture of individualism, given the importance attached to independence, self-expression, personal liberties, rights, and autonomy, or self-determination, a reigning principle in Western bioethics. Along these lines, in contrast to this culture of consumerism, we can also speak of a culture of poverty.[37]

Therefore, culture can be thought of as that hidden dimension of unwritten rules comprising values, beliefs, and behaviors. In this respect, culture operates on a subconscious level. People may uncritically assimilate prevailing values, beliefs, and practices, and, in turn, these become the norm. This hidden dimension is normative in that the tendency is to both attach a positive value to this norm and censure values that seem to oppose those norms. Accordingly, culture is learned. Through subconsciously "learning," or internalizing the norms of environment, they are taken for granted, until they are challenged. In health care, they are often dramatically challenged. For instance, health care itself encompasses the dissimilar cultures of business, medicine, nursing, patients, and faith systems. Moreover, increasing one's exposure to patients and health professionals

35 Hofstede, G. (1994). *Cultures and Organizations: Software of the Mind.* London: Harper Collins, 5.

36 Buddhist scholar David Loy argues that our uncritical faith in the "wisdom of the market," has not only fractured attempts at a covenantal or communal culture but also alienated ourselves from our own natural environment. See his *The Great Awakening: A Buddhist Social Theory* (Somerville, MA: Wisdom Publications, 2003).

37 Noted anthropologist Oscar Lewis referred to "culture of poverty" as distinct from poverty. He was especially known for his work with rural Texans, Puerto Ricans, Mexicans, Cubans, and Blackfoot Indians. See his *On Understanding Poverty: Perspectives from the Social Sciences* (New York, NY: Basic Books, 1969).

from other cultures naturally challenges all of us regarding what we've assumed to be the norm, and it *should*. The encounter with someone from another culture, with a seemingly different set of values, beliefs, and practices ought to compel people to reexamine their own assumptions, values, and beliefs. Looking outward also helps one look inward.

Layers of Culture

Again, what is culture? Georgetown University's National Center for Cultural Competence offers a comprehensive definition:

> [Culture is] an integrated pattern of human behavior that includes thoughts, communications, languages, practices, beliefs, values, customs, courtesies, rituals, manners of interacting and roles, relationships and expected behaviors or a racial, ethnic, religious or social group; and the ability to transmit the above to succeeding generations.[38]

Note especially the last phrase. There is a "transmitting" quality to culture. It is not merely a bundle of shared patterns but is entirely active in its influence on all of us. Indeed, the sustaining power of culture lies in its ongoing affect upon its members and beyond. This volume describes this transmitting power of culture, as the various cultural systems and traditions intersect with

spirituality and religion to exert their forces upon views of health, illness, and treatment.

Culture's Inner Core

The National Center for Cultural Competence's definition no doubt captures the complexity of culture, which comprises mental, linguistic, symbolic, behavioral, ideological, normative, ritual, historical, temporal, and affective elements. This complexity need not daunt us, however. When broken down, one can see that culture consists of a pattern of shared features that are both hidden and obvious. British linguist Helen Spencer-Oatey elaborates on these layers of concealed and overt manifestations. She refers to the concealed realm of culture as its "inner core."[39] This inner core consists of fundamental assumptions and values. These assumptions have to do with what a culture believes to be real and meaningful, and they are sustained through deep-rooted values.

Note the story of Kisagotami. The tale occurs in a setting that assumes the universality of suffering. Buddhists, as well as many other faith perspectives, are intensely aware of the truth that no one escapes suffering, pain, and death. "The living are few, but the dead are many." Kisagotami, however, has somehow lost sight of this perspective, so that when her son dies, she is so radically distraught that she cannot come to terms with his loss.

In turn, this elemental assumption of the universality of suffering generates the value of working to relieve others' suffering to the best of one's ability. This further evokes values of awareness, detachment,

---

38 National Center for Cultural Competence of Georgetown University. (n.d.). *Planner's Guide*. Washington, DC: Georgetown University Center for Child and Human Development. Available at: www11.georgetown.edu/research/gucchd/nccc/documents/Planners_Guide.pdf (accessed 15 Sept 2012).

---

39 Spencer-Oatey, H. (2000). *Culturally Speaking: Managing Rapport through Talk Across Cultures*. London: Continuum, 2.

and compassion. The challenge lies in how to relieve Kisagotami of her suffering. Her son is dead. He cannot be cured. However, she can be healed. Yet, she can be healed only when she awakens to the truth of the universality of suffering, frees herself from attachment to her dead son, experiences her kinship with all other living beings, and acts out of compassion for others.

In the previous chapter on spirituality and religion, one can see that a key element of spirituality fits into the cultural perspective of Kisagotami's search for meaning – spirituality entails discovering "how to live in the world." In this way, a culture's inner core is revealed through its spirituality. Spirituality conveys intimacy and connection, and these generate those deep values in the inner core of culture. Moreover, as described earlier, matters of the "sacred" have to do with addressing the fundamental question "What gives ultimate meaning to our lives?" A culture's sense of the sacred unveils that culture's inner core. A culture's deep values are its responses to the universal quest for meaning and purpose, for "ultimate concern."

At the same time, a culture's values embody that culture's ideals and the inner core manifests what a culture believes about how things "ought to be." As in the case of Kisagotami, compassion is the highest virtue for Buddhists. This comes about when people recognize their essential kinship, their solidarity, their oneness, with all other living beings. Until Kisagotami awakens to this, she will not be free from her suffering, nor can she relieve others of theirs.

Culture's Outer Layers

Spencer-Oatey goes further in enabling thought about culture. This inner core expresses itself outwardly. A culture's basic

assumptions and values generate a layer of "beliefs, attitudes, and conventions." These are expressed through teachings and beliefs that can become systematized to varying degrees. Throughout this text, these are described in the sections headed "Basic Teachings." Systematizing, as a way of putting things into some framework, certainly reflects a deep-seeded need for order. Kisagotami's story helps to see how Buddhist assumptions and values about suffering and life's transient nature lead to more formalized teachings such as the Four Noble Truths (centered on the universal truth of suffering and ways to be free from suffering and to free others) and the Three Signs of Existence – impermanence, nonsubstantiality, and suffering.

Beliefs manifest a culture's inner core of assumptions and values and are thus intended to be congruent with that inner core. Thus the Four Noble Truths reflect Buddhism's inner core. However, as with many cultural traditions and belief systems, various interpretations of the inner core may lead to varying beliefs. This is seen in the history of Buddhism. Conflicting interpretations of the Buddha's teaching produced various schools of Buddhism. Nonetheless, this does not necessarily reflect a change in Buddhism's inner core. In other words, interpretations of teachings may change, but this does not mean that the inner core is in essence altered.

According to Spencer-Oatey, beliefs, attitude, and conventions bring about another layer of "systems and institutions." These systems and institutions then express themselves through "artifacts and products" and "rituals and behavior."[40] This text describes these in the sections headed

---

40 Ibid, 6.

"Basic Practices." Here, prominent symbols and ceremonies assume a key role. For instance, Shamanism is a traditional form of healing in Native American and indigenous Australian, Pacific, and African cultures. The healer is the shaman. Healing assumes a living and interconnected relationship people have with all of nature. Its ceremonies include certain rhythmic music that reaches into the individual and collective subconscious of participants. In Kisagotami's story, note the symbolism behind the mustard seed, the forest where she left the body of her dead child, the image of the Buddha as a "doctor," and his teaching as "medicine."

Rituals, symbols, and behaviors tend to become internalized, as is the case with beliefs, so that certain practices are assumed to be the norm. We see this throughout cultural practices regarding ways to treat the body, noting spatial distance, attention to time, using or avoiding eye contact, ways of speaking, views of physical contact, and the significance of nonverbal behaviors.

Five Cautions

There are at least five cautions to consider in this discussion of culture and its role in societal expectations and experiences. First, consider the etymological root of "culture." The term comes from the Latin *colere*, which literally means "to plant," "to cultivate," "to build." Therefore, the product of what is cultivated is culture. More important, this product is always in process and constantly undergoes some transformation. Culture is, by nature, dynamic. This idea is critical for a proper understanding of culture. It should make one wary of viewing culture in general and any culture in particular in a static, reified sense. We reify when we make a "thing" or "object" of an idea that is inherently abstract and dynamic. We need to

avoid reifying cultures. The many cultures in the form of religious and spiritual traditions referred to in this book are dynamic, and they thereby experience fluctuation and modification, sometimes radical, through internal dynamics and encounters with external forces.

Second, we need to be especially watchful that we do not homogenize cultures. We must avoid casting a monolithic net over a culture, lumping all of its members into one category. Doing so ignores a culture's internal discrepancies. Within cultures, there are many subdivisions and subcultures. Not all members of a culture think alike. The same is true for religious traditions. Assuming that all Buddhists, Christians, Hindus, Jews, and Muslims, for example, conform to a specific set of beliefs and practices within their respective traditions is a fallacy. Moreover, homogenizing a culture fails to recognize a culture's similarities with other cultures.

Third, and this logically follows on from the second caution, as profoundly significant as culture is, people need to be careful not to think of culture as absolutely determinative. That is, one needs to account for individual personalities, dispositions, values, and characters. Individuals are certainly influenced by their cultures, yet that does not mean they are fully determined by their cultures. This is crucial in assessing the relationship between culture and morality. One of the biggest challenges in ethics lies in ascertaining the various sources of morality. While it is certainly the case that cultural values shape an individual's morality to varying degrees, it remains arguable whether morality is strictly defined by cultural values.

A fourth caution has to do with context. We must be careful to not overlook the importance of context in understanding culture. This is especially critical when it comes to communicating with persons from other cultures. Anthropologist Edward T. Hall, one of the first to use the term "intercultural communication," distinguished between high-context cultures and low-context cultures.[41] In high-context cultures, when individuals are communicating with each other, more importance is attached to their specific milieu and context rather than to their verbal or written messages to each other. In low-context cultures, the reverse is the case – more significance is assigned to the actual transmitted messages. This means that for certain cultures, nonverbal behavior, silence, and context play a more valuable role in communicating. This is equally true for spiritual traditions. For example, the Amish faith community is much less vocal in expressions of worship, grief, and so forth, than Pentecostal Protestant traditions.

A fifth caution lies in not equating healing with curing. The two are not the same. Our US biomedical culture emphasizes curing as a way to restore a patient to some level of medical normalcy. Healing reaches deeper and has to do with restoring inner balance, harmony, and spiritualty. One of the most profound lessons in Kisagotami's story lies in drawing the distinction between healing and curing. As you will see through the pages of this book, this becomes evident in many cultural, spiritual, and religious views of health and illness. Healing is personal and in this respect is intensely spiritual. We humans have a universal longing to be healed. In the case of Kisagotami, and this is seen in many Asian views of healing, healing can only come about when there is harmony. As the previous chapter relates, spirituality ultimately compels us to walk in harmony, whether this is harmony with nature (primal traditions), within oneself in inner peace and balance (Asian traditions), or with one God in covenant with community (monotheistic traditions). Here is the natural alliance of culture and spirituality.

Throughout this book, the authors hope that we shall all discover more common ground among cultures and religions than we may have originally thought possible. Their many distinctions are no doubt significant, but so are their similarities.

---

41 Hall, E. (1959). *The Silent Language*. New York, NY: Doubleday; Hall, E. (1969). *The Hidden Dimension: Man's Use of Space in Public and Private*. London: Bodley Head.

Spirituality and Religion: Relevance in the Clinical Setting?

As people face a serious and perhaps life-threatening illness, lots of questions often arise. Questions like "why me, why now, what will my future hold?" People often begin to question the very purpose and meaning of life. Some people question God's existence and others simply question the fairness of life and the reason for suffering. These questions might lead people down a spiritual path.[42]

We will explain why this is an important perspective shortly.

"Disease forges an especially close relationship between God and man; the Divine Presence Itself, as It were, rests on the head of the sickbed," said the late Immanuel Jakobovits, the former Chief Rabbi of the British Commonwealth of Nations.[43] The words of David Lukoff further delineate the close relationship between spiritual and physical health expressed by an overwhelming majority of the general population: "Religion and spirituality are among the most important cultural factors that give structure and meaning to human values, behaviors and experiences ... 94 per cent of patients regard their spiritual health and physical health as equally important."[44]

As the testimonies of these two individuals suggest, illness, dying and death are inextricably connected to people's spirituality and can produce emotional and spiritual crises in their lives. To acknowledge this and be willing to address the emotional and spiritual suffering people experience in a clinical setting is a significant aspect of treating the whole person. However, this concept is not novel, as the following section reveals; only its revival in the modern period is.

Rationale from Antiquity

I dare say that you have heard eminent physicians say to a patient who comes to them with bad eyes that they cannot cure the eyes by themselves, but if the eyes are to be cured the head must be treated. And again they say that to think of curing the head alone and not the rest of the body also is the height of folly. Arguing in this way, they apply their methods to the whole body and try to treat and heal the whole and the part together.[45]

42 Jeffers, S. (2001). *Finding a Sacred Oasis in Illness.* Overland Park, KS: Leathers Publishing, iii.

43 Jakobovits, I. (1975). *Jewish Medical Ethics: A Contemporary and Historical Study of the Religious Attitude to Medicine and Its Practice.* New York, NY: Block. Rabbi Jakobovits' words were cited in Post, S. G., C. M. Puchalski, and D. B. Larson. (2000). Physicians and patient spirituality: professional boundaries, competency, and ethics. *Annals of Internal Medicine,* 132(7), 578–583.

44 Lukoff, D., F. Lu, and R. Turner. (1992). Toward a more culturally sensitive DSM-IV: pyschoreligious and psychospiritual problems. *Journal of Nervous and Mental Disease,* 180(11), 673–682.

45 Jowett, B. (1924). Charmides. *The Dialogues of Plato.* Vol. 1. New York, NY: Oxford University Press. Plato's words were cited in Keung, Y. K. and R. McQuellon. (2001). When medical meets

These words were not written in modern times, but by the renowned ancient Greek philosopher Plato, who goes on to say:

> I learned these lessons when serving with the army from one of the physicians of the Thracian King Zamolxis, who said, "as you ought not to attempt to cure the eyes without the head or the head without the body, so neither ought you to attempt to cure the body without the soul. And this is the reason why the cure of many diseases is unknown to the physicians of Greece, because they are ignorant of the whole which ought to be studied also, for the part can never be well unless the whole is well. Therefore, if the head and body are to be well, you must begin by curing the soul."

Study the whole? Cure the soul? What do these mean?

The "head and the body" are studied routinely in the medical community. Psychiatry, internal medicine and the various subspecialties are accepted as standard medical practice. But according to ancients like Plato and many moderns as well, the "whole" is comprises three constituent parts, not two. Spirit, or *soul* as it is often called, is the completing element of the triad in this system of understanding personhood.

It seems logical to conclude, then, that the study of the whole should include the study of the soul in conjunction with the study of the mental and physical aspects of humankind. Is it even possible, though, to study the soul? If so, is it important to consider such a study? The following sections will provide some answers to these questions.[46]

Rationale from the Modern Period

From the medical community of the late twentieth century, Christina Puchalski, MD, one of the leading proponents of the spirituality in health movement stated, "Spirituality is the essence of what makes us human. It is important to recognize this dimension in healthcare."[47]

According to Puchalski and many other individuals who would posit the indissoluble relationship among body, mind, and spirit, attention to the spiritual dimension should be an integral component of a patient's plan of care. Now, it is highly unlikely that few in the field of medicine, whether in research or in clinical practice, would argue against the use of "best practices," which is predicated on evidence-based criteria. Why is that the case? Medicine is science, and physicians are scientists. Furthermore, in the ongoing journey to excelling in the use of best clinical practices for the benefit of patients, research in physical and mental health will continue to proliferate. However, in order to enhance patients' overall sense of well-being, the research field for an ever-increasing number of physicians has been expanded to include spiritual health as an indispensable element of evidence-based practice.

In the mid-1900s "studying the whole," to use Plato's nomenclature, became an academic exercise in prestigious university-based medical centers across the United States. At academic centers

---

spiritual. *North Carolina Medical Journal*, July/August, 62(4), 192–194, discussion 195.

46 The three previous paragraphs, although slightly different, also appear in "Spirituality and Cultural

Diversity: Innner Resources for Healing" (2008) by Steven L. Jeffers and Dennis Kenny, a chapter in *Putting Patients First: Best Practices in Patient-Centered Care*. 2nd ed. San Francisco, CA: Jossey-Bass.

47 Puchalski, C. *Institute for Spirituality in Health of Shawnee Mission Medical Center Conference*, information obtained by Steven Jeffers, 2003.

such as Duke[48,49,50] and George Washington University,[51,52] among others, physicians engage in research, writing, and speaking about the role of spirituality in physical and mental health. Even the world-renowned Mayo Clinic has physicians involved in similar initiatives.[53] The research projects in these and many other institutions are designed to scientifically determine the relationship, if one exists, between spirituality and physical/mental health.

In many of the scientific studies and clinical trials, the results have been overwhelmingly conclusive that attention to patient spirituality enhances the body's healing process, facilitates greater coping abilities and contributes to one's overall sense of well-being. People's religious or spiritual beliefs do affect how they experience various maladies.[54,55]

Rationale from Contemporary Research

Scientific studies to determine the role of spirituality in health started to emerge from the mid-twentieth-century medical community, and the results of many of these studies appeared in peer-reviewed journals. Koenig et al.[56] compiled a comprehensive review of history, research, and discussion of religion and health in a volume of 700-plus pages. One study of long-term AIDS survivors performed by Ironson et al.[57] noted a strong correlation between spirituality and a reduction in stress, a more hopeful outlook, and healthier behaviors. Another study, meta-analysis by McCullough et al.,[58] demonstrated that religious involvement reduced mortality by over 20%. Many of the scientific studies reported in the medical literature attests to the importance of the spiritual dimension in dealing with illness, dying, and death. In addition to the proliferation of literature on the subject, medical schools have started incorporating spirituality and health courses into their curriculums, and programs devoted to the study of spirituality in health have been established in university-based medical centers.[59]

48 Koenig, H. (1999). *The Healing Power of Faith*. New York, NY: Simon & Schuster. Koenig, as professor of medicine and founder of Duke's institute for spirituality and health, conducts research and writes prolifically about the relationship between spirituality and physical health.
49 Koenig, H. (2001). Religion and medicine IV: religion, physical health, and clinical implications. *International Journal of Psychiatry in Medicine*, 31(3), 321–336.
50 Koenig, H. (2001). *Spirituality in Patient Care*. Pennsylvania, PA: Templeton Foundation Press.
51 Puchalski, C. (2000). Physicians and patient spirituality: professional boundaries, competency and ethics. *Annals of Internal Medicine*, 132(7), 578–583.
52 Puchalski, C. (2001). Spirituality and health: the art of compassionate medicine. *Hospital Physician*, 37(3), 30–36.
53 Koenig, H. (2001). Religion, spirituality and medicine: how are they related and what does it mean? *Mayo Clinic Proceedings*, 76(12), 1189–1191.
54 Graber, D. and J. Johnson. (2001). Spirituality and healthcare organizations. *Journal of Healthcare Management*, 46(1), 39–50.
55 Mueller, P. S., D. J. Plevak, and T. A. Rummans. (2001). Religious involvement, spirituality, and medicine: implications for clinical practice. *Mayo Clinic Proceedings*, 76(12), 1225–1235.

56 Koenig, H. G., M. E. McCullough, and D. B. Larson. (2001). *Handbook of Religion and Health*. New York, NY: Oxford University Press.
57 Ironson, G., G. F. Solomon, E. G. Balbin, et al. (2002). The Ironson-Woods Spirituality/Religiousness Index is associated with long survival, healthy behaviors, less stress, and low cortisol in people with HIV/AIDS. *Annals of Behavioral Medicine*, 24(1), 34–48.
58 McCullough, M. E., W. T. Hoyt, D. B. Larson, et al. (2000). Religious involvement and mortality: a meta-analytic review. *Health Psychology*, 19(3), 211–222.
59 By 2005, approximately 80% of the medical schools in the United States had courses on spirituality and health in their curriculums. Institutes devoted to the study of the relationship between spirituality and health were established at Harvard, Duke, and George Washington universities, among others.

There are multiple reasons for this change in attitude toward spirituality and religion in medicine, not the least of which may be a breakdown in the current health care system with respect to its patient-centered philosophy of care. This has occurred partly as a result of increasing time pressures, fiscal responsibilities, and administrative duties, which have become an ever-increasing burden on health care providers and have usurped efforts that previously had been directed toward development of the physician-patient relationship.

A patient-centered, whole-person care approach to health care involves addressing issues and concerns that, in addition to those of the physical nature, are important to patients during illness and dying. For many patients and their families, spiritual concerns are as important as physical concerns. David Lukoff's research supports this view.

> Religion and spirituality are among the most important cultural factors that give structure and meaning to human values, behaviors and experiences ... ninety-four percent of patients regard their spiritual health and physical health as equally important.[60]

The Institute for Spirituality in Health of Shawnee Mission Medical Center (SMMC) was founded in 2002 to promote the integration of spirituality into the provision of health care. One of the first projects undertaken was a random survey of SMMC's customers in response to many physicians asking the same question: "What do our patients want from us with respect to spiritual matters?" They asked this question because of the belief that they would be better equipped to respond to spiritual needs if they had a better understanding of patients' preferences. The data are presented in detail in the Appendix at the end of this chapter. However, to summarize, the SMMC survey noted strong support among respondents for physicians discussing spiritual and religious beliefs during times of severe illness. A total of 54.5% of the respondents said "I would like my doctor to be aware of my beliefs that influence my medical decisions" and 49.2% preferred that their physicians talk with them about spiritual or religious beliefs that affect their physical health. Furthermore, 50.2% said that they would choose a doctor who responded to their spiritual or religious beliefs over one that did not. These findings are in line with the results documented by Ehman et al.[61] in a survey of 177 patients in Pennsylvania. Of the 79 patients who had beliefs that influenced their medical decisions, 74 (94%) would prefer to discuss issues with their physicians. In a survey conducted by Mansfield et al.[62] in the southeastern United States, 68.4% of the respondents reported wanting to talk about spiritual concerns if seriously ill. However, in the same study, only 3% reported that they would choose to discuss these concerns with a physician. Another survey, conducted by Maugans and Wadland[63] in Vermont, found that only

---

60 Lukoff, et al. Toward a more culturally sensitive DSM-IV.

61 Ehman, J. W., B. B. Ott, T. H. Short, et al. (1999). Do patients want physicians to inquire about their spiritual or religious beliefs if they become gravely ill? *Archives of Internal Medicine*, 159 (15), 1803–1806.

62 Mansfield, C., J. Mitchell, and D. E. King. (2002). The doctor as God's mechanic? Beliefs in the southeastern United States. *Social Science and Medicine*, 54(3), 399–409.

63 Maugans, T. and W. Wadland. (1991). Religion and family medicine: a survey of physicians and patients. *Journal of Family Practice*, 32(2), 210–213.

40% of patients would prefer to discuss religious issues with their physician. However, this question was not asked in the context of a severe illness. The disparities in these findings may be due to differences in culture between the various geographical areas or the structure of the survey questionnaires. Yet, the data does support that there is a significant percentage of patients who experience a need to discuss religious and spiritual issues in the context of medical care with their physicians.

Physician Survey

As a follow-up to the patient survey that provided answers to the question posed by physicians concerning their role in addressing patients' spiritual or religious concerns, the Institute for Spirituality in Health shifted its focus back to physicians. In order to better understand the attitudes and beliefs of the medical community at SMMC, a survey was conducted in 2004 to identify physician beliefs regarding the inclusion of religion and spirituality into the practice of medicine, the frequency of behaviors associated with those beliefs, and a description of the potential barriers to aligning beliefs with behaviors.

RESEARCH RESULTS

The entirety of the data is presented in Appendix 1. However, it is important to emphasize that approximately 85% (84.5%) of the physicians reported that spirituality or religion is an important part of their lives. Approximately 69% (69.3%) reported that a patient's faith and spirituality is relevant to their provision of care. Additionally, 80% agreed or strongly agreed with the statement that "a patient's involvement in religion or spirituality reduces morbidity and mortality." Less than a quarter of the respondents

(23.4%) reported feeling uncomfortable addressing religious or spiritual issues pertaining to medical decisions with patients. In summary, the majority of physicians in this group communicated that spirituality is important in their personal lives, is relevant to how they provide care, and adds value to their patients' lives. In addition, they are comfortable discussing spirituality with their patients.

However, when asked about behaviors associated with integrating spiritual care into their practices, a different picture emerges. Only about 28% (28.4%) of the physicians reported routinely asking patients about beliefs that impact their medical decisions (often or always). Approximately 73% (73.3%) of physicians reported never or rarely initiating a spiritual history with patients. Another 54% of physicians reported that they have never or rarely discussed with patients ways to improve their quality of life through religious or spiritual coping. Fifty-six per cent have never or rarely referred a patient for spiritual care follow-up. Less than one-third (31%) of physicians reported praying with patients with any frequency (sometimes, often, or always). The physicians' behaviors represent a significant contrast to the reported beliefs.

This disparity between physician beliefs and behaviors may be due to the barriers identified in the survey. Of the six choices of barriers provided, lack of time was identified by the greatest number of respondents (58%). Fifty-six per cent of physicians indicated that lack of experience and training in taking a spiritual history was a barrier. Correctly identifying patients who desire a discussion of spiritual issues was identified as a barrier by 51% of the respondents. Interestingly, a third of the physicians

(36.8%) reported that a concern for projecting their own beliefs onto the patients was a limiting factor in addressing spirituality.

DISCUSSION OF RESEARCH RESULTS

Despite the differences that surfaced between their beliefs and their practices, few physicians expressed personal beliefs that could be perceived as barriers to integrating spirituality into their practices. Only 14% believed that talking about spirituality is not appropriate to the physician role. Less than 12% (11.7%) believed that patients do not want to share spiritual concerns with their physicians.

Health care providers and faith community leaders have long realized that the experiences of illness, disability, dying, and death are stressful and challenging times for patients and their families. Generations of physicians have worked to ease the physical pain of their patients with the goal of arresting disease and restoring health. However, this goal has not always been met. Furthermore, physicians are often not trained to deal with patients' existential suffering. Addressing patients' suffering or spiritual distress was assumed, by some physicians, to be the exclusive role of the clergy, who themselves often receive little training in dealing with the concerns of the sick and dying. Nevertheless, throughout the centuries, when the cure was elusive, health care professionals and spiritual advisers have attempted to help people who struggle to find meaning and purpose in those difficult stages of the human condition.

Implications for Clinical Application

What, then, do the results of this research mean for physicians, other health care providers, and, most important, for patients?

Without question, it certainly supports the idea that illness, dying and death raise awareness of issues that pertain to transcendental realities and often cause crises of faith for many patients and their families. For this reason, intentionally initiating appropriate spiritual interventions is a necessity in providing quality holistic care. Therefore, the "journey to excellence" in patient care must include not only evidence-based medical practices but also evidence-based spiritual care practices.

Research into the relationship between spirituality and physical and mental health must continue. However, the research must not be an end in itself. Research needs to be applied in the clinical setting. In order to provide optimum care for patients and their families, there needs to be an increase in the number of clergy and laypeople trained in the art of providing care to the critically ill and dying. Additionally, physicians and other health care providers must become cognizant of the importance of spirituality in reducing morbidity and mortality and be willing to receive training in the art of identifying and addressing the spiritual concerns of patients. Discussing advance care planning, utilizing a spiritual history assessment tool,[64,65,66,67,68] and/or having a

---

64 Puchalski, C. and A. Romer. (2000). Taking a spiritual history allows clinicians to understand patients more fully. *Journal of Palliative Medicine*, 3(1), 129–137.

65 Lo, B., T. Quill, and J. Talky. (1999). Discussing palliative care with patients. *Annals of Internal Medicine*, 130(9), 744–749.

66 Kuhn, C. (1988). A spiritual inventory of the medically ill patient. *Psychiatric Medicine*, 6(2), 87–100.

67 Maugans, T. A. (1996). The SPIRITual history. *Archives of Family Medicine*, 5(1), 11–16.

68 Anandarajah, G. and E. Hight. (2001). Spirituality and medical practice: using the HOPE questions as a practical tool for spiritual assessment. *American Family Physician*, 63(1), 81–88.

"heart-to-heart" conversation are examples of ways to initiate dialogue with a patient about spiritual matters. A poignant example is related in a poem by Raymond Carver, reflecting a conversation between patient and physician from the patient's perspective – "What the Doctor Said."[69]

> He said it doesn't look good.
> He said it looks bad in fact real bad.
> He said I counted thirty-two of them
>   on one lung.
> Before he quit counting them
> I said I'm glad. I wouldn't want to
>   know
> About any more being there than
>   that;
> He said are you a religious man? Do
>   you kneel down
> In forest groves and let yourself ask
>   for help?
> When you come to a waterfall
> Mist blowing against your face and
>   arms
> Do you stop and ask for
>   understanding at those moments?
> I said not yet but I intend to start
>   today.
> He said I'm real sorry; he said
> I wish I had some other kind of news
>   to give you.
> I said Amen and he said something
>   else
> I didn't catch and not knowing what
>   else to do
> And not wanting him to have to
>   repeat it
> And me to have to fully digest it
> I just looked at him

> For a minute and he looked back; it
>   was then
> I jumped up and shook hands with
>   this man who'd just given me
> Something no one else on earth had
>   ever given me.
> I may even have thanked him habit
>   being so strong.

What happened here? This story illustrates the concept of caring for the whole person.

The physician engaged in a heart-to-heart conversation with the patient. He or she was "real," down-to-earth in the approach. The physician attempted to provide a means by which the patient could find answers to questions that medical science could not provide.

Conclusion

As to research in the field of spirituality in the clinical setting, conclusions drawn from much of that research confirm the importance and relevance of spirituality in patient care. However, health care professionals and the organizations to which they belong should not be satisfied in conducting research for the sake of publishing its findings, being compliant with the Joint Commission and other accrediting agencies in simply "doing things right." They might consider that they are called to a higher standard in "doing the right things" professionally, ethically, morally, and spiritually. These "right things" have been aptly described by Graber and Johnson:

> With proper consideration and caution by clinicians and managers, a truly "spiritual" healthcare organization can be developed: one that supports patients' expressions of faith; provides guidance and direction to staff

---

69 Carver, R. (1989). What the doctor said. In R. Carver. *A New Path to the Waterfall.* New York, NY: Atlantic Monthly Press, 113.

on how to discuss faith, health and meaning in illness; encourages staff and clinicians to be warm, caring and sensitive; and supports individuals (patients, families, physicians and hospital employees) search for meaning and fulfillment.[70]

Spirituality, often expressed in cultural or religious tradition, provides a personal framework for the understanding of life's purpose and meaning, the sense of well-being and the relationship with humanity and the divine. Furthermore, it is a determining factor in how individuals explain and respond to life events. Additionally, spirituality is an important element in the ability of patients, families, and health care providers to cope with illness, dying, and death.[71] The most important reason for incorporating spirituality into the patient's plan of care is that people want their spiritual beliefs acknowledged and addressed, especially in the situation of a health crisis. Therefore, spirituality has clinical relevance. Doing what is best for the patient as a "whole person" lies at the heart of providing quality medical care.

This chapter began with poignant words from a revered philosopher from antiquity, Plato. Perhaps, the words of a contemporary philosopher-physician are the perfect summary for this discussion.

Treat a disease. You win, you lose.

Treat a person. You win no matter what the outcome.

—Hunter "Patch" Adams, MD[72]

Appendix
Patient Survey
RESEARCH METHOD

An 11-item, self-administered questionnaire was developed by a small team of people comprising community volunteers, physicians, clergy, and a quality management specialist. The instrument was designed to identify patient preferences in discussing spiritual and religious beliefs in the context of receiving health care. The phrase "spiritual/religious beliefs" was used throughout the survey as an inclusive approach to respondents who may not describe themselves as religious while still maintaining some sense of spirituality. Survey questions were selected from the medical literature as well as questions of interest from local physicians.[73] A five-point scale was used with a range of strongly disagree, disagree, no opinion, agree, and strongly agree. The survey was then reviewed by a group of 20 volunteers for readability and comprehension. The survey was to be sent to people who had received inpatient care at SMMC within the previous 12 months. (The parameter of a recent inpatient stay was used to provide the respondent a reference when answering the questionnaire.) However, certain diagnoses and patient groups were excluded for privacy and sensitivity reasons (e.g., behavioral health patients, oncology patients, newborns, and pediatric patients). Additionally, demographic data was collected to assist in identifying similarities and differences in groups. (Table 1 provides a list of the survey questions and results of the research.)

70   Graber, D. R. and J. A. Johnson. (2001). Spirituality and healthcare organizations. *Journal of Healthcare Management*, 46(1), 39–50.
71   Anandarajah and Hight. Spirituality and medical practice.
72   Adams, P., M. Mylander, and S. Oedekerk. (1998).

Patch Adams. Directed by T. Shadyac. Universal City, CA: Universal Studios.
73   Koenig, H., G. R. Parkerson Jr., and K. G. Meador. (1997). Religion index for psychiatric research. *American Journal of Psychiatry*, 154(6), 885–886.

In September of 2003, the survey was mailed to 3286 individuals in SMMC's primary service areas of Wyandotte and Johnson counties in Kansas. A single mailing of the survey was sent with a cover letter explaining the purpose and importance of the survey. Of the 3286 surveys distributed, 442 were returned for a 13.5% response rate.

RESEARCH RESULTS

The survey, designed to assess personal preferences and expectations regarding the role of spirituality or religious beliefs in the physician-patient relationship, produced useful information for physicians. Approximately 88% (88.4%) of respondents reported strong agreement or agreement with the statement "Religion or spirituality is an important part of my daily life." However, many of this same group did not see a connection between their spiritual and religious beliefs and medical decisions. The percentage of patients responding affirmatively to the statement "I have spiritual/religious beliefs that influence my medical decisions" dropped to 55% (55.4%). This 33-point difference could be due to several factors, including the presence of only minor or transient medical conditions, or focus of beliefs on issues not salient to medical practice. Similarly, about 54% (54.5%) indicated, "I would like my doctor to be aware of my beliefs that influence my medical decisions."

An important issue for physicians that can be extracted from the data is identifying those patients who have spiritual or religious beliefs that impact the medical decisions and want these beliefs to be part of the physician-patient dialogue. To investigate differences in the patients who have spiritual and religious beliefs that impact medical decisions and want their physician

to be aware, the survey responses were divided into two groups: Group 1, those who do have beliefs *and* want the physician to be aware; Group 2, those who do not have beliefs that impact their medical decisions *or* do not want their physician to be aware of them. (Table 2 provides the demographic breakdown of the two groups.)

The profiles between Group 1 (n = 240), those who desire physician awareness, and Group 2 (n = 202), those who have no opinion or who would not want their physician to be aware, possessed many similarities; the two groups demonstrated no statistically significant differences in terms of age, gender, educational background, religious affiliation, or race. However, there was one statistically significant difference: attendance at religious services.

The group with no preference for physician awareness of their beliefs (Group 2) described their attendance as "never/rarely" or "a few times a year" much more often that the group preferring physician awareness (41.7% versus 11.5%, respectively). Thus, the group that would prefer for their physicians to be aware of their religious and spiritual beliefs (Group 1) was much more involved in structured religious services. Over 75% (79.4%) of respondents from that group reported attendance at religious services weekly or more than once a week. In contrast, Group 2 respondents reported this level of attendance only 50.3% of the time.

The data presented strongly suggests that patients who have spiritual or religious beliefs and want their physician to be aware of them are found in any age group, have no particular religious affiliation, but do attend religious services more frequently. Therefore, it seems safe to conclude that the best indicator for patients who have spiritual and religious beliefs that impact medical decisions is the frequency of attendance at religious services. This information could be used by the physician who picks up on a patient's reference to religious involvement during their conversations as a clue that the patient may also have beliefs that affect medical decision making.

Another interesting thing that is suggested by the research findings is the person patients prefer to discuss religious issues affecting their health. The findings showed that 28.5% of respondents would like their physicians to make referrals to clergy or other spiritual counselors for religious issues affecting their health. Surprisingly, 49.2% of respondents preferred that their physicians talk with them about spiritual or religious beliefs that affect their physical health; 54.5% desired that their physicians discuss spiritual beliefs during times of severe illness. Furthermore, 50.2% said that they would choose a doctor who responded to their spiritual or religious beliefs over one who did not. Certainly, one could anticipate that patients would prefer clergy, or other people similarly trained, to address spiritual concerns in time of illness, but the results of this survey indicate otherwise. This group of patients preferred physicians to care for not only their physical needs but also their spiritual needs.

TABLE 1 Patient Survey: Questions and Results

Survey Statement	Responses (n)	Strongly Disagree	Disagree	No Opinion	No Opinion	Strongly Agree
Religion or spirituality is an important part of my daily life	202	1.0%	0.5%	1.0%	5.9%	91.6%
I have spiritual/religious beliefs that influence my medical decisions	202	0.0%	0.0%	0.5%	26.2%	73.3%
I would like my doctor to be aware of my beliefs that influence my medical decisions	202	0.0%	0.0%	0.0%	27.2%	72.8%
I would like my doctor to discuss spiritual/religious beliefs during times of severe illness	199	3.5%	2.0%	16.6%	18.6%	59.3%
I would like my doctor to talk about spiritual/religious beliefs only if I bring up the subject	197	25.9%	8.6%	18.8%	21.3%	24.9%
I would like my doctor to talk with me about how my spiritual and/or religious beliefs affect my physical health	200	3.5%	2.0%	21.5%	25.0%	48.0%
I would like my doctor to talk with me about ways to improve my quality of life through spiritual and/or religious coping	197	9.6%	3.6%	18.8%	20.3%	47.7%
I would like my doctor to refer me to a pastor, rabbi, priest, imam, or other spiritual counselor for religious issues affecting my health	193	26.9%	7.3%	26.9%	10.4%	28.0%
I would like my doctor to pray with me	196	16.8%	3.6%	18.8%	20.3%	47.7%
I would choose a doctor who responds to my spiritual/religious needs over on who does not	201	8.0%	2.5%	13.9%	19.9%	55.7%
I would choose a hospital that responds to my spiritual/religious needs over one that does not	199	4.0%	1.0%	11.6%	19.6%	63.8%

TABLE 2 Patient Survey: Characteristics of Respondents Who Desire Physician Awareness and Those Who Do Not Want Physician Awareness of Spiritual and Religious Beliefs

Characteristics	No Physician Awareness (n = 202) (%)	Desire Physician Awareness (n = 240) (%)
Age group (years)		
18–25	3.3	1.0
26–44	30.4	26.2
45–64	22.5	26.7
65–74	18.8	14.4
75 and above	25.0	31.7
Religious affiliation		
Buddhist	0.8	2.0
Christian	90.3	94.6
Jewish	1.3	0.5
other	1.7	2.5
none	5.9	0.5
Religious attendance		
never/rarely	20.6	4.0
few times a year	21.1	7.5
monthly	8.0	9.1
weekly	41.4	57.3
more than once a week	8.9	22.1
Gender		
female	76.7	72.0
male	23.3	28.0
Race		
African American	2.5	3.5
Caucasian	91.5	92.4
Hispanic	2.5	2.5
other	3.4	1.5
Education		
some high school	3.4	3.0
high school	28.7	31.5
college	47.3	49.0
advanced degree	20.7	16.0

Physician Survey

RESEARCH METHODS[74]

The survey questions were developed from a review of medical literature and feedback from physicians who were interviewed regarding the integration of spirituality into their practices of medicine. Survey questions and research results are provided in Table 3. The statements addressing beliefs and barriers used a five-point Likert scale with the following options: strongly disagree, disagree, no opinion, agree, and strongly agree. The statements addressing behaviors used a five-point frequency scale with the following options: never, rarely, sometimes, often, and always. The survey was distributed to 430 physicians active on SMMC's staff. The survey was mailed to each physician's home address along with a cover letter explaining the purpose of the survey. A total of 129 surveys were returned for a response rate of 30%. Demographic data including gender, age, race, medical specialty, religious affiliation, attendance at religious services, and frequency of private religious activities were collected. Demographic characteristics of respondents to the survey are summarized in Table 4.

TABLE 3 Physician Survey: Questions and Results

	Sample (n)	Strongly Disagree (%)	Disagree (%)	No Opinion (%)	Agree (%)	Strongly Agree (%)
Beliefs						
There is a difference between religion and spirituality	128	1.6	2.3	8.6	36.7	50.8
A patient's involvement in religion or spirituality reduces morbidity and mortality	128	4.7	2.3	12.5	49.2	31.3
I am uncomfortable addressing issues of religion or faith with patients as they pertain to medical decisions	127	22.7	40.0	14.1	20.3	3.1
A patient's faith and spirituality are relevant to my provision of medical care	129	6.3	11.8	12.6	47.2	22.1
Religion or spirituality is an important part of my life	129	2.3	3.9	9.3	34.9	49.6

(continued)

---

74 The authors are deeply indebted to Dennis Beers, a former senior quality management analyst at SMMC, who helped create the survey instrument and who tabulated the results from returned surveys.

TABLE 3 Physician Survey: Questions and Results (*cont.*)

	Sample (n)	Strongly Disagree (%)	Disagree (%)	No Opinion (%)	Agree (%)	Strongly Agree (%)
Barriers						
I lack time to address patients' spiritual needs	128	10.2	23.4	14.1	48.4	10.2
I lack experience or training in taking a spiritual history	128	7.8	24.2	11.7	43.0	13.3
I am uncertain about how to identify patients who desire a discussion of spiritual issues	127	5.5	31.5	11.8	44.9	6.3
I am concerned that I will project my own beliefs onto patients	128	16.4	38.3	8.6	30.5	6.3
I believe that expressing spiritual concerns is not appropriate to the physician's role	129	27.9	46.5	11.6	9.3	4.7
I believe that patients do not want to share spiritual concerns with their physicians	128	21.1	43.0	24.2	9.4	2.3

		Never (%)	Rarely (%)	Sometimes (%)	Often (%)	Always (%)
Behaviors						
I ask patients about beliefs that might impact their medical decisions	127	10.2	17.3	44.1	26.0	2.4
I refer patients for spiritual follow-up	127	22.8	33.1	32.3	11.8	0.0
I discuss with patients ways to improve their quality of life through religious or spiritual coping	127	22.8	31.5	28.4	15.8	1.6
I have prayed with patients	126	36.5	31.8	19.8	11.1	0.8
I initiate a spiritual history with patients	127	45.7	27.6	19.7	7.1	0.0

TABLE 4 Physician Survey: Demographics

Characteristic	Physicians (%)
Gender	
male	64
female	36
Specialty	
internal medicine	12
family/general practice	16
surgery	20
internal medicine subspecialty	10
pediatrics	14
obstetrics and gynecology	8
psychiatry	9
emergency medicine	3
other	8
Religious affiliation	
Buddhist	1
Christian	85
Hindu	4
Jewish	7
Muslim	2
other	3
none	6
Religious attendance	
never/rarely	9
few times a year	26
monthly	18
weekly	34
more than once a week	13
Private religious activity	
never/rarely	8
few times a year	13
monthly	10
weekly	19
more than once a week	48
daily	2

Spirituality and Religion in the Clinical Setting: Pros and Cons

Does spirituality have a place in the clinical setting? That was the question posed in the title of the previous chapter. In reading that chapter, one could easily conclude that the answer was a resounding "Yes!" Not only does it make sense to "simply believe" that spirituality, religion, or faith is beneficial to one's overall sense of well-being, but scientific research has provided evidence to support such a supposition. "A majority of the nearly 350 studies of physical health and 850 studies of mental health that have used religious and spiritual variables have found that religious involvement and spirituality are associated with better health outcomes," says Paul Mueller, MD.[75] Research findings in several domains of the human experience confirm Mueller's words and continue the theme set forth earlier.

Illness

- A meta-analysis of 16 studies reported that 12 studies found religious involvement by the patient was correlated with less cardiovascular disease or death.[76]
- Heart surgery patients who are religious have 20% shorter postoperative hospital stays than nonreligious patients.[77]

Life-Limiting Illness

- One study of 1620 persons with cancer and HIV disease found that spiritual well-being predicted higher health-related quality of life, independent of physical, emotional, and social well-being.[78]
- A meta-analysis of data from 42 independent samples examining the association of a measure of religious involvement and all-cause mortality showed that religious involvement was significantly associated with lower mortality.[79]
- People who profess stronger spiritual beliefs seem to resolve their grief more rapidly and completely after the death of a close person than do people with no spiritual beliefs.[80]

Aging

- Eighteen prospective studies over the last 30 years have shown that religiously involved persons live longer.[81]
- Even after controlling for variables such

---

75 Mueller, P. S., D. J. Plevak, and T. A. Rummans. (2001). Religious involvement, spirituality, and medicine: implications for clinical practice. *Mayo Clinic Proceedings*, 76(12), 1226.
76 Ibid, 1227.
77 McSherry, E., S. Salisbury, M. Ciulla, et al. (1987). Spiritual resources in older hospitalized men. *Social Compass*, 34(4), 515–537.

78 Brady, M. J., A. H. Peterman, G. Fitchett, et al. (1999). A case for including spirituality in quality of life measurement in oncology. *Psychooncology*, 8(5), 417–428.
79 McCullough, M. E., W. T. Hoyt, D. B. Larson, et al. (2000). Religious involvement and mortality: a meta-analytic review. *Health Psycholgy*, 19(3), 211–222.
80 Walsh, K., M. King, L. Jones, et al. (2002). Spiritual beliefs may affect outcome of bereavement: prospective study. *British Medical Journal*, 324(7353), 1551–1554.
81 Mueller, et al. Religious involvement, spirituality, and medicine, 1226.

as chronic disease, disability, and smoking or alcohol use, elderly persons who attended religious services were 24% less likely than nonattenders to die during a 5-year follow-up period for 1931 older residents of Marin County, California.[82]

- Older adults who attend religious services at least once per week and who pray or study the Bible at least once per day are 40% less likely to have hypertension than those who attend services and pray less often.[83]

Coping

- Religious coping behaviors are related to better mental health.[84]
- Prayer and spirituality may improve quality of life by enhancing a person's subjective well-being by providing coping strategies, stress relief and social support.[85]
- Attachment to God was predictive of spiritual coping, which in turn was predictive of adjustment. Attachment to God provides a useful framework for understanding why individuals chose particular coping strategies.[86]

Health and Wellness

- Involvement in religious activities is associated with health-promoting behaviors (i.e., better nutrition, more exercise, use of seat belts, smoking cessation).[87]
- Those who attend religious services, at least once per week, have been shown to have stronger immune system function compared with less frequent attendees.[88]
- Those who attend religious services at least once per week maintain their physical activity significantly longer.[89]

This review of these and other scientific studies suggests that a positive correlation between spirituality and health does exist. However, not all researchers agree that there is compelling evidence to support such a relationship. Richard Sloan, PhD, Director of the Behavioral Medicine Program at Columbia-Presbyterian Medical Center in New York, and several of his colleagues note that the results of many studies have not been consistent; some have shown that religious attendance is associated with longer life, but others have not.[90] In addition, the studies tend to vary on how they define religious and spiritual activity, leading to difficulty in comparing them.[91]

82 Oman, D. and D. Reed. (1998). Religion and mortality among the community-dwelling elderly. *American Journal of Public Health*, 88(10), 1469–1475.

83 Koenig, H., K. I. Pargament, J. Nielsen, et al. (1998). Religious coping and health status in medically ill hospitalized older adults. *Journal of Nervous and Mental Disease*, 186(9), 513–521.

84 Ibid.

85 McCaffrey, A. M., D. M. Eisenberg, A. T. Legedza, et al. (2004). Prayer for health concerns: results of a national survey on prevalence and patterns of use. *Archives of Internal Medicine*, 164(8), 858–862.

86 Belavich, T. and K. Pargament. (2002). The role of attachment in predicting spiritual coping with a loved one in surgery. *Journal of Adult Development*, 9(1), 13–29.

87 Mueller, et al. Religious involvement, spirituality, and medicine, 1227.

88 Koenig, H. G., H. J. Cohen, L. K. George, et al. (1997). Attendance at religious services, interleukin-6, and other biological parameters of immune function in older adults. *International Journal of Psychiatry in Medicine*, 27(3), 233–250.

89 Idler, E. L. and S. V. Kasl. (1997). Religion among disabled and nondisabled persons: I. Cross-sectional patterns in health practices, social activities, and well-being. *Journal of Gerontology: Social Sciences*, 52(6), S294–S305.

90 Sloan, R. (1999). Religion, spirituality, and medicine [speech]. Twenty-Second Annual Freedom from Religion Foundation Convention, San Antonio, TX, November 6, 1999.

91 Sloan, R. (2000). Sounding board. *New England*

Furthermore, Sloan suggests that there are methodological flaws in the research process that make the conclusions suspect.

The first of the methodological concerns cited is *failure to control for confounding variables and covariates.* Sloan emphasizes the importance of being able to control for confounders, like behavioral and genetic differences and variables such as age, gender, education, ethnicity, socioeconomic status, and health status. Control for only a segment of confounders and variables can lead to biased and, therefore, skewed findings. For example, a large study in Alameda County, California, demonstrated that attendance at religious services reduced mortality. When controlled, though, for all relevant variables, the longevity was true for women only.[92]

A second methodological concern is *failure to control for multiple comparisons.* Sloan suggests that if you make enough comparisons, sooner or later one or two will turn out to be significant. However, the significance may only be a product of chance. If a researcher is going to measure multiple variables, she has to have control mechanisms for making adjustments in determining what constitutes an adequate level of statistical significance in any one of the variables. For example, if you are making comparisons of eight different variables, the likelihood of finding something significant increases eightfold, purely by chance.[93]

Thirdly, there is a concern about *reliance on epidemiological studies.* Much of the work in the area of spirituality and religion in medicine has used survey methods or some form of interviewing for data collection. These designs can only suggest whether religion is associated with health, not whether religion *causes* health. Sloan posits that

> even well-conducted epidemiologic studies reflect only associations at the popular level; they do not provide evidence that a recommendation to attend religious services actually leads to increased attendance, let alone better health. Evidence from epidemiologic studies must be confirmed by rigorous clinical trials.[94]

Sloan's point about the distinction between association and hard evidence that can lead to a solid conclusion is important to keep in mind. Even with the plethora of literature and data from research projects pointing to the positive effects of patient spirituality in shorter hospital stays, coping better with serious illness and dying, better health outcomes than nonreligious patients, there are several things that research has not been able to demonstrate:[95]

- God heals.
- Religious people don't get sick.
- Doctors should prescribe religious activities.
- Spirituality is the most important health factor.
- Illness is due to a lack of faith and/or participation in religious activities.

Journal of Medicine, 342(25), 1913.

92 Sloan R., E. Bagiella, and T. Powell. (1999). Religion, spirituality, and medicine. *Lancet,* 353(9153), 665.

93 Ibid, 665. [See Koenig, et al. Attendance at religious services. This study is an example of Sloan's criticism about failing to control for multiple comparisons.]

94 Sloan. Sounding board, 1914.

95 Levin, J. S. (1994). Religion and health: is there an association, is it valid and is it causal? *Social Science Medicine,* 38(11), 1375–1382. (Cited in Mueller, et al. Religious involvement, spirituality, and medicine, 1230.)

This last point is unfortunately demonstrated in the practice of some clergy and "super" spiritual people when they relate to patients that their illnesses are due to sin in their lives, not enough faith for healing, or not regularly attending worship services. Sloan's assessment of such practices led to him to conclude:

> When you suggest that religious activity is associated with better health, you implicitly suggest quite the opposite: that poor health is a product of insufficient devotion, insufficient faith.[96]

Furthermore, the research has not pointed out the potential *negative effects of spirituality* in patient well-being (i.e., the reality that unhealthy belief systems and practices can adversely affect people's health):

- Patient's perceived abandonment by God, feeling unloved by God or punished by God may be correlated with increased risk of dying.[97]
- Rejection of medical interventions for "faith healing" can lead to earlier death from often treatable diseases.
- Religious beliefs may encourage avoidance of preventive health measures such as childhood immunizations.
- Unrealistically high expectations related to beliefs may lead to isolation, stress, and anxiety.
- Refusal of appropriate medical care based on influence of faith community.[98]
- Certain forms of religiousness may

increase the risk of death (e.g., religious struggle with illness).[99]

In light of the previous discussion that offers that quantifying the role of spirituality and religion as causal to better health in a clinical setting through scientific research is not as straightforward as some might suggest, along with the prevalence of negative effects that spirituality can have on patient well-being, how then might the role of spirituality in the clinical setting be understood? Paul Mueller provides wise council:

> Even though an association between religious involvement and spirituality and better health outcomes appears valid, clinicians should be careful **NOT** to draw erroneous conclusions from research findings.[100]

He goes on to say, though, that

> discerning, acknowledging and supporting the spiritual needs of patients in a straightforward, ethical and noncontroversial manner may relieve suffering and facilitate recovery from illness.[101]

The rationale for Mueller's latter statement, along with many other researchers who think similarly, is based on the following suppositions.

- Most people have a spiritual life.
- Most patients want their spiritual needs addressed.

96 Sloan. Religion, spirituality, and medicine [speech].
97 Larson, D. and S. Larson. (2003). Spirituality's potential relevance to physical and emotional health: a brief review of quantitative research. *Journal of Psychology and Theology*, 31(1), 37–51.
98 Mueller, et al. Religious involvement, spirituality, and medicine, 1230.
99 Pargament, K. I., H. G. Koenig, N. Tarakeshwar, et al. (2001). Religious struggle as a predictor of mortality among medically ill elderly patients: a 2-year longitudinal study. *Archives of Internal Medicine*, 161(15), 1881–1885.
100 Mueller, et al. Religious involvement, spirituality, and medicine, 1230.
101 Ibid, 1232.

- Supporting a patient's spirituality may enhance coping and recovery from illness.
- Most studies have found a direct relationship between religious involvement and spirituality and better health outcomes.

The role of spirituality in health is part of the curriculum in the majority of the nation's medical schools. According to a 2008 publication of *American Medical News*, 100 of the roughly 150 medical schools in the United States offer some courses in their curricula on spirituality in medicine, and 75 of the 100 make at least one course on that subject a student requirement. Furthermore, the Association of American Medical Colleges has provided a description of spirituality as a component of its Medical School Objectives Project:

Spirituality is recognized as a factor that contributes to health in many persons. It is expressed in an individual's search for ultimate meaning through participation in religion and/or belief in God, family, naturalism, humanism and the arts. All of these factors can influence how patients and health care professionals perceive health and illness and how they interact with one another.[102]

One final word of caution should be noted, however. Even though the medical literature and various medical associations overwhelmingly support the role of spirituality in reducing morbidity and mortality, great care should be taken when incorporating spirituality into the patient's plan of care. The patient's agenda and needs are the primary foci, not those of the clinician. With the cautions outlined here in mind, we now proceed with a discussion of how to appropriately assess patients' need for spiritual care and its application in a clinical setting.

---

102 Booth, B. (2008). More schools teaching spirituality in medicine. *American Medical News*, March 10. Available at: www.ama-assn.org/amednews/2008/03/10/prsc0310.htm (accessed 5 Sept 12).

Spiritual Care in the Clinical Setting: Assessment and Application

Birth, illness, dying, and death all bring people to the threshold of what their minds can comprehend. Please consider the following three possible reactions to the discovery that individuals have been diagnosed with lung cancer.

1. "I guess I shouldn't be surprised that I have lung cancer. I have smoked for 40 years."
2. "There are some things in my life that I am not very proud of. I wonder if this disease is God's way of punishing me?"
3. "I can't believe that a nonsmoker like me got lung cancer, but I guess it happens. I'm lucky to be generally healthy and will see if that will support my healing of this disease."

In the first scenario, the patient perceived that his illness was a natural consequence of his actions. In the second scenario, the patient perceived that her disease was God's punishment for a "sinful" life. In the third scenario, the patient perceived that his condition was unjustified. Statements, questions, and resulting perceptions like these are not uncommon when people are confronted with life-threatening or life-limiting medical conditions. Ways in which individuals perceive illnesses are their attempts to answer the "why" questions and to gain some understanding about their experiences. Viktor Frankl, a Holocaust survivor, articulated this masterfully: "Man is not destroyed by suffering; he is destroyed by suffering without meaning ... In some way, suffering ceases to be suffering at the moment it finds a meaning."[103]

Rationale for Spiritual Care in a Clinical Setting

In many cases, there are no answers to the "why" questions that people ask in health care–related issues. Yet, those unanswerable questions need to be voiced in order for healing to begin. Physicians and other health care providers often listen attentively to these questions and respond with words from the heart that communicate "I don't know why ... I wish I had a satisfactory answer to that question." While this may be frustrating to admit, as medical school training is all about "fixing the problem," honesty and compassion can be very helpful to patients and their families. In contrast to those unanswerable "why" questions, though, there are questions to which there are often meaningful answers: what? and where? "What do I do now? Where do I go from here?" Physicians and other health care personnel can be valuable resources in aiding those individuals and families that feel helpless with their situation to find answers to these and similar questions. In so doing, they have been instruments in

---

103 Frankl, V. (1959). *Man's Search for Meaning*. New York, NY: Washington Square Press. Frankl's words were cited by, Rabow M, McPhee SJ. Beyond breaking bad news: how to help patients who suffer, *Western Journal of Medicine* (October, 1999), 171, 261–262.

turning a sense of hopelessness into one of hopefulness and performing a valuable spiritual care service.

The stress associated with health-related crises can stretch the limits of one's faith and personal spirituality. Health care providers can benefit their patients by recognizing the existential suffering and help them find some sense of meaning in their circumstances. The process for this begins with an assessment of how the disease is understood. Perceptions of illness, though, are varied:[104]

- illness as a *challenge* to get through
- illness as an *enemy* to fight
- illness as a *punishment* to endure
- illness as a *weakness* to overcome
- illness as a *natural consequence* to accept
- illness as a *rest* to welcome
- illness as a *value* to acknowledge
- illness as a *blessing* to embrace.

It is important to mention that perceptions of illness can change during the disease trajectory. For example, a situation initially perceived as a weakness to overcome can be subsequently understood as a rest to welcome. Similarly, what a person may see as a challenge to get through might be viewed later as a blessing to embrace.

Illness, dying, and death can be likened to a roller-coaster ride with its ups and downs. The downward slide often gives rise to crises in patient's lives. One of these can be a crisis of faith, which can produce a variety of reactions:

- sudden turn toward God
- uncharacteristic congregational involvement
- "God's will" mindset

- belief that God is powerless
- belief that God does not care
- belief that "I failed God"
- belief that God is not in control
- anger at God
- feeling distant from God
- sense of isolation from God and faith community
- withdrawal from faith community
- loss of meaning and purpose
- sense of hopelessness
- questioning the basic beliefs of one's faith
- familiar faith practices seem empty
- "why me" syndrome.

People might exhibit any of these reactions because of their struggles, and this does not necessarily indicate loss of faith, lack of faith, or dysfunctional faith. Why is this? It is not a common event in most people's everyday experience to have a loved one diagnosed with a chronic, debilitating condition, develop a life-limiting illness, or be in the process of dying. Therefore, existential and spiritual concerns could easily and justifiably surface in such difficult times. It seems logical to conclude, then, that any resultant patient and/or family reactions, which are simply symptomatic, should be understood as normal reactions in normal people to abnormal occurrences in their lives.

One of the fundamental principles of spiritual care is that spiritual growth can be stimulated during illness, dying, and death. It is during those stressful situations that health care providers have the opportunity to make significant contributions to the patient's and family's sense of well-being. Andrew Schwartz, MD, a cardiothoracic surgeon at Shawnee Mission Medical Center, stated that "the science of medicine

---

104 Kuhn, C. (1988). A spiritual inventory of the medically ill patient. *Psychiatric Medicine*, 6(2), 87–100.

looks for the cure; the art of medicine seeks to heal where there might not be a cure." The diagnostic tools for this "art of medicine" are not stethoscopes, X-ray machines, or EKG machines, but the eyes, ears, and heart.[105]

"The keys to emotional coping with serious illness and disability are frequently found within the matrix of patient spirituality," says Christina Puchalski, MD.[106] The reality of that statement gives credence to the words of Harold Koenig, MD, who suggests that addressing patient spirituality should be an integral part of the overall plan of care.[107]

Many patients are religious and use religious beliefs and practices to cope with illness. Because of this, religious beliefs often influence medical decisions, especially those made when illness is serious or critical. Many patients would like physicians to address spiritual needs and support them in this area, especially when the seriousness of illness increases. Furthermore, a growing research database indicates that in the majority of cases, religious beliefs and practices are related to better health and quality of life.

Spirituality, which helps define the ultimate meaning and purpose in life, and religion, a means by which spirituality is often expressed, do have clinical relevance. It is critical that both spirituality and religion be given serious attention by health care providers in a hospital, nursing home, or clinic to help patients and their families and loved ones trying to make some sense out of what is happening.

The remainder of this section will focus on spiritual assessment and spiritual care and providing models for their application in the clinical setting.

Principle Elements of Spirituality, Assessment, and Application of Spiritual Care

As opposed to being concerned about saying or doing the "right thing," the caregiver should focus on being fully present. This notion of "being fully present" means much more than simply being physically present; it includes having an awareness of multiple issues about which the patient might be concerned in addition to the physical – spiritual, emotional, relational, professional, financial. Asking the question, "What about this situation concerns you the most?" is one way to communicate "being fully present." The practice of spiritual care is more about "who a person is." What message does my body language convey? Do I make people feel at ease when communicating with them? Questions such as these, which provide for reflection and self-awareness, are important to improve one's effectiveness in providing holistic care to patients and their families.

It is also essential for those who want to provide spiritual care for their patients to have a basic understanding of the key principles of spirituality as they relate to medical issues in the clinical setting.

• Spirituality influences the mental and physical aspects of living and dying.

105 Yeagley, L. Living with dying. Adventist Health System Mission Conference. Information obtained in interview with Larry Yeagley at the conference, February 2004.
106 Puchalski, C. and A. Romer. (2000). Taking a spiritual history allows clinicians to understand patients more fully. *Journal of Palliative Medicine*, 3(1), 129–137.
107 Koenig, H. (2002). *Spirituality in Patient Care*. Philadelphia, PA: Templeton Foundation Press, 18–19.

- Spirituality is an ongoing issue in patient care.
- Spiritual needs can arise at any time.
- Spirituality can vary during the course of the disease process.
- Spirituality is multifaceted.
- Spirituality can be expressed and enhanced in a number of ways.

Understanding Spiritual Assessment and Spiritual Care

What is spiritual assessment? Is it acquiring information about a patient's religious tradition and utilizing that information as the criteria for providing spiritual care? Michael Zedek,[108] former senior rabbi of Temple B'nai Jehudah in Overland Park, Kansas, said: "Physicians who know a patient's religious affiliation know nothing more than a label." Similarly, T. J. Mansen related that "when it is assumed that satisfying the rites and rituals of a particular religion meets a patient's spiritual needs, interventions may become standardized rather than individualized."[109] The responses of these individuals indicate that spiritual assessment is not solely about addressing religious concerns. In order to more fully understand the meaning of spiritual assessment, it is essential to review the definition of spiritual care.

Spiritual care is recognizing and responding to the multifaceted expressions of spirituality in patients and their families. It involves compassion, presence, listening and encouragement of realistic hope and might not involve any discussion of God or religion. It also could include understanding and helping with certain theological beliefs and conflicts.[110]

As this definition of spiritual care by Drs. Anandarajah and Hight shows, a spiritual assessment should be broader in context than the narrower concentration on religious matters. This is confirmed by their definition of spiritual assessment as "the process by which health care providers can identify patients' spiritual needs pertaining to medical care." This process includes a number of elements, in addition to the religious dimension. For example, the "H" section in their HOPE questionnaire as a tool for spiritual assessment (H for hope, O for organized religion, P for personal spirituality, and E for effects on medical care) includes the question "What sustains you and keeps you going?" The answer to this question may or may not have anything to do with religion or rituals, and yet it might.

Purpose and Strategies of Spiritual Assessment

In addition to gaining an understanding of how patients perceive illness, discussed in the "Rationale for Spiritual Care in the Clinical Setting" section, other elements of the overall purpose of spiritual assessment are:

- Gain awareness of the role spirituality plays in people's lives in formulating purpose and meaning.
- Obtain useful information in providing whole-person care:

---

108 Zedek, M., interview by Steven Jeffers, Center for Practical Bioethics' Compassion Sabbath February 4, 2000.

109 Mansen, T. and S. Haak. (1996). Evaluation of health assessment skills using a computer videodisk interactive program. *Journal of Nursing Education*, 35(8), 382–383.

110 Anandarajah, G. and E. Hight. (2001). Spirituality and medical practice: using the HOPE questions as a practical tool for spiritual assessment. *American Family Physician*, 63(1), 81–88.

○ beliefs that influence treatment decisions and compliance

○ means for bolstering patient's spirits

○ grief or difficulty patient or family may have in coping with the medical condition

○ patient wishes for end-of-life care.

How does a health care provider access this pertinent information? Strategies that can be useful for conducting a spiritual assessment are:

• establish rapport and trust with patients and families

• recognize the sensitive and personal nature of spirituality, religious beliefs and end-of-life issues

• encourage the use of storytelling.

"Assessing spiritual needs is best done within a caring relationship where it feels safe enough to explore together the experience of the illness in the context of the person's life journey or story," explains nursing professor Elizabeth Johnston Taylor.[111] She goes on to say that "disclosure of a person's spirituality is seldom spontaneous; it emerges through a relationship of trust, respect and usually out of the life story."

Model for Performing Spiritual Assessment

Harold Koenig, MD, suggests that spiritual assessment tools possess certain qualities: brevity, patient-centeredness and ease of memorizing.[112] The medical and nursing literature is replete with models for performing a spiritual assessment (also referred to

as a spiritual history), some of which meet this criteria. There is the aforementioned HOPE questionnaire by Anandarajah and Hight. Others using acronyms as descriptors are the SPIRITual[113] and the FICA[114] histories. Additional assessment tools for consideration, but which do not meet the criterion of ease of memorization, are those by Stoll,[115] Kuhn,[116] Dossey and Dossey,[117] Matthews,[118] and Lo et al.[119]

The CARE[120] model chosen by the authors for this discussion meets the criteria set forth by Koenig. In fact, it was developed in response to the results of a survey on the subject of physician involvement in addressing patient spirituality. Interestingly, according to the survey results, 36% of the 130 participants reported that a concern for projecting their own beliefs onto patients was a limiting factor in inquiring about patients' spirituality.[121] Because of this concern by physicians, the CARE model avoids asking specific questions about religion and/or God. In addition, the avoidance of such questions is predicated on the assumption that not everybody is associated with a particular religion or faith community

---

111 Taylor, E. (1998). Spiritual dimensions of health care [course NURS 422], University of Southern California, Department of Nursing. Information obtained by Steve Jeffers from lectures notes shared by Dr. Taylor.

112 Koenig, *Spirituality in Patient Care*, 88.

113 Maugans, T. (1996). The SPIRITual history. *Archives of Family Medicine*, 5(1), 11–16.

114 Puchalski and Romer. Taking a spiritual history.

115 Stoll, R. (1979). Guidelines for spiritual assessment. *American Journal of Nursing*, 79(9), 1574–1577.

116 Kuhn. A spiritual inventory of the medically ill patient.

117 Dossey, B. and Dossey, L. (1998). Attending to holistic care. *American Journal of Nursing*, 98(8), 35–38.

118 Matthews, D. (1998). *The Faith Factor*. New York, NY: Penguin Group, 274.

119 Lo, B., T. Quill, and J. Talky. (1999). Discussing palliative care with patients. *Annals of Internal Medicine*, 130(9), 744–749.

120 Jeffers, S. Patients and spirituality. *The Leading Edge*, Winter, 2005, 2(1).

121 November, 2003 survey sent to approximately 450 physicians on staff at Shawnee Mission Medical Center, Shawnee Mission, KS.

(most of the other models mentioned do include questions about religion, faith, and God). Furthermore, religious people may be angry at God concerning their health issues. Thus, direct questions about God, religion, and faith may be offensive and/or detrimental to opportunities for spiritual growth in the midst of the illness.

Based on this and other information from the survey, the authors of the CARE model were intentional in keeping with the principles of the definition for spiritual care stated earlier in this chapter: *Spiritual care is recognizing and responding to the multifaceted expressions of spirituality in patients and their families. It involves compassion, presence, listening and encouragement of realistic hope and might not involve any discussion of God or religion.*

Now, we turn to a discussion of CARE, an acronym that represents a framework for addressing and attending to the multifaceted concerns of the sick and dying.
- **C**, for Comfort established and Coping skills identified
- **A**, for Assessment of needs and concerns
- **R**, for Resource identification and mobilization
- **E**, for Empowerment for hope and growth through the illness experience

The **C** refers to patient comfort and coping. Comfort relates to the relationship between patient and physician. Does the patient feel at ease with the physician? Does the patient believe that the physician cares for them as a human being, not simply someone who is being treated for a disease? Physicians can play a significant role in establishing that sense of patient comfort in their interactions by paying attention to their own body language, patterns of speech (voice inflection, pace of speech, word usage, etc.)

and overall demeanor. With respect to helping patients identify coping mechanisms, physicians can make statements and pose questions.
- I know this must be difficult for you. How have you coped with tough times in the past?
- What is the most important thing I can do for you right now?
- Tell me how I might help you get through this?

The **A** refers to assessment of needs and concerns. Patient needs and concerns may well range beyond the physical (i.e., those disease-related issues). There could be relational, professional, financial, emotional, and spiritual concerns. Asking questions is the best approach in finding out what is most troublesome to the patient about their current situation.
- What about this illness experience concerns you the most?
- Are there any specific concerns or needs you have at this time?

The **R** refers to resource identification and mobilization. The assessment portion of the process most likely identified some specific areas of concern. In response to that information, clinicians can ask for more information and address the concern themselves or recommend a person who can help in addressing the concern.
- Would you tell me more about _____?
- What did you mean when you said _____?
- Is there someone I can call for you?
- Would you like me to arrange for a chaplain, social worker, and so forth, to speak with you?

The **E** refers to empowerment. The results of this simple, yet important, dialogue with patients can help replace weakness with strength, provide reasonable hope in the face of hopelessness and assure patients that their physicians do indeed care for them.

SHARE[122] as Model for Performing Spiritual Care

In addition to utilizing the CARE model as a tool to assess a patient's perceptions of one's situation and needs as well as to then identify resources to address those needs, one can utilize the SHARE model, which offers some practical tips for providing compassionate patient-centered care.

S, FOR *SENSE* PEOPLE'S NEEDS BEFORE THEY ASK

Be aware of the signs, signals, and clues that indicate what is important to people.

- Smile and greet patients and families in a friendly manner.
- Remember the patient's name.
- Maintain eye level: sitting, standing, or kneeling to make it easy for patient to connect visually.
- Ask, "Is there anything I can do for you?"
- Use a variety of the "senses," in addition to hearing, to perceive and interpret what patients and families might not be verbalizing.
- Be aware that there may be multiple issues of concern to patients/families beyond the physical – relational, emotional, professional, financial, spiritual – and be willing to address any that may arise, if not personally then through referral.
- Look for clues from patients.

Ask yourself:
- Do my eyes communicate care and compassion or are they distant?
- Do patients feel they are seen by me or do they feel overlooked?

H, FOR *HELP OUT* PATIENTS, FAMILY, AND STAFF

Give the human touch of warmth, comfort, humor, and kindness.

- Observe and respond to signs of discomfort.
- Ask, "Is there anything specific you would like to ask me?"
- Go the "extra mile" to be helpful.
- Extend a caring hand; for many patients, "appropriate touching" says "This person really cares."

Ask yourself:
- Does my touch convey care, support, and nurturing?
- Do I speak of love, kindness, and respect through my hands?

A, FOR *ACKNOWLEDGE* PEOPLE'S FEELINGS

Let people know they are recognized and appreciated as unique individuals.

- Recognize patients' accomplishments, life experiences, talents, and family.
- Listen to patients' stories.
- Allow patients to express their feelings without being judgmental.
- Allow patients to cry and support them with sincerity.
- Allow patients to make choices; offer options for appropriate treatments and provide realistic hope.

---

122 Adapted from Adventist Health System's SHARE customer service program and *Communication with Compassion*, Adventures in Caring Foundation. Santa Barbara, CA: Win/Win Productions. Available at www.adventuresincaring.org (accessed 23 September 2012).

- Communicate concern and empathy for patients and families.
- Honor patients' faith traditions and religious practices.

Ask yourself:
- Do I recognize and appreciate the values, beliefs, and special needs and concerns of patients as individuals?

R, FOR *RESPECT* THE DIGNITY AND PRIVACY OF PATIENTS

Treat others the way we ourselves would like to be treated.
- Honor people's personal space.
- Knock before entering a patient's room.
- Guard the confidentiality of patient information.
- Show appreciation to patients for allowing you to care for them.
- Respect people's desire to retain a sense of modesty.
- Do not interject personal spiritual or religious beliefs into patient or family conversation without invitation.
- Accept patients as people; interact with patients as human beings, not as a disease.

Ask yourself:
- Do I create a patient friendly environment?
- Do I convey a caring physical presence?

E, FOR *EXPLAIN* WHAT IS HAPPENING

Communicate appropriately in a caring manner.
- Ask questions to facilitate understanding.
- Encourage patients to ask questions, even the hard ones.
- Be a good listener.
- Be focused on the patient when speaking.
- Communicate medical information in a clear and understandable manner.

- Speak using proper voice inflection, volume, and pace of speech.

Ask yourself:
- Do patients hear in my voice that I care, have time for them, and they are safe with me?

In addition to the principles stated here for providing individualized, compassionate care, the authors want health care providers to be aware of certain issues that are important to patients and their families in end-of-life situations.

These are as follows:
- dealing with regrets
- taking care of "unfinished business"
- celebrating life through storytelling
- reflecting on personal spirituality.

Interestingly, most people are not cognizant that these things are important to them because of the anxiety, confusion, and despair often associated with these situations. However, for a care provider to introduce these items in the course of a conversation and to facilitate, or at least to help to begin, a dialogue will be perceived by that patient and/or family as a treasured gift. It may also be helpful to include the five elements of relationship completion,[123] coined by Ira Byock, MD, in that conversation.
- I forgive you
- You forgive me
- Thank you
- I love you
- Goodbye

It is also noteworthy to mention the role of

---

123 Byock, I. (1997). *Dying Well: The Prospect for Growth at the End of Life.* New York, NY: Riverhead Books, 140.

silence in meeting needs of those experiencing spiritual pain. There are times when people's pain and suffering is so deep, that they are unable to vocalize their feelings. In such cases, the simple, but profound "ministry of presence" is no more greatly appreciated by hurting people than during those times of deep spiritual pain. Respecting and honoring their silence with the same is providing spiritual care. It is important to remember, this one maxim: "Spiritual care is not always about what is said, but sometimes about what is not said."

Conclusion

Patients often present themselves to physicians with the vulnerability of a child. Metaphorically speaking, they reach with arms outstretched calling out, "Help me!" They and their families are often scared, anxious and do not know where to turn for help in a health-related crisis, except to their physician. When physicians show interest in their patients' overall sense of well-being, they have empowered their patients and their families to get through the difficult experience with minimal negative effects. Furthermore, the information obtained from a spiritual assessment can enable physicians to better understand medical problems in the broad context of their patients' lives.

Spirituality is like a river flowing through every person. Unfortunately it can be dammed in times of illness, dying, and death with suffering, fear, and loneliness. However, a compassionate, caring presence can prevent the dam from forming and allow the river to continue its flow. Attention to patient spirituality is an indispensable component of quality holistic care.

American Indian Spirituality

All is Sacred

Prepared by:
Karalee L. Hawkins
American Indian Spirituality Member of the Greater
  Kansas City Interfaith Council
Shawnee, KS

Reviewed and approved by:
Jimm G. GoodTracks, MSW
Baxoge Jiwere-Nutachi (Ioway-Otoe-Missouria)
  Language Project
White Cloud, KS

History and Facts

American Indian Spirituality as an oral tradition has no identifiable point of time origin and survives through its keepers who share and pass down the ancestral teachings. More a way of life than a religion, American Indian Spirituality is a shared cultural view that understands that the good health of one's family and community is dependent upon each individual's good relationship, alignment, and harmony with *Great Spirit* and all of Creation. One is taught to observe harmony and balance in nature, and to strive for that harmony and balance in one's own life. It is believed that as one comes into harmony and balance and good relationship with *All That Is*, wellness of body, mind, spirit, and emotions will come to pass, not only for one's self but also for all of one's family, extended family kinships, and community.

Spiritual leaders, healers, and keepers of the oral tradition are recognized as such within their community and in other Native communities by their activities, their relationships, and their personal service within the community. While there are no holy books, sacred writings, or religious authorities that mandate tenets of faith for adherents to follow, the keepers of American Indian Spirituality pass down the teachings through storytelling, language, and ceremony. One does not become a keeper, spiritual leader, or healer by going to school or receiving certification or a degree. Rather than by exacting personal selection as a vocation or community position, spiritual leaders, keepers, and healers are usually the result of individual inspiration. Through prayer, the inspired individual acquires a practicing mentor for a lifelong apprenticeship. The mentor will, over the course of time, share traditional knowledge with the apprentice and the application of the knowledge for appropriate ritual and ceremony that are applied with traditional teachings and understandings of the mentor of his environment and of his Creator/Higher Power.

Though there are more than 2.5 million Americans who are descendants of the original inhabitants of this country, not all Native Americans adhere to or support traditional beliefs. For those who do, there is much regional diversity in ceremonial and healing practices. Therefore, the scope of this paper will outline, to the best of the author's ability, a shared cultural view of American Indian Spirituality and will not attempt to detail ritual or ceremonies specific to tribal orientation. There are 558 recognized tribes in 35 states in the United States. The largest tribe is the Navajo, or Diné, with an estimated population of 250 000.

Basic Teachings

From the author's experience and study of American Indian Spirituality and culture, the following are basic teachings cross-culturally accepted among Native people.

- **God, Creator, Great Spirit.** At the heart of American Indian Spirituality is belief in an *Essence of Spirit: a Higher Power*, Who is omniscient and immanent throughout the universe and Who has created all that is seen and unseen. This Essence of Spirit or Higher Power is holy and sacred and is referred to by Native people by a number of names (e.g., Creator, Great Spirit, Grandfather, All That Is, or Great Mystery). In the Ioway-Otoe-Missouria, Omaha, Ponca, Osage, Quapaw, and Kansa languages, this Essence of Spirit is called *Wakanda*. For the Lakota, it is *Wakan Tanka*. For the Cheyenne, it is *Maheo*.

- **Autonomy of the Individual.** Spirituality for a Native American is an individual choice and a family matter. There are no intermediaries between the individual and Creator. American Indian Spirituality encourages the seeker to find his or her own truth and form his or her own personal relationship with Spirit assisted by personal mentorship of an elder.

- **We are all Related and Interconnected.** American Indian Spirituality teaches that Great Spirit is immanent within all Creation and manifested and reflected in all aspects and elements of the created Earth and all its inhabitants: human, animal, fowl, plant life, the rocks, the waters, and so forth. Thus, we are all relatives as Great Spirit is manifested and reflected in us. We are all interconnected and interrelated with all aspects of Creation. As reflected in the words of Adkube Shibisha Aguwi'e (VYB), Hidatsa, as told to Jimm GoodTracks:

> There is a life force that flows through all living things – the plants, the animals, the birds, even to the smallest creatures on the ground or in the earth. Through all these living things, including us human beings, flows a life force. We have that in common with all these things and it causes us to be related to all living things as this life force is of the Sacred Creation.

- The Lakota/Dakota ceremonial prayer *"Mitakuye oyasin"* (All my relatives) is representative of the universality of the American Indian understanding of our interrelationship and interconnection with the Divine.

- **The Medicine Wheel or Sacred Circle.** The Medicine Wheel or Sacred Circle is a symbol of the cultural view that all life flows in a natural cyclical, clockwise direction as the sun rises and sets. The Medicine Wheel or Sacred Circle is used to help us relate to and understand concepts or ideas that are not physical objects.

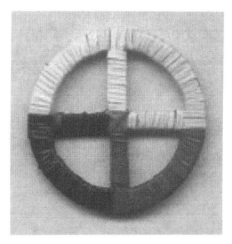

Consider the following concepts of the natural flow of the cycles of life:

○ spring, summer, autumn, winter
○ birth, growth, maturation, completion
○ sunrise, high noon, sunset, midnight
○ intention, actualization, reflection, renewal.

- Though the English language conceptualizes time as linear, with all things having a beginning and an ending, American Indian culture and language affords a circular worldview. For all that is manifest, there is (1) a perceived beginning, (2) a maturation process, (3) a time of reflection and introspection, and (4) a time of transition and release to the Great Spirit. The concept of "Indian time" is based on natural rhythms rather than minutes on a clock. For example, if one might ask a Native "How long will this take?," the response is likely to be, "Until we're done." As a general rule, it is best not to assign time limitations when Native relatives are involved in a traditional activity with their healing relative. An activity will not be hurried along. It is expected to take as much time as is necessary.

- **The Four Directions.** The Four Directions, also known as the Four Winds, are often referred to as Grandfather(s) Who is (are) immanent within all that is around us, above us and below us. These Four Grandfathers in the West, North, East, and South Directions are joined by the Fifth, Sixth, and Seventh Directions. The Fifth Direction is the "Father, Grandfather Sky" being above us. The Sixth Direction is our "Mother, Grandmother," the Earth, lying beneath us, and the Seventh Direction is the Great Spirit residing within us. Referring to Spirit as Grandfather recognizes that Spirit was here before us. (Note: Referring to Mother Earth or Father Sky, connotes the physical manifestation of the Divine; Grandmother and Grandfather refers to the spiritual essence of the Divine.)

- **All is Sacred and All is Alive.** American Indian Spirituality teaches that as God, or Great Spirit, is immanent within all that is created, all Creation is therefore sacred and alive and is to be treated with respect accordingly. All in Creation are considered *holy beings*, including humans, birds, fish, the four-legged, the trees, the stones, the clouds, and so forth.

- **The Four Aspects of Being.** All Creation has four aspects of being: physical, spiritual, emotional, and mental. In health care, American Indian Spirituality teaches that these four aspects of being need to be addressed in providing optimum health care. In modern medicine, this is called holistic. Metaphysically, Native American understanding extends these four aspects beyond the human being to all elements of Creation. A plant or a thought, for example, would be considered to have four aspects of being: physical, spiritual, emotional, and mental.

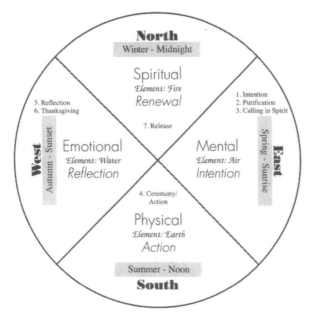

Healing is not only a one-to-one relationship, it is multidimensional. This is at the basis of the Navajo philosophy. We call it "Walking in Beauty." It is a way of living a balanced and harmonious life, in touch with all the components of one's world. This, not increased technology and more and more layers of bureaucracy, is the path we must now take to achieve better health and healing in life. The latest breakthroughs of research and methodology are stunning achievements and must be acknowledged as such, but along the way we have forgotten some of the things that heal us best – our relationships, how we live our lives, our feelings of wholeness and belonging.[124]

Depicted here is the author's understanding of the Medicine Wheel and the Cycles

---

124 Alvord, L. and E. Cohen Van Pelt. (1999). *The Scalpel and the Silver Bear*. New York, NY: Bantam Books. Quote taken from the back cover of the book. (Note: Dr. Alvord is the first woman Navajo surgeon combining traditional medicine ways with Western allopathic medicine.)

of Life. The depiction and ascription of the Four Directions that follows is not meant to reflect the belief of any particular tribal or cultural view. The author's intent is to simply convey the Native cultural view that all life is a circle and in a cyclical movement.

- *The East Direction* is the place of birth, spring, new beginnings, the new day, the place of the morning star and the rising sun. In ceremony and in Native American healing practice, it is the place where intentions are made, where Spirit is called in, sacred space is set and all is purified.

- *The South Direction* is the actualization of the intention made in the East. It is the heart of the ceremony or healing ritual. In the Circle of Life, it is the place of summer and time of day when the sun is at its highest. The seeds of intentions made in the East Direction are bearing fruit. Growth and maturation take place in the South Direction.

- *The West Direction* is the place in ceremony, healing practice, and the cycle of life when one reflects upon what has transpired in the South Direction. It is the place of autumn where one reflects upon harvest. The West Direction is a place of reflection, of prayer and thanksgiving, and the time when one prepares for completion, closure, transition, and release.

- *The North Direction* is the cycle of completion and transition of the physical form back into the Spirit World. In ceremony and in healing, it is the place of renewal, midnight, and the cycle when all that has been born has completed its full cycle and returns to the Source – Great Spirit. It is the cycle of rest, cleansing and renewal, and the "readying" for rebirth into the next cycle of life, or into the next cycle of being.

Basic Practices

- Native Americans are, by nature, quiet and reserved. All social and personal interaction springs from "Good Ways," which are referred to here as a "code of ethics," which respects all creation and ascribes each part of creation as sacred. *A Traditional Code of Ethics* (*"Good Ways"*), presented here, is one of many that have been written down and is included here as a window to understanding American Indian Spirituality as a way of life rather than a religion. "Good Ways" extend beyond the Indian community to all contacts and interactions with all human beings and to all God's creation.

- Native Americans are very careful that their conversation and actions do not cause any one to lose credibility or be made to feel disgraced or inferior. Conversation may seem to be slow and nondirect. Native people may not seem to be as forthcoming as non-Native people when answering questions or

volunteering information about their personal lives or health conditions. However, as the caregiver cultivates the practice of listening and becomes comfortable with the long pauses that may ensue, the answers to his or her questions will be forthcoming. Long pauses indicate that careful consideration is being given to the question. By careful listening, patience, and being nondirect, one may learn quite a bit.

- Anecdotes or metaphors may be used. For example, a story told about an ill neighbor may be a way of saying the patient is experiencing the same symptoms. In this way of communication, the patient is not put "on the spot" by directly speaking of his or her condition.

- There is no hierarchy of priests, elders, or spiritual persons in American Indian Spirituality. There are ceremonial leaders, elders, and medicine people who are recognized as such within their families and communities based upon their apprenticeships, experience, and/or ancestry.

- Every person is the beneficiary of prayer: family, clan, young people, the unborn, those who are sick and in need, the elders, mentors, and the leaders of nations. The individual prays first for all those other than him- or herself, praying last for self. The strength, prosperity, and preservation of the culture depend upon each individual walking in balance: physically, spiritually, mentally, and emotionally.

- Native Americans often refer to others in kinship or familial terms, rather than by name. It is considered more respectful to speak of one's nephew or grandfather than it is to refer to them by their given name. However, be aware that the kinship may be from the traditional kinship system, which would be considered as

A Traditional Code of Ethics ("Good Ways")
- Give thanks to Creator each morning upon rising and each evening before sleeping.
- Seek courage to be a better person.
- Show respect to *all life forms*: human, animal, fowl, plants, minerals, and so forth.
- Respect the wisdom of people in council. Once you give an idea, it no longer belongs to you.
- Be truthful at all times.
- Receive strangers and outsiders kindly.
- Always treat your guests with honor and consideration, providing them with food and the comfort you have available.
- The hurt of one is the hurt of all. The honor of one is the honor of all.
- All people are children of the Creator and need to be respected.
- Serve others – be useful to family, community, or nation. True happiness comes to those who dedicate their lives to the service of others.
- Observe moderation and balance in all things.
- Know the things that lead to your well-being and those things that lead to your destruction.
- Listen and follow your inner voice. Expect guidance to come in many forms (e.g., prayer, dreams, solitude, and the words and actions of others).

an extended family relationship by the national society. Also, it may be a spiritual kinship, such as is common within many Christian denominations (e.g., "Sister," "Brother," "Father").

- Finger-pointing, loud and boisterous conversation, and staring at another are considered aggressive and rude behaviors. Avoid constant eye contact as it can be considered probing and construed as being disrespectful. It is customary for Natives to look off to the side while they are talking to another – making occasional eye contact, but not staring. When one needs to indicate a direction to another, one does so with words or a nod of the head. Some older Native people may be seen to purse their lips in the direction to which they are referring.
- Interrupting conversations is considered impolite. If one desires to speak to another

already engaged in conversation with someone else, it is a show of respect to wait quietly nearby. Native Americans are aware of the person's presence. They will turn to the person when they are ready to include him or her in the conversation.

- It is very common for a Native American to practice another faith, such as Christianity, along with his or her family traditions. For many, Native American Spirituality easily integrates with other religious practices. A Native may practice some of his or her family traditions, or practice none of them.

Principles for Clinical Care

To be Indian and to die young is to be a part of a long history that from the eyes of America is unremarkable. The life expectancy for Native Americans is variously reported as between 40 and 55. To die or even to die young is not necessarily in and of itself a tragedy. But, when one group of people is dying in such great numbers while others thrive, when the people of one group die violently, or die from diseases preventable and treatable, when they die slow and painful deaths, we need to know why.[125]

Dietary Issues

- The only dietary issue may be with regard to the clan to which the Native person may belong. However, it is unlikely that clan food, such as deer or bison, would be served in the hospital.
- Check with the patient or the family members as to any special dietary needs.

General Medical Beliefs

- Delivering effective health care to members of an ethnic group depends upon acknowledgement by the health care profession that certain cultural, social, and spiritual values may exist that may not be shared or understood by the caregiver. This is especially true for the indigenous people of the United States whose oral traditions and spirituality are a way of life, no matter the degree of assimilation into the dominant culture.
- Native American medicine is holistic. For example, for a patient presenting with a physical symptom, such as a migraine headache, for example, the caregiver would consider the possible emotional, mental, and spiritual aspects of the migraine. Likewise, if a patient presents with an emotional or mental symptom, the caregiver would consider corresponding physical and spiritual aspects. Native American medicine focuses on *healing* rather than *curing*. Healing treatments are not universal but are particular to each individual.
- For Native people, the moral character of the caregiver matters. Just having a medical degree does not assure the Native that the caregiver can heal. The caregiver must also have compassion, be upright, of good character, be good to his or her family, and have balance in his or her life. It is believed by many in the Native culture that for optimum healing, the facilitator or caregiver needs to be in alignment spiritually, physically, mentally, and emotionally. Those who are mentored in Native American medicine ways learn to become clear channels for Spirit to move through, so that energetically, the patient will be comfortable in his or her presence.
- Traditional healing may be combined with the use of Western medicine.
- Allow traditional healers to perform rituals whenever requested by the patient or patient's family.
- Do not touch or casually admire ritual objects. For example, some Native people may wear a medicine bag. It should not be treated casually or removed without permission from patient or family. If it is necessary to remove it, or any other ritual object, allow a family member (if available) to accommodate. Keep the removed object as close as possible to the patient and return it as soon as possible. This also pertains to care of the body of a deceased patient.

---

125 Dr. Jennifer Lisa Vest, Assistant Professor, Teacher of Native American Philosophy, University of Central Florida, lecturing at the Fifteenth Annual Meeting of the Association for Practical and Professional Ethics, Panel: Health Disparities and Native Americans, Jacksonville, FL, Saturday, March 4, 2006.

Specific Medical Issues

- **Abortion**: Abortion is neither endorsed nor forbidden by traditional teachings; therefore, it is an individual's or family's decision.
- **Advance Directives**: Due to the history and misuse of signed documents, some Natives may be reluctant or even unwilling to sign informed consent or advance directives. Some may display hostility toward health care providers because of the history of treatment of Native Americans by non-Native Americans. Inquire as to the wishes of the family with regard to their wishes.
- **Birth Control**: Birth control is neither endorsed nor forbidden by traditional teachings, therefore it is an individual's or a couple's decision.
- **Blood Transfusions**: The use of blood products is neither endorsed nor forbidden by traditional teachings; therefore, blood transfusions are an individual's or a family's decision.
- **Circumcision**: Circumcision, as with all other medical practices, is neither endorsed nor unendorsed by traditional teachings.
- **In Vitro Fertilization**: In vitro fertilization is neither endorsed nor forbidden by traditional teachings; therefore, it is an individual's or a family's decision.
- **Stem Cell Research**: Stem cell research for therapeutic purposes is neither endorsed nor forbidden by traditional teachings; therefore, it is an individual's or a family's decision.
- **Vaccinations**: The issue of vaccinations is an individual or family consideration and is not addressed by the faith.
- **Withholding/Withdrawing Life Support**: The concept of "medically futile" is not a part of American Indian philosophy or belief. The choice to withhold or withdraw mechanical life support is an individual or family's decision.

Gender and Personal Issues

- Respect gender preferences; some Natives may prefer to be treated by one of their own gender.
- Tolerance without complaint is highly valued. Native patients may not express their pain. Perhaps, they might say to the caregiver, "I don't feel so good" or "Something doesn't feel right." If a Native patient reports feeling "uncomfortable" and is not given pain relief, he or she generally won't ask again. Offer pain medication when the condition warrants it, even if the patient does not appear to be in pain.
- Shake hands lightly and quickly. Hard handshakes are considered rude and a sign of aggressive behavior.
- Patients will generally make their own decisions. The decision-making process can also function according to kinship structure. For example, in a matrilineal family structure, women and/or their brothers would be the decision makers. (Navajo, Hopi, and Zuni tribes are examples of matrilineal societies.)

Principles for Spiritual Care through the Cycles of Life
Concepts of Living and Dying for Spiritual Support

- The cultural view among American Indians is that all life flows in a natural cyclical, clockwise direction from east, to south, to west, to north, to east again. Just as the sun rises to mid-heaven, sets, and rises again, so it is that all life cycles are viewed. Birth, growth, maturation, aging, transition, and return to the Spirit World are viewed as the natural cycles of life.

During Birth

- The birth of a child, as with all aspects of life for the Native American, is a sacred and holy event.
- Check with the mother and her family concerning any special considerations regarding the birth process.
- Some Native cultures practice birth rituals (e.g., the saving of the umbilical cord).
- As stated earlier, circumcision, as with all other medical practices, is neither endorsed nor unendorsed by traditional Native teachings.

During Illness

- The autonomous nature of the individual's relationship to the Divine would preclude a generic approach to the patient and his or her family. In the author's experience, the best spiritual support one may offer a patient is a respectful presence. There is an American Indian Spirituality concept called the *hollow bone*. As a hollow bone, the caregiver prepares to meet the needs of the patient or patient's family by emptying the self of all preconceived notions, assumptions, and so forth, thereby allowing the flow of the Divine to direct the caregiver with regard to a patient's spiritual support.
- Make no assumptions regarding the spiritual practice of a Native-looking person. Always ask if there is anything you can do, or if there is any person or religious representative the patient might want to see.
- Do not automatically ask a Native "what tribe are you from" when assessing faith beliefs. Those who wish to tell you their tribal affiliation, if they have one, will do so at their discretion.

- Refrain from indicating your own Native family ancestry should you have one. This information is considered irrelevant, personal, and not appropriate in casual conversation.
- The individual and his or her decision are of first concern; the family's is second. However, always listen respectfully to the family and ask questions carefully.
- Extended family is important, and any illness concerns the entire family.
- The family may ask to sing or pray over their sick or dying family member. They may ask if it is OK to burn cedar, sage or sweetgrass for purification. It might be asked whether the Sacred Pipe may be brought in to pray with the family. Recently a request for a bedside ceremony was honored at a nursing home for a dying Native woman. Arrangements were made by the facilitator with the social worker and staff to honor her privacy and the sacredness of the event. Willow trees were brought in to fashion an arbor over the woman's bed. A sacred pipe was filled outside the home, then brought in and prayed with during the ceremony. No actual burning of sage or tobacco took place. The drapes that hang to separate the roommates were fashioned as a "lodge" around the woman and those who had come to pray for her. Singing of the sacred songs and Native American flute filled the air. Clan foods and sacred objects lay upon the altar. After the ceremony, the group retired to the park nearby to share the sacred clan food and smoke the sacred pipe.
- The sacred pipe uses tobacco only. The prayers are made and prayed into the pinches of tobacco taken from the tobacco pouch or bowl and placed in a sacred manner into the sacred pipe. The smoke that issues from the pipe are *prayers made*

visible. Check with hospital regulations as to whether the burning of tobacco or sage, cedar, or sweetgrass is permissible for religious purposes. If not, the spiritual essence of each might be utilized by the family member or person designated by the family to lead the prayer, such as praying with a pipe not smoked (see previous bullet point).

During End of Life

- Determine with the individual and his or her family regarding their disposition toward discussion of health directives or terminal prognosis. For some, it is believed that any discussion of end-of-life issues in the company of the patient, even if unconscious, might hasten death. Others will use the information to make appropriate preparations.
- Though some Native Americans may avoid contact with the dying, others will want to be at the bedside 24 hours a day. Visitors may display a jovial attitude so as not to demoralize the patient. Mourning is usually done in private, away from the patient.
- Some family members may want to leave a window open for the soul of their loved one to leave through at his or her passing; others may orient the patient's body to a cardinal direction before death.
- Whenever possible, do not say the name of a patient who has died; instead use familial or relational language (e.g., "your mother," "your father," "your sister").
- The cutting of a lock of hair of the deceased individual may be performed as part of a year-long "soul keeping" ceremony.
- Ask the family their wishes concerning the care and disposition of personal effects: clothing, jewelry, ritual objects, and so forth.

Care of the Body

- It is important not to move the body after death until the family has authorized you to do so. Though not always practical, refrain from touching the body in any way or from closing the eyelids after the individual may appear to be physically "gone." Some Natives believe that the spirit or soul may be disturbed from his or her journey to the Spirit World and be summoned back. Other Natives believe that the deceased spirit stays nearby for up to 5 days for the soul to witness and be a part of the family preparations for their forthcoming transition to the Heavens or place of the departed.
- Some hospitals will arrange for the recently deceased to remain undisturbed in the room, lowering the room temperature to slow down the physical disintegration, if the family requests it.
- Ask if the family wishes to perform prayers, ceremony, or ritual before the body is removed.
- Cremation, embalming, and other disposition aspects of the body are individual or family decisions.
- Donation of the body for medical research is an individual or family decision.

Organ and Tissue Donation

- Organ and tissue donation are individual or family decisions. It may be preferable for a chaplain and/or nurse who are trained designated requesters to be consulted for assistance.

Special Days: American Indian Spirituality

Every day is considered as sacred as any other day. Ceremonies, activities, and events are scheduled according to clan and family traditions, and the individual spiritual needs of the family and community.

As many Native events do take place outside, Native People, when assigning ceremonial activities and events to a calendar day, will consider the lunar, solar, and stellar cycles of the heavenly bodies. For example, weather can be less favorable when the moon is new or full, so the facilitator would do his or her best to schedule the ceremony or event in between the cycles of the moon.

Ceremonies, activities, and events are planned and facilitated by family or community spiritual leaders with regard to the natural energies each season affords. Prayer Lodges are often held seasonally to give thanks and appreciation for all that was afforded by Great Spirit up to that moment in time, and to pray for the well-being and health of all the community for the season ahead. Many Natives save the telling of their sacred stories for the winter season, the time of rest and renewal. There are ceremonies to celebrate all life's passages; birth, naming, coming of age, marriage, illness, transition, memorial, and so forth.

Please note that Native people may or may not observe the traditional US holidays or holy days such as Christmas, Easter, Independence Day, and so forth. The best advice in regard to Natives is to not assume to know their spiritual nature or religion. Spirituality is a private and family matter, and, as stated earlier, a Native may practice spirituality, another faith, or none at all. If there is a need to know, it is best to ask.

Bahá'í Faith

The tabernacle of unity hath been raised; regard ye not one another as strangers. Ye are the fruits of one tree, and the leaves of one branch.

We cherish the hope that the light of justice may shine upon the world and sanctify it from tyranny.[126]

Prepared by:
Barb McAtee and David Edalati, MD
Overland Park, KS

History and Facts

The Bahá'í Faith (pronounced *Buh-high*) was founded by Bahá'u'lláh in the mid-nineteenth century in Persia (Iran). The name Bahá'u'lláh means "The Glory of God." He was born in Persia on November 12, 1817, into a noble family. He gave up a life of privilege to deliver a new message of peace and unity to humanity.[127]

According to Bahá'í teachings, religious history is a process of progressive revelation. Throughout the ages, God has progressively revealed His teachings by sending chosen messengers to gradually educate humanity. Bahá'ís call these messengers "Manifestations of God."

Bahá'u'lláh claimed to be the latest Manifestation of God for this age, in fulfillment of promises made by Abraham, Krishna, Moses, Zoroaster, Buddha, Christ, and Muhammad. According to Bahá'í belief, Manifestations of God are the founders of the world's great religions. They have been sent by a loving Creator to educate and guide humanity. They make it possible for people to know and worship God. They also provide the impetus to elevate human civilization to higher levels of achievement.

Bahá'u'lláh's claim to a direct revelation from God brought intense persecution upon him, his family, and his followers. The established clergy of Persia, the Shah of Iran, and the Ottoman Empire tried to exterminate the faith. More than 20 000 Bahá'í believers were martyred in the land of its origin. Countless more were summarily arrested and tortured, without legal recourse. Even today, persecution of Bahá'ís continues to occur in Iran and other Islamic countries.

For that reason, many Bahá'ís have moved to more tolerant places where they can openly practice their faith, educate their children, practice their professions, and

---

126 Baha'u'llah. (1988). *Tablets of Baha'u'llah Revealed after the Kitab-i-Aqdas.* Wilmette, IL: Bahá'í Publishing Trust, 164.

127 Suggestions for accuracy of information in this document were provided by the National Bahá'í Review Office.

contribute to society. The Bahá'í communities in the United States often include immigrants from the Middle East. They also include Bahá'ís from every religious, social, economic, national, and ethnic group.

Before he died in 1892, Bahá'u'lláh designated his son, 'Abdu'l-Bahá, to be the one authorized interpreter of the Bahá'í teachings and the head of the faith. This *covenant* is a unique feature of the Bahá'í Faith. It guarantees unity within the Bahá'í community and prevents schisms. It also preserves the integrity of Bahá'u'lláh's teachings.

From earliest childhood, 'Abdu'l-Bahá (whose name means "Servant of Bahá") was imprisoned with his father. Together, they were banished from Iran to Baghdad, later to Constantinople, then to Adrianople, and finally to Akká (or Acre, a prison city in what was then the land of Syria, later known as Palestine, and now the nation of Israel.) It was there that 'Abdu'l-Bahá received the first Bahá'í pilgrims from the Western world. He was released from prison in 1908. He traveled to Europe and the United States, proclaiming Bahá'u'lláh's message of unity, peace, and social justice to faith communities, peace societies, and universities.

On November 29, 1921, 10 000 people – Jews, Christians, and Muslims from all persuasions and denominations – gathered on Mount Carmel in the Holy Land to mourn the passing of 'Abdu'l-Bahá. He was eulogized as the essence of "Virtue and Wisdom, of Knowledge and Generosity." On that occasion, Abdu'l-Bahá was described by a Jewish leader as a "living example of self-sacrifice," by a Christian orator as one who led humanity to the "Way of Truth," and by a prominent Muslim leader as a "Pillar of Peace" and the embodiment of "glory and greatness."

In his will and testament, 'Abdu'l-Bahá appointed his grandson, Shoghi Effendi, to lead the faith. Using the principles and laws revealed by Bahá'u'lláh and expounded upon by 'Abdu'l-Bahá, Shoghi Effendi established the Administrative Order of the Bahá'í Faith, which includes the elected bodies of the Universal House of Justice, National Spiritual Assemblies, Regional Bahá'í Councils, and local Spiritual Assemblies. Among other duties, the Universal House of Justice legislates upon issues not specifically addressed in the Bahá'í Writings.

Other elected bodies in the Administrative Order oversee the organization of the Bahá'í community and perform administrative tasks formerly handled by clergy, because there is no clergy in the Bahá'í Faith. Shoghi Effendi did not appoint a successor. After his death, the Universal House of Justice was elected and serves as the highest ranking authority in the faith.

The Bahá'í Faith is one of the fastest-growing world religions. It is the second-most widespread faith in the world, surpassing every religion but Christianity in its geographic reach. It spread rapidly beyond its birthplace, to more than 100 000 localities around the world.

It has become a global community of 5–6 million people, from virtually every country, ethnicity, and culture. It represents more than 2100 different ethnic and tribal groups worldwide. Elected members on a local, national, and international basis administer the Faith with no clergy and no ritual.

The writings of Bahá'u'lláh, which provide guidance for Bahá'ís, would comprise about 100 volumes. They were written or dictated by him in the Persian and Arabic languages. The existence of original texts, preserved at the Bahá'í World Centre, prevents speculation about the character of the teachings because they are authentic source materials. These texts have since been translated into more than 2000 languages.

Basic Teachings

For civilization to progress, Bahá'u'lláh said that humans must act in accord with certain principles. These principles include:

- **Oneness of God**: Bahá'u'lláh said "the peoples of the world, of whatever race or religion, derive their inspiration from one heavenly Source, and are the subjects of one God."[128]
- **Oneness of Religion**: Bahá'u'lláh taught that the religions of the world are, in reality, one common faith. They originate from the same divine reality, have the same goals of bringing humankind closer to its Creator, promoting an ever-advancing civilization, and expressing a single unfolding Divine Plan. He said, "This is the changeless Faith of God, eternal in the past, eternal in the future."[129]
- **Oneness of Mankind**: Bahá'u'lláh said there is, in reality, only one race, the human race. He proclaimed, "The world is but one country, and mankind its citizens."[130]

'Abdu'l-Bahá' wrote:

The world of existence is like unto an orchard and humanity is like unto the trees. All these trees are planted in the same orchard. The world of humanity is like unto a rose garden and the various races, tongues and people are like unto contrasting flowers. The diversity of colors in a rose garden adds to the charm and beauty of the scene as variety enhances unity.[131]

- **Elimination of All Prejudices**: Bahá'u'lláh promoted mutual understanding and cooperation among nations, cultures, and people. He counseled his followers to rid themselves of all prejudice, whether based on race, ethnicity, nationality, religion, class, or gender. In *The Hidden Words*, Bahá'u'lláh wrote:

Children of Men!
Know ye not why We created you all from the same dust? That no one should exalt himself over the other. Ponder at all times in your hearts how ye were created. Since We have created you all from one same substance, it is incumbent on you to be even as one soul, to walk with the same feet, eat with the same mouth and dwell in the same land, that from your inmost being, by your deeds and actions, the signs of oneness and the essence of detachment may be made manifest.[132]

- **Independent Investigation of Truth**: Bahá'u'lláh emphasized the fundamental obligation of human beings to seek the truth and acquire knowledge. Each person has the capacity to reason and to investigate truth without prejudice. Blind allegiance, he warned, is dangerous; whereas truth, regardless of its source, has

128 Baha'u'llah. (1988). *Gleanings from the Writings of Baha'u'llah*. Translated by Shoghi Effendi. Wilmette, IL: Bahá'í Publishing Trust, 217.

129 Ibid, 136.

130 Baha'u'llah. (1991). *The Compilation of Compilations*. Vol. 1. Ingleside, New South Wales: Bahá'í Publications Australia, 67.

131 'Abdu'l-Bahá. (1918). *Divine Philosophy*. Compiled and published by Isabel Chamber Chamberlain. Boston, MA: The Tudor Press, 183. Available at: http://bahai-library.com/books/div.phil/ accessed 15 Sept 2012).

132 Baha'u'llah. (1985, reprint). *Hidden Words of Bahaullah*. Willmete, IL: Bahá'í Publishing Trust, 20.

the power to unify and to create bonds of understanding.

- **Full Equality of Women and Men**: Bahá'u'lláh said, "Women and men have been and will always be equal in the sight of God."[133] 'Abdu'l-Bahá said:

  And among the teachings of Bahá'u'lláh is the equality of women and men. The world of humanity has two wings – one is women and the other men. Not until both wings are equally developed can the bird fly. Should one wing remain weak, flight is impossible. Not until the world of women becomes equal to the world of men in the acquisition of virtues and perfections, can success and prosperity be attained as they ought to be.[134]

- **Science and Religion Must Agree**: The Bahá'í teachings stress the fundamental harmony of science and religion. Bahá'u'lláh affirmed that "This gift giveth man the power to discern the truth in all things, leadeth him to that which is right and helpeth him to discover the secrets of creation."[135] 'Abdu'l-Bahá emphasized:

  If religious beliefs and opinions are found contrary to the standards of science, they are mere superstitions and imaginations. Unquestionably, there must be agreement between true religion and science. If a question be found contrary to reason, faith and belief in it are impossible, and there is no outcome but wavering and vacillation."[136]

- **Universal Education**: Bahá'u'lláh promoted universal education and enjoined upon his followers the duty to educate children in religious truth, as well as arts and sciences, so that they can "carry forward an ever-advancing civilization." The raising and education of children to become spiritually mature adults is a fundamental purpose of family and community life. Education of children is the responsibility of the entire society.

- **Spiritual Solutions for Economic Problems**: The unity of humankind is based on justice. An unjust imbalance in economic conditions within and among nations continues to grow. 'Abdu'l-Bahá wrote, "The fundamentals of the whole economic condition are divine in nature and are associated with the world of the heart and spirit."[137]

  Furthermore, the Bahá'í teachings affirm the importance of private ownership of property, the need for private economic initiatives and just compensation based on services or products provided.

- **Establishment of a World Federalism**: The purpose of this is to provide global security, while maintaining the integrity of national and local governments, and decentralization in local decision making.

- **Establishment of One Universal Auxiliary Language**: The accomplishment of this will seek to preserve native languages and cultures.

133 Baha'u'lláh. (1991). *The Compilation of Compilations*. Vol. 2. Ingleside, New South Wales: Bahá'í Publications Australia, 379.

134 'Abdu'l-Bahá. (1976, reprint). *Bahá'í World Faith: Selected Writings of Baha'u'llah and 'Abdu'l Baha*. Wilmette, IL: Bahá'í Publishing Trust. Copyright 1943, 1956, and 1976 by the National Spiritual Assembly of the Bahá'ís of the United States, sixth printing of 1956 edition, 288.

135 Baha'u'llah. *Gleanings from the Writings of Baha'u'llah*, 194.

136 'Abdu'l-Bahá. *Bahá'í World Faith*, 240.

137 'Abdu'l-Bahá. (1982). *The Promulgation of Universal Peace*. Wilmette, IL: Bahá'í Publishing Trust, 238.

- **Establishment of a Universal System of Currency, Weights, and Measures**.

Basic Practices

- Bahá'ís are committed to spiritually transforming their individual and collective lives, to living socially moral lives, to contributing to the advancement of their communities, and to promoting the social and spiritual principles enunciated by Bahá'u'lláh. The fundamental principle of unity pervades all that they do.
- Daily prayer and reading of holy scriptures, obedience to Bahá'í law, and participation in Bahá'í community life are responsibilities of each individual.
- Since there is no clergy, people are responsible for their own spiritual growth. There are virtually no rituals or ceremonies. Bahá'ís come together to learn in "study circles," hold devotional gatherings, and once a month have a "Feast."
- The Feast is an important institution of Bahá'í community life. It is a gathering of Bahá'ís for reading of the holy word, followed by discussion of community concerns, and then by socializing and hospitality. In the Bahá'í Feast, the serving of food is kept simple. 'Abdu'l-Bahá compared the institution of the Feast to the Christian sacrament of Communion in its importance and spiritual meaning.
- Chastity before marriage is enjoined upon believers as a means of insuring a happy and lasting marital bond. Sexual activity between a husband and wife is considered wholesome. Fidelity to one's spouse is also a Bahá'í law.
- Adult Bahá'ís (15 years of age and older) are commanded to fast once a year for the duration of 19 days, between the hours of sunrise and sunset, from March 2 through March 20. Bahá'u'lláh exempted the elderly (over 70 years of age), pregnant women, women in their menstrual cycle, the sick, those who perform strenuous physical exertion, and those who are traveling. The purpose of the fast, like prayer, is to draw a person closer to God.
- Bahá'ís are required to obey the law of the land. (The only exception is that Bahá'ís are forbidden to recant their faith, even under duress by legal authorities.)
- Bahá'ís believe they should spend their time in this life as productively as possible.
  - They should engage in arts and professions that serve mankind.
  - They should pray and meditate daily.
  - They should strive to continue to learn and grow spiritually all their lives.
  - They should strive to develop their minds, continually learning about science, religion, art, history, ethics, and so forth.
  - They should cultivate virtues such as honesty, patience, love, compassion, wisdom, reliance on God, and detachment from material or emotional concerns.

Principles for Clinical Care

The contact information provided in this section can be useful for clinicians if they are unable to find answers to their concerns in the content of this chapter.

- Local and national Spiritual Assemblies can be of assistance to anyone with questions about the Bahá'í Faith and its practices. Local Assemblies can be called upon to assist Bahá'í patients and their families. Medical personnel should feel free to contact them.
- Local assemblies and Bahá'í Centers are often listed in the white pages of the

telephone book. Many also have websites. The US Bahá'í National Center can direct an inquiry to the nearest Local Assembly. The telephone number for the Bahá'í National Center in Evanston, Illinois, is +1-847-733-3400.

Dietary Issues

- There are no dietary restrictions of the Bahá'í Faith, with the exception of abstention from alcohol.

General Medical Beliefs

- **Alcoholic Beverage**: Use of alcoholic beverage and other intoxicants (which "dull the mind and numb the spirit") is forbidden for Bahá'ís. Exceptions can be made when prescribed by a physician, when appropriate for a legitimate medical condition. For example, the use of opium is strictly forbidden but opiate-derived medications, when prescribed by a physician for medical use, are permitted.
- **Suicide**: Suicide is forbidden by Bahá'í law. It prevents the soul from continuing to develop fully in this life. Bahá'í teachings indicate that there can be value to suffering. Learning to bear suffering with patience and magnanimity fosters spiritual growth. However, one should not seek to suffer. (Asceticism as a spiritual practice is forbidden.) Bahá'í law does allow a Bahá'í funeral and burial in a Bahá'í cemetery for a person who commits suicide.
- **Physicians**: Bahá'í holy writings guide the individual to seek the care of a competent physician, when needed. This would apply to all stages of life, to decisions regarding vaccination, promotion of health, nutrition, treatment of disease, medication, surgery, anesthesia, and so forth.

Specific Medical Issues

- **Abortion**: There is no specific guidance in the Bahá'í Faith that provides a definite yes or no answer to the matter of abortion.[138]
- **Advance Directives**: Patients should be reminded to complete an advance directive. Instructions in the document could include a "*do not resuscitate*" order, and a *durable power of attorney*. These are matters left to individual choice.
- **Birth Control**: Birth control is allowed if it does not involve aborting a conceptus.
- **Blood Transfusions**: There are no religious laws against blood transfusions. Individuals should make their decisions in consultation with their physicians.
- **Circumcision**: Circumcision is not a religious practice of the Bahá'í Faith. It is a matter for the parents to decide.
- **In Vitro Fertilization**: There is no specific guidance in the Bahá'í Faith that provides a definite yes or no answer to the issue of in vitro fertilization.[139]
- **Stem Cell Research**: There are different sources of stem cells. Not all stem cell research is necessarily the same. Furthermore, processes used in research and the end results vary. Considering the different factors involved, the Universal House of Justice may eventually legislate concerning this matter. At this time, they have not done so.
- **Vaccinations**: There are no prohibitions

---

138 If this subject arises, it would be prudent to consult *Lights of Guidance*, compiled by Helen Hornby, or to contact the National Spiritual Assembly at the Bahá'í National Center in Evanston, Illinois (phone: +1-847-733-3400).

139 If this subject arises, it would be prudent to consult *Lights of Guidance*, compiled by Helen Hornby, or to contact the National Spiritual Assembly at the Bahá'í National Center in Evanston, Illinois (phone: +1-847 733-3400).

regarding the vaccination of children or medical treatment for illness.

- **Withholding/Withdrawing Life Support**: Withholding or withdrawing life support is allowed in the Bahá'í Faith. It is left to the individual's conscience or choice. As with all medical decision making, the individual is encouraged to seek the opinion of a competent physician.

Gender and Personal Issues

- It is important to recognize that Bahá'ís come from widely diverse backgrounds. Cultural differences should be considered.
- While Bahá'ís are encouraged to be modest in their dress and behavior, there is no prohibition against medical treatment provided by a person of another sex or religion.
- Cleanliness is highly praised in Bahá'í holy writings. Bahá'u'lláh encouraged believers to bathe daily.

Principles for Spiritual Care through the Cycles of Life
Concepts of Living and Dying for Spiritual Support

- Life is a sacred gift.
- The soul is eternal. It attains to spiritual growth throughout its lifetime on earth and in the "world to come." After the physical body has died, the soul continues to live in another stage or state of existence. Bahá'u'lláh wrote:

Know thou of a truth that the soul, after its separation from the body, will continue to progress until it attaineth the presence of God, in a state and condition which neither the revolution of ages and centuries, nor the changes and chances of this world, can alter. It will endure as long as the Kingdom of God, His sovereignty, His dominion and power will endure. It will manifest the signs of God and His attributes, and will reveal His loving kindness and bounty. The movement of My Pen is stilled when it attempteth to befittingly describe the loftiness and glory of so exalted a station.[140]

- Experience in this physical life is important to the growth of the soul. Pain and difficulties, like joy and pleasure, contribute to one's growth and ultimate happiness.
- Death is something all must experience. It should not be feared.
- Death is the beginning of greater experiences in the life of the soul. In the *Hidden Words*, Bahá'u'lláh said:

32. O SON OF THE SUPREME!
I have made death a messenger of joy to thee. Wherefore dost thou grieve? I made the light to shed on thee its splendor. Why dost thou veil thyself there from?
33. O SON OF SPIRIT!
With the joyful tidings of light I hail thee: rejoice! To the court of holiness I summon thee; abide therein that thou mayest live in peace for evermore.
34. O SON OF SPIRIT!
The spirit of holiness beareth unto thee the joyful tidings of reunion; wherefore dost thou grieve? The spirit of power confirmeth thee in His cause; why dost thou veil thyself? The light of His countenance doth lead thee; how canst thou go astray?
35. O SON OF MAN!
Sorrow not save that thou art far from Us. Rejoice not save that thou art drawing near and returning unto Us.

---

140 Baha'u'llah. *Gleanings from the Writings of Baha'u'llah*, 155–156.

36. O SON OF MAN!

Rejoice in the gladness of thine heart, that thou mayest be worthy to meet Me and to mirror forth My beauty.[141]

Powers of the mind, including learning and memory, can be adversely affected through illness or injury. These spiritual powers will function at the optimal level after death. They can be expressed more powerfully and clearly in the next life. Written on behalf of Shoghi Effendi, letter dated April 10, 1938, to an individual believer:

You ask an explanation of what happens to us after we leave this world: This is a question which none of the Prophets have ever answered in detail, for the very simple reason that you cannot convey to a person's mind something entirely different from everything they have ever experienced. 'Abdu'l-Bahá gave the wonderful example of the relation of this life to the next life being like the child in the womb; it develops eyes, ears, hands, feet, tongue, and yet it has nothing to see or hear, it cannot walk or grasp things or speak; all these faculties it is developing for this world. If you tried to explain to an embryo what this world is like it would never understand – but it understands when it is born, and its faculties can be used. So we cannot picture our state in the next world. All we know is that our consciousness, our personality, endures in some new state, and that that world is as much better than this one as this one is better than the dark womb of our mother was.[142]

- The soul and mind of the individual will continue to grow and learn in the next stage of life beyond the physical realm.

During Birth

- Birth control is not strictly forbidden but neither is it encouraged.
- Bahá'u'lláh taught that the life of the individual soul begins at conception (with the uniting of sperm and ova).
- Rearing of children is a sacred purpose of marriage. That is not to say it is the only purpose of marriage, or that all married couples must do so. Each couple has the right to decide this matter for themselves.
- Life begins at conception. Abortion prevents an important stage in the development of the soul. Parents have the responsibility to decide, in consultation with their doctor, on the very rare occasion, if ever, that this would be an option.
- An aborted or miscarried fetus should be treated with the same respect as the body of an older person and buried in the same manner as a child or adult.
- As stated earlier, circumcision is not a religious practice of the Bahá'í Faith. It is a matter for the parents to decide.
- There is no ritual act of spiritual care that should occur in hospital at the death of a baby or a fetal demise. The parents may wish to pray, or may ask others to pray, for them and their baby.

During Illness

- Although Bahá'ís believe in the power of prayer to heal, they are to seek a knowledgeable physician to treat their illnesses. Healing prayers were revealed by Bahá'u'lláh, and written for Bahá'ís to use. Bahá'ís often pray for healing for themselves and others, while also pursuing medical treatment.

---

141 Baha'u'llah. *The Hidden Words of Baha'u'llah*, 11–12.
142 *Compilations*. (1998). Evanston, IL: NSA USA-Developing Distinctive Bahá'í Communities Guidelines For Spiritual Assemblies Office of Assembly Development, section 18.15, p. 102.

- Patients may receive comfort from the reading of Bahá'í holy books or other devotional material and/or listening to religious music.
- Patients may desire to have religious objects in their rooms – for example, a nine-pointed star, "The Greatest Name" (a stylized calligraphic rendition of Arabic words meaning *God Is All Glorious*), a picture of 'Abdu'l-Bahá, a Bahá'í prayer book, Bahá'í literature, and photographs of Bahá'í holy places.
- Many Bahá'ís are receptive to literature, prayers, and clergy of other faith traditions.
- Call the local Bahá'í Spiritual Assembly if requested by the patient or family or to facilitate the process of conflict resolution.
- An individual or family may request the presence of a member of the Bahá'í community or an individual designated by the local Spiritual Assembly.

During End of Life

- Bahá'í law specifies that the individual should write a will and testament before death. It may be helpful to ask if this document has been completed.
- Patients should be reminded to complete an advance directive. Various care issues contained within the advance directive are matters left to an individual's choice.
- Prayers on behalf of a deceased patient are seen as efficacious for progress of the patient in the spiritual journey.
- The patient's family may request the local Spiritual Assembly to send a member of the Bahá'í community to help with spiritual or emotional needs of the family.

Care of the Body

- Cremation and embalming are prohibited, unless required by law. There are no Bahá'í laws in regard to the time of burial of the body after death, but the body is usually prepared for burial within 24 hours because of the prohibition against embalming.
- The body is to be washed and shrouded in white cloth made of cotton or silk. Normally, relatives or friends of the deceased prepare the body for burial. If they are not available, it is permissible for medical staff or mortuaries to do so.
- A Bahá'í burial ring[143] should be placed upon a finger of an adult Bahá'í (the particular finger is not specified). The ring bears the inscription (usually in Arabic, but here translated to English) "I came forth from God, and return unto Him, detached from all save him, holding fast to His name, the Merciful, the Compassionate."
- The body should be placed in a casket made of crystal, stone, or wood. It should be buried within an hour's journey of the place of death. In some places, Bahá'í-owned cemeteries exist, but the body is not required to be buried in a Bahá'í cemetery. Bahá'í prayers for the dead are read at the gravesite. A memorial service can be held before or after burial, but is not required.
- Disinterment of the body should not take place, unless required by law.
- Autopsy is not prohibited by the Bahá'í Faith.

---

143 Bahá'í burial rings can be obtained through the nearest Local Spiritual Assembly. They are also available from various vendors. One popular vendor is Special Ideas, based in Heltonville, Indiana (phone: +1-800-326-1197; website: www.bahairesources.com).

- Bahá'ís may will their bodies to science. Advance planning for such donations is required by most receiving organizations. Last-minute donations are usually not possible. Once the body is no longer needed for that purpose, it should be buried in accordance with Bahá'í burial law.

Organ and Tissue Donation

- Organ and tissue donation is permitted and is an individual decision. It may be preferable for a chaplain and/or nurse who are trained designated requesters to be consulted for assistance.

Scriptures, Inspirational Readings, and Prayers

READINGS DURING ILLNESS

There are many Bahá'í books, prayers, and meditations that can be read or offered to help the patient during an illness.[144,145]

If this should be the case, how is it, thou hast observed, that whereas such slight injuries to his mental faculties as fainting and severe illness deprive him of his understanding and consciousness, his death, which must involve the decomposition of his body and the dissolution of its elements, is powerless to destroy that understanding and extinguish that consciousness? How can any one imagine that man's consciousness and personality will be maintained, when the very instruments necessary to their existence and function will have completely disintegrated?

Know thou that the soul of man is exalted above, and is independent of all infirmities of body or mind. That a sick person showeth signs of weakness is due to the hindrances that interpose themselves between his soul and his body, for the soul itself remaineth unaffected by any bodily ailments. Consider the light of the lamp. Though an external object may interfere with its radiance, the light itself continueth to shine with undiminished power. In like manner, every malady afflicting the body of man is an impediment that preventeth the soul from manifesting its inherent might and power. When it leaveth the body, however, it will evince such ascendancy, and reveal such influence as no force on earth can equal. Every pure, every refined and sanctified soul will be endowed with tremendous power, and shall rejoice with exceeding gladness.

Consider the lamp which is hidden under a bushel. Though its light be shining, yet its radiance is concealed from men. Likewise, consider the sun which hath been obscured by the clouds. Observe how its splendor appeareth to have diminished, when in reality the source of that light hath remained unchanged. The soul of man should be likened unto this sun, and all things on earth should be regarded as his body. So long as no external impediment interveneth between them, the body will, in its entirety, continue to reflect the light of the soul, and to be sustained by its power. As soon as, however, a veil

---

144 Baha'u'llah. *Gleanings from the Writings of Baha'u'llah.* Page numbers cited in text for various selections.

145 Holley, H. ed. (1923). *Bahá'í Scriptures: Selections from the Utterances of Bahá'u'lláh and 'Abdu'l-Bahá.* New York, NY: Brentano's Publishers. Page numbers cited in text for various selections.

interposeth itself between them, the brightness of that light seemeth to lessen.

Consider again the sun when it is completely hidden behind the clouds. Though the earth is still illumined with its light, yet the measure of light which it receiveth is considerably reduced. Not until the clouds have dispersed, can the sun shine again in the plenitude of its glory. Neither the presence of the cloud nor its absence can, in any way, affect the inherent splendor of the sun. The soul of man is the sun by which his body is illumined, and from which it draweth its sustenance, and should be so regarded.

Consider, moreover, how the fruit, ere it is formed, lieth potentially within the tree. Were the tree to be cut into pieces, no sign nor any part of the fruit, however small, could be detected. When it appeareth, however, it manifesteth itself, as thou hast observed, in its wondrous beauty and glorious perfection. Certain fruits, indeed, attain their fullest development only after being severed from the tree.

—*Gleanings from the Writings of Bahá'u'lláh*, 153–155

You know that the spirit is permanent and steadfast in its station and the feebleness of the sick person is due to preventing causes. Yet in fact the feebleness will never approach the spirit. For example, when you look at the lighted lamp you find it shining and radiating, but if there is something before it, then the light will be prevented, yet in its sphere it is radiating, but by the means of prevention, its light was kept from shining forth. In the same way with the person, while he is in the diseased condition the manifestation of the power and might of the spirit will be prevented and concealed on account of the means of prevention; but after the spirit leaves the body, it will appear with such power, might and superiority that all ordinary comparison is impossible. The choice, pure and holy spirits are and will be in perfect might and joy. For example, if a lighted lamp is put under an iron lantern its light will never come forth, yet it is shining just the same. Look toward the sun when it is behind the cloud, shining and gleaming in its rank, but owing to the cloud its illumination seems weak. Now suppose that this sun is the human spirit and all other things are body, and that by its light and rays, all the body is lighted and illuminated. This is so when no means of prevention will be found to veil the light. Now the appearance of the sun seems very weak behind the veil when the cloud exists; though the land is illuminated by the light of the sun, yet this light is always weak; but after the cloud passes away, the illuminations are again manifested. In the two cases, the sun was the same in its rank; likewise the sun of the souls, which is named, mentioned as, and ever will be called, the spirit.

—*Bahá'í Scriptures*, 228–229

PRAYERS DURING ILLNESS

These prayers can be offered by family, friends, clergy, and health care professionals.[146,147]

Prayers and Meditations by Bahá'u'lláh

Thy name is my healing, O my God, and remembrance of Thee is my remedy. Nearness to Thee is my hope, and love for Thee is my companion. Thy mercy to me is my healing and my succor in both this world and the world to come. Thou, verily, art the All-Bountiful, the All-Knowing, the All-Wise.

—Bahá'u'lláh, *Bahá'í Prayers*, 262

Bahá'í Prayers

O God, my God! Shield Thy trusted servants from the evils of self and passion, protect them with the watchful eye of thy loving kindness from all rancor, hate and envy, shelter them in the impregnable stronghold of Thy care and, safe from the darts of doubtfulness, make them the manifestations of Thy glorious signs, illumine their faces with the effulgent rays shed from the Dayspring of Thy divine unity, gladden their hearts with the verses revealed from Thy holy kingdom, strengthen their loins by Thine all-swaying power that cometh from Thy realm of glory. Thou art the All-Bountiful, the Protector, the Almighty, the Gracious.

—'Abdu'l-Bahá, *Bahá'í Prayers*, 135–136

O my Lord! Thou knowest that the people are encircled with pain and calamities and are environed with hardships and trouble. Every trial doth attack man and every dire adversity doth assail him like unto the assault of a serpent. There is no shelter and asylum for him except under the wing of Thy protection, preservation, guard and custody.

O Thou the Merciful One! O my Lord! Make Thy protection my armor, Thy preservation my shield, humbleness before the door of Thy oneness my guard, and Thy custody and defense my fortress and my abode. Preserve me from the suggestions of self and desire, and guard me from every sickness, trial, difficulty and ordeal.

Verily, Thou art the Protector, the Guardian, the Preserver, the Sufficer, and verify, Thou art the Merciful of the Most Merciful.

—'Abdu'l-Bahá, *Bahá'í Prayers*, 136

Dispel my grief by Thy bounty and Thy generosity, O God, my God, and banish mine anguish through Thy sovereignty and Thy might. Thou seest me, O my god, with my face set

---

146 Effendi, S. trans. (1987). *Prayers and Meditations by Baha'u'llah*. Wilmette, IL: Bahá'í Publishing Trust. Page numbers of prayers cited with selections in the text.

147 *Bahá'í Prayers: A Selection of Prayers Revealed by Bahá'u'lláh, The Báb, and 'Abdu'l-Bahá.* (1991). Wilmette, IL: Bahá'í Publishing Trust. Page numbers of prayers cited with the various selections within the text.

towards Thee at a time when sorrows have compassed me on every side. I implore Thee, O Thou Who art the Lord of all being, and overshadowest all things visible and invisible, by Thy Name whereby Thou hast subdued the hearts and the souls of men, and by the billows of the Ocean of Thy mercy and the splendors of the Daystar of Thy bounty, to number me with them whom nothing whatsoever hath deterred from setting their faces toward Thee, O Thou Lord of all names and Maker of the heavens!

Thou beholdest, O my Lord, the things which have befallen me in Thy days. I entreat Thee, by Him Who is the Dayspring of Thy names and the Dawning-Place of Thine attributes, to ordain for me what will enable me to arise to serve Thee and to extol Thy virtues. Thou art, verily, the Almighty, the Most Powerful, Who art wont to answer the prayers of all men!

And, finally, I beg of Thee by the light of Thy countenance to bless my affairs, and redeem my debts, and satisfy my needs. Thou art He to Whose power and to Whose dominion every tongue hath testified, and Whose majesty and Whose sovereignty every understanding heart hath acknowledged. No God is there but Thee, Who hearest and art ready to answer.

—Bahá'u'lláh, *Bahá'í Prayers*, 26–27

by them that long to behold Thee, not to withhold from me Thy tender mercies in Thy Day, nor to deprive me of the melodies of the Dove that extolleth Thy oneness before the light that shineth from thy face. I am the one who is in misery, O God! Behold me cleaving fast to Thy Name, the All-Possessing. I am the one who is sure to perish; behold me clinging to Thy Name, the Imperishable. I implore Thee, therefore, by Thy Self, the Exalted, the Most High, not to abandon me unto mine own self and unto the desires of a corrupt inclination. Hold Thou my hand with the hand of Thy power, and deliver me from the depths of my fancies and idle imaginings, and cleanse me of all that is abhorrent unto Thee.

Cause me, then, to turn wholly unto Thee, to put my whole trust in Thee, to seek Thee as my Refuge, and to flee unto Thy face. Thou art, verily, He, Who, through the power of His might, doeth whatsoever He desireth, and commandeth, through the potency of His will, whatsoever He chooseth. None can withstand the operation of Thy decree; none can divert the course of Thine appointment. Thou art, in truth, the Almighty, the All-Glorious, the Most Bountiful.

—Bahá'u'lláh, *Bahá'í Prayers*, 27–28

Lauded and glorified art thou, O my God! I entreat Thee by the sighing of Thy lovers and by the tears shed

Is there any Remover of difficulties save God? Say: Praised be God! He is God! All are His servants, and all abide by His bidding!

Say: God sufficeth all things above all
things, and nothing in the heavens
or in the earth but God sufficeth.
Verily, He is in Himself the Knower,
the Sustainer, the Omnipotent.

—The Báb, *Bahá'í Prayers*, 28–29

READINGS DURING END-OF-LIFE PROCESS

These selections can be read by family, friends,
clergy, and health care professionals.[148,149,150]

Therefore, you must thank God
that He has bestowed upon you the
blessing of life and existence in the
human kingdom. Strive diligently to
acquire virtues befitting your degree
and station. Be as lights of the world
which cannot be hid and which have
no setting in horizons of darkness.
Ascend to the zenith of an existence
which is never beclouded by the fears
and forebodings of non-existence.
When man is not endowed with
inner perception he is not informed
of these important mysteries. The
retina of outer vision though sensitive
and delicate may nevertheless be a
hindrance to the inner eye which
alone can perceive. The bestowals
of God which are manifest in all
phenomenal life are sometimes hidden
by intervening veils of mental and
mortal vision which render man
spiritually blind and incapable but
when those scales are removed and
the veils rent asunder, then the great
signs of God will become visible
and he will witness the eternal light
filling the world. The bestowals of
God are all and always manifest.
The promises of heaven are ever
present. The favors of God are all-
surrounding but should the conscious
eye of the soul of man remain veiled
and darkened he will be led to deny
these universal signs and remain
deprived of these manifestations of
divine bounty. Therefore we must
endeavor with heart and soul in order
that the veil covering the eye of inner
vision may be removed, that we may
behold the manifestations of the
signs of God, discern His mysterious
graces, and realize that material
blessings as compared with spiritual
bounties are as nothing. The spiritual
blessings of God are greatest. When
we were in the mineral kingdom,
although endowed with certain gifts
and powers, they were not to be
compared with the blessings of the
human kingdom. In the matrix of
the mother we were the recipients of
endowments and blessings of God,
yet these were as nothing compared
to the powers and graces bestowed
upon us after birth into this human
world. Likewise if we are born
from the matrix of this physical and
phenomenal environment into the
freedom and loftiness of the life and
vision spiritual, we shall consider this
mortal existence and its blessings as
worthless by comparison.

—*Promulgation of Universal Peace*,
89–90

148 'Abdu'l Baha. *The Promulgation of Universal Peace*.
Page number cited in text.

149 'Abdu'l-Bahá. (1976, reprint). *Bahá'í World Faith*
('Abdu'l Baha's section only). Page number cited in
text.

150 'Abdu'l Baha. (1982, reprint). *'Abdu'l Baha in
London*. London: Bahá'í Publishing Trust (UK).
Page number cited in text.

From the death of that beloved youth due to his separation from you the utmost sorrow and grief has been occasioned, for he flew away in the flower of his age and the bloom of his youth, to the heavenly nest. But as he has been freed from this sorrow-stricken shelter and has turned his face toward the everlasting nest of the Kingdom and has been delivered from a dark and narrow world and has hastened to the sanctified realm of Light, therein lies the consolation of our hearts.

The inscrutable divine wisdom underlies such heart-rending occurrences. It is as if a kind gardener transfers a fresh and tender shrub from a narrow place to a vast region. This transference is not the cause of the withering, the waning or the destruction of that shrub, nay rather it makes it grow and thrive, acquire freshness and delicacy and attain verdure and fruition. This hidden secret is well-known to the gardener, while those souls who are unaware of this bounty suppose that the gardener in his anger and wrath has uprooted the shrub. But to those who are aware this concealed fact is manifest and this predestined decree considered a favor. Do not feel grieved and disconsolate therefore at the ascension of that bird of faithfulness, nay under all circumstances pray and beg for that youth forgiveness and elevation of station.

I hope that you will attain to the utmost patience, composure and resignation, and I supplicate and entreat at the Threshold of Oneness and beg pardon and forgiveness. My hope from the infinite bounties of God is that He may cause this dove of the garden of faith to abide on the branch of the Supreme Concourse that it may sing in the best of tunes the praises and the excellencies of the Lord of names and attributes.

— 'Abdu'l-Bahá, *Bahá'í World Faith*, 379

A friend asked: "How should one look forward to death?"

'Abdu'l-Bahá answered: "How does one look forward to the goal of any journey? With hope and with expectation. It is even so with the end of this earthly journey. In the next world, man will find himself freed from many of the disabilities under which he now suffers. Those who have passed on through death, have a sphere of their own. It is not removed from ours; their work, the work of the Kingdom, is ours; but it is sanctified from what we call "time and place." Time with us is measured by the sun. When there is no more sunrise, and no more sunset, that kind of time does not exist for man. Those who have ascended have different attributes from those who are still on earth, yet there is no real separation.

— 'Abdu'l-Bahá, *'Abdu'l-Bahá in London*, 95–96

PRAYERS DURING END-OF-LIFE PROCESS
These prayers can be offered by family, friends, clergy, and health care professionals.[151]

---

151 *Bahá'í Prayers: A Selection of Prayers Revealed by*

Bahá'í Prayers

Glory be to Thee, O Lord my God! Abase not him whom Thou hast exalted through the power of Thine everlasting sovereignty, and remove not far from Thee him whom Thou hast caused to enter the tabernacle of Thine eternity. Wilt Thou cast away, O my God, him whom thou hast overshadowed with Thy Lordship, and wilt Thou turn away from Thee, O my Desire, him to whom Thou hast been a refuge? Canst Thou degrade him whom Thou hast uplifted, or forget him whom Thou didst enable to remember Thee?

Glorified, immensely glorified art Thou! Thou art He Who from everlasting hath been the King of the entire creation and its Prime Mover, and Thou wilt to everlasting remain the Lord of all created things and their Ordainer. Glorified art Thou, O my God! If Thou ceasest to be merciful unto Thy servants, who, then, will show mercy unto them; and if Thou refusest to succor thy loved ones, who is there that can succor them?

Glorified, immeasurably glorified art Thou! Thou art adored in Thy truth, and Thee do we all, verily, worship; and Thou art manifest in Thy justice, and to Thee do we all, verily, bear witness. Thou art, in truth, beloved in Thy grace. No God is there but Thee, the Help in Peril, the Self-Subsisting.

—Bahá'u'lláh, *Bahá'í Prayers*, 41–42

He is God, exalted is He, the Lord of loving-kindness and bounty!

Glory be unto Thee, O my God, the Lord Omnipotent. I testify to Thine omnipotence and Thy might, Thy sovereignty and Thy loving-kindness, Thy grace and Thy power, the oneness of Thy Being and the unity of thine Essence, Thy sanctity and exaltation above the world of being and all that is therein.

O my God! Thou seest me detached from all save Thee, holding fast unto Thee and turning unto the ocean of Thy bounty, to the heaven of Thy favor, to the Daystar of Thy grace.

Lord! I bear witness that in Thy servant Thou hast reposed Thy Trust, and that is the Spirit whereunto Thou hast given life to the world.

I ask of Thee by the splendor of the Orb of Thy Revelation, mercifully to accept from him that which he hath achieved in Thy days. Grant then that he may be invested with the glory of Thy good-pleasure and adorned with Thine acceptance.

O my Lord! I myself and all created things bear witness unto Thy might, and I pray Thee not to turn away from Thyself this spirit that hath ascended unto Thee, unto Thy heavenly place, Thine exalted Paradise and Thy retreats of nearness, O Thou who art the Lord of all men!

Grant, then, O my God, that Thy

Bahá'u'lláh, The Báb, and 'Abdu'l-Bahá. Page numbers of prayers cited with the various selections within the text.

servant may consort with Thy chosen ones, Thy saints and Thy Messengers in heavenly places that the pen cannot tell nor the tongue recount.

O My Lord, the poor one hath verily hastened unto the Kingdom of Thy wealth, the stranger unto his home within Thy precincts, he that is sore athirst to the heavenly river of Thy bounty. Deprive him not, O Lord, from his share of the banquet of Thy grace and from the favor of Thy bounty. Thou art in truth the Almighty, the Gracious, the All-Bountiful.

O my God, Thy Trust hath been returned unto Thee. It behooveth Thy grace and Thy bounty that have compassed Thy dominions on earth and in heaven, to vouchsafe unto Thy newly welcomed one Thy gifts and Thy bestowals, and the fruits of the tree of Thy grace! Powerful art Thou to do as Thou willest, there is none other God but Thee, the Gracious, the Most Bountiful, the Compassionate, the Bestower, the Pardoner, the Precious, the All-Knowing.

I testify, O my Lord, that Thou hast enjoined upon men to honor their guest, and he that hath ascended unto Thee hath verily reached Thee and attained Thy Presence. Deal with him then according to Thy grace and bounty! By Thy glory, I know of a certainly that Thou wilt not withhold Thyself from that which Thou hast commanded Thy servants, nor wilt Thou deprive him that hath clung to the cord of Thy bounty and hath ascended to the Dayspring of Thy wealth.

There is none other God but Thee, the One, the Single, the Powerful, the Omniscient, the Bountiful.

— Bahá'u'lláh, *Bahá'í Prayers*, 43–45

O my God! O Thou forgiver of sins, bestower of gifts, dispeller of afflictions!

Verily, I beseech Thee to forgive the sins of such as have abandoned the physical garment and have ascended to the spiritual world.

O my Lord! Purify them from trespasses, dispel their sorrows, and change their darkness into light. Cause them to enter the garden of happiness, cleanse them with the most pure water, and grant them to behold Thy splendors on the loftiest mount.

— 'Abdu'l-Bahá, *Bahá'í Prayers*, 45–46

O my God! O my God! Verily, thy servant, humble before the majesty of Thy divine supremacy, lowly at the door of Thy oneness, hath believed in Thee and in Thy verses, hath testified to Thy word, hath been enkindled with the fire of Thy love, hath been immersed in the depths of the ocean of Thy knowledge, hath been attracted by Thy breezes, hath relied upon his supplications to Thee, and hath been assured of Thy pardon and forgiveness. He hath abandoned this mortal life and hath flown to the kingdom of immortality, yearning for the favor of meeting Thee.

O Lord, glorify his station, shelter him under the pavilion of Thy supreme mercy, cause him to enter

Thy glorious paradise, and perpetuate his existence in Thine exalted rose garden, that he may plunge into the sea of light in the world of mysteries.

Verily, Thou art the Generous, the Powerful, the Forgiver and the Bestower.

—'Abdu'l-Bahá, *Bahá'í Prayers*, 46–47

Special Days: Bahá'í

January 20 *World Religion Day* – The aim of World Religion Day, held on the third Sunday in January, is to foster the establishment of interfaith understanding and harmony by emphasizing the common denominators underlying all religions. World Religion Day observances are dedicated toward encouraging the leaders and followers of every religion to acknowledge the similarities in each of our sacred faiths.

February 26 *Ayyám-i-Há (Intercalary Days)* – The Bahá'í calendar is made up of 19 months of 19 days each. The period of *Ayyám-i-Há* adjusts the Bahá'í year to the solar cycle. These days are set aside for hospitality, gift-giving, special acts of charity, and preparing for the Bahá'í Fast.

March 2 Nineteen-Day Fast – *Ala* (Loftiness) is the nineteenth and final month. It marks the beginning of a 19-day fast that lasts until March 20 and which prepares worshippers for the *Naw-Ruz*. Observing the fast is an individual obligation, and is binding on all Bahá'ís who have reached the age of maturity (15 years) until the age of 70. The fast is from sunrise to sunset, with complete abstinence of food and drink. Along with obligatory prayer, it is one of the greatest obligations of a Bahá'í. Shoghi Effendi, the Guardian of the Bahá'í Faith, explains:

> It is essentially a period of meditation and, of spiritual recuperation, during which the believer must strive to make the necessary readjustments in his inner life, and to refresh and reinvigorate the spiritual forces latent in his soul. Its significance and purpose are, therefore, fundamentally spiritual in character. Fasting is symbolic, and a reminder of abstinence from selfish and carnal desires.

March 20 *Naw-Ruz: Bahá (New Year)* – The *Naw-Ruz* falls on the vernal equinox, symbolizing spiritual growth and renewal. On this holiday, Bahá'ís spend time with their families during the day and feast with celebration during the evening. The first month of the Bahá'í year is *Bahá*, which means "splendor."

April 21 *Ridvan* – A 12-day festival in the Bahá'í Faith, commemorating the commencement of Bahá'u'lláh's prophethood. It begins at sunset on April 20 and continues until sunset, May 2. On the first (April 21), ninth (April 29), and twelfth days of *Riḍvan* (May 2), work and schooling is suspended. *Riḍvan* means paradise, and is named for the Garden of Ridvan, outside Baghdad where Bahá'u'lláh stayed for 12 days after the Ottoman Empire exiled him from Baghdad and before commencing his journey to Constantinople. It is the most holy Bahá'í festival and is also referred to as the "Most Great Festival" and the "King of Festivals."

May 22 *Declaration of the Báb* – The Báb (meaning "Gate") founded the Babi Faith and was the forerunner of Bahá'u'lláh. This feast is celebrated May 22–23 (from 2 hours after sunset on May 22). The Báb was the forerunner of Bahá'u'lláh. His mission was to prepare the world for the coming of Bahá'u'lláh, and he declared it on the evening of May 22, 1844. The Báb was later imprisoned and executed for his beliefs and activities.

May 28 *Ascension of Bahá'u'lláh* – May 28/29 marks the anniversary of the Ascension of Bahá'u'lláh, the Prophet-Founder of the Bahá'í Faith. The day is one of 9 holy days on which Bahá'ís suspend work and school. Bahá'u'lláh died after a brief illness in 1892 in the Mansion of Bahji outside Akká, in what is now northern Israel. After spending most of his life in exile, he was able to live his later years at Bahji in relative tranquility, and he was buried in a small stone house adjacent to the mansion. This shrine is the holiest place on earth for Bahá'ís, the place toward which they turn in prayer each day.

July 8 *Martyrdom of the Báb* – Mirza Ali Muhammad is the given name of the Báb. This major holy day is celebrated at noon and commemorates the events surrounding the death of the Báb in 1850. The Báb had many followers, but his beliefs did not meet with approval from the leaders of the state religion in Persia, and they decided he should be taken from prison and put to death by firing squad. The Báb's followers rescued the bodies, and years later the remains were buried on Mount Carmel in Israel, in a shrine that is now a place of pilgrimage for Bahá'ís worldwide. To commemorate this day, Bahá'ís read special prayers at noon, which is the time of the scheduled execution. This is also a day of rest, when Bahá'ís should not work.

October 19 *Birth of the Báb* – On October 20 of each year, Bahá'ís around the world celebrate the birth of one of the founders of their faith. Mirza Ali Muhammad was born on October 20, 1819, in Shiraz, Persia, one of the lineage of the Prophet Muhammad and destined to become the *Qa'im*, the Promised One of Islam. No portents marked his birth; he was simply a baby named Ali Muhammad.

November 11 *Birth of Bahá'u'lláh* – The Birth of Bahá'u'lláh is one of 9 holy days in the calendar that is celebrated by Bahá'ís and during which work is suspended. Bahá'u'lláh was born on November 12, 1817, in Tehran, Iran. This holy day was instituted in the book of laws, where Bahá'u'lláh first refers to four great festivals: (1) the Festival of Ridvan; (2) the Declaration of the Báb; (3) the Birth of the Báb, who is considered to be a Manifestation of God who foretold the coming of Bahá'u'lláh; and (4) the Birth of Bahá'u'lláh.

November 25 *Day of the Covenant* – The Day of the Covenant is the day when Bahá'ís celebrate the appointment of 'Abdu'l-Bahá as the Center of Bahá'u'lláh's Covenant with his followers. 'Abdu'l-Bahá stated that May 23 should under no circumstances be celebrated as his day of birth. It was the day of the Declaration of the Báb, exclusively associated with him. But as the Bahá'ís begged for a day to be celebrated as his, he gave them November 26, 180 days after the ascension of Bahá'u'lláh, to be observed as the day of the appointment of the Center of the Covenant.

November 27 *Ascension of 'Abdu'l-Bahá* – On November 28, members of the Bahá'í Faith throughout the world commemorate the passing of 'Abdu'l-Bahá, the eldest son and successor of Bahá'u'lláh. He died in his house in Haifa, which was then in Palestine, in 1921 at the age of 77. He was laid to rest in a vault adjoining that in which he had laid the remains of the Báb on Mount Carmel in 1909. Bahá'ís observe the Holy Day at 1 a.m., about the time of His death. There are no prescribed ceremonies but gatherings usually involve prayers and devotional readings.

Buddhism: General Introduction

Prepared by:
Lama Chuck Stanford
(Changchup Kunchok Dorje)
Rime Buddhist Center
Kansas City, MO

Buddhism was founded by a historical figure referred to as the Buddha, who lived and taught 2500 years ago in India. It is the world's fourth-largest religion, with about 350 million practitioners worldwide. There are an estimated 2.7 million Buddhists in the United States. To begin to understand this ancient religion, it is helpful to make some broad general statements so the reader can view it in comparison with the more familiar monotheistic faiths.

- Buddhism is a nontheistic religion.
- Buddhism has no creator gods or saviors (the Buddha himself is viewed neither as a god nor as a savior).
- Buddhism does not believe in creation (as described in the holy books of other religions).
- Buddhism is relatively free of dogma and "blind" faith.
- Buddhism both rejected and adopted certain doctrines from the Vedic tradition (later referred to as Hinduism).
- Buddhism believes man's basic nature is not only good but also in fact enlightened (*see* "Buddha Nature" in the "History and Facts" section of the two following Buddhism chapters).
- Buddhism is based more upon one's own direct experience than upon religious doctrine.

Who was this man called the Buddha? Although much myth surrounds the life of Siddhārtha Gautama, also known as *Shakyamuni* (sage of the *Shakya* clan) Buddha, he was, nonetheless, a historical person born approximately 560 BCE in an area that is present-day Nepal. While Siddhārtha is the historical Buddha, the scriptures relate that he was not the only Buddha. In fact, there were six Buddhas preceding Siddhārtha during earlier eras. Thus, he is usually referred to as Siddhārtha Buddha to distinguish him from the previous "transcendent" Buddhas. His first name was Siddhārtha (meaning "a wish fulfilled") and his family name was Gautama. So, he was also referred to as Gautama Buddha. According to the teachings, he was born into a family of nobles, and his father was the king of a clan of local people known as the *Shakyas*. Within the hereditary caste system of that time, his noble family was of the second-highest caste, known as the warrior caste. (The only higher caste was the Brahmin or priest caste.)

Similar to founders of other world religions, Siddhārtha's birth was foretold by prophets. There is considerable myth concerning the conception and birth of Siddhārtha. It is related that his mother conceived him in a dream of a six-tusked white elephant, which dissolved into her body. After a 10-month gestation period, his mother gave birth in a grove near the town of Lumbini, Nepal. It is said she gave birth from her side, and not only that he was born clean but also that he immediately stood up and took seven steps. In each of his footsteps, a lotus blossom bloomed, and he declared, "I am the greatest in the world. This is my last birth. I will put an end to the suffering of birth, old age, and death." Lumbini is one of the four major holy sites that are frequented by Buddhists on pilgrimages. The other three are (1) Bodh Gaya, India (the place where Siddhārtha received enlightenment); (2) Kushinagar, India (town near the place of the Buddha's death); and (3) Sarnath, India (on the outskirts of Varanasi), where he gave his first teaching.

Prophets of the day also predicted that Siddhārtha would become either a great king or a great spiritual leader. (He grew up studying the Vedas and the Upanishads within the Bramanical or Vedic tradition.) His father was determined to keep Siddhārtha from becoming one of the many wandering ascetics, because he wanted his son to follow in his footsteps. Therefore, to prevent him from becoming interested in spiritual matters, his father protected him from the outside world; he was never allowed to leave the palace. In order to compensate for the restrictions placed upon Siddhārtha, his father provided the finest of everything imaginable, and Siddhārtha led a hedonistic life of luxury.

Despite his father's best efforts to keep him from the outside world, Siddhārtha made four trips beyond the palace walls. What he saw on those four trips changed him (and the world) forever and are referred to as "four great sights." It is reported that he saw an *old man*, a *sick man*, a *corpse*, and a *holy man* or *wandering ascetic*. The first three sights represented that all life is characterized by suffering and impermanence – namely, old age, sickness, and eventually death. However, the holy man represented peace and liberation from these sufferings through spiritual attainment.

It is reported that Siddhārtha was married at the age of 16 (a custom of that era) and had one son. At the age of 29, he left the palace forever, determined to master spiritual practices until he overcame the suffering of the world, and he became one of the many wandering ascetics. For 6 years, Siddhārtha mastered a variety of austere practices, described by John Snelling.

> So then Siddhārtha took himself off into the jungle near Uruvela and began to submit himself to the most grueling forms of asceticism. The rationale for this was that by mortifying the body, subjecting it to the most extreme forms of privation and suffering, suffering itself could be finally overcome. He spent long periods living alone and naked in eerie forests and in charnel grounds. He slept on beds of thorns. He burned in the heat of the midday sun and suffered cold at night. At the same time, he tried to burn and crush all thoughts from his mind, and experimented with holding his breath for long periods until there were violent pains in his head and he lapsed into unconsciousness. He also starved himself into a state of extreme emaciation.[152]

After nearly dying from starvation, Siddhārtha realized that asceticism was not the answer to overcoming suffering. Finally,

---

152 Snelling, J. (1991). *The Buddhist Handbook*. Rochester, VT: Inner Traditions International, 20–21.

at the age of 35, he went to present-day Bodh Gaya, India, where he vowed to meditate under a bodhi tree until he discovered the solution to suffering – or died trying. According to the teachings, Siddhārtha meditated one night from dusk to dawn. It was during his meditation that a protagonist by the name of Mara enters the story (some might compare Mara with the Christian concept of the devil, except from the Buddhist perspective Mara is not separate from one's own mind). Mara, known as the tempter, tried every conceivable means of tempting the hero to abandon his meditative state. Despite these temptations, Siddhārtha continued undaunted. Finally, at the end of his meditation, Siddhārtha attained complete enlightenment and became the Buddha – the awakened one. It is said that he remained in this state under the bodhi tree for a period of 49 days. Since that time, Bodh Gaya has been one of the four major holy sites frequented by Buddhists on pilgrimages.

Upon attaining complete enlightenment, the Buddha came to several realizations. First, he was able to "see" his previous lives and realized that this was his last and final rebirth. Second, he fully understood the workings of karma. Third, he formulated what was to become known as the "Four Noble Truths."

Shortly after his enlightenment, while walking down a road, the Buddha encountered a man who could tell this was no ordinary human being. The man asked, "Are you a God?" The Buddha replied, "No." The man then asked, "Are you then an angel?" Again the Buddha replied, "No." Finally the man asked, "Then what are you?" The Buddha replied, "I am awake." His name, Buddha, which means "awake," became his title.

For 45 years, the Buddha traveled throughout India teaching what he learned under the bodhi tree, while a monastic community arose around him. He continued teaching until the age of 80, when it is said he died from food poisoning near the town of Kushinagar, India. The Buddha's death is referred to as his *parinirvana*, which means death after nirvana by abandoning this earthly body. Since that time, Kushinagar has been another of the four major holy sites frequented by Buddhists on pilgrimages. Nearing his death, the Buddha gave his final teaching in the *Mahaparinibbana Sutta*: "All compound things decay; work out your own salvation with diligence."

The teachings of the Buddha are expansive. However, his teachings were not initially written down but, rather, were committed to memory and transmitted in an ongoing oral tradition for generations. In approximately 250 BCE, nearly 300 years after his death, the first of several councils was held to reach agreement upon the Buddha's teachings. This was the first time the teachings of the Buddha were committed to writing. These teachings today are called "sutras." Because the teachings were an oral tradition for so many centuries, all of the sutras begin with the words "Thus have I heard ..."

These written scriptures of the Buddha exist in four great collections: (1) the Pali Canon, also known as the "Tripitaka," preserved in the Theravadan tradition; (2) the Chinese Tripitaka; (3) the *Sarvastivadins* Tripitaka (preserved in Sanskrit); and (4) the Tibetan *Kanjur* and *Tanjur*. The teachings of the Buddha on medicine are recorded in the *Four Medical Tantras*. The illustrated Tibetan version is called the *Blue Beryl*. An important sutra recited in all Buddhist communities is the *Heart Sutra*. The *Heart Sutra* is commonly chanted at different rituals as well as before teachings. The *Heart Sutra* is part of the collection of the *Prajnaparamita Sutras*, which was the Buddha's second turning of the wheel of *dharma* (*dharma* refers to the Buddha's teachings), on the topic of *shunyata* or emptiness. Most of the other sutras are sources of reference rather than practice manuals.

Even though the teachings of the Buddha found in the scriptures share doctrines such as karma and rebirth with the Vedic (Hindu) tradition, the Buddha rejected both the caste system and the Vedic belief that the priests had to conduct rituals and intercede on behalf of the practitioners. For this reason, the Buddha taught that human beings were capable of attaining enlightenment through their own efforts, just as he had done. The following principles and teachings are the core of the Buddha's instruction for a life well lived resulting in the attainment of enlightenment.

The Middle Path

The primary guiding principle for all of the Buddha's teachings was something referred to as "the middle path." This is the path that avoids extremes, which is perfectly understandable when one reflects upon the life of the Buddha who was raised in a life of privilege with every imaginable luxury. After rejecting this hedonistic life, the Buddha then set out upon a life of renunciation as an ascetic. After years of austere practices, he found this was not the answer either. So after his enlightenment, he taught the middle path of avoiding extremes.

The Four Noble Truths[153]

The Four Noble Truths were the Buddha's first teaching immediately following his enlightenment and were given at Deer Park in Benares, India. These teachings are referred to as the "first turning of the wheel of *dharma*."

1. **The First Noble Truth: The Truth of Dissatisfaction and Suffering**: The First Noble Truth describes the nature of life and one's personal experience of this impermanent, ever-changing world. All beings desire happiness, safety, peace, and comfort. They desire what is satisfying, pleasurable, joyful, and permanent. However, the very nature of existence is impermanent, always changing, and therefore incapable of fully satisfying their desire. Inevitably, people experience frustration, anger, loss, unhappiness, and dissatisfaction. Life is in constant change, and changes such as birth, old age, sickness, and death can bring dissatisfaction or suffering. Suffering may arise from being associated with people or conditions that are unpleasant, from being separated from people loved or conditions enjoyed, from not getting what is desired, or from getting what is desired then losing it. Even people's own thoughts and feelings are impermanent, constantly changing. Inevitably, all physical, emotional, and mental conditions will change. *Insight into the First Noble Truth: To overcome dissatisfaction and suffering, it is essential that we understand and accept the*

---

153 Cohen, N. Text printed on laminated cards. Reprinted with permission from Mr. Cohen. The text can also be found on the following website: http://naljorprisondharmaservice.org/pdf/FourNobleTruths.htm (accessed 15 Sept 2012).

ever-changing, impermanent nature of life; we acknowledge the presence of dissatisfaction and suffering; we understand the very nature of suffering; and we embrace suffering compassionately, without fear or avoidance.

2. **The Second Noble Truth: The Cause of Dissatisfaction and Suffering**: The Second Noble Truth refers to the arising, origin, and cause of our dissatisfaction and suffering. People desire, crave, and thirst for happiness, security, and identity in this world of impermanence. Influenced by this misperception (ignorance/delusion), individuals want life to satisfy their every craving, need, and desire. They want from life what it can never provide: constant happiness, pleasure, and security undisturbed by change or loss. When life fails to satisfy needs and desires, people experience fear, frustration, hurt, anger, pain, or suffering. Afflicted by such thoughts and emotions, they tend to speak and act in negative ways, which causes further suffering. Therefore, dissatisfaction and suffering do not come from outside of self. People cause their own suffering when they fail to realize that the impermanent nature of life is incapable of providing constant satisfaction for craving, need, and desire. The origin and cause of dissatisfaction and suffering is this misperception of reality (ignorance/delusion), self-centered desire (greed), craving, grasping, attachment to things that do not last, and negative behavior. *Insight into the Second Noble Truth: To overcome dissatisfaction and suffering, it is essential that we clearly identify the causes of this experience; we deeply feel and fully understand these causes; finally, we choose to abandon,*

remove and stop creating the causes of our suffering.

3. **The Third Noble Truth: The End of Dissatisfaction and Suffering**: The Third Noble Truth relates there is an end to dissatisfaction and suffering when people let go of, abandon, and liberate themselves from the delusion, craving and attachment that causes it. Because pain, confusion and suffering have a cause and a beginning, they also have an end. Once people understand the nature of illness, it can be cured with the right remedies. In this same way, once individuals see and understand what causes their suffering, they can bring an end to it by eliminating those causes and realizing well-being. Liberation from suffering, awakening, lasting happiness, supreme peace and perfect wisdom are possible. These qualities are the very essence and nature of one's being. They are always available within, awaiting realization. *Insight into the Third Noble Truth: When our delusion, greed, craving, attachment and negative behavior have been extinguished, what remains in this absence of suffering is the experience of Nirvana: the awakened quality of our true nature. It is essential, however, that this supreme peace and wisdom of our true nature be realized and made fully conscious by way of direct experience. For one liberated in this way in whose heart dwells peace, there is nothing to be added to what has been accomplished. This is the end of dissatisfaction and suffering – the realization of our true nature, Ultimate Reality, Nirvana.*

4. **The Fourth Noble Truth: The Path Leading to the End of Dissatisfaction and Suffering**: The Fourth Noble Truth is the Way, the Path leading to the end of

dissatisfaction and suffering. By following and practicing the Noble Eightfold Path – Right Understanding, Right Thought, Right Speech, Right Action, Right Livelihood, Right Effort, Right Mindfulness and Right Concentration – people will overcome dissatisfaction and suffering. Following this Path, also known as the Noble Middle Path, humans avoid the extremes of searching for happiness through a life of indulgence in desire and sensual pleasure, or the opposite extreme of trying to gain happiness or liberation by tormenting their bodies and minds through unreasonable, unprofitable, and painful forms of spiritual austerity (self-mortification). The Noble Eightfold Path is the Way to the end of suffering: the Middle Way that leads to peace, discernment, lasting happiness, perfect wisdom, enlightenment and Nirvana. *Insight into the Fourth Noble Truth: No matter how profound our conceptual knowledge of the Path may be, this will not be sufficient for true accomplishment. It is essential that we follow, cultivate and practice the Path with diligence, sincerity and full confidence.*

The Noble Eightfold Path

John Snelling states:

The fourth noble truth defines this path to liberation by telling us what practical steps we have to take in order to root our *trishna* (desire) and thereby create the fertile ground in which nirvana may arise. These steps are laid out in the teaching of the Noble Eightfold Path.[154]

1. Right Understanding
2. Right Thought
3. Right Speech
4. Right Action
5. Right Livelihood
6. Right Effort
7. Right Mindfulness
8. Right Concentration

Explanation of the Noble Eightfold Path[155]

1. **Right Understanding** (or Right View) is the ability to understand the nature of things exactly as they are, without delusion or distortion. If people hold wrong views, misunderstanding the nature of reality, then their thoughts, speech, actions, and plans come forth from this misunderstanding, bringing unhappiness and suffering, If people cultivate the Right View of reality, their thoughts, speech, actions, and plans come forth from this Right Understanding, bringing happiness and freedom from suffering. Imposing self-centered desires, needs, expectations, or fears onto life – being satisfied and happy when things go our way, and upset if they do not – are wrong ways of understanding. With Right Understanding, people correctly perceive the interdependent, impermanent, ever-changing nature of life. They realize lasting happiness and satisfaction do not come from anything external. In addition, they understand the wholesome, life-affirming actions that bring benefit to all beings, as well as the unwholesome, negative actions that bring suffering. Right Understanding requires full comprehension of the Four Noble Truths, which explain the nature of reality.

154 Snelling, J. (1991). *The Buddhist Handbook.* Rochester, VT: Inner Traditions International, 46.

155 Cohen. Reprinted with permission.

Through Right Understanding, people cultivate wisdom, an essential aspect of the Path.

2. **Right Thought** (or Right Intention) means people's thoughts, feelings, desires, and intentions are in complete harmony with the wisdom of life, in accordance with the way reality works. With Right Thought, thoughts and intentions are completely free from selfish desire, hostility, and cruelty. Right Thought means thinking, attitude, and motivation are rightly aligned with love, kindness, compassion, wisdom, and harmlessness, and these noble qualities are extended to all living beings. Right Thought is directly related to Right Speech and Right Action; the way people think always influences their speech and actions. Therefore, misunderstanding of reality causes wrong thinking, which gives rise to non-virtuous speech and actions which cause harm. Right Thought gives rise to virtuous speech and actions which bring happiness and benefit. When thought, desire, intention, and motivation are in harmony with Reality, the Way, the *Dharma*, this is Right Thought. Through Right Thought people cultivate wisdom, an essential aspect of the Path.

3. **Right Speech** is the ability to speak truthfully and harmlessly. Right Speech comes naturally from Right Thought, since speech is a direct expression of thoughts. Speech should never be cruel or hurtful to others. Words should not create hatred, misunderstanding, or suffering. Right Speech means people do not lie, slander, or speak in ways that create resentment, conflict, division, or disharmony among individuals or groups. Right Speech means not speaking in ways that are harsh, rude, impolite, abusive, or malicious. People refrain from idle, useless, and foolish talk or gossip. In this way, they cultivate the ability to speak the truth; they learn to use words that are friendly, gentle, benevolent, and meaningful. Right Speech means speaking kindly and wisely at the right time and place. When individuals are not able to speak in ways that are useful, kind, or uplifting, they may consider the wisdom of remaining in noble silence. Through Right Speech people cultivate ethical conduct (personal integrity), the essential foundation of the Path.

4. **Right Action** means that behavior is ethical, honorable, and responsible. Right Action comes naturally from Right Thought, since actions are a direct expression of thoughts. Being in accord with Right Action, people are always compassionate, generous, nonviolent and peaceful. They abstain from unwholesome behavior such as destroying life, taking what is not given (stealing), sexual misconduct, and dealing with others in hurtful or dishonest ways. They live a life of honesty, being always conscientious with a heart full of sympathy, desiring the welfare of all living beings. To the best of their ability, they support others in leading a peaceful, nonviolent, and honorable life as well. Through Right Action people cultivate ethical conduct (personal integrity), the essential foundation of the Path.

5. **Right Livelihood** suggests that people earn a living in an honorable and life-affirming way, free from deceit or dishonesty. They do not earn a livelihood in any way that involves harm,

cruelty, or injustice to either human beings or animals, nor do they support those who harm other beings. For example, Right Livelihood means not selling or trading in arms and lethal weapons, not selling intoxicating drinks or poisons, not killing or mistreating animals, not cheating or deceiving others, and so forth. The *dharma* of a human being is to support and assist life, embracing interconnection with all sentient beings. Being in accord with Right Livelihood means living in harmony and unity with all of life, living not just to satisfy one's own personal desires, but to compassionately serve the welfare of all beings. Through Right Livelihood people cultivate ethical conduct (personal integrity), the essential foundation of the Path.

6. **Right Effort** is the wholehearted, diligent, and energetic endeavor to train the mind and heart. People are to restrain negative feelings, thoughts and other unwholesome states of mind from arising. They are to abandon those negative feelings, thoughts, and unwholesome states of mind that have already arisen in awareness. In addition, they are to develop and maintain positive, loving, virtuous, and wholesome states of mind and heart. Right Effort means to avoid being carried away by distractions, to develop steady perseverance, making a firm, unshakable resolve to practice the *dharma*. People endeavor to express love, compassion, wisdom, and virtue in thoughts, speech, and actions. If they truly want to awaken and attain liberation from suffering, they must practice with determination. They must train the mind and heart by diligently applying the necessary effort. Through Right Effort, they cultivate mental discipline and concentration, an essential aspect of the Path.

7. **Right Mindfulness** (or Right Attention) means being attentive, mindful, and aware of bodily actions, sensations, and feelings, and the activity of the mind. Right Mindfulness means giving full attention to that which is positive, life affirming and beneficial to other beings. People are also to be mindful of that which is negative, harmful or destructive. In addition, they are to cultivate those states of mind conducive to spiritual progress. In accord with Right Mindfulness, awareness is where it should be, completely attentive to what is happening within and around in the present moment. People see things as they are, without distortion. When attention is scattered, deluded, or placed on too many things at once, thoughts, speech, or actions may become careless, which causes harm to self or others. In these situations, people can practice Right Mindfulness by embracing the painful consequences of their actions with full awareness. As individuals practice Right Mindfulness, they are steady, open, aware, present, insightful, and serene in attitude; they think, speak, and act with loving-kindness, compassion, and wisdom. Through Right Mindfulness, people cultivate mental discipline and concentration, an essential aspect of the Path.

8. **Right Concentration** is the means for training and centering the mind. Through Right Concentration, people bring their ordinarily restless, un-concentrated minds into states of tranquility and unbroken attentiveness. By training the mind through Right

Concentration, individuals extinguish the delusion, self-centered desire, and destructive thinking that rule the scattered, untrained mind. In this way, they develop serenity and mental and emotional stability to gain insight into the true nature of reality. Right Concentration leads one through the various stages of *dhyana* (meditation) into equanimity, joy, purity of mind, and attainment of the highest wisdom. Right Concentration is a fully engaged means of training the mind and heart to be completely present in each moment, without cutting oneself off from others or escaping the responsibilities of life. Through Right Concentration, people cultivate mental discipline and concentration, an essential aspect of the Path.

The Five Precepts

For ordinary people involved in worldly life, the way to implement right speech and right action is to practice the five precepts.

1. **To Abstain from Killing Any Living Creature**: Honoring and respecting all sentient beings, not acting out of hatred or aversion in such a way as to cause harm to any living being.
2. **To Abstain from Stealing**: Not taking what is not freely given, respect the rights and property of all beings in the global economy.
3. **To Abstain from False Speech**: Refrain from false speech, say only what is true and useful; speak wisely, responsibly, and appropriately. Be mindful of speech, for it can both enlighten and destroy.
4. **To Abstain from Sexual Misconduct**: Be conscious of sexual energy. It is very powerful and can be destructive. Use the energy to express compassion, love, and genuine intimacy.
5. **To Abstain from Intoxicants**: Refrain from the needless use of intoxicants. They cloud the mind and cause more pain than they cure.

These five precepts are the essential minimum needed for moral conduct. They must be followed by anyone who wishes to practice the *dharma*. On a fundamental level, these precepts are intended to avoid harming (*ahimsa*) others. Monastics (monks and nuns) not only commit themselves to these five precepts but also to 250 additional vows. Although Buddhism doesn't have anything exactly like the Jewish/Christian Ten Commandments, there is a moral basis that is considered essential to the practice of Buddhism. In fact, there is a saying in the teachings that trying to practice Buddhism without a moral basis is like trying to row a boat still tied to the dock: no matter how strenuous your efforts, you won't get anywhere.

In addition to instructional material in the writings of the Buddha, one finds prayers as well. However, since the Buddha is not considered a god, prayers are directed to the Buddha within each of us. Prayer can be conducted anywhere and everywhere and may be accompanied by the use of prayer beads or *mudras* (ritual hand gestures). Common prayers include: (1) Refuge Vow; (2) The Four Immeasurables; (3) The Seven-Limbed Prayer; (4) Offering Prayer (e.g., Mandala Offering, symbolically offering the entire universe); (5) Dedication Prayers; (6) Long Life Prayers; (7) Prayers to Honor Great Teachers; (8) Prayers to Individual Manifestations of the Buddha – or other mantras. Other prayers are recited for confession, purification, and rejoicing in or transferring merit.

As with other faith traditions of the world, spiritual leaders are important in Buddhism. However, there is no central authority figure for all of Buddhism who sets policy or ritual. The heads of the various temples and groups in specific geographic areas are the local spiritual leaders. Similarly, the heads of various schools or lineages are the leaders for larger areas (generally countries). However, even His Holiness the Dalai Lama (who is the spiritual and temporal head of Buddhism from Tibet) cannot be said to be the leader of all Tibetan Buddhism, because Bhutan's state religion is Tibetan Buddhism, but it has its own head lama.

Finally, even though Buddhism was a child of India (and the Buddha himself a child of the Vedic tradition) and it continued to flourish there until the twelfth century, the destruction of Nalanda (the most famous Buddhist University) by invaders was the event that began the decline of Buddhism in India. This decline continued for almost a century, until Buddhism was no longer viable in that country because it lacked a monastic infrastructure. However, Buddhism was not confined to its birth country, even when experiencing growth and acceptance. Between the first and tenth centuries CE, Buddhism spread along the silk route to China, where different schools of Buddhism emerged. The main schools of Mahāyāna, Theravada, and Vajrayana will be discussed in the following three chapters.

Special Days: Buddhism

There are many special or holy days held throughout the year by the Buddhist community. Many of these days celebrate the birthdays of *bodhisattvas* in the Mahāyāna tradition or other significant dates in the Buddhist calendar. The most significant celebration happens every May on the night of the first full moon, when Buddhists all over the world celebrate the birth, enlightenment, and death of the Buddha over 2500 years ago. It has come to be known as *Vesak* or Buddha Day.

Buddhist festivals are always joyful occasions. Typically, on a festival day, laypeople will go the local temple or monastery and offer food to the monks and take the Five Precepts and listen to a *dharma* talk. In the afternoon, they distribute food to the poor to make merit, and in the evening perhaps join in a ceremony of circumambulation of a *stupa* three times as a sign of respect to the Buddha, the *Dharma*, and the *Sangha*. The day will conclude with evening chanting of the Buddha's teachings and meditation.

There are two aspects to take into consideration regarding Buddhist festivals: (1) most Buddhists, with the exception of the Japanese, use the lunar calendar and (2) the dates of Buddhist festivals vary from country to country and between Buddhist traditions.

January 1 *Temple Day* – The first of January has become a special day for North American Buddhists of all schools to attend a special service in the local temple.

January 22 *Mahāyāna New Year (3 days)* – The Mahāyāna Buddhist New Year is a time of celebration and hope for the upcoming year. The event allows participants to reflect on their past and rectify the mistakes they have made. Zen, a popular form of Buddhism in the United States, is from the Mahāyāna School of Buddhism.

January/February/March/April *Chinese/Vietnamese/Korean/Tibetan New Year* – In Theravadin countries, Thailand, Burma, Sri Lanka, Cambodia, and Laos, the new year is celebrated for 3 days from the first full moon day in April. In Mahāyāna countries the new year starts on the first full moon day in January. However, the Buddhist new year depends on the country of origin or ethnic background of the people – for example, Chinese, Koreans, and Vietnamese celebrate late January or early February according to the lunar calendar, while the Tibetans usually celebrate about 1 month later. The new year begins a 15-day festival for people in these countries of all religions. Family reunions with thanksgiving and remembrance of deceased relatives take place. Traditionally, a religious ceremony honors heaven and earth.

February 15 *Nirvana Day (Mahāyāna tradition) (Theravada commemorates this event on the Vesak or Visakha Puja Day)* – Nirvana Day, also known as *Parinirvana*, is the celebration of Buddha's death when he reached total nirvana, at the age of 80. On Nirvana Day, Buddhists think about their lives and how they can work toward gaining the perfect peace of nirvana, believed to be the end of rebirth and the ultimate aim of Buddhism. Buddhists celebrate nirvana by meditating or by going to Buddhist temples or monasteries. Celebrations vary throughout the world. In monasteries, Nirvana Day is treated as a social occasion. Food is prepared and some people bring presents such as money, household goods or clothes. Some Buddhists will read passages from the *Paranibbana Sutta*, which describes the last days of Buddha, while others may reflect on those who have recently passed away.

February/March *Magha Puja (full moon of the third lunar month, so the date varies according to the lunar calendar)* – The presentation by the Buddha, 8 months after his enlightenment, at the Assembly of all existed arahants or enlightened disciples at the time, who gathered to pay their respects to the Buddha, is commemorated on this day. *Magha Puja* is an important religious festival celebrated by Thai

Buddhists on the full moon day of the third lunar month (this usually falls in February). It is a public holiday in Thailand and is an occasion when Buddhists tend to go to the temple to perform merit-making activities. *Magha Puja* day marks the four auspicious occasions, which happened nine months after the Enlightenment of the Lord Buddha at Veluvana Bamboo Grove, near Rajagaha in Northern India. On that occasion, four miraculous events coincided: (1) 1250 enlightened disciples of the Buddha spontaneously gathered, (2) every one of those enlightened disciples had been given monastic ordination personally by the Lord Buddha, (3) those disciples knew by themselves and went unannounced to meet together without any previous appointment, and (4) it was the full-moon day. The Lord Buddha gave an important teaching to the assembled monks on that day 2597 years ago (587 BCE) called the *Ovadapatimokkha*, which laid down the principles by which the monks should spread the Buddhist teachings. In Theravada tradition, this teaching has been dubbed the "Heart or Core of Buddhism"; namely, (1) avoid doing bad deeds, (2) do good deeds, and (3) purify one's mind. Therefore, Magha Puja Day is considered to be the "**Dharma Day.**"

April 8 *Hana Matsuri* – Some Buddhists, mostly from Japan, celebrate *Hana Matsuri*, the birth of Buddha on April 8. Buddhist shrines and temples around Japan fill with joyful celebrants. Processions can be seen in many places, with children dressed up in their best kimonos, chanting their way to the temple alongside decorative floats. *Hana* means flower; Buddha's birthday is a flower festival. His actual birthday is in May.

April 13–13 *Songkran* – In Thailand and many Southeast Asia countries (e.g., Laos, Cambodia), Buddhists celebrate their New Year in mid-April. Water is an important element of the festival. Statues of the Buddha are bathed in water, and people throw water at each other until everyone is soaking wet. There are boat races, parades, plays, concerts, and fireworks. People add gold leaves to a Buddha statue as an offering.

May *Visakha Puja/Vesak (full moon of the sixth lunar month, so the date varies according to the lunar calendar)* – As the moon turns full on the sixth lunar month, Buddhists worldwide enjoy the arrival of *Vesak* Day. *Vesak* Day represents a simultaneous celebration of the birth, enlightenment, and death (*parinirvana*) of the Lord Buddha. In the Theravada tradition, the three occurrences fall on the same full moon day of the sixth lunar month. The day the Buddha passed away, *parinirvana*, marks the beginning of the Buddhist Era (543 BCE), which is still being observed as the official calendar in Thailand (i.e., the year 2010 CE is 2553 BE in the Thai calendar). On December 13, 1999, the United Nations General Assembly adopted unanimously to declare *Vesak* Day as a world celebration day of the Buddha's Birth, Enlightenment, and His Passing away.

July 6 *Dalai Lama Birthday* – Observation with traditional dances, picnics, and singing. Each dalai lama is seen as the reincarnation of the predecessor and a manifestation of Avalokitesvara – the *bodhisattva* of compassion.

July 7 *Asalha Puja Day (full moon of the eighth lunar month, so the date varies according to the lunar calendar)* – Asalha Puja (known as *Asanha Puja* in Thailand) is a Theravada Buddhist festival that typically takes place in July, on the full moon of the eighth lunar month. It commemorates the Buddha's first sermon, *Dharmachakrakappawattana Sutra*, at the Deer Park, Sarnath, near Benares. The Buddha taught the Middle Path and the Four Noble Truths, to the first five disciples, one of whom became a noble disciple through attaining the "Eye of the Wisdom," therefore the founding of the Buddhist *sangha* was established. Asalha Puja Day is also considered to be the "**Sangha Day**." In Thailand, *Asalha Puja* is an official holiday. The day is observed by making offerings to temples and listening to sermons.

July 13 *Ullambana* – *Ullambana*, popularly known as the Festival of the Hungry Ghosts, is celebrated by Buddhists and Taoists in China, Korea, Japan, Singapore, and other countries. Following the Chinese Mahā yāna tradition, it falls on the fifteenth day of the seventh month of the lunar calendar. The festival evolved from a Mahāyāna sutra called *Ullambana Sutra*, supposed to have been delivered by the Buddha with reference to the suffering mother of the second chief disciple, Maha Moggallana (Mu Lian). *Ullambana* is a Sanskrit term that means "hanging upside down." Hence, it is commented that she was in purgatory undergoing the torment of being hung upside down. The Pali equivalent of the term is *Ullampana*, which means "merciful disposition." Thus, it also depicts the sympathetic attitude to be cultivated toward the departed ones.

July 18 *Dharma Day (same as the Asalha Puja Day)* – *Dharma Day* marks the beginning of the Buddha's teaching. The word *dharma* can be translated as truth and is the term used for the path to enlightenment, or the Buddhist teaching. Soon after his Enlightenment, the Buddha went to find his former disciples and share his experience with them. This event could be seen as the start of the Buddhist religion, and is what *Dharma* Day celebrates. The first teaching to the Buddha's original five disciples is known as "The First Turning of the Wheel of the *Dharma* (*Dharmachakra*)." In early Buddhism, the time around what has now become *Dharma* Day (the eighth lunar month in the traditional Indian calendar) marked the beginning of the rainy season. At this point, the Buddha and his monks and nuns would suspend their nomadic lifestyle for 3 months. They would shelter together until the monsoon season was over, using this time as a period of further meditation and reflection. At the end of this time, they would resume their traveling, passing on the Buddha's teachings to those who were interested. *Dharma* Day is now seen as a chance to express gratitude that the Buddha, and other enlightened teachers, have shared their knowledge with others. *Dharma* Day is usually celebrated with readings from the Buddhist scriptures, and is an opportunity to reflect deeply on their content.

October/November *Kathina (date varies according the lunar calendar; has to be within 1 month after the ending of rainy season retreat)* – *Kathina* is a Buddhist festival that comes at the end of *Vassa*, the 3-month rainy season retreat for Theravada Buddhists. The season during which a monastery may hold a *Kathina* festival is 1-month long, beginning after the full moon of the eleventh month in the lunar calendar (usually October or November). In order to hold a *Kathina*, a monastery must have had five monks in residence during the retreat period and only those who were present for the entire retreat are eligible to receive the robe cloth offered. It is a time of giving, for the laity to express gratitude to monks. Lay Buddhists bring donations to temples, especially new robes for the monks.

December 8 *Bodhi Day (Mahāyāna tradition) (Theravada commemorates this event on the Vesak or Visakha Puja Day)* – Bodhi Day, traditionally December 8, is the Buddhist holiday that commemorates the day that the historical Buddha, Shakyamuni or Siddhārtha Gautama, experienced enlightenment. According to tradition, Siddhārtha had recently forsaken years of extreme ascetic practices and decided to sit under a bodhi tree and simply meditate until he found the root of suffering, and how to liberate one's self from it. Traditions vary on what happened. Some say he made a great vow to Heaven and Earth to find the root of suffering, or die trying. In other traditions, while meditating he was harassed and tempted by the Hindu god Mara, Lord of Illusion. Other traditions simply state that he entered deeper and deeper states of meditation, confronting the nature of the self. Like many Buddhist holidays, traditions and observances surrounding Bodhi Day vary depending on the culture in question. However, Bodhi Day is widely seen as a reminder to Buddhists that, with the right effort and understanding, any person can become enlightened.

Date varies *Vassa (date varies; the full moons of the eighth lunar month, usually July through October)* – This day marks the beginning of the 3-month "Rains Retreat" (between the full moons of the eighth and eleventh lunar months) for monks and nuns as a time of annual retreat in Theravada Buddhism. The term originates from the time of the Buddha preventing *bhikkus* (Buddhist monks) from traveling during the rainy season of India and Southeast Asia. It is a 3-month period during which monks stay in the monastery to concentrate on the teachings of the Buddha. Male novices will also be received at this time to undertake an initial period of study.

Date varies *Pavarana (date varies; the full moons of the eleventh lunar month, usually in October)* – Pavarana is a Buddhist holy day celebrated on the full moon of the eleventh lunar month. It marks the end of the month of Vassa, sometimes called "Buddhist Lent." This day marks the end of the rainy season in some Asian countries such as Thailand, where Theravada Buddhism is practiced. On this day, each monk must come before the community of monks (*sangha*) and atone for an offense he may have committed during the *Vassa*. Most Mahāyāna Buddhists do not observe *Vassa*.

Glossary of Buddhist Terms

ahimsa: Avoidance of harm to others; nonviolence.

anatta: Concept of not self, soulless, selfless.

anicca: Concept of impermanence, a central theme in Buddhism.

arahant: Spiritual practitioner who realized the culmination of the spiritual life. Such a person, having removed all causes for future becoming, is not reborn after biological death. A fully enlightened being.

bardo: Junctures in life when the possibility of liberation or enlightenment is much greater. Common usage of the term has been as the transition between birth and death, but this is not completely accurate. There is not one but four bardos: (1) the natural bardo of this life, (2) the painful bardo of dying, (3) the luminous bardo of *dharmata* (the after-death bardo state, where the real light, or intrinsic radiance appears), and (4) the karmic bardo of becoming, commonly referred to as rebirth.

bodhicitta: Meaning "enlightened heart," this is the desire to alleviate the suffering of all beings without distinction.

bodhisattva: One who postpones the attainment of nirvana in order to work for the benefit of others.

dharma: Refers to the teachings and doctrines of the Buddha. It also refers to the truth or reality, as well as the path of practice that leads to realization of the ultimate truth.

dharmata: The after-death bardo state, where the real light or intrinsic radiance appears.

Dhyana (**Sanskrit**), *Chan* (**Chinese**), **or** *Zen* (**Japanese**): Type or aspect of meditation that ultimately leads to liberation from the cycle of birth, death, and rebirth.

ditthi: Concepts; rigidly held beliefs. It usually implies having one's own underlying personal bias associated with such concepts or beliefs.

dukkha: Suffering, dis-ease, dissatisfaction, and the focus and the first of the Four Noble Truths.

karma: A philosophical explanation of karma can differ slightly between traditions, but the general concept is basically the same. It is usually understood as a sum of all that an individual has done, is currently doing and will do. Karma is not about retribution, vengeance, punishment, or reward; karma simply deals with what is. The effects of all deeds actively create past, present, and future experiences, thus making one responsible for one's own life, and the pain and joy it brings to them and others. In religions that incorporate reincarnation, karma extends through one's present life and all past and future lives as well. Classically, the Buddha stated that "**Volition** (*intention, motivation*), O monks, I declare **is** *Karma*. Having willed (intention), man acts by deed, word, or thought." Karma simply means action. What people frequently refer to as karma is in fact **karma-vipaka**, or the consequence of past action.

karuna: Commonly summed up as wisdom tempered with compassion; more commonly, especially in Mahāyāna Buddhism, *karuna* is one of the two qualities, along with wisdom, to be cultivated on the *bodhisattva* path. *Karuna or compassion is one of the three virtues of the Buddha, besides Purity and Wisdom. It is one of the Four Holy Abidings – namely, Metta-Loving-kindness, Karuna-Compassion, Mudita-Sympathetic joy or altruistic joy, and Upekkha-Equanimity.*

koan: A story, dialogue, question, or statement in the history and lore of Zen Buddhism. Generally contains aspects that are inaccessible to rational understanding yet may be accessible to intuition. Its goal is to break away from the biased conceptual thought or duality to experience the unbiased ultimate reality or nonduality.

lama: Title for a Tibetan teacher of *dharma*; the name is similar to the Sanskrit term guru.

lojong: Often translated into English as Mind Training, this is a practice in the Tibetan Buddhist tradition based on a set of proverbs formulated in Tibet in the twelfth century by Chekawa. Practitioners undertake to connect with the world in an unconditionally positive way, and also to take full responsibility for their experience of it. The practice involves redefining, reconceptualizing, and reprogramming one's intent and way of thinking – hence, "Mind Training."

Lotus Sutra: Believed by many Buddhist adherents as the sutra that contains the quintessence of the teaching of Shakyamuni Buddha above all other scriptures.

magga: Treatment or antidote; the method for alleviating suffering is living the *Middle Path/Way* (avoiding the two extremes of sensual indulgence and self-mortification), which is attained by following the Noble Eightfold Path – the fourth Noble Truth.

Mara: Known as the tempter; some might compare Mara with the Christian concept of the devil, except from the Buddhist perspective Mara is not separate from one's own mind.

mudras: Symbolic or ritual gesture; while some *mudras* involve the entire body, most are performed with the hands and fingers.

Nam-myoho-renge-kyo: Prayer that translates as "I devote myself to the Mystic Law of cause and effect contained the Buddha's teaching" (used in Nichiren Buddhism).

Namu Amida Butsu: Prayer that translates as "I worship Amida Buddha and follow his doctrine" and is used in many Buddhist sects.

nirodha: Cure; the cessation of suffering is the achievement of nirvana, which is ultimate peace – the third Noble Truth.

nirvana: Cessation of participation in the cycle of birth, death, and rebirth; the release from bondage to karma.

Pali Canon: The standard scripture collection of the Theravada Buddhist tradition, as preserved in the Pali language; also known as the Tipitaka or Tripitaka.

paramitas: The perfection or culmination of certain virtues that are cultivated as a way of purification, purifying (karma), and helping the aspirant to live an unobstructed life, while reaching the goal of enlightenment.

parinirvana: Death after nirvana by abandoning this earthly body. The final or complete nirvana. It means the death of an arahant or fully enlightened being. The Great Decease of the Buddha.

phowa: Tibetan term for a Buddhist meditation practice that may be translated as the "practice of conscious dying," "transference of consciousness at the time of death," or "mindstream transference."

prajna (**Sanskrit**) or *panna* (**Pali**): Refers to the wisdom that is based on the direct realization of the Four Noble Truths, impermanence, dependent origination, not-self, emptiness, and so forth. It is the wisdom that is able to extinguish afflictions and bring about enlightenment.

rebirth: Preferential term in Buddhism instead of reincarnation; since reincarnation seems to imply the existence of a soul (*atman*), Buddhists, who believe in the concept of not self, soulless, or selfless (*anatman*), prefer the term rebirth, as having no true permanent "self" to be reborn. As long as one is still clinging to the sense of "self," rebirth will continue to roll on, fueled by one's own karma or past action and *tanha* or craving.

Rinpoche: Tibetan Buddhist religious or theological honorific title. Rinpoche literally means "precious one."

sadhana: Term for "a means of accomplishing something" or more specifically "spiritual practice." It includes a variety of disciplines that are followed in order to achieve various spiritual or ritual objectives.

Samma-Ditthi: Right View or Right Understanding, without any personal bias, on the Four Noble Truths and Dependent Origination/Arising.

samsara: Term for cycle of birth, death, and rebirth.

samudaya: Cause; the cause of suffering is *craving* with sensual desire, liking and disliking, in the unwholesome concepts of greed, hatred, and delusion – the Second Noble Truth.

sangha: term designating the Buddhist community or order of righteous followers treading the path toward enlightenment.

shunyata: Emptiness or voidness of inherent existence; all things and events, whether material, mental, or even abstract concepts like time, are devoid of objective, independent existence.

Sinhala: Sanskrit word for the island of Sri Lanka.

skandhas (**Sanskrit**) or *kandhas* (**Pali**): Five aggregates that categorize all individual experience – form, feeling, perception, conception or volition, and consciousness.

stupa: Religious monument that can vary in

size from a few feet to several stories in height. A relic mound, or a monument erected over the ashes of a holy person.

sutra: A scriptural narrative, especially a text traditionally regarded as a discourse of the Buddha; because the teachings were an oral tradition for so many centuries, the majority of the sutras begin with the words "Thus have I heard ...," signifying that it was originally recited by *Ananda*, the Buddha's personal attendant (as he requested the Buddha to recite whatever he taught others on each day to him). It may also imply that such sutras were not written at the later dates.

tanha: Thirst, craving for things (identified in the Second Noble Truth – the cause of suffering) that leads to suffering.

tantra: Means "continuum" or "weft" and is an entire system of spiritual practices, including meditation, used to transform the gross aspects of mind into the enlightened qualities of the Buddha's mind used for the benefit of others.

tonglen: Tibetan word for "taking and giving," it refers to a meditation practice found in Tibetan Buddhism. In the practice, one visualizes taking onto oneself the suffering of others, and giving one's own happiness and success to others. As such, it is a training in altruism in its most extreme form. The function of the practice is to reduce selfish attachment, increase a sense of renunciation, create positive karma by giving and helping, and develop loving-kindness.

Tripitaka/Tipitaka: *See* Pali Canon.

trishna **(Sanskrit) or** *tanha* **(Pali)**: Desire, craving, or wanting that leads to suffering.

tsa tsas: Molded images made of clay or plaster.

vinaya: Discipline, the regulatory framework for the Buddhist monastic community.

Mahāyāna Buddhism

*At all times I think to myself: How can I cause living beings to gain entry
into the unsurpassed way and quickly acquire the body of a Buddha?*[156]

Prepared by:
Guy McCloskey
National Advisor, Soka Gakkai International – USA
Chicago, IL

Reviewed and approved by:
Clark Strand
Contributing Editor, *Tricycle: The Buddhist Review*
Woodstock, NY

History and Facts

The Mahāyāna (Great Vehicle) stream of
Buddhism developed around the start of the
Christian era. It taught that the *bodhisattva path* of wisdom and compassionate
action for the sake of all living beings led
to Buddhahood itself, rather than the lower
state of Arhat that only gains enlightenment
for the individual practitioner. This "lower
state," sought by the original schools, was
referred to negatively by the Mahayanists
as the Hinayana, or Lesser Vehicle. The latter focused on individual liberation while
the former aimed at the enlightenment and
release from suffering of all sentient beings.
The two most prominent *bodhisattva* virtues are wisdom and compassion.

Northern Mahāyāna moved from India
to Tibet, Mongolia, Nepal, Bhutan, and
parts of China where Tantric practices dominated. Moving along the Silk Road (the
overland trade route that connected India to
Central Asia and China), Eastern Mahāyāna
was established in China, from where it
expanded to Korea, Japan, and Vietnam,

acquiring cultural accretions along the way.
With the exception of Tibetan forms, the
three most prominent schools of Mahāyāna
Buddhism found in the United States today
are as follows.

1. **Zen** (Chinese, *Chan*, Meditation)
   traces its origins to the Indian monk
   Bodhidharma during the early sixth
   century CE and is probably the most
   widely known among the Buddhist
   schools in the West. Its practice includes
   sitting with one's back straight, mindful
   of one's breathing, silencing the mind,
   with focused awareness in the here and
   now. Numerous Zen centers now exist
   in the United States, where their practice remains nondoctrinal and strictly
   meditative. Some Christians and Jews
   find the Zen experience of mindfulness
   and attentiveness compatible with their
   existing faith traditions.

2. **Pure Land** stresses an abiding faith
   in the Buddha or Other Power, and
   its core practice is the devotional
   repetition of the name of Amitabha
   (Japanese, *Amida*) Buddha in order to
   gain rebirth in the Pure Land. There is
   a paradox, since various forms of Pure

---

156 Watson, B. trans. (1993). *The Lotus Sutra.* New
York, NY: Oxford University Press, 232.

Land teaching emphasize the *bodhisattva path* to benefit all sentient beings, while at the same time stressing liberation through the salvational power of Amitabha. It is especially popular in China, where it developed in the fifth century CE, and in Japan. Pure Land teachings were intermingled with *Chan* and *T'ien-t'ai* in China and only became a distinct school under Honen (1133–1212) and his successors in Japan. Its practitioners in the United States are generally ethnic Chinese, Vietnamese, and Japanese.

3. *Nichiren* **Buddhism** is based on the *Lotus Sutra*, the quintessential Mahāyāna teaching of universal salvation through awakening to one's "Buddha nature." This form of Buddhism is based on the interpretation of the thirteenth-century Japanese monk Nichiren (1222–1282 CE). It survived primarily as a priestly tradition until the appearance of the Soka Gakkai International (SGI), which originated as a lay movement in Japan in 1930 through the efforts of a group of educators. It is today the most diverse group of Buddhists in the United States. The current organizational leader is Daisaku Ikeda. There are more than 12 million practitioners in 190 countries and territories around the world.

Basic Teachings

The lotus flower, blossoming in muddy waters, has been taken as an apt symbol of the Buddha, an enlightened being in the midst of this world of suffering. ... Translated into Chinese, the *Lotus Sutra* came to prominence in East Asia and was upheld by Buddhist adherents as the *sutra* that contains the quintessence of the teaching of Shakyamuni above all other scriptures. It was the subject of numerous commentaries across the centuries, serving also as the inspiration for various movements in religious, cultural, social, and political spheres. The *Lotus Sutra* has also been regarded as one of the four most influential religious books in the world, along with the New Testament, the Qur'an, and the Bhagavad Gita.[157]

Human beings are the temporary union of five components (Sanskrit, *skandhas*): form, perception, conception, volition, and consciousness.

1. **Form** is the physical aspect of life, including the senses with which we perceive the external world. (The other four represent the mental or spiritual aspect of life.)

2. **Perception** is the function of receiving external information through the sense organs.

3. **Conception** is the process of interpreting that information.

4. **Volition** is the will that acts based on the concepts formed.

5. **Consciousness** is the discernment that integrates the components of perception, conception, and volition.

Four Noble Truths: The Four Noble Truths were the Buddha's first teaching immediately following his enlightenment and were given at Deer Park in Benares, India. These teachings are referred to as the "first turning of the wheel of *dharma*." For a full discussion of the Four Noble Truths, *see* "Buddhism: General Introduction" chapter.

---

157 Habito, R. (2005). *Experiencing Buddhism: Ways of Wisdom and Compassion*. Maryknoll, NY: Orbis Books, 272.

1. **The First Noble Truth**: The truth of dissatisfaction and suffering.
2. **The Second Noble Truth**: The cause of dissatisfaction and suffering.
3. **The Third Noble Truth**: The end of dissatisfaction and suffering.
4. **The Fourth Noble Truth**: The path leading to the end of dissatisfaction and suffering. The Fourth Noble Truth is the Way, the Path leading to the end of dissatisfaction and suffering. By following and practicing the Noble Eightfold Path, we will overcome our dissatisfaction and suffering.

The Noble Eightfold Path:
1. Right Understanding
2. Right Thought
3. Right Speech
4. Right Action
5. Right Livelihood
6. Right Effort
7. Right Mindfulness
8. Right Concentration.

For a full discussion of the Noble Eightfold Path, *see* "Buddhism: General Introduction" chapter.
1. **Right Understanding** (or Right View) is the ability to understand the nature of things exactly as they are, without delusion or distortion.
2. **Right Thought** (or Right Intention) means one's thoughts, feelings, desires, and intentions are in complete harmony with the wisdom of life, in accordance with the way reality works.
3. **Right Speech** is the ability to speak truthfully and harmlessly.
4. **Right Action** means that one's behavior is ethical, honorable, and responsible.
5. **Right Livelihood** suggests that people earn their living in an honorable and

life-affirming way, free from deceit or dishonesty.
6. **Right Effort** is the wholehearted, diligent, and energetic endeavor to train one's mind and heart.
7. **Right Mindfulness** (or Right Attention) means being attentive, mindful, and aware of one's bodily actions, sensations and feelings, and the activity of the mind.
8. **Right Concentration** is the means for training and centering the mind.

Basic to Mahāyāna teachings, following the *Four Noble Truths* and *Eightfold Path* of traditional Buddhism (*see* "Buddhism: General Introduction" chapter), are the *bodhisattva* vows:
1. Living beings are numberless: I vow to save them.
2. Earthly desires are countless: I vow to eradicate them.
3. The teachings are endless: I vow to master them.
4. Enlightenment is supreme: I vow to attain it.

The *bodhisattva* ideal has six *paramitas*, or perfections, that allow the one aspiring to awakening (Sanskrit, *bodhicitta*) to manifest the virtues of wisdom and compassion.
1. Almsgiving or generosity
2. Ethical behavior or morality
3. Patience or perseverance
4. Effort or endeavor
5. Meditation or concentration
6. Wisdom.

• *Zen* (Chinese, *Chan*) doctrine teaches that all beings have the potential for Buddhahood but have lost sight of it through lifetimes of defilements and attachments. Meditation seeks to remove the obstacles that block the path to awakening. *Chan* claims an unbroken lineage to the historical Buddha (Shakyamuni) through the Indian monk Bodhidharma (ca. early sixth century CE).

- *Pure Land* teaching derives from the promise of the Buddha Amitabha (Japanese, *Amida*) to save all sentient beings when they "sincerely and joyfully entrust themselves" to him by calling his name. Those who recite the Buddha's name at the point of death will be met by him and taken to the Pure Land of Bliss. Inviting the infinite power of *Amida's* compassion to take over our lives relies on that Other Power, rather than self-power, to work in and through us. There are five guidelines for behavior:
  1. Listen to the teachings of Pure Land throughout one's life.
  2. Refrain from quarreling with other Buddhist schools and religions.
  3. Fully actualize the mind that sees and treats people and events with equanimity.
  4. Respect and honor life.
  5. Abandon superstitious and magical practices.

- *Nichiren* Buddhism teaches that "The heart of the Lotus Sutra is the revelation that one may attain supreme enlightenment in one's present form without altering one's status as an ordinary person. This means that without casting aside one's karmic impediments one can still attain the Buddha way."[158] Based on his study of the *Lotus Sutra*, Nichiren established the invocation (chant) of *Nam-myoho-renge-kyo* as a universal

practice to enable people to manifest the Buddhahood inherent in their lives and gain the strength and wisdom to challenge and overcome any adverse circumstances. Nichiren saw the *Lotus Sutra* as a vehicle for people's empowerment – stressing that everyone can attain enlightenment and enjoy happiness while they are alive.

Basic Practices

- *Zen* has two basic approaches to practice: (1) "Just sitting" is the gradual method followed by the Soto school, which believes that, since one is already a Buddha, sitting in quiet meditation will allow enlightenment to become manifest, and (2) the "sudden" awakening of the Rinzai branch comes from meditation on a *koan*, a paradoxical saying given by one's teacher, such as, "Who hears?" or "The sound of one hand." This form was adopted by the Japanese samurai as it emphasized blows, shouts, and witty exchanges to attain enlightenment. One's qualified teacher determines the level of one's enlightenment based on a series of questions and the response of the practitioner.

- *Pure Land* devotees maintain a Buddhist home altar enshrining an image of Amida Buddha or his name together with flowers, candles, and incense offerings. It consists of a single practice, in Japanese: the recitation of the phrase *Namu Amida Butsu*.

- *Nichiren* Buddhism has three basic elements to its practice: (1) chanting the phrase *Nam-myoho-renge-kyo* as a prayer for oneself and others; (2) studying the teachings of Nichiren; and (3) making efforts to share the teachings of Buddhism, to spread the Buddhist perspective of life's inherent dignity and potential. SGI members perform a morning and evening

---

158 Gosho Translation Committee. trans. (1999). *The Writings of Nichiren Daishonin*. Vol. 1. Tokyo, Japan: Soka Gakkai, 410.

practice that consists of chanting *Nam-myoho-renge-kyo* and reciting portions of the *Lotus Sutra*.

Principles for Clinical Care

Buddhism arose from humankind's struggle to overcome the most fundamental problems of human existence – the four sufferings of birth, aging, sickness, and death. These four conditions – though sources of pain – are inseparable from human life. Clinical care should be based on compassionate respect for human dignity and avoid any tendency to treat it as a matter of medical technology alone. Compassion means action taken to overcome the sufferings of life, together with other people. Human relations, and especially those of patient and caregiver, should be based on a model of shared responsibility and mutual respect.

Dietary Issues

- Most Asian Buddhists (except Tibetans) practice some form of vegetarianism as a matter of individual choice.

General Medical Beliefs

- Illness is a matter of disharmony between the body and the spirit and between life and its environment. Good health is judged not only on the basis of physiological diagnosis of abnormalities but also on a holistic view of life that includes spiritual elements. Since all living beings must pass through birth, old age, sickness, and death, illness is a natural component of the life cycle. Sickness helps people pioneer a more fulfilled way of living by reflecting on the meaning and dignity of life. The very process of overcoming illness tempers the body and mind and enables us to create a broader equilibrium or homeostasis.

- The great Chinese Buddhist teacher T'ien-t'ai (538–597 CE) gave six reasons for illness.
  1. First, sickness results from disharmony among the four elements – earth, water, fire, and wind – that make up the human body and correspond to the physical states: solid, liquid, thermal, and gaseous. This disharmony can result from a failure to adapt to changes in the external environment, such as the weather.
  2. Second are illnesses arising from poor dietary habits or irregular mealtimes.
  3. Third are sicknesses caused by irregular meditation, which might include insufficient sleep and exercise, making us more susceptible to illness.
  4. The fourth cause of illness is "news from demons," which can be understood as bacteria, viruses, or externally caused psychological stress.
  5. The fifth cause is the influence of malevolent forces, generally brought on by delusions arising from greed and anger, and resulting in mental illness.
  6. Sixth are sicknesses caused by karma, the cumulative effects of one's thoughts, words, and deeds over the three existences of past, present, and future.

- Medical procedures are basically a matter of individual choice based on the principle of non-harming, to both the donor and the recipient.

Specific Medical Issues

- **Abortion**: Abortion is never a good choice; although it may be determined that it is an unavoidable taking of a life for the benefit of the mother and the fetus.

- **Advance Directives**: Use of advance directives for health care planning is encouraged but is an individual choice.
- **Birth Control**: Buddhists consider the issue of birth control a matter of personal choice, which should be guided by meditation.
- **Blood Transfusions**: Blood transfusions would generally be acceptable.
- **Circumcision**: Circumcision, which is not Asian in origin, is not specifically addressed and therefore remains an individual decision.
- **In Vitro Fertilization**: In vitro fertilization would generally be acceptable.
- **Stem Cell Research**: Stem cell research for therapeutic purposes would generally be acceptable.
- **Vaccinations**: There are generally no ethical issues involved in vaccinations; their efficacy in preserving health, especially among children, gives them positive value.
- **Witholding/Withdrawing Life Support**: The point at which life support and extraordinary means should be withheld is up to the individual and should be considered from the standpoint of both viability and the dignity of the person's life.

Gender and Personal Issues

- James Coleman asserts:

  All Buddhist schools agree that the state of enlightenment the seeker strives to realize is the same in everyone regardless of gender, age, or social background. Many of the great Mahāyāna sutras tell us that this ultimate reality is beyond the realm of all dualities, which of course includes that of female and male. Moreover, since the highest ethical imperative of Buddhism is to save all beings

from suffering and the way to escape suffering is Buddhist practice, it seems absolutely incongruous that women would be denied equal access to the techniques and training necessary to that practice.[159]

- Coleman goes on to say that

  [a]lthough the point is somewhat controversial, many would argue that Western Buddhism has not only allowed the full participation of women but is itself being "feminized," that is, it is moving away from a more goal-oriented and hierarchical "masculine" approach to a softer approach that focuses more on the needs of individual members. It is also far more open to gays, lesbians, and other stigmatized groups than most traditional Western religions.[160]

- The goddess of the *Vimalakirti Sutra* instructs the great disciple Shariputra about gender differences: "… though they appear in women's bodies, they are not women. Therefore the Buddha teaches that all phenomena are neither male nor female."[161]
- Nichiren, writing in thirteenth-century Japan, asserts: "There should be no discrimination among those who propagate the five characters of Myoho-renge-kyo in the Latter Day of the Law, be they men or women"[162] and, even more strongly, "a woman who embraces this sutra not only

---

159 Coleman, J. (2001). *The New Buddhism: The Western Transformation of an Ancient Tradition*. New York, NY: Oxford University Press, 140.
160 Ibid, 218.
161 Watson, B. trans. (1997). *The Vimalakirti Sutra*. New York, NY: Columbia University Press, 91.
162 Gosho Translation Committee. *The Writings of Nichiren Daishonin*, 385.

excels all other women, but also surpasses all men."[163]

- In practical terms, though, Rita Gross states:

  I have always been puzzled by the generations of Buddhists who have taken the *bodhisattva* vow with utmost sincerity and yet have also practiced, promoted, and justified gender hierarchy and gender privilege in Buddhism. The gap between the vision and the practice of Buddhism nowhere seems wider. Someone who has taken the *bodhisattva* vow should not promote gender inequality, whether by direct action or by passively accepting the status quo.[164]

- Kenneth Tanaka has observed that

  [n]ot only do women make up a sizable percentage of membership but many of the teachers are women, particularly within the Euro-American groups. Half of the Vipassana teachers, for example, are women. Even in the more structured institution of the Soka Gakkai International, American women are taking vital leadership roles. This trend is further manifested in the San Francisco Zen Center, one of the largest organizations in the country, which in February 1996 installed Blanche Hartman as abbess, to join the ranks of two other abbots.[165]

Principles for Spiritual Care through the Cycles of Life

Humanism and respect for the dignity of each person's life remain the fundamental guidelines for caring, based on the recognition that all of life is interdependent and interconnected; that no one can be free of suffering while others are suffering.

Concepts of Living and Dying for Spiritual Support

What we call death is the total non-functioning of the physical body. Do all these forces and energies stop altogether with the non-functioning of the body? Buddhism says "No." Will, volition, desire, thirst to exist, to continue, to become more and more, is a tremendous force that moves whole lives, whole existences; that even moves the whole world. According to Buddhism, this force does not stop with the non-functioning of the body, which is death; but it continues manifesting itself in another form, producing re-existence which is called rebirth.[166]

- Illness is an opportunity to attain a higher, nobler state of life. Instead of agonizing over disease or despairing of overcoming it, one can use illness to develop a stronger, more compassionate self that can use the experience to give hope to others suffering in similar circumstances.
- Cycles of life and death can be likened to the alternating patterns of sleep and wakefulness. Just as sleep prepares us for the next day's activity, death can be seen as a state in which we rest and replenish ourselves for new life. In this light, death

---

163 Ibid, 464.

164 Gross, R. (1993). *Buddhism After Patriarchy.* Albany: State University of New York, 183–184.

165 Prebish, C. and K. Tanaka. (1998). *The Faces of Buddhism in America.* Berkeley: University of California Press, 289.

166 Rahula, W. (1974). *What the Buddha Taught.* New York, NY: Grove Press, 33.

should be acknowledged, along with life, as a blessing to be appreciated.

- Birth is a process like dying, and is repeated endlessly. Birth is the cause for death, and death is the cause for being born again. A life appearing in this world has the opportunity during the "active" phase of its existence to make positive causes that move it toward higher states and eventual enlightenment.
- Human life is dignified in and of itself and dying should manifest that dignity. Death is a certainty. Therefore, it is not whether people's lives are long or short, but how they have been lived. Even a short life can be as fruitful as a long one. The fundamental purpose of death is birth – to make a fresh start in the eternal cycle of life.

During Birth

- As stated earlier, circumcision, which is not Asian in origin, is not specifically addressed and therefore remains an individual decision.
- Rituals at birth (and neonatal death) vary with the tradition, but generally follow the practices followed by adults on a regular basis, including sutra or mantra recitation.

During Illness

- Hope and the renewed determination to recover that accompanies it are key factors in overcoming illness.
- Health care providers can inquire from the patient about any requirements, including the installation of a Buddhist altar, and be respectful of the privacy of the patient, family, and friends during any practice periods in the patient room.

During End of Life

Daisaku Ikeda offers a perspective on dying:

Buddhism establishes three categories of pain: physical; psychological – caused by loss; and existential – caused by awareness of the transitory nature of the phenomenal world. Death and the fear of death are said to be the conjunction of these three ... The first type of pain can be alleviated with the help of medical science. Social welfare systems and the combined cooperative efforts of family and the medical system can lighten psychological suffering. Overcoming existential suffering, however, is another story altogether. This is the anguish caused by our own mortality. I am convinced that a way of thinking about life and death and of triumphing over the fear and apprehension of death rooted in eternal truths is necessary. If people can internalize a spiritual view of life and death, it will enable them to overcome the despair of these three types of pain and greet the final chapter of their lives, tranquil and fulfilled.[167]

- Helping the patient call to mind the awareness that life is eternal, or that one's life is interrelated with the lives of all others, or that life is as expansive as the universe can offer spiritual comfort to those whose lives are in decline.
- Remind the patient that the ability to experience the dying process in a positive way is greatly influenced by the way one has lived. Having no regrets can enable one to freely and confidently move into the passive, intermediate phase of exist-

---

167 Ikeda, D., R. Simard, and G. Bourgeault. (2003). *On Being Human: Where Ethics, Medicine and Spirituality Converge.* Santa Monica, CA: Middleway Press, 123–124.

ence, or death, that acts as an interval between rebirths.

- Health care providers can inquire from the patient about any requirements, including the installation of a Buddhist altar, and be respectful of the privacy of the patient, family, and friends during any practice periods in the patient room.

Care of the Body

- Most Buddhists consider the essential life to have left the body following brain death, although for the Pure Land, Nichiren, and some other traditions the life force remains physically nearby for a period of time, thus allowing for prayers and rites to be offered as means of guiding the life to its next existence.
- Family members and close friends may choose to remain with the body for some time afterward.
- Cremation is the common form of handling the remains.
- Individuals may choose to donate the body for medical research.
- Autopsies may be authorized based on medical or other need to determine the cause of death.
- The physical body has no particular function after the prayers for eternal life and fortunate rebirth have been completed.

Organ and Tissue Donation

- Organ donation is an opportunity for the deceased to continue acting on behalf of other suffering beings in fulfillment of the bodhisattva vow, so it is generally supported. It may be preferable for a chaplain and/or nurse who are trained designated requesters to be consulted for assistance.

Scriptures, Inspirational Readings, and Prayers

READINGS DURING END-OF-LIFE PROCESS

These verses can be read by family, friends, or health care professionals.

Zen

Because there is nothing to be
  attained,
The *bodhisattva* relying on
  prajnaparamita has
No obstruction in his mind.
Because there is no obstruction, he
  has no fear,
And he passes far beyond confused
  imagination.
And reaches ultimate nirvana.[168]

Pure Land

When the time of their death
approaches, the Tathagata ...
Amitabha will stand before [them]
surrounded and honored by a host of
countless monks. Thereupon, having
seen the Blessed One, their thoughts
will only be thoughts of serene trust,
and forthwith they will be reborn in
the Land of Bliss.[169]

Nichiren

For one who summons up one's faith
and chants Nam-myoho-renge-kyo

---

168 *The Heart Sutra*. Buddha Dharma Education Association/BuddhaNet. Available at: www.buddha net.net/e-learning/heartstr.htm (accessed 5 Sept 12).

169 Gómez, L. O. trans. (1996). *The Land of Bliss: The Paradise of the Buddha of Measureless Light; Sanskrit and Chinese Versions of the Sukhāvatīvyūha Sutras*. Honolulu: University of Hawaii Press, 91.

with the profound insight that now is the last moment of one's life, the sutra proclaims: "When the lives of these persons come to an end, they will be received into the hands of a thousand Buddhas, who will free them from all fear and keep them from falling into the evil paths of existence." How can we possibly hold back our tears at the inexpressible joy of knowing that not just one or two, not just one hundred or two hundred, but as many as a thousand Buddhas will come to greet us with open arms![170]

170 Gosho Translation Committee. *The Writings of Nichiren Daishonin*, 216.

Theravada Buddhism

*Perishable are all conditioned things, one should
perfect one's self-awareness/mindfulness.*[171]

Prepared by:
Kongsak Tanphaichitr, MD
Chairman of the Buddhist Council of Greater St. Louis
St. Louis, MO

History and Facts

Buddhism, the term coined by Westerners, is known in the East as *Buddha-Sasana.* The Buddha himself called it *dharma-vinaya.* Buddhism is also frequently referred to as *Buddha-dharma*, or the truth or teachings taught by the Buddha.

Buddhism is the awakened way of life from ignorance of "craving" (*tanha*) and "concepts" (*dittthi*) of greed, hatred, delusion, clinging, and suffering. The Buddha taught this awakened way of life, which he discovered through his enlightenment, to liberate one's mind and free oneself (nirvana) from all the bondage, craving, and clinging to "self" that is the source of unhappiness (unsatisfactoriness, problem, stress, conflict, suffering – *dukkha*).

Buddhists take refuge in the **Triple Gem**: (1) Buddha, (2) *Dharma*, and (3) *Sangha*.

1. The **Buddha** (which means "Awakened One") was born as the crown prince of the Sakaya Dynasty of Kapilavattu (currently in southern Nepal) approximately 2600 years ago. He attained enlightenment through self-realization under the bodhi tree at Bodh Gaya, India, in 588 BCE and passed away in 543 BCE (BE, the Buddhist Era way of counting time, began with this date). The Buddha had three great virtues: (1) purity, (2) wisdom, and (3) compassion. Everyone is capable of attaining Buddhahood through practicing the path of the awakened way of life, as taught by the self-enlightened Sakayamuni Buddha.

2. ***Dharma***, the Buddha's teachings (i.e., reflection in words of the truth about the Secret of Nature or the *Ultimate Norm of the Universe*), is based upon or stemmed from the experiences of the Buddha's enlightenment. His teaching is a mass of timeless, flexible methods appropriate for different times, different places and, most important, for people's different temperaments. It is a down-to-earth method, dealing directly with one's own *body and mind*. This "down-to-earth" method of teaching can guide anyone toward enlightenment by practicing the *Middle Path*, because "Buddha Nature" or "Buddha Seed" exists in everyone, regardless

---

171 Tanphaichitr, K. (2006). *Buddhism Answers Life.* Bangkok, Thailand: Horatanachai Printing, 188. These were the last words of the Buddha.

of age, sex, race, nationality, literacy, dialect, occupation, or religious belief. The Buddha's Teaching is recorded in a 45-volume set of Pali text called the Tripitaka or Tipitaka, as well as in Thai text, and many other languages, containing 84 000 *dharma* headings. These texts comprise of three canons or "baskets" of teachings: (1) Discipline (*vinaya*); (2) Discourses – Buddha's life and teaching (*sutra*); and (3) Higher doctrine – philosohy and psycholgy of Buddhism (*Abhidharma*). *Dharma* can be summarized as follows:

○ *Ultimate of Nature* (**Four Noble Truths**): Life is suffering, yet there is a way to end suffering

○ *Law of Nature* (***pariyatti*** – **to study**): following the law of the *Three Universal Characteristics or Marks of Existence*

○ Duty according to the Law of Nature (***patipatti*** – **to practice**)

○ Benefit, Fruition, or Consequence of performing the Duty according to the Law of Nature (***pativedha*** – **to penetrate, realize**).

Patiyatti, *patipatti*, and *pativedha* are the three main "practical aspects" or the "three pillars of Buddhism" that support Buddhists in pursuing nirvana through enlightenment. The highest goal of this awakened way of life is nirvana. The various components of *dharma* will be discussed in greater detail in the next section, "Basic Teachings."

3. *Sangha* is the term designating the Buddhist community or order of righteous followers treading the path toward enlightenment. The *sangha* members (*ariya* – noble ones/disciples) are the ones who carry and pass on the torch of the Buddha's teachings to others, transmitting this awakened way of life to the followers and future generations, as well as setting themselves as living proofs to the truth of this awakened way of life.

Theravada Buddhism refers to "the teachings laid down as principles by the Elders." The word "Elders" in this context refers to those 500 *Arahant* Elders, or the fully enlightened senior monks, who participated in the First Rehearsal or Council (*Sangayana*). Theravada Buddhism means Buddhism that is based on the "First Rehearsal," which was agreed upon by the Elders and handed down from generation to generation.

Councils of other religious traditions are often convened to settle disputes about their tenets, to formulate their dogmas and establish policies in propagating their religions. The primary purpose of Buddhist Rehearsals (Councils) is to preserve the original teachings of the Buddha as accurately as possible, not allowing anyone to alter, modify, deviate, omit, or add anything to them.

The First Rehearsal convened 3 months after the Buddha's death or final nirvana (*parinirvana*) in 543 BCE, took place at the Sattapanna-guha Cave on Mount Vebhara, near the city of Rajagaha, under the auspices of King Ajatasattu. The Elder or Venerable Mahakassapa presided over this assembly of 500 fully enlightened or *Arahant* Elders; he also acted as the interrogator about the Buddha's teachings.

The teachings were originally divided by the Buddha himself into two major domains: (1) the doctrine (*dharma*), recited by Venerable Ananda, the Buddha's personal attendant, and (2) the discipline (*vinaya*), recited by Venerable Upali, who was personally praised by the Buddha as being excellent in the discipline. Once a consensus was reached on the content of a given subject, the Elders would chant it together so that the approved contents would be settled as the model for memorization and transmission later on. It took 7 months to complete this rehearsal, which was treated as settled and final.

The Buddha's teachings from this First Rehearsal had two stages of development. The former stage involved reciting the teachings orally, called *mukhapatha* or "oral transmission," and the latter stage – in the later periods – involved writing the teachings down, called *potthakaropana* or "putting down in books."

The Second Rehearsal was conducted in 443 BCE (100 BE [Buddhist Era]) at Vesali to address ten issues which deviated from the *dharma-vinaya*. This process was accomplished through the cooperation of the eight Elders, presiding over the assembly of 700 monks, with the Elder Rewatta as the interrogator and the Elder Sappakamee as the one who gave responses to those ten issues. The council was convened under the auspices of King Kalasoka and took 8 months to complete.

The Third Rehearsal was conducted in 307 BCE (236 BE) at Patlibutra (presently called Patna) to address the increasing numbers of "fake monks." Elder Moggaleeputtratissa Thera presided over the assembly of 1000 monks, which addressed this concern. The council was convened under the auspices of King Asokha, the Great. The king also sent nine Buddhist missionaries throughout his kingdom and beyond. His son, the Elder Mahindra, headed the missionary venture to Sri Lanka, where Buddhism became firmly established. Another missionary venture led by the Elders Sona and Uttara went to the Golden Peninsula or Indochina, and established Buddhism around the Phra Pathom Chedi, Nakhon Pathom, Thailand.

The Fourth Rehearsal was conducted around 83 BCE (460 BE) at the Aluvihara Monastery, Alokalena, in Sri Lanka. The Tipitaka was recited orally from 543 BCE up to the time of this council. Now, the words of the Buddha and other related matters were preserved in writing by inscribing them on palm leaves in the Pali language and incorporating those leaves into what is known as the Pali Canon. The commitment of the words to writing was to preserve, as accurately as possible, the actual words of the Buddha.

The commentaries on the Pali Canon are explanations of the text for the learner and were transmitted in *Sinhala*, when they were introduced in Sri Lanka. Around 407–457 CE (950–1000 BE), the Elders Buddhaghosa and Dhammapala, who both traveled from India to Sri Lanka, translated and compiled these commentaries back into Pali, the version being studied today.[172]

The Thai version of the Tipitaka, together with the commentaries, comprises 91 volumes of written textbooks. It serves as the reference to the original teachings by the Buddha, which has been well preserved with precise accuracy. This was demonstrated at the last International Rehearsal, the Seventh Rehearsal, in Burma or Myanmar between 1954 and 1956 (2497 and 2499 BE). Various versions of the Tipitaka in Pali from different countries were compared and were found to be exactly the same, except for a few minor misspellings.

---

172 Payutto, P. (2004). *The Pali Canon. What A Buddhist Must Know.* Bangkok, Thailand: Buddhadharma Foundation, 14–24.

Basic Teachings

The fundamental elements (heart or core) of the Buddha's teaching can be summarized in **three main principles**.

First, **avoid doing bad deeds** – *morality* – which is implemented through the *five basic moral codes* (*precepts*) for laypersons.

1. Do not kill humans and animals.
2. Do not steal.
3. Do not practice sexual misconduct.
4. Do not lie.
5. Do not drink or take any drug or intoxicant.

Theravada monks – *bhikkhus* – observe 227 precepts, including practicing celibacy, and consuming no solid food after 12 noon. Theravada female monks or nuns – *bhikkhunis* – observe 311 precepts (this female monk lineage ceased to exist in the Theravada tradition 500 years after the Buddha passed away – 43 BCE; efforts to bring back this lineage are being actively pursued in Sri Lanka). The discipline (*vinaya*) or the moral codes are basically guidelines for monks or nuns to live together peacefully and harmoniously among themselves, communities, societies, environment, and nature. Such moral precepts are basically guidelines on mannerism, personal hygiene, preventive health care, body and mind training, the way to deal with laypersons; the precepts also were restraining principles drawn up by the Buddha to prevent potential damage, whenever there were inappropriate incidents that could have jeopardized the whole *sangha* community. Even though monks and nuns come from all walks of life and different Brahmin (the ancient Hindu tradition) caste systems, they were being treated equally when they entered the monkhood or *sangha* community.

Second, **do good deeds** – practicing *mental concentration* through mind development or mental discipline. One should go beyond adherence to the listed precepts to nurture the mind with the *five basic virtues*.

*   Loving-kindness and compassion – respect others' and one's own lives.
*   Right livelihood – respect others' ownership of their possessions or belongings, not to take them as yours.
*   Restraining oneself from improper sexual behavior – respect others' bodies and rights, not to take advantage of them.
*   Speaking the truth – respect others and oneself by being truthful and honest.
*   Maintaining one's mindfulness and self-awareness, and staying away from any drug or intoxicant which would dull them.

Third, **purify one's mind** in order to gain insights and *wisdom* through practicing Insight Meditation. To accomplish this, one would transcend the worldly concept or supposition of good and evil. One would see the true nature of things and one's own body and mind as they truly are, bearing the Three Universal Characteristics of Existence of Impermanence, Imperfection, and Selfless in nature, thus gaining insights without any bias. One would be disenchanted, discerned, and would let go without any more grasping or clinging. One's mind would be liberated and free from suffering. Nirvana is being realized. This third fundamental principle of "purifying one's mind" through practicing Insight Meditation goes beyond the common teachings of avoidance in doing bad deeds and encouragement on doing good deeds which are taught in other religions. Purification of one's mind occurs through practicing the *Middle Path* as the way to end suffering through seeing the true nature of one's mind.

The effective implementation of these three fundamental principles requires mindfulness and self-awareness (*see* Insight Meditation notes later in this section).

The Four Noble (Ultimate) Truths

1. **Dukkha** (Suffering or Dis-ease – equivalent to disease): To be born is suffering. To age is suffering. To die is suffering. Departing from loved one is suffering. Not getting what one wants is suffering. Getting what one does not want is suffering. Physical ailment or mental ailment is suffering. Grief, sorrow, lamentation, or despair is suffering. In brief, the *Five Aggregates of Clinging* (i.e., the five basic components of life – namely, body, feeling, perception, thought formation, and consciousness, with craving and clinging to the "self" concept) are suffering. *Dukkha or suffering is to be comprehended.* In reality, they are but "selfless" in nature, without any true permanent entity as a real person. Realization of this truth would free one from craving, clinging, and suffering.

2. **Samudaya** (Cause of Suffering – "Cause" of disease): The cause of suffering is *craving* with sensual desire, liking, and disliking, in the unwholesome concepts of greed, hatred, and delusion. *Samudaya or the cause of suffering is to be eradicated.*

3. **Nirodha** (End of Suffering – "Cure"): The cessation of suffering is the achievement of nirvana, which is ultimate peace. *Nirodha or nirvana is to be realized.*

4. **Magga** (Path to End Suffering – "Treatment or antidote"): The method for alleviating suffering is living the *Middle Way* (avoiding the two extremes of sensual indulgence and self-mortification), which is attained by following the Noble Eightfold Path. *Magga or the Middle Path is to be developed.*

The Noble Eightfold Path

1. Right understanding/view
2. Right thought
3. Right speech
4. Right action
5. Right livelihood
6. Right effort
7. Right mindfulness
8. Right concentration

Right understanding and right thought are **wisdom**. Right speech, right action, and right livelihood are **morality**. Right effort, right mindfulness, and right concentration are mental **concentration**.

Morality (*sila*), concentration (*samadhi*), and wisdom (*panna*) are the *Threefold Trainings of Buddhism*. For laypeople, these Threefold Trainings are modified into a simpler format of generosity (*dana*), morality (*sila*), and meditation (*bhavana*).

The Three Universal Characteristics or Marks of Existence

1. *Annica* (Impermanence): This mark of existence is obscured by *continuity*.
2. *Dukkha* (Conflict, imbalance, imperfection, stress, suffering): This mark of existence is obscured by *movement, motion*.
3. *Anatta* (Not self, selfless, emptiness): This mark of existence is obscured by *cohesiveness, bundling, mass*. Nothing exists "independently" on its own (except nirvana); therefore, there is no true permanent individual or a "self" entity.

All phenomena originate from and are dependent upon causes and effects, a concept known as *Dependent Arising* or *Dependent Origination*. This concept is basically the expanded version of the Four Noble Truths and is known as the "arising" and "ceasing" pathways.

By realizing these "Three Universal Characteristics of Existence," one would also realize the true nature of things, thereby making one disenchanted. Through disenchantment, one would be discerned, and would let go. One would gain wisdom by liberating oneself from all craving and clinging. One would become totally free mentally, spiritually, and intellectually, and be in perfect harmony with oneself, with one's body and mind, with others and nature. Transcending all the worldly concepts, one would realize nirvana, the ultimate and perfect peace and happiness.

Insight Meditation

This unique concept is the practical aspect of Buddhism; it enables people to realize the true nature of all existence (Universal **Characteristics of Existence**: *anicca*, *dukkha*, and *anatta*) and to see things clearly as they truly are. This is accomplished through practicing the *Four Foundations of Mindfulness*, the method of self-observation or self-monitoring of one's own (1) body, (2) feelings, (3) mind, and (4) mental objects/events/phenomena.

The Four Foundations of Mindfulness is the supreme path to purify all beings, letting one transcend grief and sorrow, while getting rid of pain, despair, and distress. Practice of Insight Meditation allows one to accomplish the three main principles of the Buddha's teaching: (1) avoid doing bad deeds, (2) do good deeds, and (3) purify one's mind. It enables one to realize nirvana.

Nirvana: Ultimate Outcome

Nirvana frees one from suffering, death, and rebirth, as well as all other worldly bonds. *It is the common goal of spiritual practice in all branches of Buddhism.* It is departure from the cycle of *rebirths* (samsara) *and* entry into an entirely different mode of existence, beyond any concept or supposition. Basically, the selfless and purified mind unites as one with the voidness/emptiness or the background of the original universe, known as nirvana.

Achieving nirvana requires a complete overcoming of the three unwholesome roots – desire, hatred, delusion – and the cessation of active volition, mental impulse, or thought formation. Nirvana ends egoism and self-conceit. It extinguishes suffering. It means freedom from the determining effect of karma.

Nirvana is unconditioned; its characteristic marks are absence of arising, subsisting, changing, and passing away. Nirvana can be realized through enlightenment which can be achieved by practicing Insight Meditation. With continuous mindfulness and awareness of one's thought, along with insight – seeing things clearly as they truly are with pure perception and wisdom – liberation of one's mind will result. One's mind would be perfectly free from dis-ease, conflict, and suffering because there would no longer be any attachment to worldly phenomena, nor blindness by greed, hatred, and delusion. One would be perfectly free, calm, peaceful, and happy, in this state of unborn, ungrowing, undying, unchanging, and unconditioning of nirvana.

The ideal or the goal of life is nirvana. The Buddha explained nirvana to his disciples as follows:

Such state does exist.

Earth, wind, water, and fire (the
4 elements),

The Realm of the Infinity of
Space, the Realm of the Infinity
of Consciousness, the Realm of
Nothingness, the Realm of No
Memories, neither perception nor
non-perception (the 4 formless
jhanas or mental absorption),

This realm, or next realm, both the
sun, and the moon,

Do not exist in such state.

O' Monks.

I do <u>not</u> address that state as, coming,
going, or sustaining, death, or birth.

Such state is not enduring, not
ongoing, nor any clinging.

This is the end of suffering.[173]

Basic Practices

- Living a harmonious and peaceful life:
  9 months after his enlightenment, 44 years
  before the Buddhist Era (587 BCE), the
  Buddha laid down the guidelines for liv-
  ing a harmonious life.
  - Not harming others verbally.
  - Not harming others physically.
  - Disciplining oneself by observing the
    moral codes (i.e., the 227 precepts for
    monks, the 311 precepts for female
    monks or nuns, and the five precepts
    for the laity).
  - Being moderate in consumption, so

173 *Udana.* PTS (the Pali Text Society's English version
of the Tipitaka). Oxford: Pali Text Society, Ud, 81.
PTS was published by the Pali Text Society as a
series of English translations of the Tipitaka over a
period of 50 years (between 1877 and 1927). There
are 57 volumes including indexes, with a few volumes subsequently being replaced by new editions.

that one would not deprive others for
the same natural resource.
  - Dwelling in a suitable and peaceful
    environment.
  - Training one's mind to be peaceful and
    purified.
- Living one's life, for the layperson,
  according to the five basic moral codes
  (precepts):
  1. Do not kill humans and animals.
  2. Do not steal.
  3. Do not practice sexual misconduct.
  4. Do not lie.
  5. Do not drink or take any drug or
     intoxicant.
- Following the Noble Eightfold Path.
- Observing important holidays: One of
  the most important Buddhist holidays is
  a day that, in many countries, commemorates the Buddha's birth, enlightenment,
  and *parinirvana.* This day is called
  Visaka-Puja, Vesak, Wesak, and other
  variations; it occurs on the full moon of
  the sixth lunar month, in either May or
  June, depending upon the lunar calendar.
- Buddhist monks serve as the spiritual leaders in Theravada Buddhism.
  There may be minor variations among
  Theravada Buddhist monks from various
  Theravada Buddhist countries, including Thailand, Sri Lanka, Myanmar, Laos,
  and Cambodia, which would be based in
  part on the local traditions, customs, and
  beliefs rather than Buddhism itself.

Principles for Clinical Care
Dietary Issues

- Many Buddhists, especially of the
  Mahāyāna tradition, are vegetarians, but
  this is by no means universal. The Buddha
  himself was asked by one of his followers, who happened to be his rival during

their childhood, to start a new lineage of vegetarian monks. But the Buddha did not give the permission. He simply stated that monks have to be easily livable, and to eat whatever was being offered to them.

- Whether one is a vegetarian or not, does not make one be more or less wise, nor prevents one from realizing nirvana. Some masters even stated that, if being a vegetarian is the key to enlightenment, then there would be innumerable numbers of water buffaloes and rabbits that attained enlightenment. However, by being vegetarian as well as being moderate in food consumption, one may be leaner and healthier physically, which would help one to practice meditation more easily. Above all, it is the practice of the Middle Path that purifies one's mind, not the kind of food one is consuming.
- Theravada Buddhist monks have to observe certain precepts of not killing animals and plants, deeds that are punishable with equal intensity, as both are living things.
- Monks are forbidden to accept any invitation for dining if they learn that the hosts are going to slaughter animals to offer them as food, as there is an intention to kill for their (the monks') benefit.
- Monks should not consume food for pleasure, but mainly as one of the *Four Essentials of Life – namely, food, shelter, clothing, and medicine.* In fact, monks remind themselves of this fact in their morning and evening praying on a daily basis.
- One should be moderate in consumption.

A person who is always mindful,
Be moderate in food consumption.
Being less uncomfortable,

Aging would come slower.
Longevity is to be expected.[174]

The Buddha's advice led to a successful weight loss by the obese King Pasendhikosala, with improvement of his overall health, for which he was very grateful. This counsel on losing weight is timeless; modern medical practitioners are acutely aware of the fact that obesity leads to increased risk for heart attack, stroke, hypertension, heart failure, difficulty in breathing, and cancer.

General Medical Beliefs

In youth, there is aging. In health,
   there is illness. In life, there is death.
Even some may live to be 100 years
   old, yet no one can escape death.
Death would crush all lives, without
   exception.[175]

There are no forbidden rules on medical interventions in Buddhism. Modern medicine, including chemotherapy and life supporting systems, are being offered to and accepted by Buddhists and Buddhist monks without restrictions.

The **Tipitaka** or the **Pali Canon** is a very rich resource of documented evidence of how the Buddha viewed life and how "medicine" was being practiced in India over 2500 years ago.

What is a person? The Buddha viewed life or a person as a combination of body and mind. The body feels or senses pain, but it is

---

174 *Thonapaka Sutra – Samyuttanikaya Sagathavagga.* PTS (the Pali Text Society's English version of the Tipitaka). Oxford: Pali Text Society, *S I*, 82.

175 Freer L, editor. *Jara Sutra – Samyuttanikaya Mahavagga.* PTS (the Pali Text Society's English version of the Tipitaka). Volume 5 Oxford: Pali Text Society:1976; 217.

the mind that suffers, with or without pain (e.g., when one is sick or dies). The Buddha described a person as the "*Five Aggregates of Clinging*," (i.e., the five basic components of life, namely, body, feeling, perception, thought formation, and consciousness, with craving and clinging to the 'self' concept, are suffering). In reality, they are but self-less in nature, without any true permanent entity as a real person. Realization of this truth would free one from craving, clinging, and suffering. Therefore, it is of utmost importance to purify one's mind to free oneself from suffering.

Disease: The Buddha identified two kinds of illnesses – physical and mental/spiritual.

1. Physical Illness: The true nature of one's body is that it is subjected to the three Universal Characteristics of Existence: (1) impermanence (people can grow, but unfortunately grow old); (2) imperfection, stress, conflict, and suffering (cells die and are constantly being replaced by new ones); and (3) not-self, selfless, voidness, and emptiness (no one can escape death; no true control of self). The Buddha stated that all humans and animals are but companions of dis-ease, birth, aging, sickness, and death, with no exception.

2. Mental/Spiritual Illness: Because of the lack of mindfulness and self-awareness, one would not see one's own thoughts or emotions which could lead to mental disturbances, and even a nervous breakdown. The story of Patacara, who lost her whole family in 1 day, is an example of mental or spiritual despair, which subsequently resulted in a healing. Patacara's husband was bitten by a cobra; her infant was snatched away by an eagle; another young son drowned in a swift current; and her parents and brother died in a fire. As a result of these tragic events, she became insane and wandered around town, naked. One day she roamed into a hall where the Buddha was preaching. When the Buddha greeted her gently with "May mindfulness be with you, sister," she suddenly "came back to herself" with self-awareness, and was quite ashamed at being naked and immediately asked for some clothes to wear. Later on, she attained enlightenment through practicing Insight Meditation and became totally free from suffering.

Health Care: *Jeevaka-komarapat* was the physician appointed to the Court of King Pimpisara of Rajagaha, as well as the personal physician caring for the Buddha and the monks. Physicians in the time of the Buddha treated numerous types of diseases: sinus headaches, hemorrhoids, anemia, performed various types of surgical procedures. The Buddha became involved in health care as well. He personally took care of a sick monk with diarrhea who had been neglected and left lying in his own urine and feces. He set an example for the monks and advised them to care for others when they got sick, as if they were caring for him. This model of caring set forth by the Buddha resulted in the building of wards for sick monks by laypersons. It also was an example to inspire King Asokha, the Great, to build hospitals not only for the public but also for sick animals. This was the establishment of the first hospitals in the history of mankind.

Patients: The Buddha described good and bad patients as follows:

- *Bad patients* are difficult to care for because they:

- o frequently do things that would make them sick
- o do not know the limit of indulging in pleasurable things
- o do not take their medications
- o do not tell the symptoms truthfully to let their doctors know whether they are better, worse, or stable
- o do not endure any severe physical pain, but rather escape the pain by committing suicide.

- *Good patients* are easy to care for because they:
  - o frequently do things that would make them healthy
  - o know the limit of indulging in pleasurable things
  - o take their medications
  - o tell the symptoms truthfully to let their doctors know whether they are better, worse, or stable
  - o can endure severe physical pain.

Doctors/Nurses: The Buddha described good and bad health care workers as follows:
- *Doctors/nurses* who should not be allowed to take care of patients are those who:
  - o cannot prescribe the correct medications for the illness
  - o cannot differentiate agreeable from disagreeable food; they take away agreeable food, while allowing disagreeable food for the patients
  - o expect rewards from the patient and lack loving-kindness
  - o hate to clean up feces, urine, vomit, and sputum
  - o do not know how to comfort or encourage patients at times with a "pep talk."
- *Good doctors/nurses* who should take care of patients are those who:
  - o can prescribe correct medications for the illness

- o can differentiate agreeable from disagreeable food, and only give agreeable food to patients
- o treat patients with loving-kindness, without expecting any reward
- o do not mind cleaning up feces, urine, vomit, or sputum
- o can explain, guide, comfort, and at times encourage patients with a "pep talk."[176]

Specific Medical Issues

- **Abortion**: Buddhism has no restrictions on abortion but it is not recommended. The Buddha clearly stated that a birth consciousness together with the sperm and the egg are essential for conception. Therefore, any medical practice that destroys a fetus would be considered killing a living being, which is against the Buddhist ethics. Intention plays the important and key decision on this matter, following the Buddha's statement that "Volition is Karma." Therefore, therapeutic abortion with the intention to save the mother's life is generally acceptable among the Thai Buddhist community. The decision is left to the individual and varies significantly from one country to another.

- **Advance Directives**: Buddhism has no objection to advance directives as long as they have been completed with full awareness.

- **Birth Control**: Buddhism has no objection to birth control of various kinds, as long as it would not harm the lady or the man. Besides, there is no conception or an existing life form that could be harmed

---

176 Morris, R. *Anguttaranikaya Pancaka-Chankkanipata*. Volume III PTS (the Pali Text Society's English version of the Tipitaka). Oxford: Pali Text Society; 1994, 144.

in the process. If one is not ready to have a child, it is better off to practice birth control, rather than burden oneself caring for a baby or a child without a proper care, which could harm the baby, physically and mentally.

- **Blood Transfusions**: Buddhism has no restrictions on the use of blood products (e.g., blood transfusions).
- **Circumcision**: Buddhism does not subscribe to the concept of circumcision, but has no objection should the parents choose to have their babies circumcised, which is mainly for reasons of personal hygiene.
- **In Vitro Fertilization**: Buddhism has no objection to in vitro fertilization, because it does not destroy any sustainable life form; on the contrary, it promotes life.
- **Stem Cell Research**: Buddhism has no objection to stem cell research for therapeutic purposes, because Buddhism respects life. Buddhists would object to stem cell research, though, if it would cause harm to one's own life or that of others.
- **Vaccinations**: Buddhism is in favor of preventive measures, including vaccinations, which have been widely practiced in Thailand since they became available (e.g., vaccinations against smallpox, polio, typhoid, cholera, and hepatitis B virus).
- **Withholding/Withdrawing Life Support**: Withdrawing life support in medically futile situations is acceptable to Buddhists, because Buddhism sees death within life, aging within youth, and deterioration of the sense organs as a norm of life.

Gender and Personal Issues

- Women and men are fundamentally of equal dignity and value. The Buddha himself allowed females to be ordained as female monks or nuns and novices, because he saw the potential for females to attain enlightenment. He even praised female monks for their supreme qualities, similar to what he praised in male monks. Women and men can attain enlightenment with equal opportunity; they do not necessarily have to be a nun or a monk to attain enlightenment, though being a monk or nun offers a better opportunity to achieve such a goal, with less circumstantial problems in life.
- In the clinical setting, there are no gender and personal issues in Buddhism, as it teaches mutual respect for the rights of all forms of life to be treated with loving-kindness and compassion.

Principles for Spiritual Care through the Cycles of Life
Concepts of Living and Dying for Spiritual Support

O' monks. This samsara (cycle of births and deaths) is endless, either in its origin or its end.

All beings with ignorance (Avijja) as an obstacle, accompanied by craving, would roam in Samsara, without any possible realizable origin.

You all have suffered, been burned, ruined, and added to the dirt in this cemetery endlessly.

For this reason, it should be enough for you all to be disenchanted with all sorts of conditioning, enough to be dispassionate, and enough for liberation.[177]

177 *Tinakatta Sutta.* PTS (the Pali Text Society's English

- Birth, death, and birth, known as cycle of births and deaths (*samsara*) would continue to exist as long as one is still clinging to the "self" concept or ego (*atta*). The cycle of births and deaths, also known as "rebirth," is basically governed by one's own "karma," yet without an underlying permanent "self" entity. The Buddha stated that

> [o]ne is the owner of one's own karma [karma simply means "action" based upon one's intention, with its consequence or fruition known as *karma-vipaka*]. One is the heir of one's own karma. One is born out of one's own karma. One's heritage is based on one's own karma. One's refuge is rooted in one's own karma.[178]

- Buddhists do not believe in a permanent soul (*atta*), as the Buddha discovered through his enlightenment that mind or consciousness, in its true nature, is but soulless, selfless, or not-self (*anatta*).

In Buddhism, "mind" (*jitta* – mind thinks), "consciousness" (*vinnana* – consciousness perceives), and "heart" (*mano* – heart feels or senses) are synonymous. *Consciousness or mind* arises, sustains and ceases all the time (specifically as eye consciousness, ear consciousness, nasal consciousness, tongue consciousness, body consciousness, or mind consciousness) whenever it encounters the corresponding *external sense spheres* of sight, sound, smell, taste, touch or thought through the *six sense organs* (i.e., eyes, ears, nose, tongue, bodily contact, or mind).

Through **biased perception** based upon one's own **conceptual processing**, the sense of "self" would automatically arise and continue to persist and perpetuate with such process of knowing. Only through **pure perception** or **perceptual processing** with mindfulness and self-awareness, would one neutrally and directly perceive all encountered phenomena without bias or "self" concept and remain in the *Middle Path*. One would realize that the true nature of one's mind and all phenomena is basically selfless, soulless or not-self, thus continuity of such "self" phenomenon would be disruptive and cease. Without "self," there would be no more bearer to inherit the consequence of the past actions. It means the end of suffering, which can be realized by anyone, even up to the moment of death.

- Death is not to be feared. Death is but a natural phenomenon, and in fact the very part of "life." No one can escape death. It is the process of dying, not death itself, that makes people suffer.
- Illness and dying are opportunities for spiritual growth, because they actually demonstrate the reality of life: that one does not have the true power to control them. If this body truly belongs to oneself, one should be able to command it not to get sick, not to get old, and not to die. However, body and mind basically follow the *Three Universal Characteristics of Existence*, (i.e., impermanence, imperfection, and not-self). By facing and accepting illness and death with these concepts in mind, one can come to realize the true nature of life, body and mind – without clinging. Thus, by "letting go," wisdom would arise and free one from suffering.
- Goal in life is to end the cycle of births and deaths to achieve nirvana.

---

version of the Tipitaka). Oxford: Pali Text Society, S II, 179 (*Samyuttanikaya Nidanavagga*).

178 *Thana Sutta*, PTS (the Pali Text Society's English version of the Tipitaka). Oxford: Pali Text Society, A III, 72 (*Anguttataranikaya Pancaka-Chankkanipata*).

During Birth

- With the advances in medicine and health care, many ancient Thai customs and traditions for the newborns and children, originally aimed at warding off illnesses, have been abandoned.
- Monks perform ceremonial hair clippings and bless the infant to grow up healthy, usually during the first month of life when the baby is brought to the temple.
- As stated earlier, Buddhism does not subscribe to the concept of circumcision, but has no objection should the parents choose to have their babies circumcised, which is mainly for reasons of personal hygiene.
- "Loving-kindness, compassion, sympathetic joy, and equanimity" are the virtues that Buddhist parents practice, known as the *Four Holy Abiding* or the *Four Virtues of Divinity*. Buddhist parents love to be very near and close to their children, from the moment they are born until they grow up. Anything that promotes such a circumstance in the clinical setting is generally encouraged and would greatly accelerate the process of healing, or allow an invaluable opportunity for reconciliation and a peaceful departure among immediate family, close friends, and relatives.
- In the event of fetal demise, the fetus would be taken to the temple for the monks to conduct ceremonial sutra chanting to pass the merits onto the baby and offering a blessing for rebirth into a better realm. Following this, the fetus would be cremated with the ashes subsequently being spread in the river.

During Illness

- Buddhists should be encouraged to think of sickness in this way: *whenever one is sick, one should think that the disease may be curable or incurable and one may even die, while undergoing treatment. If one only thinks of being cured, one would surely suffer.*
- Monks may be invited to visit Buddhists who are sick. They would give advice and teach the patients to: clear their minds and meditate on the uncertainty of life; to see the true nature of things (body and mind); learn to "let go" so that one would not suffer; they would also bless patients to facilitate a speedy recovery.
- Frequently, Buddhists may bring a small Buddha statue or image to set up as a temporary altar or a shrine above or by the head of the patient's bed. Health care providers should allow them to do so and be sensitive to treating the Buddha statue or image respectfully. Any insult to the Buddha statue or the image would create conflict and could cause animosity toward the health care personnel.
- During illness, the Buddha advised his followers on "how to deal with pain and suffering" through having the right perspective of life, as follows:

O' monks. A worldly, who has never learned about pain and suffering, whenever encounters it, would be sad, crying, lamenting, beating his chest, mourning … He would have suffered from such feelings, namely, physical suffering and mental suffering.

O' monks. It is similar to a sharp shooter shot an arrow at a person, and then shoots him again with a second arrow. Therefore, that person would suffer from being hit with both arrows, namely, physical suffering and mental suffering.

O' monks. A Noble disciple who has learned about pain and suffering, whenever encounters it, would not be sad, not crying, not lamenting, not beating his chest, nor mourning … He would suffer only physically, but not suffer mentally … It is similar to a sharp shooter shot an arrow to the person, then shoots him again with a second arrow, but missed. Therefore, such person would suffer once from the first arrow only.[179]

- Health care providers should try to help patients to maintain their dignity during their illnesses. Thai physicians have been taught to remind themselves of the famous Buddhist proverb of "Putting yourself in their shoes" (*Attanam Uppamam Gare*), which has become the slogan of Siriraj Medical School, Mahidol University, Bangkok, Thailand. This is to remind the health care professionals to be compassionate to all patients they are taking care of and to treat them properly as if the patients were themselves, or their own parents and relatives.

During End of Life
- Buddhists generally care for and support one another during the times of severe illnesses and dying.
- It is important for Buddhists to show respect and pay their gratitude to their parents who had raised them previously, and to care for them during their illness or end of life.
- End of life is the time to reconcile with one's family, friends, and relatives, but above all with oneself – one's own body and mind.

- At or near the moment of death, a monk or monks may be invited to comfort, and give blessing to the dying person. He would advise the patient to be mindfully aware and to let go of all desire, craving, conflict, and clinging. The patient is counseled to remain mindful and aware to the very last moment of life, with a clear mind to avoid any future rebirth. Above all, he or she should realize the "selfless" nature, the true nature of his or her own body and mind, not worth clinging to.
- Relatives and friends can frequently remind the dying person to be mindful by repeatedly reciting "*Buddho*" (enlightenment) or "Don't forget to become an *Arahant*" (enlightened one). The very last moment of one's life is utmost important, as it is a great opportunity to be able to attain freedom from suffering, not only physically, but also mentally.
- Insight Meditation on the *Four Foundations of Mindfulness*, and *Mindfulness with Breathing*, and so forth, are frequently advised as a way to gain insights into seeing the true nature of oneself clearly, and to let go and free oneself from suffering.
- The Buddha specifically advised the dying persons to meditate on "mindfulness" and "self-awareness" which are the keys to realizing the truth and to letting go, ending the cycle of births and deaths (*samsara*). (Please see the section entitled "Practical Method for the Terminal Phase of Life" for the actual techniques; it is found after the "Scriptures, Inspirational Readings, and Prayers" section.)
- Health care professionals, besides keeping the family and relatives informed honestly and truthfully on the patient's status and condition, should be kind and sensitive

---

179 *Sanlatta Sutra*. PTS (the Pali Text Society's English version of the Tipitaka). Oxford: Pali Text Society, KS. 4: 139–140.

in treating the patient as a human being, not just another number in their daily routine. They may help support dying Buddhist patients by allowing their families to stay with and remain close to them. This would give them the opportunity to reconcile and forgive each other. Family members could comfort and advise the patients to clear their minds and not to worry and be concerned with their businesses or other members of their families. Such friendly environment and counseling would allow the patients to remain calm and peaceful, and be mindfully aware of their own bodies and minds, thus, providing a greater chance to end the cycle of births and deaths (*samsara*) and suffering, or, if not, to emerge into a better realm in rebirth.

- Families should be allowed to bring in audiotapes or videotapes on *dharma* teachings, chanting or praying for the patients to listen to, which would help calm the patients and clear their minds from any craving and clinging. Patients may also pray along the recorded praying, or may chant from the written texts or their own memory.

Care of the Body

- According to the Thai Buddhist tradition, the deceased's body would be cleaned and dressed by a close family member, possibly embalmed, and displayed for a brief visitation by the close relatives, friends and family. This serves as the last moment to say goodbye, ask for forgiveness, and pay respect to the person, by gently pouring scented water on the right palm of the deceased. Shortly afterward the body would then be placed in the coffin, which would be permanently sealed.
- The coffin containing the body would

be placed on an altar for a religious ceremony. During the service, monks would chant the *Abhidharma* (*the Very Truths*) *Sutras* or the Buddha's teachings to pass on the merit to the deceased, and to prompt family, friends and relatives to be mindfully aware of their own lives by witnessing the uncertainty of life, right in front of them. Such sutra chanting and memorial services may go on for 3, 5, or 7 days during the early night hours.

- Cremation is the preferred means of disposition of the body. Theravada Buddhists follow the Indian custom of burning the body at death. The Buddha's body was cremated, and this set the example for many Buddhists, even in the West. Cremation by burning the coffin containing the corpse, in total, may be done on the day that follows the religious ceremony, or at a much later date (possibly 3 months to a year), though at times even longer because the family may still be mourning the deceased. The coffin containing the body would be kept at the mausoleum at the temple until the time of cremation. This is the one indispensable service rendered to the community by the monks in Buddhist countries like Thailand. In the United States, the body may be displayed at a local funeral home, with the coffin either opened or closed. Monks are invited to recite the sutras at the funeral service for 1–2 nights, before the body is cremated at a mausoleum that handles cremation. Cremation is frequently done in certain parts of the United States: up to 50% in California, even 20 years ago, while it was only 10% in the Midwest.
- Autopsy can be done upon request, either for educational, investigational, or mandatory purposes, as there is no restriction or rule against autopsy. In fact,

the Buddha advised one to observe decaying corpses as a means of meditation on the body, to see what would happen to one's own body after death and to witness the uncertainty and selfless nature of life. In older days, certain forest monks would meditate in a cemetery on the autopsied specimens of the unattended corpses or skeletons, to observe various decaying steps and the changing nature of life.

- Many Buddhists would be willing to donate their bodies to medical schools to be used as dissecting specimens for education as an act of generosity (*dana*), one of the practical aspects of Buddhism.

Organ and Tissue Donation

- Buddhism has no objection to organ or tissue donation.
- Giving or generosity is one of the practical aspects of Buddhism. Therefore, many Buddhists donate their organs for transplantation as a way of making merit. It serves as the final merit making initiated and planned by the dead, which may generate proud moments for the family and relative in saving other lives as well. It may be preferable for a chaplain and/or nurse who are trained designated requesters to be consulted for assistance.

Scriptures, Inspirational Readings, and Prayers

- There are many written scriptures for inspirational readings in Buddhism, with the classical and original teachings by the Buddha himself being recorded in the Tipitaka, which consists of 45 volumes. Together with the commentaries, it expands into 91 volumes in the Thai version.
- There are innumerable inspirational readings in Buddhism written by great teachers of various eras up to the present time. The classical inspirational readings include the *Dharmapada* (The 423 sayings by the Buddha), the *Path of Purification* (*Visuddhimagga*), the *Questions of King Milinda*, the *Buddha-dharma*, and so forth.
- Buddhist Prayers are chanted in Pali, the official language of Buddhism; sometimes the prayers are chanted with translation into the vernacular. Examples are prayers on the Virtues of the *Buddha*, *Dharma*, and *Sangha*; verses taken from *Dharmapada*; the 38 Highest Blessings (*Mangala*); *Jinapanjara-Gatha* (verse on the Conqueror's Mansion).
- Monks would chant the morning and evening prayers on a daily basis as a part of their daily activities. Many prayers are taken from the sutras, describing the teachings by the Buddha on various topics of life, body, and mind, centering on the Four Noble Truths, the Seven Factors of Enlightenment, and so forth. There are innumerable recorded versions of such chanting by monks, readily available for the patients to listen to.

READING DURING ILLNESS

This can be read by family, friends, health care professionals, or the patients themselves.

The Supreme Attitudes (Sharing the loving kindness)

Ahang sukhito homi,	*May I be happy,*
Niddukkho homi,	*may I be free from stress and pain,*
Avēro homi,	*may I be free from animosity,*
Abyāpajjho homi,	*may I be free from oppression,*
Anīgho homi,	*may I be free from trouble,*
Sukhī attānang pariharāmi,	*may I look after myself with ease,*
Sabbē sattā sukhitā hontu,	*may all living beings be happy,*
Sabbē sattā avērā hontu,	*may all living beings be free from animosity,*
Sabbē sattā abyapajjhā hontu,	*may all living beings be free from oppression,*
Sabbē sattā anīghā hontu,	*may all living beings be free from trouble,*
Sabbē sattā sukhī attānang pariharantu,	*may all living beings look after themselves with ease,*
Sabbē sattā sabba-dukkhā pamuñcantu,	*may all living beings be free from all stress and suffering,*
Sabbē sattā laddha-sampattito mā vigacchantu,	*may all living beings not be deprived of the good fortune they have attained,*
Sabbē sattā kammassakā kamma-dāyādā kamma-yoni kamma-bandhu kamma-patisaranā,	*All living beings are the owners of their karma, heir to their karma, born of their karma, related through their karma, and live dependently on their karma.*
Yang kammang karissanti kalyānang vā pāpakang vā,	*whatever they do, for good or for evil,*
Tassa dāyādā bhavissanti,	*to that will they fall heir,*
Sabbē sattā sadā hontu,	*may all beings live happily,*
Avērā sukha-jīvino,	*always free from animosity.*
Katang puñña-phalang mai-hang,	*may all share in the blessings,*
Sabbē bhāgī bhavantu tē,	*springing from the good I have done,*
Hotu sabbang sumanggalang,	*may there be every good blessing,*
Rakkhantu sabba-dēvatā,	*may the devas (angels) protect you,*
Sabba-buddhānubhāvēna,	*by the power of all the Buddhas,*
Sotthī hontu nirantarang,	*may you forever be well,*
Hotu sabbang sumanggalang,	*may there be every good blessing,*
Rakkhantu sabba-dēvatā,	*may the devas protect you,*
Sabba-dhammānubhāvēna,	*by the power of all the Dharma,*
Sotthī hontu nirantarang,	*may you forever be well,*
Hotu sabbang sumanggalang,	*may there be every good blessing,*
Rakkhantu sabba-dēvatā,	*may the devas protect you,*
Sabba-sanghānubhāvēna,	*by the power of all the Sangha,*
Sotthī hontu nirantarang,	*may you forever be well.*[180]

180 Council of Thai Bhikkhus in the USA. Chanting text (p. 16). Available at: www.stlthaitemple.org/books/Chanting_English.pdf (accessed 15 Sept 2012).

THE PRACTICAL METHOD FOR THE TERMINAL PHASE OF LIFE

The Buddha advised those who are dying to be *mindfully aware at all times*, as follows.

Kalanya Sutra

How would a mindful monk
  be like?
A monk of this Dharma-Vinaya
  (Teaching-Discipline) constantly
  reflects on the **body** at his body as
  his norm.
He perseveres with self-awareness,
  and mindfulness, he could get rid of
  worldly liking and disliking.
He constantly reflects on the **feeling**
  at his feeling …
He constantly reflects on the **mind** at
  his mind …
He constantly reflects on the
  mental phenomenon at his mental
  phenomenon as his norm.
He perseveres, with self-awareness
  and midfilness, he would get rid of
  worldly liking and disliking.
Such is called a mindful person.

"How is a monk with self-awareness
be like?
  A monk of this Dharma-Vinaya
who would normally be aware while
stepping forward and backward.
  He is aware while looking ahead
or sideway. He is aware while
stretching and bending. He is aware
while getting dressed. He is aware
while eating, drinking, chewing, and
tasting. He is aware while defecating,
and urinating. He is aware while
walking, standing, sitting, going to
bed, waking up, talking, or remaining
silent.
  Monks, you should be

mindfully-aware, awaiting for this
moment to hear my teaching.
  If the monk with mindfulness
and self-awareness, is heedful,
persevere, and determined in this
way, whenever happy feeling arises,
he would realize that the happy
feeling has arisen within him. Yet,
such happy feeling is dependent
on other factors to exist. What is it
dependent upon to arise? It depends
on this body to arise. But this body
is impermanent, and cause-and-
effect conditioning depends on each
other to exist, so how could such
happy feeling which depends on
the impermanent body to exist be
permanent. So, he would reflect
and experience the impermanence,
disintegration, discernment,
extinguishment, and tossing back of
the body and the happy feeling.
  In doing so, he would let go of the
desirable bias for the body and the
happy feeling.
  If the monk with mindfulness
and self-awareness, is heedful,
perseveres, and is determined in
this way, whenever unhappy feeling
arises, he would realize that the
unhappy feeling has arisen within
him. Yet, such unhappy feeling is
dependent on other factor to exist.
What is it dependent upon to arise?
It depends on this body to arise.
But this body is impermanent,
and cause-and-effect conditioning
depends on each other to exist, so
how could such unhappy feeling
which depends on the impermanent
body to exist be permanent. He
would reflect and experience the
impermanence, disintegration,

discernment, extinguishment, and tossing back of the body and the unhappy feeling.

In doing so, he would let go of the undesirable bias for the body and the unhappy feeling.

If the monk with mindfulness and self-awareness, is heedful, perseveres, and is determined in this way, whenever neither-happy-nor-unhappy feeling arises, he would realize that the neither-happy-nor-unhappy feeling has arisen within him. Yet, such neither-happy-nor-unhappy feeling is dependent on other factor to exist. What is it dependent upon to arise? It depends on this body to arise. But this body is impermanent, and cause-and-effect conditioning depends on each other to exist, so how could such neither-happy-nor-unhappy feeling which depends on the impermanent body to exist be permanent. He would reflect and experience the impermanence, disintegration, discernment, extinguishment, and tossing back of the body and the neither-happy-nor-unhappy feeling.

In doing so, he would let go of the ignorantbias for the body and the neither-happy-nor-unhappy feeling.

Whenever the monk is dwelling either in happiness, unhappiness, or neither-happiness-nor-unhappiness, he clearly realizes that such feeling is impermanent, not worthy of indulgence, nor enjoyment. He

would be free from defilement, even if while dwelling in such feeling of happiness, unhappiness, or neither-happiness-nor-unhappiness.

While that monk is dwelling in the feeling at the terminal stage of his body, he would clearly realize that he is dwelling in the feeling at the terminal stage of his body. When he is dwelling in the feeling at his end-of-life, he would clearly realize that he is dwelling in the feeling at his end-of-life.

He would clearly realize that after death all feelings which are but non-pleasurable would extinguish in this world for sure.

O' monks, you would have been the same.

While dwelling in the feeling at the terminal stage of his body, he would clearly realize that he is dwelling in the feeling at the terminal stage of his body.

When dwelling in the feeling at his end-of-life, he would clearly realize that he is dwelling in the feeling at his end-of-life.

He would clearly realize that after death, all feelings which are but non-pleasurable would extinguish in this world for sure."[181]

O' monks, it is similar to a lamp which depends on the oil and the wick to burn brightly. Since it ran out of the oil and the wick, that lamp, without fuel, would extinguish.[182]

---

181 *Kalanya Sutra*. PTS (the Pali Text Society's English version of the Tipitaka). Oxford: Pali Text Society, KS 4:142–143.
182 *Kalanya Sutra*. PTS, KS 4:142–143.

Vajrayana Buddhism

We are what we think.
All that we are arises with our thoughts.
With our thoughts we make the world.[183]

Prepared by:
Teri Brody, MD
Lama Chuck Stanford
(Changchup Kunchok Dorje)
Rime Buddhist Center
Kansas City, MO

History and Facts

Vajrayana or Tibetan Buddhism is perhaps the richest and most colorful of the three schools of Buddhism. This school incorporates the teachings of the other two schools, including an emphasis on the *bodhisattva* (an enlightened being who has not yet reached final enlightenment who works for the benefits of others) ideal. Vajrayana Buddhism is also known by the names mantrayana, secret mantra, adamantine vehicle, diamond-like vehicle, indestructible vehicle, ultimate vehicle, or *tantrayana*. With respect to this latter name, "tantra," Tibetan Buddhism is rich with its many mystical and magical practices called *tantra*. The earliest *tantric* teachings appeared in India around the sixth century CE.

Tantric Buddhism has a myriad of spiritual practices called *sadhanas*, individual spiritual practices related to a particular deity. Tibetan Buddhism has a plethora of such deities, each for a specific purpose.

These deities are not gods in the Western sense and, therefore, are not prayed to or worshipped, but are more like the patron saints in Catholicism. These deities are psychological representations for different states of mind. For example, *Avalokitesvara* or Kwan Yin represents compassion; *Manjushri* represents wisdom; and *Vajrakilaya* is for removing obstacles. There are also many more.

Prior to Buddhism's arrival in Tibet, the country's indigenous, widespread religion was Bon – a shamanistic, nature-based religion that views the world as divided between good and evil forces. The first attempt to bring Buddhism to Tibet was in the seventh century by King Songtsen Gampo. Now, one of the reasons for the lateness of Buddhism in coming to Tibet is the country itself. Tibet is the highest country on the planet. For this reason, it is often referred to as "the ceiling of the world." It was protected on three sides by high mountains and was considered an inhospitable place to live. For these reasons Tibet remained isolated for many centuries.

---

183 *Dhammapada*. (1993). Boston, MA: Shambhala Publications, 1.

King Gampo was believed to be an incarnation of the *bodhisattva* of compassion known as *Avalokitesharva* (Sanskrit) or *Chenrezig* (Tibetan). He built the first Buddhist temple in Tibet known as the *Jokhang*, which still stands today in Tibet's capital city of Lhasa. It wasn't until the eighth century when King Trisong Detsen brought the Indian saint, Padmasambhava, to Tibet that Buddhism began to flourish. It is believed that Padmasambhava overcame negative energies that had been preventing Buddhism from taking root in Tibet. Padmasambhava built Samye, the first monastery in Tibet. By the time of the Chinese invasion of 1959, there were over 6000 monasteries in Tibet.

As Vajrayana Buddhism spread from India to Tibet, a number of different schools (or sects) emerged. Although some cross-fertilization has always occurred between these schools, each has its own distinctive character. The schools with the greatest influence on the Tibetan Buddhism practiced in the West today are Nyingma, Kagyu, Gelugpa, and Sakaya.

- **Nyingma** (*nyeeng-mah*): This tradition is the oldest school of Tibetan Buddhism (its name means the "Ancient Ones"). Padmasambhava founded this tradition and established Samye, the first monastery in Tibet, in the eighth century. Among the many lamas responsible for introducing the Nyingma lineage to the West are Dilgo Khyentze Rinpoche (1910–1991), a major teacher of *lamas* from all traditions; Tarthang Tulku, who established the Tibetan Nyingma Meditation Center and the Odiyan Retreat Center in California; Namkhai Norbu Rinpoche, who lives in Italy and teaches regularly in the United States; and Sogyal Rinpoche, head of the worldwide Rigpa centers and author of the popular *Tibetan Book of Living and Dying*.

- **Kagyu** (*kah-gyew*): The previous head of the Kagyu tradition, the Sixteenth Karmapa (1923–1981), visited the United States on a number of occasions and dedicated his main center, Karma Triyana Dharmachakra, in Woodstock, New York. After passing away in Chicago, his incarnation was born in Tibet and escaped to India in 2000; his many centers in the West now eagerly await his return. Other Kagyu lamas who have established centers and taught extensively in the West include Kalu Rinpoche (1905–1989), widely considered one of the greatest Vajrayana meditation masters of the twentieth century; Thrangu Rinpoche; and Lama Lodu of the Kagyu Droden Kunchab center in San Francisco.

- **Gelugpa** (*gay-look-pa*): Atisha, who came to Tibet from India in 1042, started this tradition. Numerous lamas have represented this school in the West, including the late tutors of the Dalai Lama. Other notable lamas from this tradition who have had a great impact on the West include Geshe Wangyal (1901–1983), who founded centers in Freewood Acres and Washington, New Jersey; Geshe Lhundrup Sopa, retired professor at the University of Wisconsin; and Lama Thubten Veshe (1935–1984) and Thubten Zopa Rinpoche of the Foundation for the Preservation of the Mahāyāna Tradition.

- **Sakya** (*sah-kyah*): Was founded in the late eleventh century by Drogmi, a famous scholar and translator who had studied at the Vikramashila University. The current head of the Sakya tradition, the Sakya Trizin, speaks fluent English and has taught and traveled widely in the West. Among the other Sakya lamas who have been active in the United States are Deshung Rinpoche (1906–1987), Jigdal Dagchen Rinpoche of the Sakya Tegchen Choling center in Seattle, and Lama Kunga of Kensington, California.

Vajrayana Buddhism is primarily practiced in Tibet, Mongolia, and Japan, but today it is also practiced in the United States.

Basic Teachings

- In the Buddhist approach, life and death are seen as one whole, where death is the beginning of another chapter of life. The entire continuum is divided into four different, constantly changing transitional realities called bardos. Bardos are junctures in life when the possibility of liberation or enlightenment is much greater. Common usage of the term has been as the transition between birth and death, but this is not completely accurate. There is not one, but four bardos: (1) the natural bardo of this life; (2) the painful bardo of dying; (3) the luminous bardo of *dharmata* (the after-death bardo state, where the real light, or intrinsic radiance appears); and (4) the karmic bardo of becoming, commonly referred to as rebirth.
- **Spiritual Leaders**: In Tibetan Buddhism, great emphasis is placed upon the teacher or *lama*. The *lama* is viewed as not only a spiritual guide but also an actual embodiment of the Buddha himself. It is considered of utmost importance to have a teacher who will guide a person along the path.

The Middle Path

The primary guiding principle for all of the Buddha's teachings was referred to as the Middle Path. This path avoids extremes, which is perfectly understandable when one reflects upon the life of the Buddha who was raised in a life of privilege with every imaginable luxury. After rejecting the hedonistic life, the Buddha then set out upon a life of renunciation as an ascetic. After years of austere practices, he found this was not the answer either. So after his enlightenment, he taught the Middle Path of avoiding extremes.

The Four Noble Truths[184]

The Four Noble Truths were the Buddha's first teaching immediately following his enlightenment and were given at Deer Park in Benares, India. These teachings are referred to as the "first turning of the wheel of *dharma*." For a full discussion of the Four Noble Truths, *see* "Buddhism: General Introduction" chapter.

1. **The First Noble Truth**: The truth of dissatisfaction and suffering.
2. **The Second Noble Truth**: The cause of dissatisfaction and suffering.
3. **The Third Noble Truth**: The end of dissatisfaction and suffering.
4. **The Fourth Noble Truth**: The path leading to the end of dissatisfaction and suffering. The Fourth Noble Truth is the Way, the Path leading to the end of dissatisfaction and suffering. By following and practicing the Noble Eightfold Path – Right Understanding, Right Thought, Right Speech, Right Action, Right Livelihood, Right Effort, Right Mindfulness, and Right Concentration – we will overcome our dissatisfaction and suffering.

---

184 Cohen, N. Reprinted with permission. Available at: http://naljorprisondharmaservice.org/pdf/ FourNobleTruths.htm (accessed 15 Sept 2012).

The Noble Eightfold Path

1. Right Understanding
2. Right Thought
3. Right Speech
4. Right Action
5. Right Livelihood
6. Right Effort
7. Right Mindfulness
8. Right Concentration

For a full discussion of the Noble Eightfold Path,[185] *see* "Buddhism: General Introduction" chapter.

1. **Right Understanding** (or Right View) is the ability to understand the nature of things exactly as they are, without delusion or distortion.
2. **Right Thought** (or Right Intention) means one's thoughts, feelings, desires, and intentions are in complete harmony with the wisdom of life, in accordance with the way reality works.
3. **Right Speech** is the ability to speak truthfully and harmlessly.
4. **Right Action** means that one's behavior is ethical, honorable, and responsible.
5. **Right Livelihood** suggests that people earn their living in an honorable and life-affirming way, free from deceit or dishonesty.
6. **Right Effort** is the wholehearted, diligent, and energetic endeavor to train one's mind and heart.
7. **Right Mindfulness** (or Right Attention) means being attentive, mindful, and aware of one's bodily actions, sensations and feelings, and the activity of the mind.
8. **Right Concentration** is the means for training and centering the mind.

---

185 Cohen. Reprinted with permission.

The Five Precepts

For ordinary people involved in worldly life, the way to implement right speech and right action is to practice the five precepts. These five precepts are the essential minimum needed for moral conduct. They must be followed by anyone who wishes to practice the *dharma*. On a fundamental level, these precepts are intended to avoid harming (*ahimsa*) others. For a full discussion of the Five Precepts, *see* "Buddhism: General Introduction" chapter.

1. To abstain from killing any living creature
2. To abstain from stealing
3. To abstain from false speech
4. To abstain from sexual misconduct
5. To abstain from intoxicants

Basic Practices

- To become a Buddhist practitioner, an individual must have faith in the Buddha, his doctrine, and the *sangha* (community of practitioners) and choose to take refuge in all three (known as the three jewels).
- There is a saying in Tibetan monasteries that one should study:
  ○ the ethics of the Hinayana
  ○ the philosophy of the Mahāyāna
  ○ the meditation of the Vajrayana.
- In Tibetan Buddhism there are basically two approaches to spiritual practice – *sutra* and *tantra*.
  1. *Sutra* refers to the study of the teachings of the Buddha.
  2. *Tantra* means "continuum" or "weft" and is an entire system of spiritual practices, including meditation, used to transform the gross aspects of mind into the enlightened qualities of the Buddha's mind used for the

benefit of others. An important aspect of *tantra* is the transcendence of the duality of gender. Incorporating both the masculine aspect of *karuna* or compassion and the feminine aspect of *prajna* or wisdom are considered essential characteristics of supreme yoga *tantra*.

- In Vajrayana there are thousands of *bodhisattvas* that each has a specific purpose of enlightened activity. For example, Chenerzig is the *bodhisattva* representing *compassion*; Manjushri is the *bodhisattva* representing *wisdom*; Medicine Buddha is the *bodhisttava* representing *healing*, and so on. Each of these *bodhisattvas* has a specific *sadhana* practice (text) that includes recitation of the liturgy, meditation, visualization, and mantra all for the purpose of generating the associated enlightened quality of mind. The *sadhana* practice would be more powerful, though, if the practitioner had previously received the associated empowerment (authorization, teaching, and blessing by a qualified *lama*).

- An important aspect of Vajrayana Buddhism is having the proper motivation for one's spiritual practice. One's motivation should not be for the benefit of one's self but, rather, it should be for the benefit of others. This *bodhisattva* ideal of putting others' needs ahead of one's own along with *bodhichitta* is considered essential. *Bodhichitta*, which means "enlightened heart," is the desire to alleviate the suffering of all beings without distinction. There are various practices used for generating this kind of limitless compassion or universal altruism. While space does not allow a detailed explanation of each of these, they include the *lojong* teachings and *tonglen* practice

(exchanging self for others). Another method used for generating *bodhichitta* is by contemplating that because of karma and rebirth, all beings have been our mother in a past life. As our mother they were incredibly kind to us. They carried us for 9 months, gave birth to us, cared for us, fed us, and loved us just as our mother in this lifetime has done. Therefore, we should be kind to every being everywhere. No one is excluded. We should be kind and wish only happiness even to our enemies, because they too were our mother in a past life.

Principles for Clinical Care

It has been said that all of the Buddha's teachings are healing, since they all are concerned with recognizing and responding to the cessation of suffering for all sentient (feeling) beings. The Buddha described this fundamental principle in a medical analogy that is repeated in all the forms of Buddhism. Four basic motivations necessary for the practice of *dharma* are listed in the *Mahaparinirvana Sutra*: (1) to consider the teacher as a doctor, (2) to consider oneself as sick, (3) to consider the teaching as medicine, and (4) to consider practice of the teaching as medicine. The Buddha had a great influence on the *Ayurvedic* (an ancient system of medicine originating in India) medical system that existed in India at the time of his teaching, and this modified *Ayuryeda* was spread, along with Buddhism, throughout Asia.

In terms of matters of health, illness, and for most individual concerns, the most important person is the Buddhist figure that the individual considers his or her teacher and/or the head of the *sangha* (a group of spiritual practitioners). This would be the person who would be contacted if an individual became seriously ill, had a birth, or was in the process of dying. Even if these people were not in close proximity to the affected individual, they could perform prayers and rituals. Any member of the *sangha* could do the Medicine Buddha practice with or for the affected person. As mentioned earlier, the practice would be more powerful, though, if the practitioner had previously received the associated empowerment (authorization, teaching, and blessing by a teacher).

As Mahāyāna Buddhism developed, which emphasized compassion and working for the end of suffering of all beings, the devotional worship of the Medicine Buddha became prevalent. As an example of how integral medicine became with Buddhism, medicine became one of the five major subjects monks were required to study and master.

Dietary Issues

- Traditional Buddhist or *Ayurvedic* medicine considers nutrition very important because food is one of the few things that can directly affect the humors (*see* "General Medical Beliefs" section for discussion of this).
- A diversity of food types is best, avoiding overeating of any one food type.
- In general, it is said that eating a healthy amount of heavy and light food according to one's digestive ability is important. An individual needs to observe the energy level after eating (sluggish or energetic); if the stomach feels comfortable, heavy or full; whether one has gas, rumbling sounds, loose stools or constipation; and watch how different foods affect these factors.
- A vegetarian diet is encouraged, although

the majority of the population enjoys meat.

- It is best to avoid alcohol; if it is ingested it should be in very moderate amounts, certainly less than what is necessary for intoxication.
- It is best to eat hot foods morning and evening; a cold meal may be taken at lunch. Hot boiled water taken after a meal is believed to aid digestion.
- Food should be eaten in reasonable amounts, in regularly spaced meals to avoid hunger or overeating. One should be mindful to eat slowly, taking at least 20 minutes for a meal (the approximate time it takes for the brain to become aware of digesting food). According to the Tibetan tradition, when the appropriate amount of food is eaten, half the volume of the stomach should be filled with solid food, one-quarter with fluid, and one-quarter should remain empty.

General Medical Beliefs

- Euthanasia is not permissible in any way according to a precept in the *vinaya* (Buddhist monastic code) that prohibits the intentional killing of a human being.[186]
- Disease is considered a sign of imbalance in an individual's life and, oftentimes, this involves a lack of attention to spiritual issues.
- Mind is the essential cause of all illness in Buddhist thought. The mind resides in

---

186 Should any monk intentionally deprive a human being of life, or look about for a knife-bringer (to help him end his life), or eulogize death, or incite (anyone) to death saying "My good man, what need have you of this evil, difficult life? Death would be better for you than life," – or who should deliberately and purposefully in various ways eulogize death or incite (anyone) to death: he is also who is defeated (in religious life), he is not in communion.
— *Vinaya*, vol. 3, p. 72

the heart (not in the brain), and it is the state of consciousness at any one particular moment in time. It is the summation of all inner impulses, thoughts, fears, desires, aspirations, emotions, reactions, and sensitivities to everything. An individual's state of awareness, inner attitudes, and intentions all contribute to that individual's perception of the world.

- The primary cause of all suffering and disease is ignorance. Ignorance is not seeing or not recognizing how things truly exist. Ignorance manifests itself as the three negative states of mind (called the three poisons), which are desire, hatred, and closed-mindedness. These mental states in turn evolve into the three humors: wind, bile, and phlegm, respectively. These humors are subtle energies that circulate throughout the body and act as physiologic processes. They govern the body's physiology, psychology, and physiopathology via control of the functions and interactions of the five elements (fundamental energies of the universe), which compose the humors themselves, the body, as well as all other parts of the universe. The elements are fire, earth, water, space, and air. Each of the elements and the humors has defining characteristics and individual functions. The humors each concentrate in a specific part of the body (wind is located around the genital organs, hips, and waist), travel via specific pathways (wind travels via the bones, ears, pores of the skin, colon, and heart). Each humor is linked to certain emotional characteristics (wind with lust, desire, and attachment), and disturbances in each humor result in specific symptoms (with wind these include stretching, sighing, and overtalking). The three humors are constantly interacting together within

the body and are interdependent. As long as they remain in balance, the immune system is not compromised, and people are able to resist disease and manifest good health.

- Disease has no external cause, although bacteria, viruses, spirits, and so forth, may act as external conditions for disease. Disease is caused by people's self-cherishing ignorance, anger, attachment, and other delusions, and by the negative actions motivated by these negative thoughts.

- Diseases/disorders are classified into four types: (1) karmic, (2) secondary to spirits, (3) current lifetime or immediate, and (4) superficial disorders.

1. **Karmic** diseases result from negative past actions in previous lives. Since the cause is purely spiritual, the treatment must be also; regular medicines won't be helpful. Only a *lama* or high spiritually developed person can determine spiritual causes. If patients do not respond to usual medical treatment, it may be helpful to have them consult with such an individual.

2. **Spirits** are one of the main causes of psychiatric disorders. They are generally treated with religious medicines and rituals in combination with herbal medicines, mantras and traditional mantra pills. Unless the spirit is subdued by spiritual methods, no therapy will be curative.

3. **Current lifetime** diseases comprise the major category, result from humeral imbalances caused by actions in an earlier part of one's life and require medical intervention. Generally, spiritual practices such as disclosing past ill deeds, engaging

in virtuous activities to lessen their force, and developing an intention to refrain from such deeds in the future must be employed with medications.

4. **Superficial** disorders are self-terminating and don't necessarily require medical treatment since they are self-limiting. They generally result from improper intake of food or unhealthy behavior patterns and resolve when these are corrected.

- **There is a holistic approach to all four classes of disorders, both in diagnosis and treatment**; spiritual or lifestyle considerations are almost always an integral part of medical therapy.

- Western medicine is well accepted and may be preferred for life-threatening illnesses.

- If death is imminent, further testing or blood draws or unnecessary monitoring such as of intake and output, frequent blood pressure checks, and so forth, should be stopped so as not to disturb the patient.

Specific Medical Issues

- **Abortion**: Abortion is considered unacceptable because it harms the consciousness that is believed to have entered the zygote at the time of conception and carries with it the consequence of negative karma. Again, because Buddhism has no moral absolutes, such decisions are left to the individual. However, it is interesting to note that His Holiness the Dalai Lama in 1992 said, "There might be situations in which, if the child will be so severely handicapped that it will undergo great suffering, abortion is permissible. In general, however, abortion is the taking of life and is not appropriate. The main factor is motivation." On another occasion His Holiness said regarding abortion, "I think abortion should be approved or disapproved according to each circumstance."

- **Advance Directives**: Buddhists encourage the use of advance directives in health care planning.

- **Birth Control**: There are no prohibitions in the Buddhist teachings regarding contraception. Buddhism places great value on the sanctity of human life. Therefore, contraception methods that rely upon the killing of the fertilized egg and/or preventing its implantation would be considered unacceptable because they harm the consciousness that is believed to have entered the zygote at the time of conception.

- **Blood Transfusions**: Buddhists endorse the use of blood transfusions and donation of blood because they demonstrate the virtue of compassion.

- **Circumcision**: Circumcision is neither encouraged nor prohibited and, therefore, would be left to the discretion of the parents.

- **In Vitro Fertilization**: Buddhists support in vitro fertilization; however, it is an individual decision.

- **Stem Cell Research**: There is no consensus among Buddhists concerning stem cell research for therapeutic purposes; it is an individual decision.

- **Vaccinations**: Buddhism has no official position on vaccinations, but would encourage them as important to the health of the community; it is, however, an individual decision.

- **Withholding/Withdrawing Life Support**: A terminally ill patient, who has suffered for a long time, may choose to withhold food and/or medical treatment; however, this decision must be made by the patient him- or herself and not by the family or by the physician.[187] Unless the patient has left instructions concerning end-of-life care through verbal instructions, a written advance directive, and/or a living will, then withholding or withdrawing life support is discouraged.

Gender and Personal Issues
- As a generalization, people from traditional Buddhist countries tend to be much more modest than Westerners.
- Western Buddhists will expect the privacy that is commonplace in US society. The same would be true with personal hygiene issues.
- Personal preference would determine the desired gender of the medical provider.

Principles for Spiritual Care through the Cycles of Life

The Buddha revealed how disease and the contemplation of suffering can enlarge people's sympathies, motivate them on the spiritual path, and ultimately free them from compulsive behavior based on ignorance, greed, and aggression. Ultimately, the goal is not only to restore mind-body health and internal balance but also to remove subtle physical and mental defilements that obscure the Buddha nature. If people are able to address the karmic conditioning that limits their patterns of thought and action,

they will be able to progress on the spiritual path of wisdom and compassion that results in healing. Individuals accomplish this through meditation on the etiology of suffering and the inseparability of all of life; in so doing, they recognize and gradually eliminate the fundamental ignorance that is the cause of all disease. The process discussed here is very important especially for people with long-term illnesses and/or the dying. The facilitation of this happening, however, requires specially trained Buddhists.

Concepts of Living and Dying for Spiritual Support
- Impermanence is a major Buddhist tenet. Nothing remains unchanged. Difficult periods as well as ones of good fortune will inevitably change.
- People should see illness as an opportunity to develop loving kindness, compassion, and wisdom, as well as working on correcting the imbalance.
- Death is a part of life; death cannot be separated from life. Death is treated as a normal and natural event; death is quite ordinary, the natural result of birth.
- Death is not to be feared.
- Dying is an opportunity to come to terms with one's whole life.
- Dedicating one's life in death, for the sake of enlightenment for all sentient beings, decreases one's own suffering and makes death more meaningful.
- Suffering results from trying to hold onto something. In situations involving pain, suffering is related to how attached a person is to the pain and discomfort that is being experienced. The more the individual focuses on the pain and discomfort, the deeper the suffering. Distraction works at a certain level for a period of

---

187 If one who is sick ceases to take food with the intention of dying when medicine and nursing care are at hand, he commits a minor offence (*dukkata*). But in the case of a patient who has suffered a long time with a serious illness, the nursing monks may become weary and turn away in despair thinking "when will we ever cure him of this illness?" Here it is legitimate to decline food and medical care if the patient sees that the monks are worn out and his life cannot be prolonged even with intensive care.
—*Samantapasadika*, vol. 2, p. 467

time, but what is more useful is acknowledging the pain, and seeing it for what it is: an unpleasant sensation. To be really successful in dealing with suffering, one has to give up the struggle and the emotional labels attached to pain (e.g., "the unbearable pain" or anything like this that changes pain to suffering). Trained hospital staff as well as loved ones can help by gently encouraging patients to examine their pain in this way. A guided meditation that brings loving-kindness and compassion into areas of pain can also be very helpful.

- Buddhism believes in rebirth, and a person's state of mind at the time of death can greatly influence the quality of the next rebirth.
- Another very important concept in Buddhism is karma. Every thought, every word spoken, and every action has a corresponding result. This result will manifest itself in this life or some future one. Any event can be an extremely complicated mixture of many karmas ripening together. The effect of one's actions depends primarily on the motivation or intention. How an individual thinks and acts inevitably changes the future, including future lives. Past actions have created this life. Therefore, times of suffering, for example, are not punishment for some past action, but the natural consequence of previous actions. The individual is not to blame self, since he or she did not directly create the cause, but one does live the consequence of those actions. Pain is simply the effect or fruition of past karma. In Tibet, it is said that suffering "is a broom that sweeps away all our negative karma." What this means is that people need to take personal responsibility for all their actions, realizing they can choose

whether they will have future suffering or happiness. It also helps one look to future lives rather than maintaining an attitude of "this life is all that matters." How people deal with a current illness or the suffering associated with it could have great consequence in future lives.

During Birth

- Birth is viewed as only one of a continuation of the endless cycle of rebirths.
- Buddhists believe that a human rebirth is very valuable because only humans have the ability to free themselves from delusions and unhealthy thoughts and activities. Additionally, humans have the great potential to help end suffering in other sentient beings. So, the birth of a being with such potential is a terrific occasion for the birth family, but also for the human community who can also benefit from this person's life.
- Previously in Tibetan culture children were almost always born at home under the supervision of a female medical practitioner (most often a midwife) who is also a mother. However, today it is more common for childbirth to take place within a hospital. Immediate contact with the mother's body and breast-feeding are important.
- Blessing of the newborn is a wonderful celebration in Buddhism. The exact enactment varies with the culture, but all involve prayers seeking the blessings of the Buddha, *Dharma*, and *Sangha*. Auspicious prayers for the child to have a long life that is beneficial for all living beings are also recited. These ceremonies would be conducted by one or both of the parent's spiritual teachers if possible, or a seasoned monk or nun. If neither is available, then a senior member of the *sangha*

would be called. If none of those are available, the parents could perform the blessing while visualizing their teacher or one of the manifestations of the Buddha in front of them. Health care professionals would not be appropriate choices for leading this ceremony unless they were Buddhists. It is important to note that this ceremony is a blessing, but it does not impart a religion on the child

- Another common Buddhist ceremony for the newly born is a naming ceremony. Again, the exact procedure will vary with the sect or school of Buddhism represented by the individual performing it as well as that of the family. It may also vary according to the personal preferences of the same individuals. The person conducting this would be the same as with the blessing ceremony already mentioned. Generally speaking, naming ceremonies involve prayers to Green Tara, a form of the Buddha that is associated with health, wealth, and human relationships, to protect and bless the infant. It can also involve prayers for the child's enlightenment as quickly as possible. Prayers for the protection and guidance of the family and community members could follow as well as refuge vows to the Buddha, *Dharma*, and *Sangha* by the family and guests. Additionally, any special requests such as great spiritual attainment and good health and long life to all the child's family and friends may follow.
- The death of an infant or child, although recognized as particularly difficult for the family, would be handled in the same manner as if it was an adult. It might be emphasized that the deceased had very little karma to "play out" in this life and may well be destined to a very fortunate next birth. It is important for the family

to refrain from thoughts and feelings of either attachment or antagonism toward the deceased. At least expression of such thoughts and feelings should be avoided. Mourning and weeping by survivors can cause the deceased to experience darkness, frightening sounds, and painful feelings as they journey through the bardo (or transition state before rebirth). Since the mind of the deceased may wander about for weeks after death, the thoughts and emotions of survivors may influence the next rebirth. So, as much as possible, for as long as possible, especially loved ones and family should try to maintain positive thoughts and memories of the deceased and behave accordingly. Health care members involved in the care of the deceased or family members could help by reminding them that this death is not the end of their loved one. Life will continue. Rejoicing in positive memories will generate healing energies for the family and friends and spiritual support for the deceased. Rather than dwelling on sadness, survivors should be encouraged to focus on prayers and meditations.

During Illness

- The three most important aspects of healing are faith (in the medical approach and the prescribed medicines), compassion, and morality.
- Compassion is a key tenet of Buddhism, and illness gives all those involved a chance to strengthen and express it. The patient, the healer, the family, and anyone associated with the ill person should practice compassion.
- Friends, family, or health care providers can assist by meditating with the patients, listening attentively, and providing an unbiased sounding board.

- Setting up a small shrine in patients' rooms or placing pictures of the Buddha, possibly the Medicine Buddha, and their spiritual teacher may also facilitate their practice of meditation.
- Several specific meditation practices could be especially helpful and could be done by the patient alone or with family, friends, or members of the medical care team. *Tonglen* meditation, for example, could be very beneficial.
- The practice of *tonglen* meditation is particularly helpful for situations where a person wants to relieve the suffering of self or others. This practice of giving and receiving helps people to open themselves up to others and their suffering by intentionally destroying the self-grasping, self-cherishing, and self-absorption of their own ego, which is the root of all human suffering and the root of all hard-heartedness. *Tonglen* awakens compassion by reversing the usual practice of avoiding suffering and seeking pleasure. It can be done for the ill, the dying, the dead, or for those with any type of pain – mental or physical. *Tonglen* can be done as a formal or informal, so it is available at all times. *Tonglen* is a means of making one's own suffering more meaningful and, thus much more tolerable. The well-known American nun Pema Chodron states that by providing a means of relating directly with one's own suffering, *tonglen* becomes a doorway to well-being for self and others.
- Physicians need to be attentive and open; patients often feel that the doctor could "fix them" if they (the doctor) would pay attention to patients' concerns.
- A relaxed state of mind will be the most beneficial for patients; to accomplish this, patients need to be counseled in addressing their fears and encouraging them to let go of hopes of predetermined and possibly unrealistic outcomes.
- Letting go of attachments is an important concept in Buddhism. Patients need to be reminded of the need to avoid attachments during the illness. This should only be done by a *lama* or family member.
- *Sangha* members may want to perform the Medicine Buddha or Guru Yoga practice with patients.
- Listening to *dharma* tapes or CDs or reading scriptures or texts could also be beneficial to patients.
- Visitation by family and friends is generally welcomed but may need to be limited to prevent overtiring patients or trespassing too much on their privacy.
- Being able to keep prayer beads (*malas*) on their person during procedures where they will not get in the way may also be comforting to patients.
- It is helpful if Buddhist patients can have a serene, comfortable setting: for example, a private room.
- Being direct, open, and honest in communication with the patient may be most helpful of all.
- Additional suggestions for health care workers include:
  o When visiting the patient, turn your pager and cell phone to vibrate.
  o The quality of mind of the health care worker is also very important. Before entering the room, take a deep breath in order to clear your own mind and relax.
  o Take and make phone calls outside the room.
  o During each visit, try to spend a few minutes in silence, perhaps saying a prayer from your own religion.
  o Ensure the altar is kept clean and in the patient's line of vision.

○ Suggest the patient play audio tapes, or make use of other multimedia sometime during the day, to support his or her religious practice.

○ Contact the religious teacher and family as death approaches.

During End of Life

- Many Buddhists will refuse any medication that might cloud their minds such as pain medicines because a clear mind or consciousness facilitates the likelihood of recognition during death. However, more options are becoming available for pain control that do not affect consciousness; this is very important since fear of pain is one of the main fears of the dying.

- If a person has been on narcotics prior to the death process, tolerance of many of the medicine's effects develops so consciousness may not be affected. This information needs to be discussed and explained in detail by the medical practitioner so the dying person can make an informed decision about medications at the time nearest to death.

- Lama Zopa Rinpoche states that pain control that helps the person think is good, but pain control medications should not be used to treat mental anguish in the patient or family.

- Health care providers need to be aware that working out bad karma is prevented if the dying person is sedated before death.

- Buddhism considers one's state of mind at the time of death as having a great influence on rebirth. It is very important not to disturb the person near death more than is absolutely necessary, no matter if this is for tests, medications, answering questions or addressing family and friends. The most worthwhile thing anyone can do

for the dying person is to inspire them to think of others with loving kindness and compassion. As Lama Zopa Rinpoche explains, dying while thinking of benefiting others makes the person naturally happy and makes their death meaningful.

- If the dying people are suffering, encourage them to pray to whomever they believe in and ask that the suffering help alleviate the suffering of all others. Knowing that their suffering is not being wasted but has meaning for so many others will give the dying strength and compassion.

- As death becomes imminent, it is considered beneficial to read the ancient text *Tibetan Book of the Dead* to the dying person. This can be done by a *lama* or family member or even played from a CD.

- Listening to "chants for the dying" available on CD is also considered beneficial as one nears death.

- At death, a person enters one of the four bardo states called the "bardo of becoming." The longest duration of this state is 49 days and extends from the time of death until rebirth. The outstanding feature of this bardo is the predominant role of the mind. Interestingly, it is reported that people experience a judgment scene or life review during this bardo, in which they view all their thoughts, words, and actions from the previous life. The judgment is primarily for the purpose of determining if people can forgive themselves for doing, saying, and thinking what they did. It is also clear that what is ultimately important is the underlying motivation behind each of those things. It is during this bardo also that those still living can help the deceased. As rebirth gets closer, people begin to crave a material body more and more. There are a multitude of signs that indicate the realm into which they are to be reborn. If they are aware of these and their meaning, or if they are guided by a living person, they can sometimes determine or perhaps prevent rebirth, primarily by controlling desire, anger, and ignorance in this bardo. The teachings emphasize continuous opportunities for a fortunate rebirth in one of the Buddha realms or a human rebirth if they are well guided by their previous spiritual practice or knowledgeable living practitioners.

- A serene, comfortable, spiritual environment is highly desirable; the aim is to make the dying person and anyone visiting peaceful and unafraid of death or its trappings. A private room away from the nurse's station, if the person is in an institutional setting, should be requested near the time of death so disturbances can be kept to a minimum.

- The dying person needs to be approached and treated in a direct, open, natural manner; common sense and humor are the two pillars of this type of communication. Do not interrupt the person when they feel comfortable enough to express their innermost thoughts and do not offer unsolicited advice. Don't take things too personally; it must be remembered that the dying person is losing everything and may react with anger at the closest target.

- It is very important for family, friends, and health care workers to be honest with the patient. People need to know they are dying so they can address concerns such as apologies for regretted actions, preparing family for life after their death, saying goodbyes, details of desired funeral arrangements, and the large number of more business type or perfunctory things that need to be accomplished.

- The dying person needs to be encouraged to let go of all they hold dear and can't take with them. This includes family as well as material possessions. Attachments are causes of stress and fear.

- It is very important that the dying person absolve himself or herself of any regretted action. This can be accomplished by admitting the wrong acts, apologizing sincerely, and then imagining that the whole process is resolved, forgiven, and purified. These worries are a burden people do not want to carry to the next life.

- Patients should be encouraged to keep performing their usual spiritual practices. If they do not have one that they feel comfortable doing as death nears, it is important to help them to find a new one. It is also important to keep the shrine or any religious items clean and in the patient's direct line of vision.

- Favorite music or *dharma* talks may also be appreciated by the patient.

- A dying person's teacher should be notified when death is near, if at all possible. If he or she is unavailable, senior students or trained *sangha* members may be helpful.

- Simple meditation techniques and/or chanting mantras can calm the mental state of the patient as well as purify negative karma; these can be done with or for the patient by family, friends, or knowledgeable health care workers.

- Quiet meditation together is preferable to unnecessary conversation.

- It is important to know who the patient wants to have in attendance at the time of death and if there are circumstances in which those in the room should be asked to leave (e.g., if they become too emotional).

- Home-cooked food may be very appreciated by the dying patient as well as favorite articles of clothing.

- The patient may prefer certain bodily positions if able to perform spiritual practices, such as sitting up with legs crossed.
- Patients may prefer to lie on the right side, especially near death, since this was the position of the Buddha at his death.
- It is considered acceptable for a dying patient who has suffered a long time to decline food and medical care, if the patient sees that such care will only prolong his or her suffering and that death is imminent and inevitable.
- After clinical death has occurred it is customary to leave the body undisturbed for up to 3 days. This is because it is believed that the subtle consciousness (the essence that will be reborn) can remain in the body after clinical death has occurred. This, of course, presents challenges to health care workers for whom it is customary to immediately send the body to the morgue. State laws vary about the handling of a corpse. Cases are known where hospitals in the United States have complied with the family wishes by leaving the body undisturbed for up to 3 days.
- A practice known as *phowa* (transfer of consciousness) can be performed by a trained *lama* to facilitate the leaving of the subtle conscious from the deceased's crown charka. The *lama* can then advise the hospital staff when this has occurred and only then should the body be taken to the morgue. After that time, the body is considered only an empty shell to be disposed of properly.
- Immediately following death, the chant of *Sukhavati* is then recited (*see* "Scriptures, Inspirational Readings, and Prayers" section). This can be can be done by a *lama*, or, if none is available, family members can recite the chant for the deceased.
- A small shrine is erected with a picture of the deceased (to be burned later), along with flowers, a candle, and some incense. The shrine can be set up either in the family's home or at the Buddhist Center and should be left up for 49 days. During the 49 days, friends and family should be encouraged to do the meditation practice of *tonglen* in an effort to assist the deceased with any difficulties in going through the bardo experience. (It is believed that on the 49th day the deceased experiences rebirth.) It is believed that "letting go" will actually aid the deceased on the journey and to cling or to be overly attached may impede the progress through the bardo. On precisely the 49th day following the person's death, the ritual process is repeated, including reciting the Sukhavati chant. Then, the photo of the deceased is burned.

Care of the Body

- While the body may only be an empty shell, it is important for health care workers to always remember to treat the body with care and respect, which will be appreciated by the family.
- Whether the body will be embalmed, or if burial or cremation is chosen, is an individual family matter. However, most Buddhists choose cremation and generally do not use embalming fluids.
- Many Asian groups consider the corpse "dirty" or "contaminated" and thus untouchable. Therefore, tradition or family preference may determine if family members choose to wash the body as a final act of respect and intimacy or if medical personnel will perform this service.
- Some Tibetans collect remains such as nails, hair, and ashes to have blessed and placed inside statues, *tsa tsas* (molded

images made of clay or plaster) or *stupas* (a *stupa* is a religious monument that can vary in size from a few feet to several stories in height. *Stupas* customarily contain the remains of a great teacher, along with many mantras and *tsa tsas*. A *stupa* is a representation of the Buddha's enlightened mind).

- If it is determined legally necessary to have an autopsy it would be allowed in any Buddhist group.
- Donation of the body for medical research is an individual decision; the patient must have made their wishes for this known prior to death; this is not a decision to be made by the family.

Organ and Tissue Donation

- Most Buddhists believe that the merit of donating organs and/or tissue is appropriate if done strictly out of compassion to relieve the suffering of another sentient being, and not for any monetary support.
- Organ/tissue donation is basically an individual choice; the patient must have made their wishes for donation of organs or tissue known prior to death; this is not a decision to be made by the family. It may be preferable for a chaplain and/or nurse who are trained designated requesters to be consulted for assistance.

Scriptures, Inspirational Readings, and Prayers
DAILY MEDITATION PRACTICE

Refuge (3 times)
In the Buddha Dharma and Sangha,
I go for refuge until enlightenment is
  reached.
May my generosity and
  accumulations of merit
Bring benefit to all beings, and

may beings actualize perfect
Buddhahood.

Four Immeasurables (3 times)
May all beings be endowed with
  happiness;
May all beings be free from suffering;
May all beings never be separated
  from happiness;
May all beings abide in equanimity,
  undisturbed by the eight worldly
  concerns.
(Repeat three times, then say:)

For as long as space endures,
and for as long as living beings
  remain,
until then may we, too, abide to dispel
  the misery of the world.

The Seven Limbed Prayer
Reverently, I prostrate with my body,
  speech and mind
And present clouds of every
  type of offering, actual and
  mentally-transformed.
I declare all my negative actions
  accumulated since beginningless
  time
And rejoice in the merits of all holy
  and ordinary beings.
Please remain until samsara ends
And turn the wheel of Dharma for
  sentient beings.
I dedicate the merit created by
  myself and others to the great
  enlightenment.

Brief Mandala Offering
This ground, anointed with perfume,
  strewn with flowers,
Adorned with Mount Meru, four
  continents, the sun and the moon:

I imagine this as a Buddha-field and offer it.
May all living beings enjoy this pure land!

The objects of my attachment, aversion and ignorance –
Friends, enemies, strangers – and my body, wealth, and enjoyments;
Without any sense of loss, I offer this collection.
Please accept it with pleasure and bless me with freedom from the three poisons.
IDAM GURU RATNA MANDALAKAM NIYATAYAMI
E-Dum Guru Ratna Men-Da-Lakum Neeya-Taya-Mee

MEDITATION SESSION 20 MINUTES OR LONGER

Dedication of Merit (3 times)

By this merit may all obtain omniscience
May it defeat the enemy wrongdoing
From the stormy waves of birth, old age, sickness and death
From the oceans of samsara, may I free all beings.

Medicine Buddha Mantra

Recite the short or long mantra of the Healing Buddha, either 7, 21, or 108 times

Short: TADYATHA OM BHEKHANDZYE BHEKHANKZYE MAHA BHEKHANDZYE (BHEKHANKZYE)/RADZA SAMUDGATE SVAHA. (Bracketed syllable is optional)

Long: OM NAMO BHAGAVATE BHEKHANDZYE/GURU BAIDURYA/PRABHA RADZAYA/TATHAGATAYA/ ARHATE SAMYAKSAM BUDDHAYA/TADYATHA/ OM BHEKHQANDAYE (BHEKHANDZYE)/RADZA SAMUDGATE SVAHA. (Bracketed syllable is optional)

Chenrezig Mantra of Compassion

Recite the mantra of Chenrezig 7, 21, or 108 times.

OM MANI PADME HUM

Vajrasattva Practice (Purification Practice)

Refugee and Engendering Bodhicitta: I go for refuge until enlightenment to the Buddha, Dharma, and Sangha. May, I through the merit gained by generosity and so on, accomplish Buddhahood for the sake of all beings. (3 times)

Visualization: On the crown of my head, on a lotus-moon seat, is Vajrasattva, white in color and wearing all the ornaments. He has one face and two arms; in his right hand, he holds the Vajra and in the left hand, the bell; he sits in cross-legged posture. Visualize rays of light emanating from Vajrasattva's heart center, invoking the assembly of absolute knowledge deities who absorbed into him. We meditate on Vajrasattva's essence, the union of all the rare and sublime jewels.

Then recite: Vajrasattva, please purify and remove all harmful actions, obscurations of the mind, faults, and transgressions, which I and all other beings limitless as space have accumulated. After this prayer, in Vajrasattva's heart center, on a moon disc, the letter HUNG appears, surrounded by the hundred syllable mantra; from the syllables an uninterrupted stream of nectar arises, flows from his form, enters through the opening in the crown of my head, fills my body and purifies my harmful actions, obscurations of the mind, faults and transgressions.

Long mantra recitation:
Om Benzar Sato Samaya, Manu Palaya/Benzar Sato Deno Patita/ Dridho Me Bawa/Suto Khayo Mei Bawa/Supo Khayo Mei Bawa/Anu Rakto Me Bawa/Sarwa Siddhi Mei Pra Yatsa/Sarwa Karma Su Tsa Me/Tsi Tam Shri Yam Kuru Hum,/ Ha Ha Ha Ha Ho/Bagawan/Sarwa Tathagata/Benzar Ma Mei Muntsa/ Benzi Bhawa Maha Samaya Sato/Ah
   (3 times)

Short mantra recitation:
OM VAJRASATTVA HUM (108 times)

Afterwards join the palms at the heart: Confessional Prayer: Protector! Through ignorance and delusion, I have not kept my commitments and have broken them. Lama, Protector, give me refuge. O Lord of beings, Holder of the Vajra, who possesses the true nature of compassion, I take refuge in you. I openly admit all the Vajrayana commitments of body, speech, and mind – which

I have not fulfilled and have also broken, whether they are primary or secondary commitments. Grant me your blessings so that I am purified, and all harmful actions, obscurations of the mind, faults and transgressions are removed.

DEATH AND THE SUKHAVATI CEREMONY

Chant of Sukhavati
HRI
In the profundity and brilliance of
   dharmakaya
The compassion of Avalokitesvara
   arises.
In the magnificent and victorious
   vision
We proclaim the Jnana of Amitabha.
You are in the state of simplicity and
   you are free from fetters.
You have actually attained the
   fundamental enlightenment.
Please look upon us.
Forgive us our confusion.
Forgive us that we have been misled
   by the samsaric world.
I make offerings to you
I rejoice in your virtues
I request you to remain in our world
   and continue to turn the wheel of
   dharma.

Namo Amitabhaya
Samaya Tistuam
Please accept drinking water, flowers,
   incense, light, perfume, food, and
   music.
I praise your magnificent wisdom and
   power.
You can liberate all sentient beings
   with one glance of your prajna and
   upaya.

I request you to liberate the sentient beings who have passed and departed from their physical lives.

May they be released from their samsaric fetters and attain liberation at once.

If not so, may they attain a good human birth which is free and well favored.

If this is not possible, may they be freed from the lower realms.

I aspire to and worship your vision and your vow so that this particular sentient being (our brother/sister _____) and all other sentient beings may be liberated from the fetters and klesas, so that they may begin to overcome their mental obstacles and begin to understand the notion of egolessness.

May they be free from the ayatanas.

May they attain a state of liberation.

May the merit of the sangha provide eternal companionship for them

May the blessings of the teacher lead them on their journey.

May their relatives and companions proceed with them on their journey.

Namo Amitabhaya HRI.

Christianity: General Introduction

You shall love the Lord your God with all your heart, with all your soul and with all your mind ... You shall love your neighbor as yourself. On these two commandments hang all the law and the prophets.[188]

Prepared by:
Steven L. Jeffers, PhD
Director, Institute for Spirituality in Health, Shawnee Mission Medical Center
Shawnee Mission, KS

Reviewed and approved by:
Molly T. Marshall, PhD
President and Professor of Theology and Spiritual Formation
Central Baptist Theological Seminary
Shawnee, KS

Unlike the general introductions to other religious traditions/denominations (e.g., Anabaptist, Catholicism, Quakers) in this book, the general introduction to Christianity conforms to the same format of the individual faith-specific chapters. The rationale for that is much of the content in the various sections of many Christian traditions is virtually the same as found in this general overview of the world's largest religion. Furthermore, it was provided as a model to the authors of the denominationally specific chapters, with instructions to feel free to incorporate any appropriate material into their respective documents. Many, in fact, did so.

History and Facts

Christianity is a monotheistic religion based on the life and teachings of an itinerant Jewish preacher and miracle worker by the name of Jesus who was born in Palestine in

about 6 BCE. Detailed information about his adult life is recorded in the Christian scriptures in a literary genre called gospel, which means "good news." The following information is found in the gospel writings. During his earthly ministry, Jesus' teachings were mostly considered as anti-establishment by the majority in the Jewish community. Even so, great crowds of people thronged to him, but they came primarily for miracles of healing and out of curiosity; fewer came to receive his teachings. After a brief 2- or 3-year period of public ministry when he was approximately 33 years of age, Jesus was in Jerusalem for the Jewish celebration of Passover. At the beginning of the week, he was hailed as a king by the masses. By midweek, public sentiment was turned against him at the instigation of the Jewish religious leaders. Subsequently, he was arrested, tried by a religious body and Roman civil authorities, convicted of blasphemy and inciting insurrection, sentenced to death, executed by crucifixion, and buried in a borrowed tomb. It is what happened

---

188 Matt. 22:37, 39 (New Revised Standard Version).

3 days later that served as the catalyst for the beginning of this new religion: his resurrection from the dead.

The new faith tradition began in Jerusalem following Jesus' resurrection, according to the author of another document in the scriptures, the "Acts of the Apostles," which chronicles a theological history. The writer intimates, though, that this religious movement was perceived by the Roman government and general public as simply a sect of Judaism, because the early converts, who were Jewish, retained their identity as Jews. However, many within the Jewish community viewed this new group as a serious threat and launched an intense persecution against the "Way" (nomenclature of the sect in the early sections of Acts), having many arrested and actually killing others. As a result of this persecution, many members of the new religion fled Jerusalem into other parts of Palestine and into Syria. It was at Antioch in Syria that the people of the "Way" were first called "Christians," a designation that remains to the present day. Interestingly, one of the "Way's" chief persecutors was a highly educated and widely respected rabbi by the name of Saul, who later became known as the Apostle Paul, and it was the Christian community in Antioch that "ordained" him as the minister to spread its message of "good news" throughout the Roman world.

With respect to the New Testament scriptures already mentioned, the first written documents contained therein are attributed to the Apostle Paul, according to many biblical scholars. Thirteen letters in the New Testament are believed by many to have been written by him. Later New Testament writings include the four gospels, which relate the life and teachings of Jesus, other letters, a chronicle of early Church history

from its birth through the early 60s CE, and a document called an apocalypse, which means "revelation." These New Testament writings portray Jesus as the Savior of the world, the promised messiah of Judaism reflected in the Hebrew scriptures. A central message of that collection of writings was a belief that Jesus was the incarnation of God who taught a life of compassion, self-giving, humility, and the importance of inclusive community.

In the following few centuries, Christianity became increasingly identified with the Roman government and concerned with codifying its organizational structure and doctrine, as a reaction to "heretical" teachings. During the reign of Emperor Constantine, the capital of the empire was moved to Constantinople, and the Church established councils that produced creeds as official statements of the Christian Faith that were both Catholic (universal) and Orthodox (meaning right worship or praise). Five early centers of the Christian Church developed (Rome, as primary see, Constantinople, Jerusalem, Antioch, and Alexandria). In the fifth century, a Latin text of scripture was produced by St. Jerome, and St. Augustine became a great spokesperson for Christianity in the wake of the demise of the Roman Empire. Eventually, a schism occurred between the Church in Rome (the Roman Catholic Church or "The West") and Constantinople and the other early centers of the Church (the Orthodox Church or "The East").

During the early Middle Ages (also known as the Dark Ages), Christianity in the West became more focused upon other-worldly concerns. Because of poverty, ignorance, exploitation of labor, and poor health conditions in Europe, life for the common people had lost much of its savor and the other-worldly claims of Christianity become paramount.

The sixteenth century was a period of tremendous upheaval for the Catholic Church. A series of internal reformation efforts were lead by Martin Luther, John Calvin, and others. These reformers were reacting against church authoritarianism and the church's propagation of a "works-oriented" mode of salvation as opposed to belief in and acceptance of Jesus as Savior and Lord. Some of these early reformers' principles listed here remain foundational for the churches founded by them.

- All Christians are able to communicate with God without the mediation of clergy.
- Scripture is more central to the faith than the traditions of the church.
- Salvation and heavenly hope are the result of one's faith rather than through one's actions, although Christian practices issue forth from an experience of grace.

Today, Christianity could be understood not so much as a single religion but, rather, as a family of religions that vary widely by culture, as well as by diverse beliefs and sects. Broadly speaking, though, the Christian Church can be divided into three main branches:

1. Roman Catholicism
2. Orthodox Christianity (mainly Eastern, Russian, Oriental Orthodoxy)
3. Protestantism (many denominations and the most diverse).

These three modern-day segments of the Christian Church are reflective of the fragmentation that occurred during the history of the early Christian Church. Even though there are multiple traditions and a vast array of differing beliefs among the various Christian groups, there is a core of fundamental beliefs that most share in common.

Basic Teachings

Many Christians will affirm the content of the ancient *Apostles' Creed*, which is a brief statement of faith attributed to the early Church.

The Apostles' Creed

I believe in God, the Father almighty,
   creator of heaven and earth,
I believe in Jesus Christ, His only
   Son, our Lord.
Who was conceived by the power of
   the Holy Spirit;
Born of the virgin Mary;
Suffered under Pontius Pilate;
Was crucified, died, and buried.
He descended into hell (or the realm
   of the dead).
On the third day he rose again.
He ascended into heaven and is
   seated at the right hand of the
   Father.
He will come again to judge the living
   and the dead.
I believe in the Holy Spirit,
The holy catholic (universal) church,
The communion of saints,
The forgiveness of sins,
The resurrection of the body and the
   life everlasting. Amen.[189]

Many Christians will also affirm:
- All humans are fallen from an original state of innocence and are bent toward

---

189 Guilbert, C. (Custodian of the *Standard Book of Common Prayer*). (1990). *The Book of Common Prayer*. New York, NY: Oxford University Press, 96.

actions (i.e., sins) that disconnect them from God and others.

- All humans deserve just punishment for misdeeds.
- Humans can be rescued (i.e., saved) from just punishment through faith in the death, burial, and resurrection of Jesus.
- The final destination for those who have been saved from the consequences of their misdeeds is heaven, which is communion with God and all the redeemed in a state of peace, justice, and perfect love.
- The final destination of those who are not saved is hell, a state of punishment and disconnectedness from God and the saved. Opinions differ as to whether or not hell is eternal.
- Christians affirm the Bible, or Holy Scriptures, which is a compilation of 66 different books written over a thousand-year period. These writings contain wisdom sayings, history, poetry, social commentary, and devotional literature from ancient Semitic Jewish, Hellenistic Jewish, and early Christian authors. Some Christians also include additional books from Hellenistic Jewish culture called the Apocrypha. The number of these books varies according to the different traditions.

Basic Practices

- Christians value communal worship, and will gather often on Sundays as well as at other times to hear preaching, study scripture, sing hymns, and pray.
- The sharing of one's faith (evangelism) is of great importance in many denominations. Some of the ways it is communicated is through loving actions, talking about personal spiritual experiences, reading scriptures, distributing informational tracts, and discussions of doctrinal positions.
- The Lord's Supper, also called Holy Communion or Eucharist (meaning "thanksgiving"), is a powerful ordinance (sacrament or ritual). It is a liturgical reenactment of the crucifixion, death, burial, and resurrection of Jesus, in which Christians eat bread (to commemorate the broken body of Jesus) and drink wine or grape juice (to symbolize Jesus' shed blood). This can be done during communal worship or in other settings and is usually administered by ordained clergy.
- Prayer, meditation, and scripture are the fundamental spiritual practices for many Christians. The many forms of these practices include reading and/or silent contemplation upon scripture or doctrinal beliefs and prayers of various kinds – petition, healing, repentance for unethical thoughts and actions, praise, worship, and thanksgiving to God.
- Mission work is important to Christians. These acts of service may include working for social justice with marginalized peoples, charitable giving to provide food, building and educational programs for the poor, volunteerism, and so forth. Mission work is also an intentional witness to one's faith through proclamation and teaching.
- Infant baptism, practiced by some traditions, especially emphasizes the action of God in the life of the child. This tradition places a great responsibility upon the church community to raise the child to make responsible ethical and spiritual decisions and to influence the child to choose to follow God through the process of Confirmation, (summation of specific religious training – usually in early teens).
- Believer's baptism, practiced by some

traditions, emphasizes waiting until the child is old enough to make an informed decision with respect to his or her relationship to God. Thus, the responsibility is upon the action of the individual in choosing to follow the ways of God, albeit not without influence from family, friends, and faith community. Most of these traditions will also practice infant dedication, which includes the church community as an integral part of the faith-journey of the child.

- Christening is the ceremonial act that includes naming of the child. It can be an official part of the ceremony of baptism or combined with infant dedication.

Principles for Clinical Care
Dietary Issues

- Some Christians of many denominations are vegetarians for health reasons.
- Some Christian traditions observe kosher food restrictions. These will be discussed in the appropriate denominationally affiliated chapters (e.g., Seventh-Day Adventists).
- While many Christians have no dietary restrictions with respect to their religious beliefs, it is best to consult each tradition's chapter concerning dietary practices.

General Medical Beliefs

- Most Christians believe that God is the ultimate source of all life, health, and healing.
- Most Christians refer to God as the Great Physician.
- Most Christians affirm the validity of traditional Western medical procedures in the treatment of illness and disease.

Specific Medical Issues

- Most Christian traditions teach on the importance of the use of **advance directives** in health care preplanning.
- Christian groups have differing opinions about certain medical procedures and practices such as **abortion, birth control, circumcision, in vitro fertilization, stem cell research** for therapeutic purposes, **vaccinations,** and **blood transfusions.** These will be discussed in the appropriate denominationally affiliated chapter (e.g., Catholic, Jehovah's Witnesses).
- **Withholding/Withdrawing Life Support**: In medically futile cases this does not violate teachings of Christian faith. It is an individual decision.

Gender and Personal Issues

- Christianity as a faith tradition has no prescriptions or proscriptions with respect to gender and personal issues. Any deviations from this will be discussed in the specific denominational chapter(s).

Principles for Spiritual Care through the Cycles of Life
Concepts of Living and Dying for Spiritual Support

- Life is sacred.
- Death is something all must experience and should not be feared.
- Death is perceived by some Christians as sleep, a time of peaceful comfort until the Second Coming of Jesus. Others perceive that Christians are "with Christ," though not in the final resurrection state.
- The soul and spirit of the deceased ascend to heaven at the moment of death, according to most traditions.
- Resurrection of the physical body and the reunion of spirit, soul, and body in some

form will happen at the Second Coming of Jesus. Humanity, all living creatures and the entire cosmos will be healed and restored to a state of perfection.

During Birth

- Christening or baptism may be requested by family for a baby, living or deceased. The chaplain or clergy should be consulted for assistance.
- Christians in Western societies may request circumcision for male infants for cultural, not religious, reasons.

During Illness

- Patients may receive comfort from the reading of scriptures or other devotional material, listening to religious music, watching televised worship services of their own or a similar tradition. Patients may request Holy Communion. The chaplain or clergy should be consulted for assistance.
- Patients may receive comfort from healing prayers. These can be offered by health care professionals. Patients from some traditions, however, may ask for healing prayer to be connected with "anointing with oil" or the "the laying on of hands." The chaplain or clergy should be consulted for assistance for these requests.
- Patients may request baptism. In the clinical setting, sprinkling is an acceptable mode of baptism, even for traditions that practice immersion. The chaplain or clergy should be consulted for assistance.

During End of Life

- Patient or the family may request baptism. The chaplain or clergy should be consulted for assistance.
- Patient or the family may request Holy Communion. The chaplain or clergy should be consulted for assistance.
- Patient or family may request Anointing of the Sick, Prayers for the Dying, or Last Rites. The chaplain or clergy should be consulted for assistance.
- Family may wish to view the body of the deceased in the hospital room or the chapel. A nurse and chaplain should be consulted for assistance.
- Family may request prayers for the deceased. These can be offered by chaplains, the clergy, family, friends, and health care professionals.

Care of the Body

- Disposition and embalming are individual decisions. Cremation is now the choice of many Christians. The chaplain and the funeral home director should be consulted for assistance.
- Autopsy is an individual decision unless required by law. The chaplain and/or nurse should be consulted for assistance.
- Donation for medical research is an individual decision. The chaplain and/or nurse should be consulted for assistance. Advance planning for such donations is required by most receiving organizations. Last-minute donations are usually not possible.

Organ and Tissue Donation

- Organ and tissue donation is permitted and is an individual decision. It may be preferable for a chaplain and/or nurse who are trained designated requesters to be consulted for assistance.

Scriptures, Inspirational Readings, and Prayers

READINGS DURING ILLNESS

These can be read by family, friends, clergy, and health care professionals. (All scripture quotations are from the New Revised Standard Version.)

The Lord is my shepherd I shall not want.
He makes me lie down in green pastures; he restores my soul.
He leads me in right paths for his name's sake.
Even though I walk through the darkest valley, I fear no evil;
for you are with me; your rod and your staff – they comfort me.
You prepare a table before me in the presence of my enemies;
you anoint my head with oil; my cup overflows.
Surely goodness and mercy shall follow me all the days of my life,
and I shall dwell in the house of the Lord my whole life long.

—Psalm 23

We know that all things work together for good …
For I am convinced that neither death, nor life, nor angels, nor rulers, nor things present, nor things to come, nor powers, nor height, nor depth, nor anything else in all creation, will be able to separate us from the love of God in Christ Jesus our Lord.

—Rom. 8:28a, 38–39

READINGS DURING END-OF-LIFE PROCESS

These can be read by family, friends, clergy, and health care professionals. (All scripture quotations are from the New Revised Standard Version.)

I am the resurrection and the life. Those who believe in me, even though they die, will live, and everyone who lives and believes in me will never die.

—John 11:25–26

Do not let your hearts be troubled.
Believe in God, believe also in me.
In my Father's house there are many dwelling places. If it were not so, would I have told you that I go to prepare a place for you?
And if I go and prepare a place for you, I will come again and will take you to myself, so that where I am, there you may be also.

—John 14:1–3

PRAYER DURING END-OF-LIFE PROCESS

This prayer can be offered by family, friends, clergy, and health care professionals.

Holy and Merciful Father,
We thank you for the gift of your Son, Jesus, whom you sent to die that we might live. We thank you also that you raised Him from the dead, and that He is seated with you in heaven. We acknowledge that you are the Lord of Life and the Lord of Death. We ask that you send your holy angels to escort our brother/sister_____ through death into

your presence. Give our brother/
sister_____ peace and comfort
the family who will be saddened by
the loss.

In Jesus' precious name, we pray.
Amen.

Anabaptist Traditions: General Introduction

Prepared by:
Kathryn Goering Reid, MEd, MDiv
Executive Director, Association of Brethren Caregivers
Agency of the Church of the Brethren
Elgin, IL

Anabaptism began as a sixteenth-century Christian reform movement in Europe which attempted to restore the New Testament church.[190] "Anabaptist" is a term derived from two Greek words: *ana* (a preposition translated into English meaning "again") and *baptizo* (a verb transliterated into English meaning "to baptize") or "one who rebaptizes." The Anabaptists themselves did not like the term because they did not consider infant baptism to be a valid baptism. In addition, this term focuses attention on baptism as the major issue and de-emphasizes questions about the nature of the church and church-state relationships which were their basic concern. They preferred simply to be called *Brethren* or in the Netherlands, *Doopsgezinde* (baptism-minded).

The major roots of the Anabaptist movement include (1) Ulrich Zwingli, the Church reformer in Zurich who emphasized the direct study of scriptures instead of church tradition; (2) the revolutionary peasant movements of the fifteenth and sixteenth centuries, which can be seen in the communalism of modern-day Hutterite communities; and (3) the thought and practice of medieval mystics and ascetic monastic communities, which resulted in a strong emphasis on conversion, discipline, and the pure church. Early movement leaders included Conrad Grebel (ca. 1498–1526) and Feliz Mantz (ca. 1500–1527), both students of Zwingli, Hanx Denck (ca. 1500–1527), Hans Hut (d. 1527), and Michael Sattler (ca. 1490–1527). Menno Simons (1496–1561) became the most visible leader among the Dutch Anabaptists.

Menno Simons listed the "true signs by which the Church of Christ may be known" summarizing Anabaptist faith: (1) unadulterated, pure doctrine, theology rooted in the Bible; (2) scriptural use of the sacraments, rejecting the mass, infant baptism and the other five sacraments of Roman Catholicism; (3) obedience to the Word (discipleship); (4) unfeigned, brotherly love (love in all relationships); (5) a bold confession of God and Christ (missionary zeal); and (6) a willingness to suffer for the sake of Christ.

The following groups are often considered Anabaptist: the Mennonites, Brethren in Christ, Amish, and the Hutterites. Scholars do not agree about the degree of Brethren (Church of the Brethren, Brethren Church, Old Order Brethren, Dunkers) indebtedness to sixteenth-century Anabaptism. However, leaders of the eighteenth-century Brethren movement had some contact with Swiss Anabaptists in the German Palatine

---

190 Dyck, C. (1983). Anabaptism. *The Brethren Encyclopedia*. Philadelphia, PA: Brethren Press, 28–29.

and in Switzerland. In North America, Brethren contact with the Mennonites has been extensive. Belief and practice overlap, notably in a common desire to restore New Testament practices.

Amish

To you, O Lord, I lift up my soul.[191]

Prepared by:
Linda L. Graham, PhD(c), APRN, BC
Indiana University–Purdue University Fort Wayne
Department of Nursing;

James A. Cates, PhD, ABPP, Diplomate in Clinical
  Psychology
Amish Youth Vision Project, Inc.
Topeka, IN;

and various Amish clergy and community leaders
  (due to their humility, they prefer to remain
  anonymous)

History and Facts

There are numerous subgroups of Amish including the Old Order, New Order, Andy Weaver, Beachy, Schwartzentruber, and many others. The Old Order Amish make up 90% of the horse-and-buggy-driving Amish world. (*The majority of health care providers will come into contact with Old Order Amish.*) The subgroups primarily diverge in their emphases on separating from the world, reliance on the community as opposed to self or government, and humility. The differing sects also vary in their degree of "separation" from the world, and so forth, and actually form a continuum of Plain Peoples. The Old Order Amish now number approximately 231 000 in the United States and Canada. As with all "Plain Peoples," of which the Amish are one, their beliefs are biblically grounded and similar to many Protestant Christians.

The Amish split with other members of the Anabaptist ("rebaptizer") movement in 1693. In the late 1600s, Jakob Ammann, a young Anabaptist Swiss elder, urged the church to become more consistent in its practice of "shunning" unrepentant members. Eventually, he and his followers separated, beginning what is now known as the Amish church. Many Amish accepted William Penn's offer of religious tolerance in Pennsylvania, the first of several waves of migration to this country from Europe.

In the twenty-first century, the horse-and-buggy-driving Amish use no outside electricity sources to their homes, and a plain and prescribed style of dress and grooming for both men and women. (However, their "rejection" of advanced technology is an overstatement, as will be discussed shortly.) The Amish diverged from their neighbors in the past 100 years with the explosion of technology, making their resistance to modernity the most obvious difference. However, in years past, particularly during periods of war and enforced enlistment, their pacifist stance has been a source of greater concern for the community at large.

Amish church government is community based, although Old Order churches are united by a fundamental set of beliefs.

---

191 Quote provided by James Cates, coauthor of this chapter.

The *Ordnung*, or rules for living, vary greatly from community to community, but remain similar and unite diverse groups. Yielding to the *Ordnung* is considered an imitation of Christ, who willingly submitted to God, even to the point of death. It prescribes, among other activities of daily life, color and style of clothes, and the order of worship; it proscribes divorce, military service, and jewelry. Nevertheless, over the years, differences in beliefs have divided the Amish, so that currently the various subgroups all vary on the continuum of acceptance or rejection of technology.

Basic Teachings

- All humans are fallen from an original state of innocence and are bent toward actions (i.e., sins) that disconnect them from God and others.
- All humans deserve just punishment for misdeeds.
- Humans can be rescued (i.e., saved) from just punishment through faith in the death, burial, and resurrection of Jesus.
- The final destination for those who have been saved from the consequences of their misdeeds is heaven, which is communion with God and all the redeemed in a state of peace, justice, and perfect love.
- The final destination of those who are not saved is hell, a state of punishment and disconnected-ness from God and the saved.
- Amish affirm the Bible, or Holy Scriptures, which is a compilation of 66 different books written over a thousand-year period. These writings contain wisdom sayings, history, poetry, social commentary, and devotional literature from ancient Semitic Jewish, Hellenistic Jewish, and early Christian authors. Some

Christians also include additional books from Hellenistic Jewish culture called the Apocrypha. The number of these books varies according to the different traditions. (The Amish rely on the core 66 books.)

- Amish take 1 Pet. 2:9 literally ("But ye are a chosen generation, a peculiar people"); they should be different from the world.
- Amish maintain a fatalistic belief in God's will; all things work together for good, even apparent tragedies.
- Humility is emphasized; certain types of pride (e.g., in physical appearance or in accomplishments) are seen as significant sins.
- Because the "assurance of salvation" could be seen as pride, one hopes for salvation, but it cannot be assured.
- Public confession of significant sins is made before the church.
- Children are taught the acronym "JOY": Jesus first, Others in between, Yourself last. This captures the sense of community that Amish teach as essential to their faith.
- Church hierarchy (bishops, ministers, and deacons) are nominated by the church, but chosen by "lot," consistent with the practice of choosing a disciple after the death of Judas, the betrayer of Jesus.
- Because of the strong emphasis on community over autonomy, Amish spirituality is marked by both implicit and explicit rules of living. To an outsider, these appear culturally based, but for the Amish themselves, these rules are an integral part of their theology.
- Amish do not use icons of any kind; they take the prohibition against "graven images" very seriously (one of the reasons they avoid photos of themselves).
- Amish people are a hierarchical/patriarchal society; bishop, minister, deacon is

the church hierarchy; husband/father is the hierarchy within the family, but subordinate to the church hierarchy.

- The bishop's degree of authority varies between and within Amish groups.
- The greatest authority rests in the *Ordnung* (codified rules for living) and in the beliefs of the community, which vary from settlement to settlement.

Basic Practices

- Amish separate themselves from the world; individuals and settlements vary in the level of "distance" that involves.
- Amish do enjoy humor and teasing that is light and in good taste.
- Church leaders are chosen by lot; but the lot is believed selected by God. Church leadership is a position for life; there is no pay, and duties are in addition to all other duties as an Amish father, husband, and worker.
- Church meets biweekly; on alternate weeks, members visit other churches with family or friends.
- Churches meet in homes – basements, barns, or outbuildings. Members rotate responsibility for the service, as well as wooden benches carried in a wagon from home to home.
- Church services last approximately 3 hours, followed by a meal and fellowship; men and women sit separately during the service.
- Closed communion is celebrated in the spring and fall; all church members must be "in agreement" – that is, all controversy and disagreement must be forgiven before communion is taken.
- A bishop may serve one or two churches; each church may have several ministers and one deacon.

- The size of a church is determined by the number of families who can comfortably fit in a home. As the church grows too large, the group separates and another church is formed.
- Children are taught a German dialect in the home, and English as they enter school (although many learn English in the home from older siblings). Although "Pennsylvania Dutch" is often considered *the* language, there are actually several dialects among Amish groups.
- Amish practice adult believer's baptism; adolescents are allowed a period of exploration in the world called rumspringa before making a decision about church membership.
- For those baptized into the church and who fail to repent/confess sins, a form of "shunning" is practiced; this practice stems from the Anabaptist Dordrecht Confession of 1632.
- "Shunning" or excommunication varies by group; it can last a specified time, until the individual repents, or in the case of severe transgressions, for a lifetime.
- Amish practice pacifism; during periods of national draft, Amish affirm conscientious objector status.
- Level of pacifism varies by settlement, but may extend to reporting certain crimes to police, lawsuits, and legal redress for wrongs.
- *Martyrs Mirror* is a book found in almost every Amish home. It includes many stories of the deaths of Amish and Anabaptists who were martyred for the faith. It also helps affirm the pacifism of Amish beliefs, by encouraging a passive resistance to the world.
- Amish children attend school through the eighth grade, a special dispensation successfully argued in the United States

Supreme Court in the 1970s. Further schooling is considered unnecessary to their way of life. Children attend either Amish parochial schools or public schools; the decision rests, in part, on the affluence of the settlement, and in part on the decision of the parents. More and more children attend Amish schools.

- Amish children generally perform at a level equal or better than non-Amish children on standardized tests of achievement in parochial schools.
- Amish prefer "hands-on" work; traditionally farmers, more now work in factories, home shops, carpentry, construction, and cottage industries because of the limited availability of farmland. A strong work ethic is fundamental to their religious beliefs as well.
- Amish pay federal, state, and local taxes; whenever possible, many exempt themselves from medical insurance and social security benefits. The cost of medical care for an individual is shared by the family, extended family, church, settlement, and multiple settlements, broadening the circle as needed to pay increasing amounts.

Principles for Clinical Care
Dietary Issues
- No specific dietary restrictions are reflected in the Amish faith.
- With some heritable disorders (see "During Birth" section), there may be a need for a special diet.
- Food-sharing is an important nurturing practice in the Amish culture, a support in times of joy and sorrow.
- Amish tend to prefer simpler foods. They often can be fruits and vegetables from their own gardens.

General Medical Beliefs
- Amish are at risk for several genetic diseases.
- Farming and buggy accidents are also prevalent.
- Amish are open to state-of-the-art technology in medical settings.
- The Amish rely heavily on alternative and complementary medical practices (e.g., herbs, reflexology, massage, and irology).

Specific Medical Issues
- **Abortion**: Amish do not support abortion.
- **Advance Directives**: Amish do not normally provide advance directives.
- **Birth Control**: As a general rule, the Amish church does not support the use of contraceptives or surgical procedures as a means of birth control. That said, surveys and information provided by the Amish themselves suggest that a significant minority use some form of birth control to limit the number of births, or to delay the first pregnancy after marriage. The primary reported means of birth control is the male condom; the least prevalent but still reported means are vasectomies and tubal ligations. Female barrier methods as the primary means are less frequently reported than male condoms, but do appear to be used.
- **Blood Transfusions**: Amish do accept blood transfusions and organ transplants. Amish often donate blood.
- **Circumcision**: In general, the Amish support the practice of circumcision. However, it is an individual decision.
- **In Vitro Fertilization**: Amish generally do not practice in vitro fertilization.
- **Stem Cell Research**: Amish would oppose stem cell research because of its

identification with abortion; as other options for stem cell harvesting emerge, attitudes may change.

- **Vaccinations**: The majority of Amish accept vaccinations for children, although this varies by settlement. Vaccinations in adults (such as for influenza) are even more variable, but may be accepted for the elderly or at-risk patients if recommended by a physician.
- **Withholding/Withdrawing Life Support**: Amish families decide on a family-by-family basis regarding withholding/withdrawing life support. Generally, unnecessarily prolonging life is discouraged. Amish have a fatalistic attitude ("God's will"), and the realities of cost to the community may mean a resistance to extensive procedures, tests, and life-prolonging or costly interventions.

Gender and Personal Issues
- Amish maintain a greater level of modesty than the dominant culture; however, they are open to opposite gender health care workers.
- In the home setting, both genders may provide health care, but the majority is likely to be provided by women and younger children.
- Amish women traditionally wear a hair covering at all times; with different groups this may be the prayer bonnet or, in more casual circumstances, a scarf. However, a woman's hair covering should be removed only as an absolute necessity.

Principles for Spiritual Care through the Cycles of Life
Concepts of Living and Dying for Spiritual Support
- Life on earth is service to others.

- Suffering is a source of learning; it draws one closer to God.

During Birth
- The majority of Amish women receive prenatal care; they also use herbs and oils as alternative and complementary care.
- Birth may occur in a hospital, birthing center, or in the home; home and birthing centers are common.
- Delivery may be completed by a physician, master's prepared midwife, or lay midwife (Amish or non-Amish).
- The husband is routinely with the wife at delivery.
- Children are highly valued; consistent with a fatalistic view, the medical and physical condition of the child at birth is seen as God's will.
- Contraception is not supported by beliefs, although a reduction in family size among Amish in recent years suggests some form of planning.
- Average family size for the Old Order Amish is seven children; if the first delivery in the hospital is uncomplicated, the mother is more likely to opt for "low-tech" births at home for the next child or children.
- If a newborn is ill, physically challenged, or dies, the Amish believe it is God's will, but a clinician can appropriately express sorrow and concern for the loss or hardships ahead. Quiet concern and empathy will be appreciated.

During Illness
- Amish in inpatient settings will often have large numbers of visitors; their presence is a reflection of caring and support.
- Amish also accept home health care services from nurses and nurse assistants.
- Parents generally stay with children.

- It is perfectly acceptable to ask visitors to step out of the room during procedures, or for a period of time. The Amish themselves are usually concerned that they are not in the way.
- English is a second language, particularly for children until they start school.
- During periods of extreme stress or severe illness, Amish may revert to Dutch dialect in speech. (They are also likely to speak to one another in Dutch). An interpreter may be necessary at this point; family or friends can help in this regard.
- Amish will often appear attentive to what is being said by non-Amish, but will miss significant pieces of information. Particularly under stress, they will not request that information be repeated, and are unfamiliar with English "idioms." It may be helpful to ask the patient to repeat the information. To avoid embarrassing the patient, ask that he or she do so to make sure the clinician was clear in giving the information.
- At times, a wife will prefer that her husband handle questions, or a young adult will prefer that his or her parents handle questions. The clinician will be more likely to observe this through the interaction than be able to ask specifically for a primary spokesperson.
- Amish tend to speak with more deliberation than non-Amish; particularly with medical issues and under stress, they may search for "English equivalents" to Dutch words to make their meaning clear, or simply be too fatigued or ill to do so. Again, asking to have the information repeated may be helpful.
- Amish accept spiritual support from non-Amish spiritual leaders to varying degrees, as with all individuals. However, because of the emphasis on community, their greatest spiritual support is likely to come from groups of visitors who often include their clergy.
- One can always ask whether the support of the hospital chaplain would be welcomed; many will say yes.
- No prayers are said aloud except in church.
- A health care worker can pray silently with an Amish patient and family.
- Physical touch is limited, other than physical care; Amish tend not to be physically affectionate, except in periods of intense emotionality.
- It remains important to respect the physical boundaries Amish place; kindness and nurture may need to stop short of efforts at physical intimacy.
- Amish may at times seem unemotional and flat; this can be their way of keeping "distance."

During End of Life
- Amish prefer to die in the home, if at all possible.
- Amish do accept hospice care.
- Specific rites (e.g., anointing) may occur prior to death; this varies with settlements and families.
- Anointing is performed by a bishop as death nears. The anointing serves as a forgiveness of sins, both known and unknown; the forehead, and sometimes the hands, may be anointed while the bishop and patient pray silently.
- Church leaders and some lay members provide counsel about a variety of issues, including fear of death, ability to let go of life, caring for those left behind, and so forth.
- Funeral rites are simple, but very specific.
- Although salvation cannot be assumed because "assurance" can be perceived as

pride, the *hope* of salvation is present at death.

Care of the Body

- In the hospital, nursing staff handle care of the body. At home, family and friends handle care of the body. Viewing of the body occurs at the home.
- The practices of the hospital are generally accepted; there is no prescribed or proscribed ritual for preparation for transport or covering of the body.
- Someone is always present with the body once it has been returned to the home.
- Burial occurs quickly, usually within 2–3 days; graves are simply marked and are rarely revisited.
- Flowers and ornamentation are not used, nor are death anniversaries traditionally marked. Flowers in the hospital room are possible, but uncommon. Cards are more common – some patients may receive literally hundreds.
- Burial is the means of disposition.
- Cremation is not an option.
- Embalming is routinely practiced.
- The body is never donated for medical research.
- Autopsies are considered invasive and disturbing, although the Amish will generally not intervene if they are legally required; also, they are willing to allow it if an autopsy will aid others.

Organ and Tissue Donation

- Although there is no faith prohibition, the donation of organs or tissues may be a novel idea.

- As with all novel ideas, it will need to be discussed thoroughly; decision making is a slow, careful process among the Amish. Although decisions can be made rapidly if necessary, it is a courtesy to give time to discuss such decisions with extended family and church leaders. Therefore, presenting the option as soon as possible is important. It may be preferable for a chaplain and/or nurse who are trained designated requesters to be consulted for assistance.

Scriptures, Inspirational Readings, and Prayers

- Amish may have favorite hymns; some from the *Ausbund*, a hymnal used in their service, normally sung only there. Others are German-language hymns and more widely familiar Protestant hymns sung at other functions.
- The Amish pray silently before (and for some groups, after) meals.
- Amish read the Bible and choose their own favorite scriptures; some are integral to their faith and are well known to all Amish. The Amish are familiar with the Bible in Luther's German.
- Health care providers can encourage Amish patients to read the Bible but are discouraged from reading and especially interpreting scriptures to Amish patients.

Brethren in Christ

[A]ccording to the truth that is in Jesus, you were taught ... to put off your old self, which is being corrupted by its deceitful desires; to be made new in the attitude of your minds; and to put on the new self, created to be like God in true righteousness and holiness.[192]

Prepared by:
Samuel M. Brubaker, MD, FACS
Lay Church Member and Former Denominational
  Board Member
Elizabethtown, PA

Reviewed and approved by:
Don McNiven
General Secretary of the Brethren in Christ Church
Grantham, PA

History and Facts

The Brethren in Christ emerged as a Christian religious society in the late 1770s. It was one of the first to emerge in North America with no organizational ties to established Christian denominations in Europe. The founders were persons of Swiss/German descent with religious roots in the Anabaptist movement of Europe, but they found new spiritual energy in the movement called Pietism, prominent among some German Christian groups.[193] For nearly a century, they were informally known as "River Brethren," a name that reflected their initial location near Pennsylvania's Susquehanna River. The name Brethren in Christ was chosen by the United States congregations of the group during the Civil War, when they needed to register their society as a nonresistant organization whose members should be, for reasons of conscience, exempt from military duties.[194]

Although the spirituality of the early Brethren in Christ was shaped by Pietism, their lifestyle retained much of the Anabaptist heritage, which was deeply ingrained in many of them by several centuries of Anabaptist family histories. That lifestyle was supported by their Pietistic spirituality. Because these were rural, mostly agricultural, people they felt that advanced education was not necessary, and that, indeed, it may undermine the faith of the one pursuing education. Therefore, higher learning was discouraged.

Understandably, the posture of separatism formed a backdrop against which their lives were conducted. They remained organizationally separate from the established Christian denominations, which they regarded as being compromised to earthly powers or insufficiently committed to Christian discipleship. They avoided participation in matters of the general public,

---

192 Eph. 4:21–24 (New International Version).
193 Wittlinger, C. (1978). *Quest for Piety and Obedience.* Nappanee, IN: Evangel Press, 3–20.

---

194 Ibid, 27.

such as office holding, voting, and military service, choosing rather to serve the good of their neighbors by personal and churchly assistance as the neighbor had need. The self-concept of being pilgrims and strangers in this life was strong, as it had been among their European Anabaptist forebears, and was a significant characteristic of the group for about 150 years. Regardless of the costs of disfavor with the wider society and of any attendant personal discomfort or inconvenience, the assurance of Divine approval in this life and the hope of life eternal with God in the next, sustained them and lent an underlying joy to their earthly pilgrimage. The fellowship of other persons of compatible spirituality and similar lifestyle supported the individual during times of difficulty.

They did not regard themselves to be owed anything from the Almighty. Whatever favorable fortune or health they enjoyed was regarded as a gracious gift from God. Unfavorable circumstances, such as famine, war, and especially ill-health, were consequences of the imperfection into which the whole earthly system had fallen, consequences that were likely to impact godly persons as long as they were in this life. Such a mindset, combined with the fact that medical science was minimally developed, produced an approach to illness that might be described not as fatalism but, rather, as resignation after what was humanly possible had been done. Prayers for healing by Divine intervention were common, frequently with the attitude of "thy will be done." A better life awaited the believer after physical death occurred.

The first physician known among the Brethren in Christ, Dr. W. O. Baker,[195]

became a convert to the group in early adulthood. He practiced medicine in Ohio from 1855 to approximately 1915. That he was elected minister and eventually bishop over several congregations (as was the organizational pattern at the time) indicates that, at least in northeast Ohio, the Brethren in Christ people of the mid-nineteenth century were accepting of persons whose profession was the healing art. In the early 1900s, this same Dr. Baker, now a senior clergyman and local bishop, was chosen for 5 consecutive years by the annual General Conference to serve as Moderator. This would suggest that the wider group of Brethren in Christ (scattered in various states such as Pennsylvania, Ontario, Ohio, and Kansas) also were accepting of physicians and their efforts at healing. However, it would not be until the 1920s that a person of Brethren in Christ heritage would enter medical school. There is record to suggest that, even then, some persons were uncomfortable with one of their own entering upon a career of advanced education and medical practice.

The Brethren in Christ embraced major change in the 1950s and decades following. Higher education became common. Alternate service as conscientious objectors during World War II had opened the minds of many to wider dimensions of human need, and the possibilities of ministering to those needs. The separatist mindset of earlier generations became modified by motivation to serve humankind by engagement in the world. Missionary projects in Africa and India had been underway for 5 decades. Now, scores of young Brethren

---

195 Heisey, D. (2004). *Healing Body and Soul: The*

Life and Times of Dr. W. O. Baker. Grantham, PA: Brethren in Christ Historical Society, 504–505. Dr. Heisey has written an extensive biography, detailing the career of Baker as physician and clergyman.

in Christ entered the healing arts, many of them serving in mission hospitals and clinics. In the early twenty-first century, there are many Brethren in Christ persons practicing or teaching the healing arts, in various settings.

Along with changing attitudes toward education and practicing the healing arts, changes have come in understanding of illness and in seeking interventions to overcome or modify illness. The sense of separatism of earlier generations has been mostly replaced by an attitude of constructive engagement, motivated by a strong service ethic. The separatist lifestyle is no longer evident among Brethren in Christ members in the early twenty-first century, but strong remnants of the basic beliefs of the early generations persist in the belief systems of current members. These core beliefs are a source of hope which sustains believers through the vicissitudes of earthly life.

Basic Teachings

- The resurrection of Jesus Christ validates Jesus' claims for Himself and the Apostolic teachings about him. In Jesus Christ, the Almighty has given to humankind the fullest and best revelation of Divine nature, and of the Divine will for humans.
- The scriptures of the Old and New Testaments are Divinely inspired and form a reliable guide for belief and for behavior. Since Jesus Christ is the best and fullest revelation of the Deity, any content of the Old Testament that seems at variance with Jesus' teachings is regarded to be resultant from human failings or the earlier stages of progressive Divine revelation, and has become superseded by Jesus.

Through Jesus, the moral intent of the Old Testament has become possible.
- Persons become qualified for church membership not by birth but by personal assent to the historic, apostolic Christian beliefs about Jesus Christ, and by declaration of intent to live by Jesus' teachings as the church understands them.
- The church is to be separate from governmental control and support, should not use the power of government to achieve churchly goals, and should not compromise its commitment to Jesus' teachings for the sake of compliance with the goals or efforts of earthly government. From their beginnings, the Brethren in Christ regarded military service to be inconsistent with the teachings of Jesus; their current Articles of Faith and Doctrine assert the same belief. Therefore, many members have served their fellow citizens and humanity as conscientious objectors to war.
- Baptism is reserved for persons who have made a choice to accept Christian doctrine as understood by the group, and is the believer's testimony to that belief.
- Believers are to conduct their earthly lives in a manner consistent with God's revelation of his will and ways through Jesus and the Apostles, as recorded in the Christian New Testament.
- God extends attention and care toward the individual.
- Brethren in Christ believe that the spirit of a person lives on after physical death, and that the physical body is a temporary "house of clay" (2 Cor. 4:7) in which the spirit has residence.
- Brethren in Christ believe that eternal destiny is sealed when earthly life ends, and leave to God the determination of destiny.

- Eternal happiness awaits those who pursue godly living empowered by faith in Jesus Christ, or eternal disappointment, possibly misery, for those who reject faith in Jesus Christ.

Basic Practices

- Corporate worship is important. Weekly gatherings of the congregation – varying between 50 and 500-plus individuals – are for many the religious high point. These gatherings usually occur in church buildings. They include singing, scripture readings, prayers, preaching, and Eucharist, all intended to help the worshipper to focus attention on the attributes of God, the person and work of Jesus Christ, and the characteristics of living directed by the teachings of scripture. Inherent in the sharing of the worship experience is a strong sense of fellowship and interpersonal support.
- Small gatherings, usually fewer than 12 persons, for fellowship, study, and prayer are common. These groups gather in homes, at a schedule mutually convenient, and function without clergy. Study of the Bible, often using expository materials, is a major focus.
- Personal and family prayers and devotional time are encouraged. These practices vary greatly between individuals; they frequently include reading of a variety of Christian literature.
- The focus of religious devotion is toward the Deity, and with concern how to live according to God's ways revealed in the scripture. National interests are of concern, and often the subject of prayer, but are not a primary focus. Officially, the denomination disapproves the display of a national flag in its sanctuaries.

- Baptism is administered to believers of age sufficient to give personal affirmation of belief in Jesus Christ and intent to live in His ways. The mode of baptism is trine (three times) immersion, with exceptions made for persons of physical incapacity.
- Living as a Christian includes performing and/or supporting ministries to serve human needs, especially needs otherwise unmet. This frequently means serving in ministries to people affected by poverty, to the disadvantaged, to the disenfranchised. The service efforts may be conducted in the servant's home community, or may take the servant to distant places. The servants frequently work as volunteers. Many Brethren in Christ prefer to direct their charitable giving toward aiding the disadvantaged rather than toward philanthropic projects benefiting those less needy.
- Evangelism is important to the Brethren in Christ. This means spreading and explaining the good news about Jesus Christ, to people who have not yet assented to it, or, especially to people who have not heard it before. Evangelism is often combined with various service ministries, thus presenting a holistic ministry toward the needs of people served.
- Washing one another's feet, an act symbolizing love, humility, and servanthood, as modeled by Jesus, has been a practice from the beginning. Many congregations observe this practice at least once yearly, usually on Maundy Thursday.
- Anointing with oil in supplication for physical healing is a traditional practice, still observed by many Brethren in Christ. The rite is usually administered by clergy, although may be performed by a lay leader if desired by the supplicant.

Principles for Clinical Care
Dietary Issues

- The basic concept of dietary issues is that, during life on earth, the body of the Christian believer is the temple of the Holy Spirit (1 Cor. 6:19). From this flows the teaching that the Christian should avoid damaging that "temple" by indulging in use of substances harmful to the body. Thus, use of tobacco and recreational drugs, and intoxication by alcohol, are generally regarded to be sinful deeds.
- Dietary excess is regarded to be a health issue which has ethical impact varying with the individual. Moderate use of alcoholic beverages is generally disapproved, but a few tolerate it without moral scruple.
- Moderation is upheld as a virtue in all dietary considerations.
- The Brethren in Christ as a group do not advocate vegetarianism. Individuals may be vegetarian, or observe dietary limitations, but not on basis of group religious proscription. Dietary restrictions prescribed in the Old Testament are regarded as neither normative nor required for Brethren in Christ believers.

General Medical Beliefs

- The healing professional is generally regarded as a human agent through whom God works. Health care professionals will frequently hear themselves affirmed as assisting God in the healing process.
- The health care worker may be reminded by the patient or family that the worker is being upheld in the prayers of the support group.
- Favorable outcomes will frequently be attributed to the working of Divine healing powers mediated through natural recovery processes and the efforts of skilled humans.

- The response to illness, health care, and mortality varies according to the personality and temperament of each individual.
- Brethren in Christ members will often interpret surprisingly favorable medical outcomes unexpected by health professionals to be miracles flowing from the gracious help of a beneficent God.
- Health care professionals might also experience situations where the belief in special Divine intervention leads the believer to claim miraculous healing from a serious condition even after diagnostic procedures reveal no existent malady or a condition of minor consequence. Although some professionals may be inclined to regard such claims as intellectually dishonest, they can be more helpful to the Brethren in Christ patient by affirming that all health and healing rely on factors and powers beyond human knowledge or control.
- The Brethren in Christ do not prohibit surgical interventions.
- When unexpected disastrous events bring the prospect of sudden death of a healthy person, they accept vigorous interventions within the reasonable judgment of professionals. They commonly desire to have "everything possible" done to prolong the life of the loved one.

Specific Medical Issues

- **Abortion**: The Brethren in Christ Articles of Faith and Doctrine (1992) cites Church disapproval of induced abortion. Brethren in Christ couples will likely not entertain advice that a pregnancy with anticipated fetal problems be aborted.
- **Advance Directives**: It is common for Brethren in Christ members to enact

formal advance directives, by which they decline for themselves extreme life-extending measures whenever they should come to a terminal illness or permanently comatose state.

- **Birth Control**: Most families practice family planning, including contraception in any of its numerous forms: contraception is not regarded to be prohibited by the Christian scriptures.
- **Blood Transfusions**: The Brethren in Christ have no prohibitions against transfusion of blood products.
- **Circumcision**: Circumcision is regarded to be a medical issue, without religious significance to believers whose normative guide is the New Testament (1 Cor. 7:19).
- **In Vitro Fertilization**: Modern technologies of in vitro fertilization and use of donor genetic material are acceptable to some, but there is general caution related to the frequent byproduct of unused embryos and the attendant ethical dilemmas surrounding their disposition.
- **Stem Cell Research**: The Brethren in Christ have not issued a specific statement regarding stem cell research. As with modern techniques of treatment of infertility, so also would most Brethren in Christ be open to the benefits of new scientific developments, but would be hesitant to support any research that required the destruction of human embryonic life. Other avenues of stem cell research would not likely evoke disapproval of Brethren in Christ members.
- **Vaccinations**: The Brethren in Christ have no formal declaration or statement of guidance regarding vaccinations. Most members will gratefully accept vaccination for its acknowledged benefits, although a few may decline for reasons other than religious dogma.

- **Withholding/Withdrawing Life Support**: In general, however, the Brethren in Christ may as individuals tend to be conservative in regard to aggressive interventions. This is an individual matter, not in any way directed by group mandates.

Gender and Personal Issues

- Most Brethren in Christ feel that a healthy concept of body permits professional care, even intimate care, by persons of either gender, while they subscribe to traditional concepts of modesty and privacy. There is no religious teaching otherwise.
- Brethren in Christ religious teachings strongly affirm that proper respect of other persons includes maintenance of modesty and respect of privacy in all situations. The definition of modesty and privacy varies considerably among individuals.

Principles for Spiritual Care through the Cycles of Life
Concepts of Living and Dying for Spiritual Support

- The assurance of Divine approval in this life, and the hope of life eternal with God in the next.
- Unfavorable circumstances, such as famine, war, and especially ill-health, were consequences of the imperfection into which the whole earthly system had fallen, consequences which were likely to impact godly persons as long as they were in this life.
- Coupled with the belief that all events of life, even physical suffering, are used by God for His higher purposes, this deep trust in God's benevolence sustains the believer through difficulty.

- A better life awaited the believer after physical death occurred.

During Birth

- Life is regarded as a sacred gift from God, to be cherished and protected prior to as well as after birth of the child.
- The Brethren in Christ do not baptize their infants.
- Naming is usually accomplished without ceremony.
- As stated earlier, circumcision is regarded to be a medical issue, without religious significance to believers whose normative guide is the New Testament (1 Cor. 7:19).
- The denomination has not rendered official statements regarding modern methods of treating infertility.
- Parents commonly present young children for a religious ceremony called "child dedication," in which the parents publicly implore Divine blessing for the child, present the child to God to be used in Divine purposes, and commit themselves to nurture the child in the ways of Christian beliefs and living. The congregation also, in this ceremony, pledges to maintain a social and spiritual environment supportive to the parents' aspirations for the child.
- The Brethren in Christ Articles of Faith and Doctrine (1992) cites Church disapproval of induced abortion. Brethren in Christ couples will likely not entertain advice that a pregnancy with anticipated fetal problems be aborted. They will rather depend upon the grace of God and the sustaining support of understanding fellow believers in the accepting of risk for the sake of faithful obedience to Christian teachings as they understand them.

- The Brethren in Christ will be open to genetic counseling.
- Most families practice family planning, including contraception in any of its numerous forms: contraception is not regarded to be prohibited by the Christian scriptures.
- Brethren in Christ crave the recovery of sick infants, and deeply grieve the death of an infant, just like all parents. However, they believe in the moral innocence of young children, and thus do not entertain fears about the eternal destiny of a deceased infant. They usually can readily be comforted by caring and supportive health workers.

During Illness

- The Brethren in Christ frequently solicit the support of friends in the form of prayers for healing.
- The ritual of anointing with oil and laying on of hands is common, usually conducted by ordained clergy. This ritual usually occurs in home or house of worship, but may be conducted in hospital settings when circumstances warrant.
- The patient may desire Christian communion, especially if the illness has necessitated absence from a group gathering where the rite was observed.
- The Brethren in Christ do not decline the spiritual input of friends or clergy affiliated with other Christian denominations, although they may be unable to relate closely to spiritual ministries based upon strongly liturgical traditions.
- Prayers are usually spontaneous, and offered audibly. These religious exercises are commonly conducted by clergy or lay leaders such as deacons, but will frequently be conducted by any friend inclined to lead in spiritual input.

During End of Life

- When faced with terminal prognosis, the Brethren in Christ appreciate the hospice concepts of supportive care, and welcome the assistance of professionals engaged in this aspect of health care.
- Brethren in Christ members appreciate the visitation of clergy, and their assistance in resigning life to the Divine will.
- When unexpected disastrous events bring the prospect of sudden death of a healthy person, they accept vigorous interventions within the reasonable judgment of professionals. They commonly desire to have "everything possible" done to prolong the life of the loved one.
- It is common for Brethren in Christ members to enact formal advance directives, by which they decline for themselves extreme life-extending measures whenever they should come to a terminal illness or permanently comatose state.
- The Brethren in Christ do not offer prayers for the dead.
- Brethren in Christ offer prayers of thanks for the life of the departed, and commit the soul (spirit) to the mercy of God.
- Brethren in Christ offer prayers for the sustenance of the bereaved.

Care of the Body

- When the life has ended, the body is to be respected, but is regarded as destined to return to the dust from which it was formed (Gen. 3:19).
- Many Brethren in Christ will permit autopsy on the basis that it may yield information beneficial to the health of others.
- A small minority of Brethren in Christ members has become accepting of cremation, but traditional burial remains the preference of most.

- A small minority of Brethren in Christ are open to donating their bodies to medical science.
- Most Brethren in Christ members prefer to have a visible body presentable for viewing by mourners at a funeral.

Organ and Tissue Donation

- A small minority of Brethren in Christ members are open to organ and tissue donation. It may be preferable for a chaplain and/or nurse who are trained designated requesters to be consulted for assistance.

Scriptures, Inspirational Readings, and Prayers

Brethren in Christ members will commonly keep a personal copy of the Christian Bible close at hand in the hospital setting. They enjoy a wide range of inspirational, faith-building inputs, including many passages from the Christian scriptures, especially the Psalms, the words of Jesus Christ, or the New Testament epistles. Also used are readings from devotional or inspirational authors, and many hymns, of both historic vintage and recent composition. Personal preference and request will often be the basis of the choice. Some examples of favorites for many Brethren in Christ members are provided here.

HYMNS DURING ILLNESS[196]

Savior, like a shepherd lead us; much
  we need thy tender care
In thy pleasant pastures feed us, for
  our use thy folds prepare.

---

196 *Hymns for Praise and Worship.* (1984). Nappanee, IN: Evangel Press. Page numbers of songs are cited within the text.

Blessed Jesus, blessed Jesus, thou
hast bought us, thine we are.
We are thine, do thou befriend us, be
the guardian of our way.
Keep thy flock from sin, defend us,
seek us when we go astray.
Blessed Jesus, blessed Jesus, hear, oh
hear us when we pray.
Early let us seek thy favor, early let us
do thy will.
Blessed Lord and only Savior, with
thy love our bosoms fill.
Blessed Jesus, blessed Jesus, thou
hast loved us, love us still.

— Dorothy A. Thrupp, 1779–1847
(p. 459)

O holy Savior, friend unseen, since on
thine arm thou bid me lean,
Help me throughout life's changing
scene by faith to cling to thee.
What tho' the world deceitful prove,
and earthly friends and hopes
remove;
With patient uncomplaining love, still
would I cling to thee.
Tho' faith and hope are often tried, I
ask not, need not, aught beside;
So safe, so calm, so satisfied, the soul
that clings to thee.
Blest is my lot, what-e'er befall; what
can disturb me, who appall,
While as my strength, my rock, my
all, Savior, I cling to thee?

— Charlotte Elliott, 1789–1871
(p. 447)

He leadeth me! O blessed thought!
O words with heavenly comfort
fraught!
What-e'er I do, wher-e'er I be, still 'tis
God's hand that leadeth me.
Sometimes 'mid scenes of deepest
gloom, sometimes where Eden's
flowers bloom,
By waters still, o'er troubled sea, still
'tis his hand that leadeth me.
Lord, I would clasp your hand in
mine, nor ever murmur nor repine,
Content whatever lot I see, since 'tis
your hand that leadeth me.
And when my task on earth is done,
when, by your grace, the vict'ry's
won,
E'en death's cold wave I will not flee,
since God through Jordan leadeth
me.
Refrain: He leadeth me, he leadeth
me, by his own hand he leadeth me!
His faithful foll'wer I would be, for by
his hand he leadeth me.

— Joseph H. Gilmore, 1834–1918
(p. 391)

READINGS DURING ILLNESS

These can be read by family, friends, clergy,
and health care professionals. (All scripture
quotations are from the New International
Version.)

I lift up my eyes to the hills – where
does my help come from?
My help comes from the Lord, the
Maker of heaven and earth.
He will not let your foot slip – he who
watches you will not slumber;
Indeed, he who watches over Israel
will neither slumber nor sleep.
The Lord watches over you – the

Lord is your shade at your right
hand;
The sun will not harm you by day,
 nor the moon by night.
The Lord will keep you from all harm
 – he will watch over your life;
The Lord will watch over your
 coming and going both now and
 forevermore.

—Psalm 121

The Lord is my shepherd, I shall not
 be in want.
He makes me lie down in green
 pastures,
He leads me beside quiet waters, he
 restores my soul.
He guides me in paths of
 righteousness for his name's sake.
Even though I walk through the
 valley of the shadow of death
I will fear no evil, for you are with
 me; your rod and your staff, they
 comfort me.
You prepare a table before in the
 presence of my enemies.
You anoint my head with oil; my cup
 overflows.
Surely goodness and love will follow
 me all the days of my life,
And I will dwell in the house of the
 Lord forever.

—Psalm 23

HYMNS FOR THE END-OF-LIFE PROCESS[197]

All the way my Savior leads me; what
 have I to ask beside?
Can I doubt his tender mercy, who
 through life has been my guide?
Heav'nly peace, divinest comfort,
 here by faith in him to dwell!
For I know what-e'er befall me, Jesus
 doeth all things well.

All the way my Savior leads me,
 cheers each winding path I tread,
Gives me grace for ev'ry trial, feeds
 me with the living bread.
Though my weary steps may falter
 and my soul athirst may be,
Gushing from the rock before me, lo!
 A spring of joy I see.

All the way my Savior leads me:
 O the fullness of his love!
Perfect rest to me is promised in my
 father's house above.
When my spirit, clothed immortal,
 wings its flight to realms of day,
This my song through endless ages:
 Jesus led me all the way.

—Fannie J. Crosby, 1820–1915
(p. 439)

Sing the wondrous love of Jesus, sing
 his mercy and his grace;
In the mansions bright and blessed
 He'll prepare for us a place.
While we walk the pilgrim pathway,
 clouds will overcast the sky;

---

197 *Hymns for Praise and Worship*. Page numbers of
songs are cited within the text.

But when trav'ling days are over, not
a shadow, not a sigh.
Let us then be true and faithful,
trusting, serving ev'ry day;
Just one glimpse of him in glory will
the toils of life repay.
Onward to the prize before us! Soon
his beauty we'll behold
Soon the pearly gates will open, we
shall tread the streets of gold.
Refrain: When we all get to heaven,
what a day of rejoicing that will
be!
When we all see Jesus, we'll sing and
shout the victory.

—Eliza Hewitt, 1851–1920 (p. 532)

READINGS DURING END-OF-LIFE PROCESS

These can be read by family, friends, clergy,
and health care professionals. (All scripture
quotations are from the New International
Version.)

God is our refuge and strength, an
ever present help in trouble.
Therefore we will not fear, though
the earth give way and the
Mountains fall into the heart of
the sea.
Though its waters roar and foam,
and the mountains quake with their
surging.
There is a river whose streams make
glad the city of God,
the holy place where The Most High
dwells.
God is within her, she will not fall;
God will help her at break of day.
Nations are in uproar, kingdoms fall;
he lifts his voice, the earth melts.

The Lord Almighty is with us; the
God of Jacob is our fortress.

—Psalm 46:1–7

How lovely is your dwelling place,
O Lord Almighty!
My soul yearns, even faints, for the
courts of the Lord;
My heart and my flesh cry out for the
living God.
Even the sparrow has found a home,
and the swallow a nest for herself,
Where she may have her young – a
place near your altar,
O Lord Almighty, My King and my
God.
Blessed are those who dwell in your
house; they are ever praising you.
Blessed are those whose strength is
in you, who have set their hearts on
pilgrimage.
As they pass through the valley
of Baca, they make it a place of
springs; the autumn
rains also cover it with pools.
They go from strength to strength, till
each appears before God in Zion.
For the Lord God is a sun and shield;
the Lord bestows favor and honor;
No good thing will he withhold from
those whose walk is blameless.
O Lord Almighty, blessed is the man
who trusts in you.

—Psalm 84

Do not let your hearts be troubled.
Trust in God, trust also in me.
In my Father's house are many rooms;
if it were not so I would have told

you. I am going there to prepare a place for you.

And if I go and prepare a place for you, I will come back and take you to be with me that you also may be where I am. You know the way to the place where I am going.

—John 14:1–3

Listen, I tell you a mystery: We will not all sleep, but we will all be changed – in a flash, in the twinkling of an eye, at the last trumpet. For the trumpet will sound, and the dead will be raised imperishable, and we will be changed. For the perishable must clothe itself with the imperishable, and the mortal with immortality. When the perishable has been clothed with the imperishable, and the mortal with immortality,

Then the saying that is written will come true:

"Death has been swallowed up in victory."

"Where, O death, is your victory? Where, O death, is your sting?"

The sting of death is sin, and the strength of sin is the law. But thanks be to God! He gives us the victory through our Lord Jesus Christ.

—1 Cor. 15:51–55

Church of the Brethren

Continuing the Work of Jesus – Peacefully, Simply, Together.[198]

Prepared by:
Kathryn Goering Reid, MEd, MDiv
Former Executive Director, Association of Brethren Caregivers
Former Associate General Secretary
Church of the Brethren
Elgin, IL

History and Facts

The Church of the Brethren grew out of the Pietist movement of seventeenth and eighteenth centuries. Pietism advocated renewal of the church through the renewal of individuals and emphasized spirituality, lifestyle, and fellowship. While most Pietists sought to renew the church from within, some Pietists (the Radical Pietists) separated themselves from the state churches. The Brethren movement dates its birth to 1708, when the first Brethren baptism took place at Schwarzenau, Germany. Eight men and women, all of whom had been members of state churches, formed the new group. Their leader was Alexander Mack.

Because of persecution and economic hardship, the Brethren relocated to colonial Pennsylvania. The first group arrived in 1719 and by 1730 most were in America. In both Europe and America, the Brethren often lived in the same areas as the Anabaptists. It is unclear as to how much the early Brethren were influenced by the Anabaptists. Some scholars understand the Brethren as combining Pietist and Anabaptist thought.

As the United States grew, Brethren spread across the country. Often, they followed the same migration pattern as other German-speaking groups. By 1858, there was a Brethren congregation in California. Throughout most of the 1800s, Brethren sought to remain separated from the larger society. They wore a prescribed dress, built simple meetinghouses, and continued to speak German at home and in worship. With the coming of the twentieth century, Brethren began to participate in movements such as temperance and foreign missions, and they became less ethnic and sectarian. In 1908, the Brethren changed their official name from German Baptist Brethren to Church of the Brethren. During the first half of the twentieth century, foreign missions became the great work of the Brethren, with major mission fields in India, China, and Nigeria. After World War II, Brethren became known for their service work and began such programs as Heifer International (a program to develop livestock in depressed economies), International Christian Youth Exchange, and Brethren Volunteer Service.

---

198 Quote provided by Kathryn Goering Reid, author of this chapter.

Concerning church polity (i.e., organizational governance structure), the ultimate legislative authority in the Church of the Brethren is the Annual Conference, which is made up of representatives from local congregations. The Conference has created several agencies to carry out its programs. These include the General Board, the Brethren Benefit Trust, the Association of Brethren Caregivers, and On Earth Peace. Local congregations have a great deal of autonomy. They choose their own leadership (including pastors), determine how much they want to give to denominational programs, and maintain control over their property. Congregations are organized into 23 districts that hold their own yearly meetings and provide local services to more than 1000 congregations, with a total membership of 130 000.

Basic Teachings

Seeking to pattern themselves after the primitive church, the early Brethren took the New Testament as the guide for their faith and practice. All Brethren beliefs and practices are rooted in their understanding of the church as a community, rather than a group of individual Christians. Today, this is still the Brethren understanding. While much of Brethren theology is the same as mainstream Protestantism, the Brethren do emphasize certain beliefs and practices.

- Love feast, which combines communion with a fellowship meal and feet-washing.
- Nonresistance, which leads some to active peacemaking and conscientious objection to military service.
- Service, which leads Brethren to participate in programs to relieve hunger, provide health care, and improve the lives

of others in the United States and other parts of the world.

- Believers' baptism, whereby infant baptism is rejected in favor of a conscious decision to follow Jesus.
- The simple life, which calls Brethren to resist the temptations of the consumer-oriented society and to treat creation with respect.
- Anointing for healing based on James 5:13–16.
- Non-creedal, whereby Brethren remain open to discovering new biblical truths.

Basic Practices

- Brethren value communal worship, and will gather on Sundays and at other times to hear preaching, study scripture, sing hymns, and pray.
- The sharing of one's faith (evangelism) is of great importance in many denominations. Some of the ways it is communicated is through loving actions, talking about personal spiritual experiences, reading scriptures, distributing informational tracts, and discussions of doctrinal positions.
- The Lord's Supper, also called Holy Communion or Eucharist (meaning "thanksgiving"), is a powerful ordinance (sacrament or ritual). It is a liturgical reenactment of the crucifixion, death, burial, and resurrection of Jesus, in which Christians eat bread (to commemorate the broken body of Jesus) and drink wine or grape juice (to symbolize Jesus' shed blood). This can be done during communal worship or in other settings and is usually administered by ordained clergy.
- Prayer, meditation, and scripture are the fundamental spiritual practices for many Brethren. The many forms of these

practices include: reading and/or silent contemplation upon scripture or doctrinal beliefs and prayers of various kinds – petition, healing, repentance for unethical thoughts and actions, praise, worship, and thanksgiving to God.

- Mission work is important to Brethren. These acts of service take the forms of – working for social justice with marginalized peoples, charitable giving to provide food, building, and educational programs for the poor, volunteerism, and so forth. Mission work is also an intentional witness to one's faith through proclamation and teaching.

- Christening is the ceremonial act that includes naming of the child. It can be an official part of the ceremony of baptism or combined with infant dedication.

- All Brethren practice the unique ministry of love feast, which at its core, reflects the understanding that Brethren are servants of each other, called to minister to each other after the model of Jesus. Love feast is a reflective worship service of prayer, scripture, and singing that includes feet-washing, a simple meal, and communion.

- The care of the local congregation is given to two major categories of leadership – ministers and deacons. While many Brethren ministers have graduate-level seminary training, others are called from within the congregation receiving guidance and learning from within the church. Ministers of the church are called to preaching, to administration of the ordinances, and to the spiritual care of the congregation. Deacons are called to care for the physical needs of the members, to visit the sick, to help in administering the ordinances, to ministry of reconciliation and facilitating unity among members. Pastors and deacons, as well as congregational members, will visit those who are ill. Deacons are also responsible for providing for those who are in financial need.

- Brethren believe that all have sinned and fallen short of the glory of God, and that without the freely given salvation none is worthy to come into the God's presence. Therefore, it is incumbent on all to "build up the body of Christ," seeking unity and reconciliation among all. This calls for a commitment to the study of the Bible, prayer to live out the balanced vision, and openness to the movement of the Holy Spirit.

- Brethren believe that all biblical teaching and faith must be incorporated and consistent with a Christian's daily living. Therefore, the Brethren emphasize prayer and devotional life, silence and solitude, fasting, study of scripture, and worship to strengthen one's spiritual life.

- Baptism is by trine immersion (i.e., three times) of an individual at the age of responsibility and understanding.

- Anointing for healing, rather than being a last rite, is a biblical ordinance that recognizes that God is firmly in control of all aspects of life. It is an invitation to God to take part in the healing process and a dedication of ourselves as partners in the healing process. The rite is for those who are sick physically, emotionally, or spiritually and is intended for wholeness as well as curing. Anointing may be practiced by pastors, deacons, or members of the congregation.

Are any among you suffering? They should pray. Are any cheerful? They should sing songs of praise. Are any among you sick? They should call for the elders of the church and have them pray over them, anointing them with oil in the name of the Lord. The prayer of faith will save the sick, and the Lord will raise them up; and anyone who has committed sins will be forgiven.

—James 5:13–15 (New Revised Standard Version [NRSV])

Principles for Clinical Care
Dietary Issues
- The Church of the Brethren has no dietary restrictions with respect to religious beliefs.

General Medical Beliefs
- Brethren believe that God is the ultimate source of all life, health, and healing.
- Brethren believe that human life is a gracious gift from God who loves us.
- Most Brethren affirm the validity of traditional Western medical procedures in the treatment of illness and disease.

Specific Medical Issues
- **Abortion**: The Church of the Brethren opposes abortion because the rejection of unborn children violates the love by which God creates and nurtures human life.
- **Advance Directives**: The Church of the Brethren encourages and supports individuals to use advance directives in health care planning.
- **Birth Control**: Brethren have no prohibitions against the use of birth control.
- **Blood Transfusions**: Brethren have no prohibitions against the use of blood products.
- **Circumcision**: Brethren in Western societies have requested circumcision for male infants for cultural, not religious, reasons.

- **In Vitro Fertilization**: Brethren have no prohibitions against in vitro fertilization.
- **Stem Cell Research**: The Church of the Brethren has no official position on stem cell research for therapeutic and curative use. Individuals in the Church of the Brethren may have some cultural opposition in more conservative areas.
- **Vaccinations**: The Church of the Brethren does not have an issue with vaccinations. Any decisions about vaccination are left to individuals.
- **Withholding/Withdrawing Life Support**: Withholding/withdrawing life support in medically futile cases does not violate the teachings of the Church of the Brethren. It is an individual decision.

Gender and Personal Issues
- The Church of the Brethren as a faith tradition has no prescriptions or proscriptions with respect to gender and personal issues.

Principles for Spiritual Care through the Cycles of Life
Concepts of Living and Dying for Spiritual Support
- Life is a sacred gift of God, to be lived with thanksgiving.
- Physical death, the natural and inevitable end of physical life, is a mystery.
- The integrity of the processes of life that God has created is to be respected; birth and death are part of these processes.
- Biblical faith directs us to claim the love and power of God in our living, our dying, and our anticipation of life after death.
- Spiritual growth can come from facing suffering and death honestly.
- The Brethren, out of commitment to the Lord Jesus Christ, the study of

the scriptures, and life together, have developed traditions that continue to guide them in dying and death. Brethren seriously and joyfully embrace the understanding that death is the door to eternal life with God. Brethren are called to live in readiness because the exact timing and circumstances of death are not ours to determine. A consistent life of faithfulness and obedience to God, not deathbed conversion, is the way to prepare for death.

During Birth

- As stated earlier, Brethren in Western societies have requested circumcision for male infants for cultural, not religious, reasons.
- Baptism for believers only is an important tenet of the Church of the Brethren. Therefore, babies are never baptized. However, families will request a dedication service (as part of a Sunday morning worship service) to commit themselves to raising the child in a Christian home and to dedicate the child to God. In this practice, the congregation offers their support in the spiritual life of the family.

During Illness

- Patients may receive comfort from the reading of scriptures or other devotional material, listening to religious music, watching televised worship services of their own or a similar tradition.
- Patients may receive comfort from the use of hymns, whether praying the words of favorite hymns or singing hymns with people. Many prayers and hymns can be found in *Hymnal: A Worship Book*, published by the Church of the Brethren and the Mennonites.
- Patients may receive comfort from healing

prayers. These can be offered by health care professionals. Patients may ask for healing prayers to be connected with anointing with oil for healing. Chaplains, deacons, or ministers should be consulted for assistance with these requests.

During End of Life

- In the Brethren tradition, the family of faith has often gathered around those who were dying and grieving with ministries of care and support. The church community, past and present, offers spiritual support through anointing, special times of prayer, compassionate presence, and practical assistance, such as preparation of food and, in rural settings, help with seasonal tasks.
- Patients or the family may request anointing with oil. Chaplains, deacons, or ministers should be consulted for assistance.
- Patient or the family may request communion. Chaplains, deacons, or ministers should be consulted for assistance.
- Family may wish to view the body of the deceased in the hospital room or the chapel. A nurse and chaplain should be consulted for assistance.
- Family may request prayers for the deceased. These can be offered by a chaplain, ministers, family, friends, and health care professionals.

Care of the Body

- Disposition and embalming are individual decisions. The chaplain and the funeral home director should be consulted for assistance.
- Autopsy is an individual decision unless required by law. The chaplain and/or nurse should be consulted for assistance.
- Donation for medical research is an

individual decision. The chaplain and/or nurse should be consulted for assistance. Advance planning for such donations is required by most receiving organizations. Last-minute donations are usually not possible.

- Brethren have no inherent objection to cremation. However, there may be some cultural opposition in more conservative areas, but it is widely practiced in the denomination.
- Burial is the most common method of disposition.

Organ and Tissue Donation

- The Church of the Brethren encourages congregations, institutions, and members to:
  - inform and educate themselves by taking advantage of resources with their region as to organ and tissue donation
  - support and encourage individuals to be in discussion with ministers and family as to their wishes regarding the use of their organs and/or tissue for transplantation upon death
  - encourage and support individuals to include within their Advance Medical Directives instructions as to their wishes for organ and tissue donation – this may include the signing and carrying of a Universal Organ Donor Card
  - support those living donors who, with prayerful consideration, make an organ or tissue gift, provided that such a gift does not deprive the donor of life itself nor the functional integrity of his or her body.
- It may be preferable for a chaplain and/or nurse who are trained designated requesters to be consulted for assistance.

Scriptures, Inspirational Readings, and Prayers

READINGS DURING ILLNESS

These can be read by family, friends, ministers, and health care professionals. (All scripture quotations are from the NRSV, unless otherwise noted.)

The Lord is my shepherd I shall not
  want.
He makes me lie down in green
  pastures; he restores my soul.
He leads me in right paths for his
  name's sake.
Even though I walk through the
  darkest valley, I fear no evil;
For you are with me; your rod and
  your staff – they comfort me.
You prepare a table before me in the
  presence of my enemies;
You anoint my head with oil; my cup
  overflows.
Surely goodness and mercy shall
  follow me all the days of my life,
And I shall dwell in the house of the
  Lord my whole life long.

—Psalm 23

Do not fear, for I have redeemed you;
  I have called you by name, you are
  mine.
When you pass through the waters,
  I will be with you; and through the
  rivers, they shall not overwhelm
  you; when you walk through fire
  you shall not be burned, and the
  flame shall not consume you.
For I am the Lord your God, the
  Holy One of Israel, your Savior.

—Isa. 43:1b–3a

READINGS DURING ANOINTING FOR HEALING

The thought of my affliction … is
wormwood and gall!
My soul continually thinks of it and is
bowed down within me.
But this I call to mind, and therefore I
have hope:
The steadfast love of the Lord never
ceases, his mercies never come to an
end;
they are new every morning; great is
your faithfulness.
"The Lord is my portion," says my
soul, "therefore I will hope in him."

—Lam. 3:19–24

READINGS DURING END-OF-LIFE PROCESS

These can be read by family, friends, ministers, and health care professionals. (All scripture quotations are from the NRSV, unless otherwise noted.)

What then are we to say about these
things? If God is for us, who is
against us? He who did not withhold
his own Son, but gave him up for all
of us, will he not with him also give us
everything else? Who will bring any
charge against God's elect? It is God
who justifies. Who is to condemn? It
is Christ Jesus, who died, yes, who
was raised, who is at the right hand
of God, who indeed intercedes for us.
Who will separate us from the love of
Christ? Will hardship, or distress, or
persecution, or famine, or nakedness,
or peril, or sword?

No, in all these things we are more
than conquerors through him who
loved us. For I am convinced that
neither death, nor life, nor angels, nor
rulers, nor things present, nor things
to come, nor powers, nor height,
nor depth, nor anything else in all
creation, will be able to separate us
from the love God in Christ Jesus our
Lord.

—Rom. 8:31–35, 37–39

But we do not want you to be
uninformed, brothers and sisters,
about those who have died, so that
you may not grieve as others do
who have no hope.
For since we believe that Jesus died
and rose again, even so, through
Jesus, God will bring with him
those who have died.

—1 Thess. 4:13–14

PRAYERS DURING ILLNESS OR END-OF-LIFE PROCESS

These prayers can be offered by family, friends, clergy, and health care professionals.

The Lord's Prayer
Our Father which are in heaven,
Hallowed be thy name.
Thy kingdom come.
Thy will be done in earth, as it is in
heaven.
Give us this day our daily bread.
And forgive us our debts, as we
forgive our debtors.
And lead us not into temptation, but
deliver us from evil:

For thine is the kingdom, and the
power,
and the glory, forever. Amen.

—Matt. 6:9–13 (Authorized [King
James] Version)

Prayer before Surgery

Heavenly Father, we pray that you
will watch over our (brother/sister)
during this time of surgery. We pray
boldly for calmness and peace, for
healing, for restoration to wholeness.
We pray that you will bring healing
directly to the body, through the
action of your Holy Spirit. Knowing
that you work through the hands
of healers, we pray that you will
guide the hands of doctors, nurses,
technicians, and others involved in
this surgery. Watch over friends and
family both near and far. These things
we pray in your Son's name. Amen.

—Frank Ramirez[199]

HYMN SUGGESTIONS FOR ILLNESS

Move in Our Midst

Move in our midst, thou Spirit of
God.
Go with us down from thy holy hill.
Walk with us through the storm and
the calm.
Spirit of God, go thou with us still.[200]

My Life Flows On

My life flows on in endless song,
above earth's lamentation.
I catch the sweet, though far off hymn
that hails a new creation.
No storm can shake my inmost calm
while to that Rock I'm clinging.
Since love is Lord of heav'n and
earth, how can I keep from
singing?[201]

Amazing Grace

Amazing grace! How sweet the
sound, that saved a wretch like me!
I once was lost, but now am found,
was blind, but now I see.[202]

HYMN SUGGESTIONS FOR END-OF-LIFE PROCESS

When Peace Like a River

When peace, like a river, attendeth
my way,
When sorrows like sea billows roll,
Whatever my lot, though hast taught
me to say,
it is well, it is well with my soul.[203]

Softly and Tenderly Jesus is Calling

Softly and tenderly Jesus is calling,
calling for you and for me.
See, on the portals he's waiting and
watching, watching for you and for
me.
Come home, come home! You, who
are weary, come home."
Earnestly, tenderly Jesus is calling,
calling, "O sinner, come home!"[204]

199 ©1998 Association of Brethren Caregivers. *Deacon Manual for Caring Ministries*, 297. Used by permission.
200 ©1950 Church of the Brethren General Board. *Hymnal: A Worship Book.* (1992). Elgin, IL: Brethren Press, 418. Used by permission.
201 *Hymnal: A Worship Book*, 580.
202 Ibid, 143.
203 Ibid, 336.
204 Ibid, 491.

Move in Our Midst

Move in our midst, thou Spirit of
God.
Go with us down from thy holy hill.
Walk with us through the storm and
the calm.
Spirit of God, go thou with us still.[205]

Amazing Grace

Amazing grace! How sweet the
sound, that saved a wretch like me!
I once was lost, but now am found,
was blind, but now I see.[206]

God Be with You

God be with you till we meet again;
By his counsels guide, uphold you,
With his sheep securely fold you;
God be with you till we meet again.[207]

Steal Away

Steal away, steal away, steal away to
Jesus!
Steal away, steal away home, I ain't
got long to stay here.
My Lord, he calls me, he calls me by
the thunder;
the trumpet sounds within my soul;
I ain't got long to stay here.[208]

---

205 ©1950 Church of the Brethren General Board.
   Hymnal: A Worship Book, 418. Used by permission.
206 Ibid, 143.

207 Ibid, 431.

208 Ibid, 612.

Hutterites

*If there is no private property in heaven, there should be
none either among God's people here on earth.*[209]

Prepared by:
Rod Janzen, PhD
Professor of History, Fresno Pacific University
Fresno, CA

History and Facts

The Hutterites are a communal Christian group with roots in the sixteenth-century Anabaptist movement. The Hutterites became the dominant religious faction in the Anabaptist community in Austria and were named after early leader, Jacob Hutter. The Hutterites are mainstream Anabaptists in their emphasis on believer's baptism, pacifism, church discipline, and Christian discipleship, but they also believe that Christians should not own private property. They believe that the communally organized Early Church as portrayed in the book of Acts, chapters 2, 4, and 5, was inspired by the Holy Spirit on the Day of Pentecost. They believe that true Christianity is communal Christianity; that life on earth should be lived now as it will ultimately be lived in heaven.

The Hutterites have lived communally almost continuously since 1528. Experiencing extensive persecution from Roman Catholics, Protestants, and Muslims, they established communities in various parts of Eastern Europe in the sixteenth, seventeenth, eighteenth, and nineteenth centuries, until they immigrated en masse to the Dakota Territory in the 1870s. Today, there are about 48 000 Hutterites living in 471 colonies. These are located in the states of North and South Dakota, Montana, Washington, and Oregon (in the United States) and the provinces of Manitoba, Saskatchewan, Alberta, and British Columbia (in Canada). There is also one colony in Japan and one in Nigeria.

The Hutterites are presently divided into four different groups or *Leute*, which are for the most part endogamous and have slightly varying religious and cultural practices that are sometimes difficult for outsiders (non-Hutterites) to see. All Hutterites place great emphasis on hundreds of special sermons – the *Lehren* – that were written primarily in the seventeenth century. These are the only sermons delivered in Hutterite church services. The sermons provide unified biblical interpretation and are the foundational source for the group's *Ordnungen* (community rules) that govern all aspects of life. Each colony of 60–150 people is financially independent.

---

209 Quote provided by Rod Janzen, author of this chapter, as remembered from a speech by H. Decker in 1988.

Major contemporary challenges include high land prices, low market prices for agricultural products (most Hutterite colonies rely on farming operations), the attraction of new technologies and media (the Hutterites, unlike the Old Order Amish, use the most up-to-date technology), as well as being the target of often successful evangelistic efforts undertaken by conservative evangelical religious groups. Increasing numbers of young people are being enticed by high wages and a more individualistic way of life outside the colony. However, the Hutterites continue to grow in terms of members, with an average family size of about eight (including parents) and a relatively high retention rate (75%–80%).

Basic Teachings
- All the standard orthodox teachings of "Christianity" apply (e.g., belief in the Trinity and the *Apostles' Creed*).

The Apostles' Creed
I believe in God, the Father almighty,
  creator of heaven and earth,
I believe in Jesus Christ, His only
  Son, our Lord.
Who was conceived by the power of
  the Holy Spirit;
Born of the virgin Mary;
Suffered under Pontius Pilate;
Was crucified, died, and buried.
He descended into hell (or the realm
  of the dead).
On the third day he rose again.
He ascended into heaven and is
  seated at the right hand of the
  Father.
He will come again to judge the living
  and the dead.
I believe in the Holy Spirit,

The holy catholic (universal) church,
The communion of saints,
The forgiveness of sins,
The resurrection of the body and the
  life everlasting. Amen.

- The Bible is the central foundation for the Hutterite Church. Hutterites recognize the Apocrypha (additional books – for example, the books of the Maccabees, which are also recognized by Roman Catholic and Orthodox Christians) as an important part of the Bible.
- Hutterites take Acts 2, 4, and 5 literally ("Now the company of those who believed were of one heart and soul, and no one said that any of the things which he possessed was his own, but they had everything in common" [Acts 4:32]). Unlike Christians of most denominations, they believe in community of goods.
- Emphasis is placed on humility and *Gelassenheit* (yielding oneself to God *through* other members of the church community).
- Plain uniform dress is a Christian witness against egotism and materialism.
- There is no complete assurance of salvation.
- Church discipline is applied with regard to moral infractions. Those who repent confess serious sins publicly to other members of the church community.
- Believer's baptism is a basic tenet.
- Young people do not typically join the church until their early to mid-twenties, often directly preceding marriage.
- Closed communion (i.e., only baptized members of the community can participate) is observed once a year.
- Ministers are nominated democratically by male members. Final selection,

however, is in the hands of God, via the casting of lots.

- Hutterite society is patriarchal, and women do not vote. Nevertheless, women have extensive influence over decision making behind the scenes.
- The Hutterite *Ordnungen* (community rules) guide behavior.
- Hutterites found their faith on a literal interpretation of the Bible.
- Biblical exegesis is undertaken through the Hutterite sermons (*Lehren*), which are considered Spirit-guided interpretations of Bible passages.
- The *Chronicle of the Hutterian Brethren* is an internal history that includes stories of early Anabaptist and Hutterite martyrs and much theological interpretation.
- The Hutterite *Confession of Faith*, written by Hutterite elder Peter Riedemann, in 1540, provides theological guidance for the community.
- The sermons (*Lehren*) and Peter Riedemann's Confession of Faith (recently translated into English) are the primary ways in which the Bible is interpreted.

Basic Practices
- Hutterites believe that they should live in separation from the world.
- Church services are held daily, right before the evening meal, and twice on Sundays. Many colonies have separate church structures; others meet in school buildings.
- Church services last from 20 minutes (daily services) to 90-plus minutes (on Sunday morning).
- Each colony has a senior and assistant minister, who share speaking and counseling responsibilities while also participating in other colony work responsibilities.

- The Hutterite first language is *Hutterisch*, an Austrian/Tyrolean dialect, which is the language used most often in daily conversation. All Hutterites also speak English fluently and are somewhat conversant in German (which is studied daily in "German School" sessions and is the language used during church services).
- Most Hutterite children attend public schools through at least grade 8, but they are taught separately on the colony grounds. Some colonies have private schools and an increasing number have their own credentialed schoolteachers. More and more Hutterite young people are completing secondary school.
- Most Hutterites farm but an increasing number of colonies have developed small manufacturing enterprises.
- The Hutterites pay local, state/provincial, and federal taxes.
- Hutterites pray before and after every meal and snack time.
- Hutterites engage in very little evangelism, believing that God has called them to serve as exemplary models of the communal order that all Christians will experience when they arrive in heaven. In turn, they do not like to be evangelized or confronted with non-Hutterian interpretations of the Bible or the Christian faith.

Principles for Clinical Care
Dietary Issues
- There are no specific dietary restrictions based on theological principles.
- Meals are generally eaten together in the colony dining hall with Hutterite women preparing the food on a rotational schedule.
- Each colony has a special cook to prepare meals for the ill and for postnatal

mothers. For those with special health problems and/or dietary needs, meals are brought to individual homes.

- Hutterites have large gardens at each colony, which provide a significant percentage of the fruits and vegetables that are consumed.

General Medical Beliefs

- Hutterites are susceptible to some genetic diseases due to marriage primarily within the ethno-religious group.
- Farm accidents cause a significant number of injuries, as is the case with most rural families.
- Hutterites are open to state-of-the-art medical technologies.
- There is a heavy reliance on alternative medical practices and natural medical remedies (e.g., the use of herbs, oils, and mineral and vitamin supplements, or trips to Mexico for alternative treatments).
- Many Hutterites donate blood regularly.
- Hutterites expect care givers to explain procedures and options, and may consider alternative treatments. Be sure to ask what vitamins, herbs, and supplements they are taking or plan to take.

Specific Medical Issues

- **Abortion**: Abortion is unacceptable unless the life of the mother is endangered.
- **Advance Directives**: Use of advance directives in health care preplanning is an individual decision.
- **Birth Control**: Hutterites do not believe in birth control unless it is recommended by a medical doctor. If a contraceptive medical procedure is suggested, it is almost always women who undergo the operation. Very few Hutterite men have had vasectomies. Some Hutterites mention obtaining diaphragm prescriptions

and condoms. When married couples use these devices for birth control or health purposes, minsiters are consulted and a physician's recommendation is required.

- **Blood Transfusions**: Hutterites accept blood transfusions and organ transplants.
- **Circumcisions**: There is no Hutterite position on circumcision. It is an individual choice.
- **In Vitro Fertilization**: Hutterites are opposed to in vitro fertilization.
- **Stem Cell Research**: Hutterites have no official position on stem cell research for therapeutic purposes.
- **Vaccinations**: Most Hutterites accept all vaccination requirements since, at most colonies, the childen attend public schools. They have no position against vaccinations.
- **Withholding/Withdrawing Life Support**: Withholding/withdrawing life support in medically futile cases is an individual decision made in consultation with a physician.

Gender and Personal Issues

- Hutterites reflect a greater level of modesty than the predominant culture. While they accept care workers of the opposite gender, if necessary, for many health problems they would be more communicative with care workers of the same gender.
- Hutterites strongly prefer not to talk about pregnancy and childbirth in front of their children and young unmarried adult members. They also prefer to keep the news of their own pregnancy – or lack thereof – a complete secret for as long as possible.
- Hutterites are used to a quiet atmosphere. Because most colonies do not allow televisions in the houses, they find it very difficult to sleep when a television is on in

the same room. Most would have the same difficulty with having a radio on as well.

- Hutterites do not like to leave their members alone in hospitals. As much as possible, they try to keep someone with them day and night, especially if they are young or elderly.
- On the colony, both genders provide health care, but the majority is provided by women.
- Hutterite women are taught to pray with their heads covered, and so wear a head covering at all times. A woman's covering should be removed only as an absolute necessity.

Principles for Spiritual Care through the Cycles of Life

Concepts of Living and Dying for Spiritual Support

- Life on earth is service to others.
- Suffering is a source of learning; one can draw closer to God through it.
- Hutterites believe that there is a God-given reason for illness and any suffering that accompanies illness.

During Birth

- The majority of women receive prenatal care.
- Most births occur in hospitals; very few births occur in the home.
- Delivery is usually completed by physicians; sometimes by a Hutterite midwife.
- Hutterite husbands are usually with their wives at delivery.
- Children are highly valued; physical and intellectual attributes and conditions are believed to be God-given.
- Medical contraception is generally not accepted unless advised by a physician for medical reasons.

- Informal family planning appears to be occurring, as indicated by a falling Hutterite birth rate.
- Abortion is unacceptable unless the life of the mother is endangered.
- There are no specific rituals that accompany the birth of a child.

During Illness

- Hutterites who are ill receive many empathetic visitors.
- Hutterites accept home health care services from nurses and medical assistants.
- If children are hospitalized, parents usually stay with them.
- English is a second language for Hutterites. Children under the age of 6 are thus not usually fluent in English. If you know German, you may be able to communicate. Here is a simplified pronunciation of some common words:
  - Water – *vosser*
  - Pain – *vay-ah*
  - Hungry – *hoon-greech*
  - Do you want to urinate? – *Villst du bee-schen?*
- Hutterites may accept spiritual mentoring from hospital chaplains but their greatest spiritual support comes from Hutterite visitors, including colony ministers.
- Children may be comforted by spiritual support from colony German teachers, who, on the colony, provide Biblical instruction to boys and girls starting when they are 5 years old and continuing until they are baptized.
- Health care workers should feel free to pray alongside Hutterite family members and friends.
- Flowers in hospital rooms are becoming more common; many cards are also received.

During End of Life

- Hutterites prefer to die at home, on the colony grounds if at all possible.
- Hospice care is accepted.
- Hutterite ministers visit terminally ill members regularly and encourage reflection on personal lives, the confession of sins, and so forth. Ministers and others provide counsel on a variety of issues including the fear of death, the ability to let go of life, and caring for those left behind.
- The funeral service is an important event, attended by hundreds of friends and relatives. This is not only a time of mourning but a recognition of the more beautiful life in heaven that the dead is now experiencing.
- The hope of salvation (though not assured) is present if the individual was a baptized and committed member of the Hutterite community.
- Hutterites attend many more funerals than most non-Hutterites.

Care of the Body

- In the hospital, nursing staff superintend the care of the body. At home, family and friends play this role. Viewing of the body occurs at home, on the colony grounds.
- The practices of hospitals are generally accepted; there is no prescribed or proscribed ritual for preparation for transport or covering of the body.
- Burial after embalming is the means of disposition; cremation is not an option.

- Someone is always present with the body after it has been returned to the colony.
- Burial occurs within 2–3 days; graves are simply marked in colony cemeteries.
- Hutterites accept autopsies only if they are legally required.
- Bodies are not donated for medical research.

Organ and Tissue Donation

- Organs and tissues are sometimes donated but this is a new idea/practice. It needs to be discussed thoroughly with family members and Hutterite ministers. It may be preferable for a chaplain and/or nurse who are trained designated requesters to be consulted for assistance.

Scriptures, Inspirational Readings, and Prayers

- The Hutterites sing spiritual songs from three different German-language hymn books. They are also familiar with many English gospel hymns. Singing may be highly comforting to the sick.
- At the time of a serious illness or nearing death, the person stricken is given the opportunity to personally select a favorite hymn or passage of scripture. If the person is incoherent, this choice is made by a close family member. But, there is no specific passage or hymn that is necessarily more likely to be used than any other.

Mennonites

I will both lie down and sleep in peace; for you alone,
O Lord, make me lie down in safety.[210]

Prepared by:
The Reverend Robert J. Carlson, DMin
Overland Park, KS

Reviewed and approved by:
The Reverend Dorothy Nickel Friesen
Conference Minister, Western District Conference
Mennonite Church USA
Newton, Kansas

History and Facts

Mennonite congregations are in the "family" of Christianity. They look to the New Testament and the life of Jesus, the Christ, as a source for life and practice. They date their origins to the time of the Protestant Reformation.

In the first quarter of the sixteenth century there was considerable unrest in the educated community and among the illiterate peasants. In many principalities in central Europe, there was much uneasiness about the oppression by the ruling classes in league with the Church (Roman Catholic Church).

In Zurich, Ulrich Zwingli also challenged the Church and its practices, and was able to persuade the civil authorities to allow some reforms in church practices. In the 1520s, there were a number of others who shared Zwingli's unease with current practices such as the law that required the baptism of children in order to place them on the tax rolls and to put them in the Church at birth; forcing people to pay a church tax

to support clergy they did not choose and whose behavior might be less than holy; having to listen to sermons that were long theological discourses (in Latin) that had nothing to do with their day-to-day lives; being forced to take up arms to fight the neighboring provinces that were "Lutheran" or "Catholic."

Instead, these Swiss Brethren became interested in studying the New Testament in the original Greek, trying to follow what they believed were the teachings of Jesus, relying on one another to help them understand God's love and how to live. Early on, they decided to baptize one another as a symbol of their decision to follow Christ regardless of the risks.

This placed them at odds with the state-sanctioned practice of baptism. They were called "rebaptisers" ("Ana-baptists"). Their practice was condemned by the authorities and their gatherings were declared "illegal." Even Ulrich Zwingli, who had shared many of their concerns, felt that the risk of chaos in the countryside was too great, and he came to judge and condemn their actions and their fellowship.

---

210 Ps. 4:8 (New Revised Standard Version).

These Anabaptists are the theological and spiritual ancestors of Mennonites today.

In Northern Holland in the 1530s, a Roman Catholic Priest named Menno Simons resigned from the Church and joined the movement. Although condemned by the authorities and having to live as a fugitive, he wrote and encouraged different groups of Anabaptists in central Europe. His teaching was about spiritual community: mutual aid; sharing of resources; sister/brotherhood among believers; support to widows, their children and the poor; simple lifestyle; nonresistance; nonviolence; peacemaking; and the servanthood stance of faithfulness.

This teaching and instruction had a great influence on the development of Anabaptist thought and practice. His commentary of Matthew 25 speaks to Mennonites today: "True evangelical faith cannot lie dormant. It clothes the naked. It feeds the hungry. It comforts the sorrowful. It shelters the destitute. It serves those that harm it. It binds up that which is wounded. It has become all things to all people."[211]

Persecution forced the Anabaptists from their homes, out of the cities and into the countryside. Ultimately, some of them fled central Europe. The earliest of the Swiss Anabaptists found their way to the "protections" of the New World, especially to Pennsylvania. Some of them arrived in the American colonies in the first part of the 1700s.

In the first 100, some 4000 Anabaptists lost their lives, mostly by burning or drowning at the hands of Protestant or Catholic authorities. Since then, there have been waves of migration, mission work, and growth.

In the New World, Menno's name was attached to these Anabaptists; they were called "Mennists." Later, they accepted the label and it became the name, Mennonite.

Today worldwide, there are more than a million Anabaptists/Mennonites. There are some 300 000 in the United States. These USA Mennonites are represented in over 40 different "Conferences." Because of a strong "congregational" autonomy, they may reflect different styles of worship, clothing, or "separation from the world" (counterculture). Groups that wear a peculiar garb (women's head covering, men with beards, men not wearing ties, dressing in black or subdued colors) might be called "Old Order Mennonites." They may be confused with Amish, but generally these Mennonites will use modern vehicles and make use of electricity while maintaining a conservative lifestyle that is different from mainstream culture.

The majority of Mennonites in the United States are located in the East and the Midwest, but that is rapidly changing. Mennonites are increasingly multicultural and are scattered from Los Angeles to Miami. Nearly 20% are Hispanic, African American, or Asian.

The three largest groups are the Mennonite Church in the United States, The Mennonite Brethren Church (a few people in these two groups wear a special garb), and the Old Order Amish.

(The Church of the Brethren has common roots in Switzerland and Central Europe but is not affiliated with the Mennonite Church except for the joint publication of a hymnal).

Most Mennonite groups cooperate in disaster and relief efforts worldwide

---

211 Quoted by Hostetter, N. (1997). *Anabaptist-Mennonites Nationwide USA*. Morgantown, PA: Masthof Press, 2.

through the Mennonite Central Committee and Mennonite Disaster Service.

Basic Teachings

- Anabaptists and Mennonites, for the most part, accept the basic creeds of the Christian Church.
- Mennonites (like the Protestant Reformers Luther and Zwingli) emphasize the authority of the scripture, salvation by grace through faith, and the priesthood of all believers.

  In addition, the Anabaptists accented the work of the Holy Spirit, a life of obedient discipleship, the practical fruits of conversion in daily life, accountability to a body of believers, adult (or believers) baptism, the rejection of oaths and violence, and in some measure, social separation from the larger society.[212]

- One of the prominent Mennonite scholars in the twentieth century summarized what he called the "Anabaptist Vision." It remains a vision statement for most Mennonites today. He saw three foci:
  1. A radical obedience to the teachings of Christ that transforms the behavior of individual believers.
  2. A new concept of the church as a voluntary body of believers, accountable to one another and separate from the larger world.
  3. An ethic of love that rejects violence in all spheres of human life.[213]

- Due in part to the congregational system of church organization, there may be considerable variation in practice in the carrying out of these themes.
- Mennonites recognize that personal sin can be the cause of suffering and illness, but this is not the dominant cause of suffering of the community where ancestors died for their "faithfulness." Instead, Mennonites have a cosmic or systemic sense of sin and its relationship to suffering. The Confession of Faith from a Mennonite perspective says, "Through sin, the powers of domination, division, destruction, and death have been unleashed in humanity and all of creation."[214] Given this understanding of sin, most Anabaptists can assume a relationship between suffering and sin, without an individual sufferer's culpability.[215]
- The Mennonite Confession of Faith (1995) says: "We believe that everything belongs to God, who calls the church to live in faithful stewardship of all that God has entrusted to us, and to participate now in the rest and justice which God has promised."[216] Mennonites have a strong tradition of responsibility for taking care of one's emotional, physical, and psychological health. Congregational programs often emphasize lifestyles consistent with health and wholeness.

The Recovery of the Anabaptist Vision. Scottdale, PA: Herald Press.

214 *Confession of Faith in a Mennonite Perspective.* (1995). Scottdale, PA: Herald Press, 31, 32.

215 Kotva, J. (2002). *The Anabaptist Tradition: Religious Traditions and Healthcare Decisions.* Chicago, IL: Park Ridge Center for the Study of Health, Faith, and Ethics.

216 *Confession of Faith in a Mennonite Perspective,* 77.

212 Kraybill, D. and C. Hostetter. (1944). *Anabaptist World USA.* Scottdale, PA: Herald Press, 2001, 23, 24.

213 Bender, H. S. *The Anabaptist Vision* [pamphlet, 44 pp]. Scottdale, PA, Herald Press. Also see "The Anabaptist Vision" (1957), in Hershberger, G. F. ed.

Basic Practices

Since Mennonites have a decentralized authority system, practices may vary greatly from congregation to congregation.

One writer describes Mennonite practices as "Anabaptist Habits."[217] These Seven Habits are as follows: (1) Discipleship, (2) Community, (3) Mutual Aid, (4) Simplicity, (5) Integrity, (6) Service, and (7) Peacemaking. This forms an outline list of practices. (The outline is Dr. Kraybill's, but the comments are the author's.)

1. **Discipleship**: Mennonites ask themselves, "How do I follow Jesus Christ?" They expect daily life to demonstrate a commitment to ethical and compassionate behavior. They emphasize connections between faith, words, and actions. Baptism, generally in the teen years, marks a personal commitment to be a Christ follower.

2. **Community**: Mennonites value community and shared relationships. Building community is a positive response to the indifference of modern culture. They seek to live in peace with all. They believe that the collective welfare is as important as individual welfare. Gathering in a congregation is a tangible expression of that community, so the percentage of members who attend church regularly is fairly high. The ritual of Communion is celebrated as a "Memorial" but also as a participation in a shared life as followers of Christ. Congregational singing is a representation of community as well. A few congregations do not use any musical instruments and sing a cappella. Most congregations use musical accompaniment, but sing in harmony.

3. **Mutual Aid**: Mennonites look out for one another. Congregations are very often caring communities, and they come together to help one another when someone is economically, physically or emotionally wounded. Larger groups have been organized for mutual aid and support, and for situations larger than could be handled by one congregation.

4. **Simplicity**: Mennonites tend to reject practices that are ostentatious or self-aggrandizing. They tend to focus on basics and essentials, on caring for what they have. This sometimes sets them apart from the "mainstream culture."

5. **Integrity**: Mennonites believe in honesty in practice and behavior. They try to behave in ways that are truthful and dependable. They believe their "word should be as good as a bond."

6. **Service**: Mennonites frequently are engaged in charitable activities and projects that serve others and the community. Many people spend 1 or 2 years in a "Service Unit," which is a community project in the United States or overseas. Many are involved in relief activities such as disaster relief, compassionate care, and rebuilding efforts. Some congregations have a ritual foot washing, as a symbol of caring for one another.

7. **Peacemaking**: Most Mennonites oppose war, and many have refused military service and served in an "Alternative Service." Mennonites believe they are called to a ministry of reconciliation. They also may be involved in peace-building, in victim-offender reconciliation, and programs that emphasize Restorative Justice.

---

217 Kraybill, D. (1997). Anabaptist Habits. Lecture at Bethel College Mennonite Church, North Newton, KS, October 26, 1997.

Principles for Clinical Care
Dietary Issues
- There are no special dietary concerns for most Anabaptist/Mennonite believers.
- Food is often important as an expression of community and associated with special ethnic memories. The *More-with-Less Cookbook* is a favorite resource for many Mennonites.

General Medical Beliefs
During World War II, conscientious objectors served in public mental hospitals. As a result, they developed a passion to create better psychiatric facilities and thus, a half-dozen small psychiatric facilities were built and operated by Mennonites. The concern for the treatment of the mentally ill is a legacy of that effort.

Mennonites have also operated general medical facilities, and have an active Association of Healthcare Institutions and Services. A number of Mennonites have entered the health professions.

Mennonites do not oppose health insurance and even operate several different health care insurance and mutual aid associations. However, some conservative Mennonite groups may exempt themselves from medical insurance (even from Mennonite-controlled programs) and from social security benefits. The cost of health care for the individual, then, may be shared by the whole community, in an ever-widening circle as needed to pay the increasing amounts.

- There are no special medical issues or practices unique to Mennonites.
- Many Mennonites believe that there is a spiritual component to healing and that God is on the side of healing. The purpose of this healing, however, is not personal physical comfort, but to enable an individual to take their place to love God and to "serve our neighbor as a witness to God's in-breaking kingdom."[218]
- In decision making, Mennonites are likely to want to consult with other members of their spiritual family as well as their biological family, depending on local practices in the congregation.

Specific Medical Issues
- **Abortion**: Most Mennonites would truly grieve an abortion and the circumstances that made it necessary.
- **Advance Directives**: As a faith tradition Mennonites have no official position on advance directives. However, some Mennonites will have completed advance directives and other end-of-life care documents.
- **Birth Control**: Mennonites have no specific policies regarding birth control. They recognize that marriage "is meant for sexual intimacy, companionship, and the birth and nurture of children."[219]
- **Blood Transfusions**: Mennonites have no restrictions regarding organ transplants, organ donations, use of blood transfusions, or blood products.
- **Circumcision**: Circumcision is common for males, but is not considered a religious practice.
- **In Vitro Fertilization**: While there are no official statements regarding in vitro fertilizations, there is cautious acceptance of the practice. In general, Mennonites recognize that children are a gift from God and the care and teaching of children is a major opportunity to show Divine love. Therefore, they would support

---

218 Kotva. *The Anabaptist Tradition.*
219 Confession of Faith in a Mennonite Perspective, article 19.

reproductive technologies, as long as the practices and procedures do not diminish human dignity. They would be reluctant to support surrogacy.

- **Stem Cell Research**: Individuals and congregations would differ on stem cell research for therapeutic purposes, but clearly they would not support practices that encourage abortion or that would be focused on destroying God-given life.
- **Vaccinations**: Among Mennonites, there are no doctrinal statements against vaccination directed toward preservation of health. Occasionally, the personal practices of some families may resist the government incursion into areas of personal responsibility for healthy behavior.
- **Withholding/Withdrawing Life Support**: Many Mennonites recognize that "stewardship of life" means "stewardship of the dying process," as well. Thus, many Mennonites would be open to discussions of withholding/withdrawing treatment in medically futile situations.

Gender and Personal Issues

- Mennonites may have personal preferences but there are no recommendations regarding the gender of health care workers.

Principles for Spiritual Care through the Cycles of Life
Concepts of Living and Dying for Spiritual Support

- Mennonites believe that the purpose of life is to love God through service and love of fellow human beings. They also believe that the culmination of life is being gathered to God to await God's final victory, "the end of this present age

of struggle, the resurrection of the dead, and a new heaven and a new earth."[220]

- Death in its own time is not a defeat, but the culmination, the fulfillment of life. It is often an occasion of gathering to celebrate the good life of a faithful disciple. An untimely death, though, is more difficult to experience and will occasion more dependence on the community, and a greater need for support from others in the congregation.
- Mennonites believe that "nothing can separate us from the love of God which we have seen in Christ Jesus" (Rom. 6:38–39).
- Hope to be with God provides comfort at death's separation.
- Funerals tend to be less formal than Catholic or other Protestant services. The service usually includes a gathering of the community, often with singing, scripture, prayer, a sermon, and sharing memories of the deceased. Memorial services are increasingly common in place of a funeral. Memorial service or funerals at the church are most often accompanied by a shared meal.

During Birth

- Children are considered "a gift from God."[221] There is no specific ritual to welcome a new birth.
- Hospital delivery is more common than home delivery. There are no prohibitions against midwifery. (Amish sisters and brothers often make use of home births and midwives.)

---

220 *Confession of Faith in a Mennonite Perspective.* Summary Statement, item 27.
221 General Conference of Mennonite Brethren Churches. (2000). *Confession of Faith: Commentary and Pastoral Application.* Winnipeg, MB: Kindred Productions, 115.

- As stated earlier, circumcision is common for males but is not considered a religious practice.
- The congregation or community welcomes new children and considers them a part of the fellowship even though they are not baptized until later. Sometimes after a birth, there is a service of "dedication" in which the congregation and the parents commit to teach and raise the child to love and serve God. This may take place at any time in the first couple of years of life.
- As stated earlier, most Mennonites would truly grieve an abortion and the circumstances that made it necessary.
- They would also grieve a stillborn or a miscarriage. Often in these circumstances, a pastor would be welcomed to offer a prayer of commitment at the bedside. Occasionally, there would be a special service in the congregation to recognize and share the grief and loss.
- In the case of a complicated delivery, or a physically challenged or ill newborn, a pastor's visit and support from the congregation would usually be welcomed. Mennonites have an association to help congregations share in the care and growth of a handicapped child. This consulting service for families with disabilities can be reached through the Mennonite Health Services.
- Most Mennonite groups would support "genetic" counseling where genetic diseases are possible.

During Illness

- Most Mennonites welcome spiritual care and counsel from a competently trained caregiver. However, like most patients, there is a special appreciation for someone from their own congregation. In case of a city hospital, a local Mennonite pastor may be called on to provide care for someone who has traveled some distance for medical resources.
- Mennonites welcome the reading of scripture.
- Mennonites welcome prayers for healing, comfort, and solace.
- Scriptural anointing, or laying-on-of-hands are usually welcome. Preferably, this should involve the Mennonite pastor or other members from the congregation.
- When the congregation is close enough, Mennonites can expect others of the congregation to visit and or share a vigil with immediate family members.
- In difficult times or in times of joy, music is often dear to Mennonite hearts. Mennonites are often invited to sing together even at a bedside.

During End of Life

- Mennonites accept hospice care.
- Many Mennonites recognize that "stewardship of life" means "stewardship of the dying process," as well. Some will have completed advance directives and other end-of-life care documents.
- There are no specific rituals to perform at the end of life.
- Many Mennonites will want as many family members to be as close as possible.
- Family members may want to have a time of privacy with the deceased, to pray and share memories.

Care of the Body

- The practices of the hospital are generally accepted; there is no prescribed ritual for preparation, covering, or transport of the body.
- Embalming is routinely practiced.
- Cremation is an option for some.

- There is no prohibition regarding autopsy.
- Mennonites have no "last rites" or ritual traditions with regard to the body.
- Donating a body for medical research is a choice for some. There are no official statements about this choice.

Organ and Tissue Donation

- Organ donation is an option in appropriate cases. It may be preferable for a chaplain and/or nurse who are trained designated requesters to be consulted for assistance.

Scriptures, Inspirational Readings, and Prayers

- Scriptures from the New Testament are often the greatest comfort. Of course, Psalm 23 is a revered treasure for all Christians.

READINGS DURING ILLNESS

These can be read by family, friends, clergy, and health care professionals. (All scripture quotations are from the New Revised Standard Version.)

The Lord is my shepherd I shall not
   want.
He makes me lie down in green
   pastures; he restores my soul.
He leads me in right paths for his
   name's sake.
Even though I walk through the
   darkest valley, I fear no evil;
for you are with me; your rod and
   your staff – they comfort me.
You prepare a table before me in the
   presence of my enemies;
you anoint my head with oil; my cup
   overflows.
Surely goodness and mercy shall
   follow me all the days of my life,

and I shall dwell in the house of the
   Lord my whole life long.

— Psalm 23

When Jesus had crossed again in the boat to the other side, a great crowd gathered around him; and he was by the sea. Then one of the leaders of the synagogue named Jairus came and, when he saw him, fell at his feet and begged him repeatedly, "My little daughter is at the point of death. Come and lay your hands on her, so that she may be made well, and live." So he went with him.

And a large crowd followed him and pressed in on him. Now there was a woman who had been suffering from hemorrhages for twelve years. She had endured much under many physicians, and had spent all that she had; and she was no better, but rather grew worse. She had heard about Jesus, and came up behind him in the crowd and touched his cloak, for she said, "If I but touch his clothes, I will be made well." Immediately her hemorrhage stopped; and she felt in her body that she was healed of her disease. Immediately aware that power had gone forth from him, Jesus turned about in the crowd and said, "Who touched my clothes?" And his disciples said to him, "You see the crowd pressing in on you; how can you say, 'Who touched me?'" He looked all around to see who had done it. But the woman, knowing what had happened to her, came in fear and trembling, fell down before him, and told him the whole truth.

He said to her, "Daughter, your faith has made you well; go in peace, and be healed of your disease."

While he was still speaking, some people came from the leader's house to say, "Your daughter is dead. Why trouble the teacher any further?" But overhearing what they said, Jesus said to the leader of the synagogue, "Do not fear, only believe." He allowed no one to follow him except Peter, James, and John, the brother of James. When they came to the house of the leader of the synagogue, he saw a commotion, people weeping and wailing loudly. When he had entered, he said to them, "Why do you make a commotion and weep? The child is not dead but sleeping." And they laughed at him. Then he put them all outside, and took the child's father and mother and those who were with him, and went in where the child was. He took her by the hand and said to her, "Talitha cum," which means, "Little girl, get up!" And immediately the girl got up and began to walk about (she was twelve years of age). At this they were overcome with amazement. He strictly ordered them that no one should know this, and told them to give her something to eat.

—Mark 5:21–43

As he approached Jericho, a blind man was sitting by the roadside begging. When he heard a crowd going by, he asked what was happening. They told him, "Jesus of Nazareth is passing by." Then he shouted, "Jesus, Son of David, have mercy on me!" Those who were in front sternly ordered him to be quiet; but he shouted even more loudly, "Son of David, have mercy on me!" Jesus stood still and ordered the man to be brought to him; and when he came near, he asked him, "What do you want me to do for you?" He said, "Lord, let me see again." Jesus said to him, "Receive your sight; your faith has saved you." Immediately he regained his sight and followed him, glorifying God; and all the people, when they saw it, praised God.

—Luke 18: 35–43

HYMNS[222] AT TIME OF ANOINTING

There's a Wideness in God's Mercy
There's a wideness in God's mercy,
like the wideness of the sea.
There's a kindness in God's justice,
which is more than liberty.

For the love of God is broader
than the measures of the mind,
and the heart of the Eternal
is most wonderfully kind.

If our love were but more simple
we should rest upon God's word,
and our lives would be illumined
By the presence of our Lord.

O Healing River
O healing river send down your
  waters,

222 Hymn texts from *Hymnal: A Worship Book*. (1992). Elgin, IL: Brethren Press. Hymns can be found in the hymnal by looking in the table of contents, where the titles are listed in alphabetical order.

Send down your waters, upon this land.
O healing river send down your waters,
And wash the blood off the sand.

This land is parching, this land is burning,
No seed is growing in the barren ground.
O healing river, send down your waters,
O healing river send your waters down.

Let the seed of freedom awake and flourish,
Let the deep roots nourish, let the tall stalks rise.
O healing river, send down your waters,
O healing river, from out the skies.

Oh Have You Not Heard

Oh, have you not heard of that beautiful stream that flows through the promised land?
Its waters gleam bright in the heavenly light, and ripple o'er golden sand.

Its fountains are deep and its waters are pure, and sweet to the weary soul.
It flows from the throne of Jehovah alone! O come where its bright waves roll.

This beautiful stream is the river of life! It flows for all nations free.
A balm for each wound in its water is found; O sinner, it flows for thee!

Oh, will you not drink of this beautiful stream, and dwell of its peaceful shore?
The Spirit says: Come, all you weary ones, home, and wander in sin no more.

A seek that beautiful stream, O seek that beautiful stream.
Its waters, so free, are flowing for thee, O seek that beautiful stream.

There is a Balm in Gilead

There is a balm in Gilead to make the wounded whole,
There is a balm in Gilead to heal the sin-sick soul.

Sometime I feel discouraged and think my work's in vain, but then the Holy Spirit revives my soul again.
If you cannot preach like Peter, if you cannot pray like Paul, You can tell the love of Jesus and say, "He died for all."

There is a balm in Gilead to make the wounded whole,
There is a balm in Gilead to heal the sin-sick soul.

READINGS DURING END-OF-LIFE PROCESS

These can be read by family, friends, clergy, and health care professionals. (All scripture quotations are from the New Revised Standard Version.)

I am the resurrection and the life. Those who believe in me, even though they die, will live, and

everyone who lives and believes in
me will never die.

—John 11:25–26

Do not let your hearts be troubled.
Believe in God, believe also in me.
In my Father's house there are many
dwelling places. If it were not so,
would I have told you that I go to
prepare a place for you? And if I
go and prepare a place for you, I
will come again and will take you to
myself, so that where I am, there you
may be also.

—John 14:1–3

I consider that the sufferings of
this present time are not worth
comparing with the glory about to
be revealed to us. For the creation
waits with eager longing for the
revealing of the children of God;
for the creation was subjected to
futility, not of its own will but by the
will of the one who subjected it, in
hope that the creation itself will be
set free from its bondage to decay
and will obtain the freedom of the
glory of the children of God. We
know that the whole creation has
been groaning in labor pains until
now; and not only the creation, but
we ourselves, who have the first
fruits of the Spirit, groan inwardly
while we wait for adoption, the
redemption of our bodies. For in
hope we were saved. Now hope that
is seen is not hope. For who hopes
for what is seen? But if we hope for

what we do not see, we wait for it
with patience.

—Rom. 8: 18–25

Now I would remind you, brothers
and sisters, of the good news that
I proclaimed to you, which you in
turn received, in which also you
stand, through which also you are
being saved, if you hold firmly to the
message that I proclaimed to you –
unless you have come to believe in
vain.

For I handed on to you as of
first importance what I in turn had
received: that Christ died for our sins
in accordance with the scriptures,
and that he was buried, and that
he was raised on the third day in
accordance with the scriptures, and
that he appeared to Cephas, then
to the twelve. Then he appeared to
more than five hundred brothers and
sisters at one time, most of whom are
still alive, though some have died.
Then he appeared to James, then to
all the apostles. Last of all, as to one
untimely born, he appeared also to
me. For I am the least of the apostles,
unfit to be called an apostle, because
I persecuted the church of God. But
by the grace of God I am what I am,
and his grace toward me has not been
in vain. On the contrary, I worked
harder than any of them – though it
was not I, but the grace of God that
is with me. Whether then it was I or
they, so we proclaim and so you have
come to believe.

Now if Christ is proclaimed as
raised from the dead, how can some

of you say there is no resurrection of the dead? If there is no resurrection of the dead, then Christ has not been raised; and if Christ has not been raised, then our proclamation has been in vain and your faith has been in vain. We are even found to be misrepresenting God, because we testified of God that he raised Christ – whom he did not raise if it is true that the dead are not raised. For if the dead are not raised, then Christ has not been raised. If Christ has not been raised, your faith is futile and you are still in your sins. Then those also who have died in Christ have perished. If for this life only we have hoped in Christ, we are of all people most to be pitied.

But in fact Christ has been raised from the dead, the first fruits of those who have died. For since death came through a human being, the resurrection of the dead has also come through a human being; for as all die in Adam, so all will be made alive in Christ. But each in his own order: Christ the first fruits, then at his coming those who belong to Christ. Then comes the end, when he hands over the kingdom to God the Father, after he has destroyed every ruler and every authority and power. For he must reign until he has put all his enemies under his feet. The last enemy to be destroyed is death. For "God has put all things in subjection under his feet." But when it says, "All things are put in subjection," it is plain that this does not include the one who put all things in subjection under him. When all things are subjected to him, then the Son himself will also be subjected to the one who put all things in subjection under him, so that God may be all in all. Otherwise, what will those people do who receive baptism on behalf of the dead? If the dead are not raised at all, why are people baptized on their behalf? And why are we putting ourselves in danger every hour? I die every day! That is as certain, brothers and sisters, as my boasting of you – a boast that I make in Christ Jesus our Lord. If with merely human hopes I fought with wild animals at Ephesus, what would I have gained by it? If the dead are not raised, "Let us eat and drink, for tomorrow we die." Do not be deceived: "Bad company ruins good morals." Come to a sober and right mind, and sin no more; for some people have no knowledge of God. I say this to your shame.

But someone will ask, "How are the dead raised? With what kind of body do they come?" Fool! What you sow does not come to life unless it dies. And as for what you sow, you do not sow the body that is to be, but a bare seed, perhaps of wheat or of some other grain. But God gives it a body as he has chosen, and to each kind of seed its own body. Not all flesh is alike, but there is one flesh for human beings, another for animals, another for birds, and another for fish. There are both heavenly bodies and earthly bodies, but the glory of the heavenly is one thing, and that of the earthly is another. There is one glory of the sun, and another glory of the moon, and another glory of the stars; indeed, star differs from star in glory.

So it is with the resurrection of the dead. What is sown is perishable, what is raised is imperishable. It is sown in dishonor, it is raised in glory. It is sown in weakness, it is raised in power. It is sown a physical body, it is raised a spiritual body. If there is a physical body, there is also a spiritual body. Thus it is written, "The first man, Adam, became a living being"; the last Adam became a life-giving spirit. But it is not the spiritual that is first, but the physical, and then the spiritual. The first man was from the earth, a man of dust; the second man is from heaven. As was the man of dust, so are those who are of the dust; and as is the man of heaven, so are those who are of heaven. Just as we have borne the image of the man of dust, we will also bear the image of the man of heaven.

What I am saying, brothers and sisters, is this: flesh and blood cannot inherit the kingdom of God, nor does the perishable inherit the imperishable. Listen, I will tell you a mystery! We will not all die, but we will all be changed, in a moment, in the twinkling of an eye, at the last trumpet. For the trumpet will sound, and the dead will be raised imperishable, and we will be changed. For this perishable body must put on imperishability, and this mortal body must put on immortality. When this perishable body puts on imperishability, and this mortal body puts on immortality, then the saying that is written will be fulfilled: "Death has been swallowed up in victory." "Where, O death, is your victory? Where, O death, is your sting?"

The sting of death is sin, and the power of sin is the law. But thanks be to God, who gives us the victory through our Lord Jesus Christ. Therefore, my beloved, be steadfast, immovable, always excelling in the work of the Lord, because you know that in the Lord your labor is not in vain.

—1 Cor. 15:1–58

HYMNS AT TIME OF DEATH

The King of Love My Shepherd Is
The King of love my shepherd is,
  whose goodness fail-eth never.
I nothing lack if I am his, and he is
  mine forever.

Where steams of living water flow my
  ransomed soul he lead-eth.
And, where the verdant pastures
  grow with food celestial feed-eth.
In death's dark vale I fear no ill with
  thee, Lord, beside me;
Thy rod and staff my comfort still,
Thy cross before to guide me.
And so through all the length
  of days
Thy goodness fail-eth never.
Good Shepherd, may I sing thy praise
within thy house forever.

Lift Your Glad Voices
Lift your glad voices in triumph on
  high,
For Jesus hath risen and we shall not
  die.
Vain were the terrors that gathered
  around him,
And short the dominion of death and
  the grave.

205

He burst from the fetters of darkness
that bound him,
Resplendent in glory, to live and to
save.
Loud was the chorus of angels on
high,
The Savior hath risen, and we shall
not die.

Glory to God, in full anthems of
joy;
The being he gave us, death cannot
destroy.
Sad were the life we may part with
tomorrow,
If tears were our birthright, and
death were our end.

But Jesus hath cheered the dark
valley of sorrow,
And bade us, immortal, to heaven
ascend.
Lift then your voices in triumph on
high,
For Jesus hath risen, and we shall not
die.

Come, Come Ye Saints

Come, come ye saints, no toil nor
labor fear but with joy wend your
way.
Though hard to you the journey may
appear, grace will be as your day.
We have a living Lord to guide, and
we can trust him to provide.
Do this and joy your hearts will swell:
All is well! All is well!

We'll find the rest which God for us
prepared, when at last he will call.
Where none will come to hurt or
make afraid, he will reign over all.
We will make the air with music ring,

shout praise to God our Lord and
King.
Oh, how we'll make the chorus swell:
All is well! All is well!

Take Thou My Hand, O Father

Take thou my hand, O Father, and
lead thou me, until my journey end-
eth eternally.
Alone I will not wander one single
day.
Be thou my true companion and with
me stay.

O cover with thy mercy my poor,
weak heart!
Let every thought rebellious from me
depart.
Permit my child to linger here at thy
feet, and fully trust thy goodness
with faith complete.

Though naught of they great power
may move my soul, with thee
through night and darkness I reach
the goal.
Take, then, my hand, O Father, and
lead thou me, until my journey end-
eth eternally.

Children of the Heavenly Father

Children of the heav'nly Father safely
in his bosom gather.
Nestling bird nor star in heaven such
a refuge e'er was given.

God his own doth tend and nourish,
in his holy courts they flourish.
From all evil things he spares them, in
his mighty arms he bears them.

Neither life nor death shall ever from
the Lord his children sever.

Unto them his grace he show-eth, and
their sorrows all he knoweth.

Though he giv-eth or he tak-eth, God
his children ne'er forsak-eth.
His the loving purpose solely to
preserve them pure and holy.

For All the Saints
For all the saints, who from their
labors rest, who thee by faith before
the world confessed,
Thy name, O Jesus, be forever
blessed. Alleluia, alleluia!

Oh, blessed communion, fellowship
divine!
We feebly struggle, they in glory
shine, yet all are one in thee, for all
are thine. Alleluia, alleluia!

The golden evening brightens in the
west.
Soon, soon to faithful servants cometh
rest.
Sweet is the calm of paradise the
blessed. Alleluia, alleluia!

But lo! There breaks a yet more
glorious day; the saints triumphant
rise in bright array, the King of
glory passes on his way. Alleluia,
alleluia!

From earth's wide bounds, from
ocean's farthest coast, through gates
of pearl streams in the countless
host, singing to Father, Son and
Holy Ghost, Alleluia, alleluia!

Catholic Traditions: General Introduction

Prepared by:
Robert E. Johnson, PhD
Professor of Christian Heritage, Central Baptist Theological Seminary
Shawnee, KS

The term "catholic" means "general" or "universal" and thus connotes the universal Church in contrast to local Christian communities. Following the schism between the Eastern and Western churches in the eleventh century CE, the Western Church tended to refer to itself as "catholic" and the Eastern Church adopted the term "orthodox." In a general sense, the term "catholic" refers to those Churches who claim a continuous historical tradition of belief and practice that dates to the New Testament Apostles. This claim of authority derived from an unbroken Apostolic tradition distinguishes this body of Christians from Protestant Christians, who place ultimate authority in the Bible as interpreted according to principles derived from the sixteenth-century Reformation. The principal Church bodies designated by the term "catholic" today are Roman Catholics, Eastern Catholics (often referred to as Uniates), and Old Catholics. Sometimes, the Anglican Churches are included in this categorization as well.

Old Catholics consist of several small groups of national Churches that separated from Rome for a variety of reasons. The Old Catholic Church in the Netherlands severed relations with the papacy over Jansenism and related concerns in the early eighteenth century. The German, Austrian, and Swiss Old Catholic Churches refused to accept the decrees of the First Vatican Council regarding papal infallibility and the universal ordinary jurisdiction of the pope. The Polish National Catholic Church and the Yugoslav Old Catholic Church resulted from national church movements among Poles in the United States and among the Croats. Since 1932, these Churches have been in communion with the Church of England. Distinctives of their theology and practice include:

- adherence to the doctrines of the *Declaration of Utrecht* (1889)
- recognition of the authority of the first seven Ecumenical Councils
- allowance of clergy marriage
- worship conducted in vernacular languages
- Eucharist observed in both kinds.

Eastern Catholic Churches are often referred to as Uniate Churches (a term given by their opponents and generally rejected by Eastern Catholic Churches). The dates when these Churches entered into communion with Rome vary, and practices can vary according to the conditions agreed upon at the time of their union. In most cases they:

- keep their own languages, rites, and canon law
- are allowed Communion in both kinds
- practice infant baptism by immersion
- permit clergy to marry.

Since 1991, these communions have been governed by a code of canon law for all Uniate Churches. Among Churches included in this communion are (1) of the Antiochene rite: the Maronite Churches, the Syrian churches under the Patriarch of Antioch, and the Malankarses Churches; (2) of the Chaldean rite: the Armenian Churches under the Patriarch of Cilicia, the Chaldean churches, and the Malabarese Churches; (3) of the Alexandrian rite: the Coptic Churches and the Ethiopian Churches; and (4) of the Byzantine rite: the Ukrainian Churches, the Hungarian Churches, the Serbian Churches in Croatia, the Podcarpathian Ruthenian Churches, the Romanian Churches, and the Melkite Churches, certain of the Bulgar Churches, and certain of the Greek Churches. Eastern Rite Catholics include about 15 million adherents.

Roman Catholicism refers to the beliefs and practices of Christians and church bodies in communion with the pope in Rome. This church traces its lineal descent from the Western Catholic Church of the Middle Ages, but emphasizes an Apostolic Succession of leadership originating with the Apostle Peter. Structurally, it is an organized hierarchy of bishops and priests headed by the pope.

Catholic theology and practice may be summarized as follows.
- Acknowledgement of the bishop of Rome as the Supreme Pontiff and authority, who serves as Christ's representative on earth and as the successor of the Apostle Peter.
- God's grace and blessings are mediated to believers through members of the Church's hierarchy via the seven sacraments (baptism, confirmation, marriage, ordination, penance, extreme unction, and the Mass).
- The Mass stands at the center of liturgical life and is a re-presentation of Christ's passion, death, and resurrection.
- In the Eucharist, the bread and wine become the real Body and Blood of Christ according to a process called transubstantiation.
- Attendance at Mass is expected on Sundays and Feasts of Obligation.
- While not obligatory, many Catholics choose to practice extra-liturgical exercises such as praying the Rosary and the Stations of the Cross.

Vatican Council Two initiated major reforms which included more open relationships with non-Catholic Churches, simplification of the liturgy, a greater role for bishops acting as an episcopal college, and the celebration of liturgical worship in the vernacular. Although these reforms emphasized the Mass as the central act of Christian devotion, devotion to saints continues to be an important dimension of spirituality for many Catholics. In addition, numerous orders of monks, friars, canons regular, and nuns continue to fill significant functions in the life and ministry of the Roman Catholic Church.

The Catholic traditions presented in the next two sections are Eastern Rite Catholic Church and Roman Catholicism.

Eastern Rite Catholic Church

We believe that through His passion, death and resurrection,
we will gain eternal life.[223]

Prepared by:
Paul Hura, MD
Overland Park, KS

Reviewed and approved by:
The Reverend James Bankston
St. Nicholas Ukrainian Catholic Cathedral
Chicago, IL

History and Facts

Although most members of the Roman Catholic Church follow a discipline, ritual, and canon law that developed in the early years of the diocese of Rome, others adhere in these matters to their own centuries-old traditions. These are the Eastern Rite Churches or Uniate churches, such as the Ukrainian, Maronite, Chaldean, and Ruthenian. Largest among these Eastern Rite Churches is the Ukrainian Greco-Catholic Church (UGCC), which has its origins in the ancient nation of Kyivan-Rus (or Rus-Ukraine). As such, describing the UGCC serves as an example of Eastern Rite Catholic Churches in general, save for the individual variations that exist among them. The term "Greco" simply means that its origins in terms of liturgy, spirituality, canon law, and so forth, are from the Greek (or Byzantine) tradition.

Christianity was adopted in Ukraine in the year 988 by Volodymyr, the Grand-Prince of Kyiv. Through the centuries and because of many various stresses, Eastern Christianity (made up of the four Patriarchates of Constantinople, Alexandria, Antioch, and Jerusalem) became estranged from Western Christianity which was led by the Patriarch in Rome. The separation, or Great Schism (usually said to have been final in the year 1054), resulted in the Roman Catholic Church and the Orthodox Churches breaking communion. The Ukrainian Orthodox Church was among the Orthodox communion. In 1596, part of the Ukrainian Orthodox Church hierarchy reestablished ecclesial communion with the Roman Catholic Church through the Treaty of Brest-Litovsk. This group today is known as the Ukrainian Greco-Catholic Church.

The UGCC was subject to persecution both under Tsarist rule and more recently under Atheistic Communism. In 1946, the pseudo-Synod of L'viv declared that the UGCC was dissolved and ceased to exist. However, the faithful laity and clergy went underground and continued to courageously practice their faith and uphold their union to the Catholic Church. When communism disintegrated in the early 1990s, a strong and vibrant UGCC came out into the open. Its strength surprised many who had thought that it had truly ceased to exist and

---

223 Quote provided by Rev. Bankston.

its survival under communism stands as a testimony to the courage and faithfulness of those who maintained their church during that period.

Basic Teachings

- The central creedal statement of the Ukrainian Catholic Church is the Nicean-Constantinopolan Creed formulated at the first and second Ecumenical Councils of Nicea (325 CE) and Constantinople (381 CE). It is recited at every Divine Liturgy in the Byzantine Liturgical tradition.

I believe in one God, the Father, the Almighty, maker of heaven and earth, of all that is seen and unseen.

I believe in one Lord, Jesus Christ, the only Son of God, eternally begotten of the Father. Light from Light, true God from true God, begotten, not made, one in being with the Father. Through Him all things were made. For us men and for our salvation He came down from heaven: by the power of the Holy Spirit He was born of the Virgin Mary, and became man. For our sake he was crucified under Pontius Pilate; he suffered, died and was buried. On the third day He rose again in fulfillment of the Scriptures; He ascended into heaven and is seated at the right hand of the Father. He will come again in glory to judge the living and the dead, and His kingdom will have no end.

I believe in the Holy Spirit, the Lord, the giver of life, who proceeds from the Father. With the Father and the Son He is worshiped and glorified. He has spoken through the Prophets.

I believe in one, holy, catholic and apostolic Church. I acknowledge one baptism for the forgiveness of sins. I look for the resurrection of the dead, and the life of the world to come. Amen.[224]

- The UGCC shares the common faith of Eastern and Western apostolic Christianity, which holds that there are seven Mysteries (or Sacraments):
  1. Baptism (for infants and adults)
  2. Chrismation (or Confirmation)
  3. Holy Eucharist
  4. Reconciliation (or Confession)
  5. Crowning (or Marriage)
  6. Holy Anointing (or Anointing of the sick)
  7. Holy Orders.
- **Spiritual leaders**: All the faithful share in the "Royal Priesthood" of Jesus Christ. However, following the example of Jesus and His selection of the Apostles, the Catholic Church, including the UGCC, has an exclusively male-ordained diaconate, presbyterate, and episcopate. Religious orders exist for both men and women, nonetheless. Religious orders for men include the Basilians, Redemptorists, and Studites; religious orders for women include the Sisters of St. Basil, Sister Servants of Mary Immaculate, and Sisters of St. Joseph.

Basic Practices

- **Liturgy**: The UGCC's worship is highly liturgical. The primary form of worship

---

224 Guilbert, C. (Custodian of the *Standard Book of Common Prayer*). (1990). *The Book of Common Prayer*. New York, NY: Oxford University Press, 326–327.

is the Divine Liturgy. This is the common work or common action of God's people – clergy and laity alike – who come together to praise and worship God while thanking Him for His many gifts and blessings; to publicly proclaim the Good News of the risen Christ while awaiting His Second Coming; to partake of the Eucharist – the very Body and Blood of Jesus Christ – which is offered to the faithful for the forgiveness of their sins and unto life everlasting; and to manifest God's Kingdom in this world. The two most commonly celebrated versions of the Divine Liturgy are the Liturgy of Saint John Chrysostom, celebrated on most Sundays and feasts; and the Liturgy of Saint Basil the Great, celebrated on Lenten Sundays, the feast of Saint Basil, and several other occasions.

○ *The Liturgy of the Word*: The first portion of the Divine Liturgy, the Liturgy of the Word, revolves around the proclamation of the Good News of Jesus Christ as revealed in the Holy Scriptures. The opening doxology, "Blessed is the Kingdom of the Father, and of the Son, and of the Holy Spirit," reminds people that, in worship, they are entering the kingdom of God. During the Great Litany, people pray for the various needs which confront them in their daily lives. The Antiphons joyfully express praise through the singing of the psalms, while the Hymn to Christ, the Only-begotten Son of God, is the acknowledgement of Jesus Christ as true God, true man, and the Savior of all. The Little Entrance is the solemn invitation to worship the risen Christ. The Tropar and Kontak proclaim the theme of the day's Liturgy. By singing the Trisaglon, "Holy God, Holy and Mighty One, Holy and Immortal One,

have mercy on us," individuals glorify the Holy Trinity. Following these introductory hymns, the Holy Scriptures are proclaimed. The Prokeimen is a responsorial psalm chanted by the reader and the people. It prepares one for the Epistle Lesson, taken from the New Testament epistles or the Acts of the Apostles, which generally emphasizes a particular aspect of Christian life. The Alleluia consists of psalm verses separated by the singing of "Alleluia," which means "Praise the Lord." The Gospel Lesson, the public proclamation of the Word of God, is taken from the gospels of Saints Matthew, Mark, Luke, and John. After the Gospel, people hear the Sermon, during which the priest reflects upon the Good News of Jesus Christ as it applies to their daily lives.

○ *The Liturgy of the Eucharist*: Having been nourished by the Word of God, people now turn their attention to the central mystery of the Faith, the death and resurrection of Jesus Christ, by celebrating the Liturgy of the Eucharist. The word Eucharist literally means "thanksgiving"; hence, by receiving Christ's Body and Blood in the Eucharist, people offer God the ultimate expression of thanks. During the Liturgy of the Eucharist, the Great Entrance is performed while the Cherubic Hymn is chanted. Gifts of bread and wine are brought in procession to the altar where they will be offered to God. People are invited to "Lay aside all earthly cares so that we may receive the King of all." The Peace is affirmation of Christ's presence and love as individuals praise the Trinity "with one mind and one heart." The Creed is the proclamation of the common faith in the Trinity. The

Eucharistic Canon recalls the institution of the Eucharist. People celebrate the love God shared through the death, resurrection, and ascension of Jesus Christ, and people joyfully anticipate His Second Coming. During the Consecration, the people call upon the Holy Spirit to change their gifts of bread and wine into the very Body and Blood of Christ. The Commemorations enable individuals to prayerfully remember all for whom their gifts are being offered. In the Lord's Prayer, people approach God as their heavenly Father. The Elevation, during which the priest raises the Body of Christ before the eyes of the faithful, is an expression of the conviction that God alone is holy. The climax of the Liturgy is the reception of the Eucharist. People enter into a common union with Him and with His People as they "taste the fountain of immortality." Having been nourished with the Body and Blood of Christ, individuals render thanks to God for bestowing His heavenly Spirit upon them. They are then invited to "depart in peace, In the Name of the Lord," in order to publicly proclaim all that they have received and experienced during the Divine Liturgy; to pray for salvation and guidance during the Closing Prayer which the priest offers in the midst of the people; and to receive the Lord's blessing, proclaimed by the priest, by venerating the holy cross.

o *The Liturgy in our Lives*: The end of every Divine Liturgy prepares people for the beginning of the next! If they strive to live and apply all that has been experienced in public worship, their lives become an inseparable part of the Liturgy and the Liturgy becomes an inseparable part of their lives. Having placed themselves in the very presence of God, they are no longer children of this world, but inheritors of the Kingdom of God and recipients of everlasting life. There are many other services that one may encounter. The most common would be Vespers, Matins, and the Liturgy of the Presanctified Gifts (celebrated during Lent).

- **Fasting**: There are four fasts during the Liturgical Year in the churches of the Byzantine Tradition. These are (in order from the beginning of the Church Year):
  1. Philip's Fast (from November 15 until December 24) in preparation for the feast of the Nativity;
  2. The Great Fast, from sunset on Cheese-fare ("Forgiveness") Sunday until sunset on the Friday before Flowery Sunday, in preparation for the Feast of the Resurrection of Jesus Christ (Pascha); the dates will vary based on the lunar calendar.
  3. Peter's Fast, from sunset on the Feast of All Saints (always the first Sunday after Pentecost) until sunset on June 28, in preparation for the Feast of Saints Peter and Paul (June 29);
  4. The Fast of *Theotókos* (God-bearer – that is, Mary the mother of God), from sunset on July 31 through sunset on August 14, in preparation for the Feast of the Dormition of the Theotókos (August 15).

- In addition, some Ukrainian Catholics fast every Wednesday and Friday during the rest of the year, except for a few periods of relief.

Jesus fasted and taught His disciples to fast (Matt. 6:16–18). The purpose of fasting is to gain mastery over oneself and to conquer the passions of the flesh. Fasting helps people become liberated from dependence on the things of this world in order to concentrate on the things of the Kingdom of God. Fasting gives power to the soul to avoid giving in to temptation and sin. People do not fast because it pleases God, for as the hymns of the Great Fast remind us, "the devil also never eats" (Lenten Triodion). People do not fast with the idea that hunger and thirst can somehow serve as "reparation" for sins. Such an understanding is never given in the scriptures, which relate that the only "reparation" for the sins of humankind is the crucifixion and death of the Lord Jesus Christ. Salvation is God's free gift (Rom. 5:15–17 and Eph. 2:8–9). People fast so that the free gift of salvation in Jesus Christ might produce great fruits in their lives, and so that they might more effectively serve God who loves and has saved them in Jesus Christ and the Holy Spirit.

A concept of fasting, reduced to legalistic measuring, is contrary to authentic Eastern Christian understanding of fasting. For example, a legalistic approach to fasting would be concerned with the amounts of food ("one main meal; two smaller meals, which, together, do not equal one main meal"). The Eastern Christian understanding of fasting or abstaining has less to do with the amounts of food consumed than with the kinds of foods consumed. An authentic Eastern Christian understanding makes any distinction between "fast" and "abstinence" obsolete. The spirit of abstinence goes beyond merely refraining from certain kinds of foods, to refraining even from activities which may lessen one's awareness of God's presence (e.g., entertainment). Accordingly, people have an obligation to seek out ways to apply the authentic meaning and spirit of abstinence in their Christian lives. Any of the fasting periods during the Church Year are opportunities for grace through self-denial and prayer. Fasting periods are not just times to "give up" something. Rather, they are opportunities to take on new challenges for personal growth in Jesus Christ. There might be something in people's lives that isn't quite right that they would like to change for the better (this is the fundamental meaning of the word repentance – a turning). Fasting helps people focus on making such changes.

An important part of the religious instruction of the young includes a correct, and authentic, meaning of fasting (abstinence). This is not an easy task in a materialistic society. As with all religious education, the example of adults serves as a powerful model and form of encouragement. Abstinence (fasting) helps to strengthen the will and promote self-discipline. For the youth, discipline learned through fasting (abstinence) is felt to help them meet greater life-challenges which will surely be encountered.

Principles for Clinical Care
Dietary Issues
- Eastern Rite Catholics have no dietary restrictions with the exception of fasting during designated holidays and not eating meat on Fridays (if one chooses to follow the strictest of year-long fasts). Exceptions to fasting include pregnant women, children under twelve years of age, adults above 64 years of age and people who are ill or otherwise cannot tolerate the physical stress of a fast.

General Medical Beliefs

- Medical science is valued, but advances in such science need to be grounded in basic principles of morality and with respect for the human person as made in the image of God.
- Care for the person throughout life – from conception to natural death – is necessary.
- The Church opposes euthanasia.

Specific Medical Issues

- **Abortion**: The Church opposes abortion for any reason, even if the question of the mother's life is at stake. The unborn child's survival and health is paramount.
- **Advance Directives**: The Church recognizes the value of and encourages the use of advance directives in health care planning.
- **Birth Control**: The Church forbids all forms of artificial birth control and suggests using natural methods of family planning only if necessary.[225]
- **Blood Transfusions**: Blood transfusions are allowed.
- **Circumcision**: Circumcision is not a religious requirement; it is an individual decision.
- **In Vitro Fertilization**: The Church opposes all forms of in vitro fertilization.
- **Stem Cell Research**: Stem cell research, as it pertains to the use of elements of a human embryo that may lead to the destruction of that embryo, is prohibited.
- **Vaccinations**: Vaccinations are allowed and encouraged in Eastern Rite Catholicism according to the recommendations of the local governments of the respected region or country.

---

225 www.east2west.org/doctrine.htm#Contracption (accessed 9 Sept 2012).

- **Withholding/Withdrawing Life Support**: The use of extraordinary means to artificially prolong life when death is imminent and certain is not required; it is an individual choice.

Gender and Personal Issues

- Eastern Rite Catholics have no prescriptions or proscriptions with respect to gender and personal issues, as far as appropriate medical treatment is concerned.

Principles for Spiritual Care through the Cycles of Life
Concepts of Living and Dying for Spiritual Support

- Life is sacred from conception to natural death.
- Death is a natural part of the life cycle and comes to everyone.
- Death is not something to be feared but is a transition to another existence.
- The resurrection is affirmed.
- Christ's triumph over sin and death is the guarantee of our own resurrection.

During Birth

- The Church encourages Baptism to occur by 3 months of age.
- When a child dies before it is baptized, a formal funeral does not take place. Instead, the child is buried with a simple ceremony that includes "prayers to the angels."
- As stated earlier, circumcision is not a religious requirement; it is an individual decision.

During Illness

- Patients may receive comfort from the reading of scriptures or other devotional material, listening to religious music, watching televised worship services of their own or a similar tradition. Patients may request Holy Communion. The chaplain or clergy should be consulted for assistance.

- Patients may receive comfort from healing prayers. These can be offered by health care professionals. Some patients, however, may ask for healing prayer to be connected with "anointing with oil" or the "the laying on of hands." The chaplain or clergy should be consulted for assistance for these requests.

During End of Life

- The Sacrament of Extreme Unction (also known as Last Rites) is administered by the priest to patients at end of life. It can be repeated if an apparent recovery was made that results in a subsequent decline of health.
- Family and friends often remain with the dying patient offering prayers and support for the patient and themselves.
- Patient or family may request the presence of a member of the clergy.
- Patient or family may request Baptism. The chaplain or clergy should be consulted for assistance.
- Patient or family may request Holy Communion. The chaplain or clergy should be consulted for assistance.

Care of the Body

- The Church allows for either cremation or burial; it is an individual decision.
- Embalming is an acceptable practice; it is an individual decision unless required by law.
- The Church allows for the body to be donated for medical research; it is an individual decision.

- The Church allows autopsies to be performed.

Organ and Tissue Donation

- Postmortem organ and tissue donations are allowed, with the caveat that death must be certain to have occurred.
- It is an individual decision. It may be preferable for a chaplain and/or nurse who are trained designated requesters to be consulted for assistance.

Scriptures, Inspirational Readings, and Prayers

Readings and prayers in this section are the same as those in the "Roman Catholicism" chapter.

READINGS DURING ILLNESS

These can be read by family, friends, clergy, and health care professionals. (All scripture quotations are from the New American Bible.)

I lift up my eyes toward the
mountains; whence shall help
Come to me? My help is from the
Lord, Who made heaven and earth.

May He not suffer your foot to slip;
May He slumber not who guards
you.
Indeed He neither slumbers nor
sleeps, the guardian of Israel. The
Lord is your guardian;

The Lord is your shade; He is beside
you at your right hand.
The sun shall not harm you by day
nor the moon by night.

The Lord will guard you from all evil;
He will guard your life.

The Lord will guard your coming and your going, both now and forever.

—Psalm 121

You who dwell in the shelter of the Most High, Who abide in the shadow of the Almighty,
Say to the Lord, "My refuge and my fortress, my God, in whom I trust."

For he will rescue you from the snare of the fowler, from the destroying pestilence.
With his pinions he will cover you, and under his wings you shall take refuge; His faithfulness is a buckler and a shield.
You shall not fear the terror of the night nor the arrow that flies by day, nor the pestilence that roams in the darkness, nor the devastating plague at noon.

Though a thousand fall at your side, ten thousand at your right hand, near you it shall not come.
Rather with your eyes shall you behold and see the requital of the wicked, because you have the Lord for your refuge;

You have made the Most High your stronghold.

—Ps. 91:1–9

PRAYERS DURING ILLNESS

These prayers can be offered by family, friends, clergy, and health care professionals.

Jesus, you suffered and died for us;
You understand suffering;
Teach me to understand my suffering as You do;
To bear it in union with You;
To offer it with You to atone for my sins and to bring Your grace to souls in need.
Calm my fears; increase my trust.
May I gladly accept Your holy will and become more like You in trial.
If it be Your will, restore me to health so that I may work for your honor and glory and the salvation of all. Amen.

Merciful Lord, you know the anguish of the sorrowful, you are attentive to the prayers of the humble. Hear your people who cry out to you in their need, and strengthen their hope in your lasting goodness. We ask this through Christ our Lord. Amen.

Prayer to Mary

Mary, health of the sick;
be at the bedside of all the world's sick people;
Of those who are unconscious and dying;
of those who have begun their last agony;
of those who have lost hope of a cure;
of those who weep and cry out in pain;
of those who cannot have care because they have no money;
of those who seek vainly on their beds for a less painful position;
of those who pass long nights sleepless;
of those who are worried by a family in distress;

of those who must renounce
cherished plans for the future;
of those, above all, who do not believe
in a better life;
of those who rebel and curse God;
of those who do not know that Christ
suffered like them and for them!

Memorare

Remember, most gracious Virgin
Mary, that never was it known
that anyone who fled to your
protection, implored your help,
or sought your intercession was
left unaided. Inspired by this
confidence, I fly to you. Virgin of
virgins, my mother. To you do I
come, before you I stand, sinful
and sorrowful. Mother of the Word
Incarnate, despise not my petitions,
but in your mercy hear and answer
me. Amen.

READINGS DURING END-OF-LIFE PROCESS

These can be read by family, friends, clergy,
and health care professionals. (All scripture
quotations are from the New American
Bible.)

The Lord is my shepherd, I shall not
want. In verdant pastures He gives
me repose;
beside restful waters He leads me,
He refreshes my soul.
He guides me in right paths for his
name's sake.

Even though I walk In the dark
valley I fear no evil;
for you are at my side with your
rod and your staff that give me
courage.

You spread the table before me In the
sight of my foes;
you anoint my head with oil; My cup
overflows.
Only goodness and kindness Follow
me all the days of my life;
And I shall dwell in the house of the
Lord for years to come.

—Psalm 23

Praised be God, the Father of our
Lord Jesus Christ, the Father
of Mercies and the God of all
consolation! He comforts us in all
our afflictions and thus enables us
to comfort those who are in trouble
with the same consolation as we
have received from Him. As we
have shared much in the suffering
of Christ, so through Christ
do we share abundantly in His
consolation.

—2 Cor. 1:3–5

PRAYERS DURING END-OF-LIFE PROCESS

These prayers can be offered by family,
friends, clergy, and health care professionals.

The Blessing of Aaron

The Lord bless you and keep you;
The Lord make his face to shine upon
you,
and be gracious to you; the Lord lift
his countenance
upon you, and give you peace.

Prayer for God's Presence

O God, my Lord, Come to me,
comfort me, console me. O God,
you are my light in the darkness.

You are my warmth in the cold.
You are my happiness in sorrow.

Eternal Rest
Eternal rest grant unto him/her
and let perpetual light shine upon
   him/her.

May he/she rest in peace. Amen.
May his/her soul and the souls of all
   the faithful departed,
through the mercy of God, rest in
   peace. Amen.

Roman Catholicism

I recognized that there is nothing better than to be glad and to do well during life.[226]

Prepared by:

The Reverend Jerry L. Spencer, MA, BCSM, BCBT, BCETS, BCECR
Catholic Priest, Holy Name Church
Chaplain, The University of Kansas Hospital
Kansas City, KS

History and Facts

The Catholic Church began with the preaching and ministry of Jesus Christ and the twelve Apostles. Christianity was developed and promulgated through the preaching, letters, and missionary journeys of Saint Paul and its utilization of the Roman model of transportation and governance. The Church's governing body began with the designation of Saint Peter as the "Rock upon whom Christ would build His Church" (Matt. 16:18) with bishops as successors of the Apostles. Saint Peter was the Bishop of Rome and, thus, the first Pope with the present Pope Benedict XVI as his 265th successor. Catholicism came to the New World in the western hemisphere with the discovery of the Americas by Christopher Columbus in 1492. The Church was established in North and South America by missionaries from Spain, Portugal, France, Ireland, and Italy. Today, the leadership of the Church in America consists of the United States Conference of Catholic Bishops (USCCB) nationally and the bishops in their respective dioceses.

Officially, the fall of the Roman Empire occurred in 476 CE. Saint Benedict and his monastic movement was a stabilizing force in the midst of chaos for the rural Church. The Franciscans, Dominicans, Carmelites, and Augustinians developed an urban ministry for the Church.

The Chalcedonian Ecumenical Council in 451 unfortunately divided those accepting this council continuing as the early Christian Church and those not accepting it becoming known as the Monophysites or Oriental Orthodox. It has more recently been acknowledged that both hold a similar theological understanding even though being on opposing sides of this Ecumenical Council. Dialogue continues concerning this split to the present day.

A further tragic event among the five centers of the Christian Church of the Ecumenical Councils was the Great Schism between Rome (the primary see now known as the Roman Catholic Church or "The West") and Constantinople, along with the other three early centers of Christianity – Jerusalem, Alexandria, and Antioch (known as the Orthodox Church or "The East") – in 1054. The Emperor Constantine had moved

---

226 Eccles. 3:12 (New American Bible).

the capital of the empire to Constantinople in the fourth century. From this point on, these ecclesiastical centers of Rome and Constantinople were in increasing conflict, resulting in their eventual split. Several unsuccessful attempts were made following this split toward restoration. Though the mutual anathemas were lifted in 1969 between the Roman Catholic and Orthodox Churches, full communion has sadly not yet been restored. What follows is the unfolding history of the Roman Catholic Church.

The Crusades were the collective name given to the various "holy wars" that were launched during the Middle Ages with the aim of recovering the Holy Land from Islamic domination or to defend Christendom from attack.

On October 31, 1517, Martin Luther posted his 95 theses on the door of the castle church at Wittenberg, Germany, which led to the start of the Protestant Reformation.

Other reformers, such as John Calvin and Ulrich Zwingli, advanced the initiatives of Luther. It was during the reign of Henry VIII (1491–1547) that England broke with the Church.

On December 13, 1545, 30 bishops met for the first session of the Council of Trent. It took 18 years for Trent to complete its work, and it defined key doctrines of the Church. Trent began the Counter-Reformation with leadership by saints like Saint Ignatius of Loyola, and Carmelite saints Teresa of Avila and John of the Cross.

Saint Peter's Basilica was built on Vatican Hill over an ancient burial ground, traditionally accepted as the site where the body of Saint Peter was placed after his crucifixion. The construction process took over a century (the corner was laid on April 18, 1506, and the building was consecrated on November 18, 1626). The first Vatican Council (held between December 8, 1869, and September 1, 1870) lasted briefly and was interrupted by the Franco-Prussian War. It was adjourned by the pope indefinitely, never officially ended and never reconvened. However, it declared the doctrine of papal infallibility and enhanced the potential for papal ministry in the Church. Pope John XXIII opened the Second Vatican Council on October 11, 1962. The purpose of the Council was "an updating" that would be a pastoral response of the Church to a need for spiritual renewal and ecumenical progress toward Church unity.

Basic Teachings

- The Church is the Mystical Body of Christ and consists of the hierarchy (ordained clergy) and the laity.
- Preeminent among all written sources in Tradition is the Holy Bible, revered and treasured as the Word of God. Ongoing amplification and clarification of Church teaching (doctrine) is done by Papal writings, Ecumenical councils, Special Synods and approved theological and biblical scholars.
- Catholics believe in the teachings of the *Nicene Creed* and *Apostles' Creed*.

The Nicene Creed

I believe in one God, the Father almighty, maker of heaven and earth, of all things visible and invisible.

I believe in one Lord Jesus Christ, the Only Begotten Son of God, born of the Father before all ages. God from God, Light from Light, true God from true God, begotten, not made, consubstantial with the Father; through him all things were made.

For us men and for our salvation

he came down from heaven, and
by the Holy Spirit was incarnate of
the Virgin Mary, and became man.
For our sake he was crucified under
Pontius Pilate, he suffered death
and was buried, and rose again on
the third day in accordance with the
Scriptures. He ascended into heaven
and is seated at the right hand of the
Father. He will come again in glory to
judge the living and the dead and his
kingdom will have no end.

I believe in the Holy Spirit, the
Lord, the giver of life, who proceeds
from the Father and the Son, who
with the Father and the Son is
adored and glorified, who has spoken
through the prophets.

I believe in one, holy, catholic
and apostolic Church. I confess one
baptism for the forgiveness of sins
and I look forward to the resurrection
of the dead and the life of the world
to come. Amen.[227]

The Apostles' Creed

I believe in God, the Father almighty,
creator of heaven and earth,
I believe in Jesus Christ, His only
Son, our Lord. Who was conceived
by the power of the Holy Spirit;
born of the virgin Mary; suffered
under Pontius Pilate; was crucified,
died, and buried.
He descended into hell. On the third
day He rose again. He ascended
into heaven and is seated at the
right hand of the Father. He will

come again to judge the living and
the dead.
I believe in the Holy Spirit, the
holy catholic (universal) church,
the communion of saints, the
forgiveness of sins, the resurrection
of the body and life everlasting.
Amen.

Christological Teachings of Early Councils

- **Nicea (325 CE):** Jesus Christ is the Son of God by nature and not by adoption. He is "begotten," not made, consubstantial with the Father.
- **Ephesus (431 CE):** Since the one who was born of Mary is divine, Mary is rightly called "Mother of God."
- **Chalcedon (451 CE):** Jesus Christ, Son of God, is true God and true man. His divine and human natures remain together without confusion, change, division, or separation.
- **Second Constantinople (553 CE):** There is only one person – a divine person – in Jesus Christ. The human acts of Jesus are also attributed to His divine person.

Basic Practices

- Prayer, meditation, the reading of sacred scripture, and celebration of the Mass are important spiritual practices for many Catholics. The many forms of these practices include reading and/or silent contemplation upon scripture or doctrinal beliefs and prayers of various kinds – petition, healing, repentance for unethical thoughts and actions, praise, worship and thanksgiving to God.
- Social Justice is important to Catholics. These acts of service take the forms of – working for social justice with marginalized peoples, charitable giving to

227 Guilbert, C. (Custodian of the *Standard Book of Common Prayer*). (1990). *The Book of Common Prayer.* New York, NY: Oxford University Press, 326–327.

provide food, building, and educational programs for the poor, volunteerism, and so forth. Mission work is also an intentional witness to one's faith through proclamation and teaching.

- The sharing of one's faith is communicated through loving actions, talking about personal spiritual experiences, reading scriptures, and discussions of doctrinal positions.
- Catholics value Sacred Liturgy, and will gather on Sundays and at other times to hear preaching, study scripture, sing hymns and pray, receive the sacraments.
- The principal form of Catholic worship is the celebration of the Eucharist, the Holy Sacrifice of the Mass.
- The sacred liturgy also includes the seven sacraments:
  1. Baptism for infants and adults
  2. Reconciliation (confession) throughout life
  3. Holy Communion throughout life
  4. Confirmation at an appropriate age
  5. Matrimony when appropriately prepared
  6. Holy Orders: Deacon, Priest, Bishop
  7. Anointing of the Sick in time of illness, accident or old age.
- Celebration of the Mass is obligatory on all Sundays and designated Holy Days.
- Sacramental objects and devotions are used in personal life and prayer (e.g., the Rosary, Stations of the Cross, religious medals and pictures).

Principles for Clinical Care
Dietary Issues
- Catholics have no dietary restrictions with the exception of fasting and not eating meat on certain days.
- The Catholic Church asks its members

between the ages of 18 and 59 years to fast on Ash Wednesday and the Fridays of Lent. Those older than 14 years of age are to abstain from meat on these days as well. Some medical conditions could excuse one from these obligations.

- Catholics are to fast 1 hour before receiving Holy Communion. The sick need only to fast for 15 minutes and medicines, whether liquid or solid, may be taken at any time.

General Medical Beliefs
- Catholics believe that God is the ultimate source of all life, health, and healing.
- Jesus Christ is referred to as the Divine Physician.
- Catholics accept most traditional Western medical procedures and respect alternative modalities of medical care.

Specific Medical Issues
- **Abortion**: The Church has been opposed to abortion for centuries and remains so today. Persons who procure or perform an abortion can incur serious ecclesiastical (i.e., Church) penalties. Abortion is not acceptable for birth control, sex selection, or convenience.
- **Advance Directives**: The Catholic Church endorses the use of advance directives; it encourages that the information provided be complete and adequately reflects the wishes of the patient concerning health care. The Church also recommends that the documents be reviewed periodically and updated as needed.
- **Birth Control**: The Catholic Church is opposed to any method of artificial contraception. The use of natural family planning is allowed in certain circumstances.
- **Blood Transfusions**: The Catholic

Church has no objections to the use of blood products; many Catholic churches sponsor blood donation drives.

- **Circumcision**: Circumcision is not a religious requirement; it is an individual decision.
- **In Vitro Fertilization**: The Catholic Church is opposed to in vitro fertilization and birth control.
- **Stem Cell Research**: Reproductive cloning is not morally permissible. While the Catholic Church has affirmed the effort to improve therapeutic options by the use of adult stem cells, even to the extent of generating organ replacements, it opposes the use of embryo stem cells for either reproductive or therapeutic purposes. (*See* following point, "Vaccinations")
- **Vaccinations**: Vaccinations against disease have enhanced the health of much of humanity. Vaccines are produced from natural and synthetic sources but some have moral implications in their procurement and production. Vaccines have been produced from various cell lines, but Directive 66 of the Ethical and Religious Directives for Catholic Health Care Services (ERD 2009) states: "Catholic health institutions should not make use of human tissue obtained by direct abortions for research or therapeutic purposes (ERD 2009)."[228] However, new methods have recently been proposed to obtain plurupotent stem cells similar to those in human embryos, while avoiding creating and destroying human embryos.

- **Withholding/Withdrawing Life Support**: Withholding/withdrawing life support in medically futile cases is permitted. Artificial nutrition and hydration are important elements in these decisions as well. One is not obliged to use extraordinary means in preserving life, but there should be a presumption in favor of providing nutrition and hydration for all patients, including patients who require medically assisted nutrition and hydration, so long as this is of sufficient benefit to outweigh the burden involved to the patient (ERD 2009).[229]

Gender and Personal Issues

- Catholicism has no prescriptions or proscriptions with respect to gender and personal issues, as far as appropriate medical treatment is concerned.
- Surgical sterilization is not permitted.
- Human sexuality is an integral part of human nature and deserves the utmost respect. Sex change surgery should only be done after thorough discernment and requisite counsel.

Principles for Spiritual Care through the Cycles of Life
Concepts of Living and Dying for Spiritual Support

- Life is sacred and deserves respect throughout.
- Death is the passage of the soul or life principle into eternity.

---

228 United States Conference of Catholic Bishops. Ethical and Religious Directives for Catholic Health Care Services, Fifth Edition. p 33. 2009. Available at: www.usccb.org/issues-and-action/human-life-and-dignity/health-care/upload/Ethical-Religious-Directives-Catholic-Health-Care-Services-fifth-edition-2009.pdf (accessed 6 Sept 2012).

229 United States Conference of Catholic Bishops. Ethical and Religious Directives for Catholic Health Care Services, Fifth Edition. p 31. 2009. Available at: www.usccb.org/issues-and-action/human-life-and-dignity/health-care/upload/Ethical-Religious-Directives-Catholic-Health-Care-Services-fifth-edition-2009.pdf (accessed 6 Sept 2012).

- Resurrection of the physical body and reunion of body and soul (spirit) will happen at the end of time at the Second Coming of Jesus. The entire cosmos will be transformed and restored to a state of perfection.

During Birth

- Baptism is normally administered shortly after birth and immediately when in danger of death. While usually done by a priest or deacon, it can be done by any layperson, Catholic or non-Catholic, using ordinary water and saying, "I baptize you in the name of the Father and of the Son and of the Holy Spirit" while pouring the water on the baby's head.

During Illness

- Patients may receive comfort from the reading of sacred scriptures or other devotional material, listening to religious music, watching televised worship services of their own or a similar tradition. Patients may request Holy Communion. Chaplain or clergy should be consulted for assistance.
- Patients may receive comfort from healing prayers. These can be offered by health care professionals. Patients from some traditions, however, may ask for healing prayer to be connected with "anointing with oil" or the "the laying on of hands." The chaplain or clergy should be consulted for assistance for these requests.
- Priests and bishops can offer the Sacraments of Reconciliation and the Anointing of the Sick. Laypeople can offer prayer, counsel and act as Extraordinary Ministers of the Eucharist, bringing Holy Communion to the sick and homebound.

During End of Life

- Patient or family may request Baptism. The chaplain or clergy should be consulted for assistance.
- Patient or family may request the Sacraments of Reconciliation, Holy Communion (Viaticum) and the Anointing of the Sick. A priest is required for Reconciliation and Anointing of the Sick. If the person is unresponsive, these sacraments can be administered "conditionally." Conditionally can refer to uncertainty that death has occurred or that, while unresponsive, there is the presumption that patients or their families would want the sacraments administered.
- Last Rites are prayers at the time of death.

Care of the Body

- Patients or families may choose either full body burial or cremation. Remains cannot be scattered on land or at sea. Cremation is permitted for economic, cultural, and practical reasons
- Embalming is an acceptable practice among Catholics and may be required in some cases.
- Autopsies may be performed and, in some cases, are mandated by law.
- Donation for medical research is an individual decision. The chaplain and/or nurse should be consulted for assistance. Advance planning for such donations is required by most receiving organizations. Last-minute donations are usually not possible.

Organ and Tissue Donation

- Organ and tissue from living donors is permitted and anatomical gifts may be given by cadaveric donors. Accurate and appropriate definitions of death need to be followed. Brain and cardiopulmonary death are commonly accepted in clinical practices. It may be preferable for a chaplain and/or nurse who are trained designated requesters to be consulted for assistance.

Scriptures, Inspirational Readings, and Prayers

READINGS DURING ILLNESS

These can be read by family, friends, clergy, and health care professionals. (All scripture quotations are from the New American Bible.)

I lift up my eyes toward the
  mountains; whence shall help Come
  to me?
My help is from the Lord, Who made
  heaven and earth.

May He not suffer your foot to slip;
  May He slumber not who guards
  you.
Indeed He neither slumbers nor
  sleeps, the guardian of Israel.

The Lord is your guardian; The Lord
  is your shade; He is beside you at
  your right hand.
The sun shall not harm you by day
  nor the moon by night.

The Lord will guard you from all evil;
  He will guard your life.
The Lord will guard your coming and
  your going, both now and forever.

—Psalm 121

You who dwell in the shelter of
  the Most High, Who abide in the
  shadow of the Almighty,
Say to the Lord, "My refuge and my
  fortress, my God, in whom I trust."
For he will rescue you from the snare
  of the fowler, from the destroying
  pestilence.
With his pinions he will cover you,
  and under his wings you shall take
  refuge; His faithfulness is a buckler
  and a shield. You shall not fear the
  terror of the night nor the arrow
  that flies by day, nor the pestilence
  that roams in the darkness, nor the
  devastating plague at noon. Though
  a thousand fall at your side, ten
  thousand at your right hand, near
  you it shall not come. Rather with
  your eyes shall you behold and see
  the requital of the wicked, because
  you have the Lord for your refuge;
  You have made the Most High your
  stronghold.

—Ps. 91:1–9

PRAYERS DURING ILLNESS

These prayers can be offered by family, friends, clergy, and health care professionals.

Jesus, you suffered and died for us;
You understand suffering;
Teach me to understand my suffering
  as You do;
To bear it in union with You;
To offer it with You to atone for my
  sins and to bring Your grace to souls
  in need.
Calm my fears; increase my trust.
May I gladly accept Your holy will
  and become more like You in trial.
If it be Your will, restore me to health

so that I may work for your honor
and glory and the salvation of all.
Amen.

Merciful Lord, you know the anguish
of the sorrowful, you are attentive to
the prayers of the humble.
Hear your people who cry out to you
in their need, and strengthen their
hope in your lasting goodness.
We ask this through Christ our Lord.
Amen.

Prayer to Mary
Mary, health of the sick; be at the
bedside of all the world's sick
people;
Of those who are unconscious and
dying; of those who have begun
their last agony;
of those who have lost hope of a cure;
of those who weep and cry out in
pain;
of those who cannot have care
because they have no money;
of those who seek vainly on their beds
for a less painful position;
of those who pass long nights
sleepless; of those who are worried
by a family in distress; of those who
must renounce
cherished plans for the future; of
those, above all, who do not
believe in a better life; of those who
rebel and curse God; of those who
do not know that Christ suffered like
them and for them!

Memorare
Remember, most gracious Virgin
Mary, that never was it known that
anyone who fled to your protection,
implored your help, or sought

your intercession was left unaided.
Inspired by this confidence, I fly to
you. Virgin of virgins, my mother. To
you do I come, before you I stand,
sinful and sorrowful. Mother of the
Word Incarnate, despise not my
petitions, but in your mercy hear and
answer me. Amen.

READINGS DURING END-OF-LIFE PROCESS
These can be read by family, friends, clergy,
and health care professionals. (All scripture
quotations are from the New American
Bible.)

The Lord is my shepherd, I shall not
want. In verdant pastures He gives
me repose;
beside restful waters He leads me,
He refreshes my soul.
He guides me in right paths for his
name's sake.

Even though I walk In the dark valley
I fear no evil;
for you are at my side with your rod
and your staff that give me courage.

You spread the table before me In the
sight of my foes;
you anoint my head with oil; My cup
overflows.
Only goodness and kindness Follow
me all the days of my life;
And I shall dwell in the house of the
Lord for years to come.

Psalm 23

Praised be God, the Father of our
Lord Jesus Christ, the Father

of Mercies and the God of all consolation! He comforts us in all our afflictions and thus enables us to comfort those who are in trouble with the same consolation as we have received from Him. As we have shared much in the suffering of Christ, so through Christ do we share abundantly in His consolation.

—2 Cor. 1:3–5

PRAYERS DURING END-OF-LIFE PROCESS

These prayers can be offered by family, friends, clergy, and health care professionals.

The Blessing of Aaron

The Lord bless you and keep you;
The Lord make his face to shine upon you,
and be gracious to you;
the Lord lift his countenance upon you,
and give you peace.

Prayer for God's Presence

O God, my Lord, Come to me, comfort me, console me. O God, you are my light in the darkness. You are my warmth in the cold. You are my happiness in sorrow.

Eternal Rest

Eternal rest grant unto him/her and let perpetual light shine upon him/her.
May he/she rest in peace. Amen.
May his/her soul and the souls of all the faithful departed,
through the mercy of God, rest in peace. Amen.

The Church of Jesus Christ of
Latter-Day Saints (Mormon)

Through serving others, people can experience joy and draw closer to God.[230]

Prepared by:
The Public Affairs Department of The Church of Jesus Christ of Latter-Day Saints
Salt Lake City, UT

History and Facts

When Jesus Christ lived on the earth, He organized His Church so that all people could receive His gospel and return one day to live with God, the Father of all creation. After Jesus Christ ascended to heaven, His apostles continued to receive revelation from Him on how to direct the work of His Church. However, after the apostles were killed, members changed the teachings of the Church that Jesus Christ had established. While many good people and some truth remained, this "Apostasy," or general falling away from the truth, brought about the withdrawal of priesthood (the power and authority to act in God's name) from the earth. The apostle Peter prophesied that Jesus would restore His Church before His second coming (see Acts 3:19–21).

In the spring of 1820, a 14-year-old boy named Joseph Smith went into a grove of trees near his home in Palmyra, New York, and prayed to learn which church he should join. In answer to his prayer, God the Father and His Son Jesus Christ appeared to him, just as heavenly beings had appeared to prophets like Moses in biblical times. Smith learned that the Church originally organized by Jesus Christ was no longer on the earth.

Joseph Smith was chosen by God to restore the Church of Jesus Christ to the earth. During the next ten years, Smith was visited by other heavenly messengers, translated the Book of Mormon, and received authority to organize the Church. The Church was organized in Fayette, New York, on 6 April, 1830, under the leadership of Joseph Smith.

As of 2011, this worldwide church organization has close to 14 million members.

The official name of the church is The Church of Jesus Christ of Latter-Day Saints, Jesus Christ being the central figure of all worship. The nickname *Mormon* is given to members, stemming from a belief that the Book of Mormon is another testament of Jesus Christ and the word of God. While it's acceptable to refer to members of The Church as Mormons, the official church name is appreciated in reference to the Church itself.

---

230 Quote provided by the authors of this chapter.

Basic Teachings

- God is the Heavenly Father of all human beings. He loves His children and wants them to return to Him.
- Jesus Christ is the Son of God. He is the Savior of all people. He redeems all from death by providing the resurrection. He saves individuals from sin as they repent, pray and ask Him for forgiveness.
- Through Christ's atonement – His sacrifice, death, and resurrection – all people can return to live with God if they keep His commandments.
- The Holy Ghost (also called Holy Spirit) helps individuals to recognize truth.
- The first principles and ordinances of the gospel are faith in Jesus Christ, repentance, baptism and receiving the Gift of the Holy Ghost.
- The Church of Jesus Christ has been restored to the earth.
- The priesthood authority (the power and authority to act in God's name) exists in His Church today, just as it did in the original Church.
- Both the Bible and the Book of Mormon are the word of God and are equally regarded as holy scripture.
- God reveals His will to prophets today, just as He did in antiquity.
- Life has a sacred purpose.
- Families can be together forever.
- Through serving others, people can experience joy and draw closer to God.
- The Church of Jesus Christ of Latter-Day Saints has a living prophet who receives direct revelation from God. Through prayer, all of God's children can grow closer to Jesus Christ and discover what choices will bring the most happiness into their lives and the lives of their families.

Basic Practices

- **Sabbath Observance**: Church members set Sunday aside as the Sabbath, or the Lord's Day – a day to worship God and rest from their labors. After attending worship services, members often spend the remainder of the day quietly at home, visiting family or friends and doing acts of service.
- **Temple Ordinances**: Temples are houses of the Lord, the most sacred structures on the earth. Temples should not be mistaken for chapels where members of the Church participate in Sunday worship services. In temples, Church members participate in ordinances designed to unite their families together forever and help them return to God. When a man and woman are married in the temple they are bound together for eternity. Children and parents can also be sealed for eternity. In the temple, Church members can also perform the necessary ordinances, such as baptism and eternal marriage, for ancestors, friends and loved ones who have passed away.
- **Baptism and Confirmation**: The Lord commands that all are to be baptized by one having priesthood authority: children at age 8 or adults when they commit to join the Church of Jesus Christ. Baptism symbolizes the death, burial, and resurrection of Jesus Christ. When a person is baptized, he or she is fully immersed in water – just as Jesus was – to wash away sins. After baptism, an individual is confirmed a member of the Church through a blessing by priesthood leaders and receives the Gift of the Holy Ghost. At baptism a person's sins are literally washed away and the person is made clean.
- **Priesthood Ordination**: The Church has a lay priesthood, with no professional

clergy. The priesthood of The Church of Jesus Christ of Latter-Day Saints is the power and authority of God delegated to man on earth. This includes the authority to preach, perform ordinances, and direct the functions of the Church. Based on worthiness and age, men progress through various levels within the priesthood.

○ The lower Aaronic Priesthood is conferred upon faithful male members beginning at age 12, and includes the offices of deacon, teacher and priest. Aaronic Priesthood holders are able to baptize, prepare and offer the sacrament (communion) to church members during Sunday worship services, visit and provide service to members in their homes and collect contributions for the poor.

○ The Melchizedek Priesthood, the higher of the two priesthood levels, includes the commonly held offices of elder and high priest and is conferred upon worthy male members aged 18 and over. Men who hold the Melchizedek Priesthood are able to bless the sacrament, give blessings of healing and ordination and bless those who are recently baptized with the Gift of the Holy Ghost.

- **Family Home Evening**: One evening each week, usually on Mondays, Church members gather their families together for spiritual instruction and activities such as playing games, doing service projects and conducting weekly planning meetings. Families are encouraged to use this time to grow closer together.

- **Missions**: Young men and women generally serve voluntary missions for the Church when they are between 19 and 21 years of age. Missionaries devote this time in their lives to serving Jesus Christ and spreading His gospel around the earth. Though their main objective is teaching the gospel of Jesus Christ to those who are interested, they also teach free English classes in many foreign countries, help the disabled and volunteer in genealogical research centers. Retired seniors are also encouraged to serve missions. As there is no paid ministry in the Church, missionaries serve from 18 months to 2 years, while being supported by themselves or their family.

- **Fasting**: On the first Sunday of each month, Church members abstain from food or drink for two meals for the purpose of increasing their spirituality. They spend that time praying, reading the scriptures, attending church and otherwise strengthening their relationship with God. They donate the money saved from those meals – and more, if possible – to the Church to assist the poor and needy.

- **Welfare and Humanitarian Efforts**: The gospel of Jesus Christ teaches that people should bear one another's burdens (see Gal. 6:2). Throughout the world, when communities suffer major disasters and face difficulties beyond their ability to meet, the Church is prepared to offer assistance contributed by its members. The aid helps people who are in need, without regard to religious affiliation, ethnicity or nationality. Church members distribute food, provide assistance in times of disaster, teach self-reliance, and fund and encourage projects that benefit stricken communities.

- **Women's Organization**: The Relief Society is one of the largest women's organizations in the world. Women in the Church participate in weekly meetings to learn about the gospel and associate with one another. Additionally, they serve members of their communities and participate in global service projects such as knitting clothing, making quilts, cooking meals for the sick, gathering food and clothing to send to Third World countries or areas in disaster. The Society helps women become better wives, mothers, and friends by learning more about Jesus Christ.

- **Youth Activities**: The Church encourages young men and women to receive education and volunteer in their communities. They're also taught to use clean language, dress modestly, and be kind to others. The Church has a curriculum for youth aged 12–18 years that includes achievement activities, spiritual instruction, and sports programs. This curriculum teaches youth how to avoid alcohol, drugs, inappropriate materials, and spiritually harmful behavior.

Principles for Clinical Care
Dietary Issues

- **The Word of Wisdom**: The body is a precious gift from God. To help keep bodies and minds healthy and strong, God gave a law of health to the Prophet Joseph Smith in 1833. This law is known as the Word of Wisdom. In addition to emphasizing the benefits of proper diet and physical and spiritual health, God has spoken against the use of tobacco, alcohol, coffee, tea, and illegal drugs. God promises great physical and spiritual blessings to those who follow the Word of Wisdom. Today, the scientific community promotes some of the same principles that a loving God gave to Joseph Smith nearly two centuries ago.

General Medical Beliefs

- A healthy lifestyle promotes a sense of well-being. Exercise, eating, and sleeping

properly all contribute to happiness and wellness.

- Modern medicine is a gift of God and should be used to cure diseases. Members are encouraged to seek the best medical care possible. When severe illness strikes, members should exercise faith in the Lord and seek competent medical assistance. However, when dying becomes inevitable, it should be seen as a blessing and a purposeful part of eternal existence. Members should not feel obligated to extend mortal life by means that are unreasonable. These judgments are best made by family members after receiving wise and competent medical advice and seeking divine guidance through fasting and prayer.

Specific Medical Issues

- **Abortion**: Members must not submit to, perform, encourage, pay for, or arrange for an abortion. The only possible exceptions are when: pregnancy resulted from rape or incest, a competent physician determines that the life or health of the mother is in serious jeopardy, or a competent physician determines that the fetus has severe defects that will not allow the baby to survive beyond birth.

- **Advance Directives**: The Church has no official position on the use of advance directives in health care planning. It is an individual decision.

- **Birth Control**: It is the privilege of married couples who are able to bear children to provide mortal bodies for the spirit children of God, whom they are then responsible to nurture and rear. The decision as to how many children to have and when to have them is extremely intimate and private and should be left between the couple and the Lord.

- **Blood Transfusions**: Whether or not to participate in blood transfusions is a decision left up to the individual and his or her family members.
- **Circumcision**: Circumcision of male infants is not a religious requirement; it is a decision for individual families.
- **In Vitro Fertilization**: In vitro fertilization using semen from anyone but the husband or an egg from anyone but the wife is strongly discouraged. However, this is a personal matter that ultimately must be left to the judgments of the husband and wife, with responsibility for the decision resting solely upon them.
- **Stem Cell Research**: The Church has no official position on stem cell research for therapeutic purposes. It is an individual decision.
- **Vaccinations**: The Church has issued no official statement on vaccinations but would encourage them as contributing to the overall health of the general community. However, it is an individual decision.
- **Witholding/Withdrawing Life Support**: Allowing death to occur is permissible when death is the inevitable and a natural outcome. The measures taken to postpone it would rob the dying person of the ability to experience satisfaction with the quality of his or her life.

Gender and Personal Issues
- Hospital workers may provide health care for members of the opposite sex.

Principles for Spiritual Care through the Cycles of Life
Concepts of Living and Dying for Spiritual Support
- Life does not begin at birth, nor does it end at death. Children of God have a divine nature and a divine destiny. They lived with Him as spirit sons and daughters before they were born. God sent them to earth to receive a physical body and gain the experiences they need to return to Him. Because Jesus Christ overcame death, they too will live again to see their families and loved ones.
- Death is not the end. There is no need to fear death. Death is really a beginning – another step forward in the Heavenly Father's plan for His children.
- When life on earth ends, the physical body will die, but each person's spirit will not. At death, the spirit will go to the spirit world, where the spirit will continue to learn and progress.
- Death is a necessary step in progression, just as birth is. Some time after death, the spirit and body will be reunited – never to be separated again. This is called resurrection, and it was made possible by the death and resurrection of Jesus Christ.

During Birth
- The Church of Jesus Christ does not practice infant baptism. Little children do not need baptism because they are not capable of committing sin. Members are baptized into the Church at 8 years of age, the age at which Church members believe a person is spiritually mature enough to discern right from wrong.
- Babies are given a special blessing shortly after birth where they are blessed with what attributes God would wish them to have to help them during their life. This blessing is given through the guidance of the Spirit by someone who holds the priesthood, which in many cases is the infant's father or another priesthood holder close to the family. Only worthy Melchizedek Priesthood holders can

perform this blessing and is normally conducted on the first Sunday of the month in a church building, though it can take place in a home or hospital if necessary.

- As stated earlier, circumcision of male infants is not a religious requirement; it is a decision for individual families.

During Illness

- Blessing of the sick: Just as in New Testament times, those who are sick may call upon priesthood holders for a special blessing of healing (see James 5:14). The person is first anointed on his or her head with a few drops of olive oil that has been consecrated for the blessing of the sick. Priesthood holders then lay their hands upon the person's head, seal (or confirm) the anointing, and pronounce a blessing through the authority of the priesthood. If a person is not healed, it is not a reflection of the person's faith, but rather God's will concerning the individual. Illness is not punishment for sins. Healing of the spirit may often take place in the absence of physical healing.
- Priesthood holders and women in the Relief Society alike can be called on in times of need to give spiritual support to the sick, depressed or lonely.
- Patients may receive comfort from reading scriptures or other devotional material and listening to religious music.

During End of Life

- Allowing death to occur is permissible when death is the inevitable and natural outcome and the measures taken to postpone it would rob the dying person of the ability to experience satisfaction with the quality of his or her life.
- Funerals: Members of The Church of Jesus Christ of Latter-Day Saints conduct funerals similar to traditional Christian funerals. A Latter-Day Saint funeral is usually directed by the local congregational leader (the bishop) and held in a chapel. The tone of the funeral is generally peaceful, reflecting the religious belief that families can be reunited after this life. Funerals are conducted with a spirit of hope and sometimes joy. Family and friends grieve for their loss, but they know that they will be with their loved ones again. This understanding brings great comfort.

Care of the Body

- How bodies are cared for after death is a decision for the individuals and their family members.
- Disposition and embalming are decisions for the individual's family.
- Autopsy is a decision for the individual's family.
- Donation for medical research is a decision for the individual and his or her family.

Organ and Tissue Donation

- Organ and tissue donation is a decision for the individual and his or her family. It may be preferable for a chaplain and/or nurse who are trained designated requesters to be consulted for assistance.

Scriptures, Inspirational Readings, and Prayers

READINGS DURING ILLNESS

These can be read by family, friends, and health care professionals. (Scripture quotations are from the Authorized [King James] Version and the Book of Mormon.)

I ... would speak unto you that are pure in heart. Look unto God with firmness of mind, and pray unto him with exceeding faith, and he will console you in your afflictions, and he will plead your cause.

—Jacob 3:1
(Book of Mormon)

Wherefore, ye must press forward with a steadfastness in Christ, having a perfect brightness of hope, and a love of God and of all men. Wherefore, if ye shall press forward, feasting upon the word of Christ, thus saith the Father: Ye shall have eternal life.

—2 Nephi 31:20
(Book of Mormon)

Therefore may God grant unto you, my brethren, that ye may begin to exercise your faith unto repentance, that ye begin to call upon his holy name, that he would have mercy upon you; yea, cry unto him for mercy; for he is mighty to save. Yea, humble yourselves, and continue in prayer unto him.

—Alma 34:17–19 (Book of Mormon)

I will not leave you comfortless: I will come to you.

—John 14:18 (The New Testament)

Peace I leave with you, my peace I give unto you: not as the world giveth, give I unto you. Let not your heart be troubled, neither let it be afraid.

—John 14:27 (The New Testament)

Are not five sparrows sold for two farthings, and not one of them is forgotten before God? But even the very hairs of your head are all numbered. Fear not therefore: ye are of more value than many sparrows.

—Luke 12:6–7 (The New Testament)

INFORMATION ON PRAYER

Anyone can pray. Prayer is one of the greatest blessings people have. It allows them to communicate with their Heavenly Father and to seek His guidance in all matters, big or small. He is always willing to listen to individuals' deepest feelings and concerns. People simply need to open up their hearts and speak to Him. Prayers will always be answered at a time and in a way that Heavenly Father knows will help the most. Praying as a family helps people to overcome challenges and grow closer together. Prayer is the desire of an individual and can be spoken or unexpressed.

A prayer follows four basic steps:
1. Address God as "Father in Heaven" or "Heavenly Father."
2. Thank Him for the things for which you are grateful ("I thank thee for …").
3. Ask Him for what you need ("I ask thee …").
4. Jesus is the Mediator (see 1 Tim. 2:5; 1 John 2:1) between people and the Heavenly Father, so close the prayer by saying, "In the name of Jesus Christ, Amen."

The Church has no recited prayers except for the two sacrament prayers for the bread and water. In communicating with God, people should feel like they can ask for what they need in their particular circumstances. The Lord answers all prayers in His own way and in His own time.

Community of Christ

*Community of Christ is a worldwide Christian denomination dedicated to
the pursuit of peace, reconciliation, and healing of the spirit with a mission to
"proclaim Jesus Christ and promote communities of joy, hope, love, and peace."*[231]

Prepared by:
Wallace B. Smith
Former President, Community of Christ Church World Headquarters
Independence, MO

History and Facts

Community of Christ traces its origins to
the Latter Day Saint movement founded by
Joseph Smith Jr. in 1830 in Palmyra, New
York. As a young man, Smith had what he
described as significant religious experiences, resulting in the Book of Mormon
being produced. This work of scripture
became the primary missionary tool of
the church in its early years. The church
spread westward with the expansion of the
American frontier, first into the Western
Reserve in Kirtland, Ohio, and later to
Independence, Missouri, where it sought to
create a religious and social community as
a base for spreading the gospel message to
the world. When conflicts with Missourians
forced them to move into Illinois, the Saints
established the city of Nauvoo. After Joseph
Smith and his brother Hyrum were assas-
sinated in June of 1844, the church split
into factions. The largest group migrated to
Utah territory under leadership of Brigham
Young. Several smaller groups in the

Midwest reorganized in 1860 under Joseph
Smith III, son of the founder. It is this group,
known for 140 years as the Reorganized
Church of Jesus Christ of Latter Day
Saints that changed its name in the year
2000 to become Community of Christ. The
denomination has grown into a worldwide
communion of over 255 000, with headquarters in Independence, Missouri. The
church's current mission statement is: We
proclaim Jesus Christ and promote communities of joy, hope, love, and peace.

Basic Teachings

The Church affirms the content of the
ancient *Apostles' Creed*, which is a brief
statement of faith attributed to the early
Christian church.

The Apostles' Creed

I believe in God, the Father almighty,
  creator of heaven and earth,
I believe in Jesus Christ, His only
  Son, our Lord.
Who was conceived by the power of
  the Holy Spirit;

---

231 Quote provided by Dr. Wallace Smith, author of this
  chapter.

Born of the virgin Mary;
Suffered under Pontius Pilate;
Was crucified, died, and buried.
He descended into hell (or the realm of the dead).
On the third day he rose again.
He ascended into heaven and is seated at the right hand of the Father.
He will come again to judge the living and the dead.
I believe in the Holy Spirit,
The holy catholic (universal) church,
The communion of saints,
The forgiveness of sins,
The resurrection of the body and the life everlasting. Amen.

- All humans are fallen from an original state of innocence and are bent toward actions (i.e., sins) that disconnect them from God and others.
- All humans deserve just punishment for misdeeds.
- Humans can be rescued (i.e., saved) from just punishment through faith in the death, burial, and resurrection of Jesus.
- The final destination for those who have been saved from the consequences of their misdeeds is heaven, which is communion with God and all the redeemed in a state of peace, justice, and perfect love.
- The final destination of those who are not saved is hell, a state of punishment and disconnected-ness from God and the saved. Opinions differ as to whether or not hell is eternal.
- Community of Christ affirms the Bible, or Holy Scriptures, which is a compilation of 66 different books written over a thousand-year period. These writings contain wisdom sayings, history, poetry, social commentary, and devotional literature from ancient Semitic Jewish, Hellenistic Jewish, and early Christian authors.
- No creedal statement is required. A common phrase is "All truth."
- The sacraments of the church are: baptism, confirmation, Holy Communion, marriage, blessing of children, anointing of the sick, ordination to priesthood, evangelists' blessing.
- In addition to the Bible, the Book of Mormon and the Book of Doctrine and Covenants are viewed as scripture.
- All persons are given gifts and abilities to enhance life and become engaged in Christ's mission. Some are called to particular responsibilities in various priesthood offices.
- Spiritual healing is a gift of the Spirit. It is most efficaciously mediated through the prayer of faith, accompanied by the anointing of the sick with consecrated oil and the laying on of hands by ordained elders.
- Community of Christ doctrine affirms that God loves all persons equally and unconditionally. All have great worth and should be respected as creations of God with basic human rights.

Basic Practices

- Christians value communal worship, and will gather on Sundays and at other times to hear preaching, study scripture, sing hymns, and pray.
- The sharing of one's faith (evangelism) is of great importance. Some of the ways it is communicated is through loving actions, talking about personal spiritual experiences, reading scriptures, distributing informational tracts, and discussions of doctrinal positions.

- Holy Communion is an integral part of worship, usually on the first Sunday of the month. Communion is open to all who confess Jesus Christ. Holy Communion (also referred to as The Lord's Supper or Eucharist, which means "thanksgiving"), is a powerful sacrament. It is a liturgical reenactment of the crucifixion, death, burial, and resurrection of Jesus, in which Christians eat bread (to commemorate the broken body of Jesus) and drink wine or grape juice (to symbolize Jesus' shed blood). This can be done during communal worship or in other settings and is usually administered by ordained clergy.
- Prayer, meditation, and scripture are the fundamental spiritual practices for many Christians. The many forms of these practices include reading and/or silent contemplation upon scripture or doctrinal beliefs and prayers of various kinds – petition, healing, repentance for unethical thoughts and actions, praise, worship, and thanksgiving to God.
- Mission work is important to the Community of Christ. These acts of service take the forms of working for social justice with marginalized peoples, charitable giving to provide food, building, and educational programs for the poor, volunteerism, and so forth. Mission work is also an intentional witness to one's faith through proclamation and teaching.
- The sacrament of baptism is by immersion at the age of accountability (ages 8 or older). This emphasizes waiting until a child is old enough to make an informed decision with respect to his or her relationship to God. Thus, the responsibility is upon the action of the individual in choosing to follow the ways of God, albeit not without influence from family, friends, and faith community.

- Infant blessing is a ceremonial act which may include naming of the child. It is not, however, part of the ceremony of baptism.
- Social action and pursuit of peace and justice for all people is encouraged.

Principles for Clinical Care
Dietary Issues
- No specific dietary restrictions are practiced by Community of Christ, although the use of alcohol and tobacco is strongly discouraged.

General Medical Beliefs
- Scientific medical practices are gifts of wisdom of God and should be utilized to the fullest extent when available.
- Acts of "active" euthanasia are opposed, including situations in which the patient requests death at the hands of family members, medical personnel, or others.

Specific Medical Issues
- **Abortion**: Abortion is acceptable in certain unusual circumstances, but only after counseling and other alternatives has been fully discussed by all parties at interest.
- **Advance Directives**: If there is an advance directive, living will, or durable power of attorney for health care indicating the wishes of the terminally ill person, the family should be sufficiently informed to participate cooperatively in end-of-life decisions.
- **Birth Control**: The Community of Christ has no proscriptions on its use.
- **Blood Transfusions**: The Community of Christ has no reservation in regard to blood transfusions.
- **Circumcision**: Circumcision of male infants is optional.

- **In Vitro Fertilization**: The Community of Christ has no reservation in regard to in vitro fertilization and birth control.
- **Stem Cell Research**: No statement on stem cell research has been made by the church.
- **Vaccinations**: The Community of Christ has no objections to vaccinations on religious grounds. Conversely, the church encourages them as part of a general good stewardship of health.
- **Withholding/Withdrawing Life Support**: Allowing death to occur is permissible when death is the inevitable and natural outcome and the measures taken to postpone it would rob the dying person of the ability to experience satisfaction with the quality of his or her life.

Gender and Personal Issues
- Community of Christ as a faith tradition has no official statements with respect to gender and personal issues beyond the assertion that all persons are of great worth and equally loved by God.

Principles for Spiritual Care through the Cycles of Life
Concepts of Living and Dying for Spiritual Support
- Life is sacred.
- Life exists as a unity or wholeness of body, mind, and spirit.
- The love of God sustains us in sickness and in health.
- The experience of death is universal, but not final. The Christian witness of the resurrection expresses the belief that death does not frustrate the purpose for which God created humankind. "Death is swallowed up in victory" (1 Cor. 15: 54).
- At the time of death the spirits of all, as

soon as they are departed the bodies, are taken home to the God who created them to await resurrection.
- Although we do not know the nature of the "body" that will be brought forth by the power of God, we accept the Apostle Paul's affirmation that the body we lay down in death will not be the body that comes forth in the resurrection.

During Birth
- Infants are born innocent and do not require baptism.
- As stated earlier, circumcision of male infants is optional.
- Infant blessing may be requested by the family for a baby, living or deceased. The chaplain or clergy should be consulted for assistance.

During Illness
- Patients may receive comfort from the reading of scriptures or other devotional material, listening to religious music, watching televised worship services of their own or a similar tradition. Patients may request Holy Communion. The chaplain or clergy should be consulted for assistance.
- Patients may request baptism. In the clinical setting, sprinkling is an acceptable mode of baptism, even for traditions that practice immersion. The chaplain or clergy should be consulted for assistance.
- Reassure the patient that illness is not punishment for sins.
- Make sure that the patient understands that healing of the spirit may take place, even in the absence of physical healing.
- Counsel the patient that failure to achieve physical healing is not evidence of lack of faith.
- Prayer, with or without anointing and

laying on of hands by the elders, may be offered.

During End of Life

- The terminally ill have a right to dignity.
- Baptism or Holy Communion is not a necessity, but may be requested. The chaplain or clergy should be consulted for assistance.
- If there is an advance directive, living will, or durable power of attorney for health care indicating the wishes of the terminally ill person, the family should be sufficiently informed to participate cooperatively in end-of-life decisions.
- Allowing death to occur is permissible when death is the inevitable and natural outcome and the measures taken to postpone it would rob the dying person of the ability to experience satisfaction with the quality of his or her life.
- The family may wish to view and/or spend time with the deceased in the hospital room. Medical personnel and a chaplain should be consulted for assistance.
- Prayer or scripture readings may be requested by the family.

Care of the Body

- Disposition and embalming are individual decisions. Cremation is now the choice of many members of the Community of Christ. The chaplain and the funeral home director should be consulted for assistance.
- Autopsy is an individual decision unless required by law. The chaplain and/or nurse should be consulted for assistance.
- Donation for medical research is an individual decision. The chaplain and/or nurse should be consulted for assistance. Advance planning for such donations is required by most receiving organizations.

Last-minute donations are usually not possible.

Organ and Tissue Donation

- There are no religious prescriptions or proscriptions regarding organ and tissue donation.
- Organ and tissue donation is an individual decision. It may be preferable for a chaplain and/or nurse who are trained designated requesters to be consulted for assistance.

Scriptures, Inspirational Readings, and Prayers

- There are no required readings or prayers for the seriously ill or dying.
- The patient or family may request a specific scripture be read or that a prayer be offered. A chaplain or clergy may assist in this, but it is not required.
- All scriptures and prayers of "Christianity" apply.

READINGS DURING ILLNESS

These can be read by family, friends, clergy, and health care professionals. (All scripture quotations are from the Revised Standard Version.)

To thee, O Lord, I lift up my soul … Make me to know thy ways, O Lord; teach me thy paths. Lead me in thy truth, and teach me, for thou art the God of my salvation; for thee I wait all the day long. Be mindful of thy mercy, O Lord, and of thy steadfast love, for they have been from of old.

—Ps. 25:1, 4–6

The Lord is my light and my salvation; whom shall I fear? The Lord is the stronghold of my life; of whom shall I be afraid? ... Hear, O Lord, when I cry aloud, be gracious to me and answer me! ... Hide not thy face from me. Turn not thy servant away in anger, thou who hast been my help. Cast me not off, forsake me not, O God of my salvation! ... Wait for the Lord; be strong and let your heart take courage; yea, wait for the Lord!

—Ps. 27:1, 7, 9, 14

Be merciful to me, O God, be merciful to me, for in thee my soul takes refuge; in the shadow of thy wings I will take refuge, till the storms of destruction pass by. I cry to God Most High, to God who fulfills his purpose for me. He will send from heaven and save me, he will put to shame those who trample on me. God will send forth his steadfast love and faithfulness!

—Ps. 57:1–3

I lift up my eyes to the hills. From whence does my help come? My help comes from the Lord, who made heaven and earth. He will not let your foot be moved, for he who keeps you will not slumber. Behold, he who keeps Israel will neither slumber nor sleep.

—Ps. 121:1–4

READINGS DURING END-OF-LIFE PROCESS

These can be read by family, friends, clergy, and health care professionals. (All scripture quotations are from the Revised Standard Version.)

Therefore, since we are justified by faith, we have peace with God through our Lord Jesus Christ. Through him we have obtained access to this grace in which we stand, and we rejoice in our hope of sharing the glory of God. More than that, we rejoice in our sufferings, knowing that suffering produces endurance, and endurance produces character, and character produces hope, and hope does not disappoint us, because God's love has been poured into our hearts through the Holy Spirit which has been given to us.

—Rom. 5:1–5

If for this life only we have hoped in Christ, we are of all men most to be pitied. But in fact, Christ has been raised from the dead, the first fruits of those who have fallen asleep. For as by a man came death, by a man has come also the resurrection of the dead. For as in Adam all die, so also in Christ shall all be made alive ... Lo! I tell you a mystery. We shall not all sleep, but we shall all be changed, in a moment, in the twinkling of an eye, at the last trumpet. For the trumpet will sound, and the dead will be raised imperishable, and we shall be changed. For this perishable nature must put on the imperishable, and this mortal nature must put on immortality … O death, where is thy victory? O death, where is thy sting? The sting of death is sin, and the power of sin is the law.

But thanks be to God, who gives us the victory through our Lord Jesus Christ.

—1 Cor. 15:19–22, 51–53, 55–57

Jehovah's Witnesses

*This good news of the kingdom will be preached in all the
inhabited earth for a witness to all the nations.*[232]

Prepared by:
James N. Pellechia
Associate Editor, Watch Tower publications
International Offices of the Watch Tower Society
Brooklyn, NY

History and Facts

Jehovah's Witnesses are members of a worldwide Christian religion whose pulpits are "doorsteps in neighborhoods." As a united body of preachers more than 1 200 000 strong across the United States, and numbering upward of 7 313 000 in 236 lands and organized into more than 105 298 congregations, the Witnesses have no paid clergy or class distinctions of clergy and laity. All baptized members are viewed as ordained ministers. Each one actively shares with others information about God, whose name is Jehovah, and about his Son, Jesus Christ. The name Jehovah's Witnesses was adopted in 1931. Previously, they were known as International Bible Students. They view first-century Christianity as their model. Their modern history can be traced back to shortly after the Civil War ended.

In 1872 at Allegheny near Pittsburgh, Pennsylvania, Charles Taze Russell began a Bible class that met regularly to study the scriptures about God's Kingdom and the Second Coming of Christ Jesus. Not many years after that, similar groups of students of the Bible, having these same interests, were organized into congregations throughout the United States and in other countries as well. In July 1879, the first issue of the magazine *Zion's Watch Tower and Herald of Christ's Presence* (now the *Watchtower*) was released. In 1881, Zion's Watch Tower Tract Society was formed, and in 1884, it was incorporated with Russell as president. The Society's name was later changed to Watch Tower Bible and Tract Society of Pennsylvania. In 1909, the corporate headquarters were transferred from Pittsburgh to its present location in Brooklyn, New York. That same year, an associate nonprofit corporation was formed, a New York corporation now known as Watchtower Bible and Tract Society, Inc. In other lands, associate corporations were formed, such as International Bible Students Association in Great Britain and in Canada. The year 1910 saw more than 1000 newspapers in the United States and Canada regularly carrying sermons written by C. T. Russell. By 1914, the number of congregations worldwide was 1200.

---

232 Matt. 24:14 (New World Translation).

During the 1930s and 1940s, Witnesses in Germany and other European countries became targets of Nazi persecution; thousands lost their lives, and ten thousand spent many years in Nazi torture camps and prisons. Canada, England, and other parts of the British Empire also persecuted the Witnesses. From 1940 to 1944, more than 2500 violent mob assaults were noted in the United States alone. From the 1930s to the 1940s there were many arrests of Witnesses for their public preaching work, and court cases were fought in the interest of preserving freedom of speech, press, assembly, and worship. In the United States, appeals from lower courts resulted in the Witnesses' winning 43 cases (now 52) before the Supreme Court of the United States. Similarly, favorable judgments have been obtained from high courts in other lands. Concerning these court victories, Professor C. S. Braden, in his book *These Also Believe*, said of the Witnesses: "They have performed a signal service to democracy by their fight to preserve their civil rights, for in their struggle they have done much to secure those rights for every minority group in America."[233]

The worldwide organization is directed by a multinational Governing Body made up of longtime Witnesses who serve at the international offices in Brooklyn, New York. The Governing Body uses nonprofit legal entities to supervise global evangelizing, organize conventions and schools for the volunteer ministry of the Witnesses, and publish materials for Bible education. The volunteer work of Jehovah's Witnesses centers around each congregation, which

is often made up of between 50 and 200 members. Each congregation is supervised by a body of elders. About 20 congregations form a circuit, and about 10 circuits are grouped into a district. Congregations receive periodic visits from traveling elders who provide additional training in the volunteer work.

Basic Teachings

- **God**: There is only one true God, the Creator of all things. His name is Jehovah and his outstanding qualities are love, justice, wisdom, and power.
- **Jesus**: He is the Son of God. Jesus came to earth from heaven and sacrificed his perfect human life as a ransom. His death and resurrection made salvation to eternal life possible for those exercising faith in him. He is now King of God's heavenly Kingdom, which will soon bring peace to the earth. Jesus never claimed equality with God and thus is not part of a Trinity.
- **The Bible**: It is God's infallible, inspired Word. Some portions of the Bible are to be understood figuratively, or symbolically.
- **Sin, Death, and Resurrection**: Death is a result of sin inherited from the first man, Adam, who chose to disobey God. The original sin was a deliberate disobedient act of eating from "the tree of the knowledge of good and bad." The dead are conscious of nothing. According to God's will for the individual, in the resurrection the person is restored in either a human or a spirit body and yet retains his personal identity, having the same personality and memories as when he died. A limited number of the dead, 144 000, are resurrected to heaven and become corulers with Jesus Christ in God's Kingdom. In the future, God through Jesus will

---

233 Braden, C. (1950). *These Also Believe*. New York, NY: MacMillan, 382. Also, see *Judging Jehovah's Witnesses: Religious Persecution and the Dawn of the Rights Revolution*, by Shawn Francis Peters, 2000 (University Press of Kansas, Lawrence, KS).

resurrect the rest of the dead to an earthly paradise.

- **Judgment**: Jesus is God's appointed Judge who determines what each one's future will be. Those judged as righteous will be given everlasting life. Those judged as unrighteous will not be tormented but will die and cease to exist.
- **Baptism**: This act of complete immersion symbolizes one's dedication to God. This step is taken by those of responsible age who have made an informed decision.
- **Marriage**: Jehovah's Witnesses view marriage as a serious, lifelong commitment. They look to the Bible for guidance in resolving marital problems in a loving and respectful way. Scripturally, divorce may be obtained on the grounds of marital unfaithfulness. Separation is acceptable in extreme situations, such as those involving willful nonsupport or physical abuse.
- **Respect for Authority**: Jehovah's Witnesses believe that it is their Christian responsibility to be model citizens. For this reason, they honor and respect governmental authority. Only on those rare occasions when a government demands what is in direct conflict with what God commands do Jehovah's Witnesses decline to comply.
- **God's Kingdom**: It is the heavenly Kingdom for which Jesus taught all his followers to pray. Soon, it will become the one government over all the earth and will solve mankind's pressing problems. The Bible does not give a date for these events, but it provides evidence to show that we are living in the last days of this troubled world. The Kingdom of God is in the hands of Jesus Christ. With Jesus will be 144 000 anointed followers who will rule with him as priests and kings over the earth for 1000 years.
- **Earth**: The earth will never be destroyed or depopulated but will become a peaceful paradise.
- **Neutrality**: Following the examples set by Jesus and the first-century Christians, Jehovah's Witnesses do not share in the politics or wars of any nation. They firmly believe that they must "beat their swords into plowshares" and not "learn war anymore" (Isa. 2:4). At the same time, Jehovah's Witnesses recognize the authority of nations to raise armies and defend themselves, and they do not interfere with what others choose to do.

Basic Practices

- Jehovah's Witnesses value communal worship, and will gather on Sundays and at other times to hear preaching, study scripture, sing hymns, and pray.
- The sharing of one's faith (evangelism) is of great importance to each Jehovah's Witness. Some of the ways it is communicated is through house-to-house visits, loving actions, talking about personal spiritual experiences, reading scriptures, distributing informational tracts, and discussions of doctrinal positions.
- Prayer, meditation, scripture, attending religious services, and evangelism are the fundamental spiritual practices for Jehovah's Witnesses. The many forms of these practices include house-to-house witnessing, reading, and/or silent contemplation upon scripture or doctrinal beliefs and prayers of various kinds – petition, repentance for unethical thoughts and actions, praise, worship and thanksgiving to God.
- *The Lord's Supper or Memorial of Christ's Death*: This is the most important religious observance of the year for Jehovah's

Witnesses. It is celebrated annually. Not all who attend partake of the communion meal, but only those few who believe they have been called by God to become future corulers with Christ in the heavens do.

- *Baptism*: Complete water immersion is performed by a minister of Jehovah's Witnesses and is a symbol of one's dedication to God. Candidates for baptism must be of responsible age and have made an informed decision; hence, baptism is not conducted for infants.
- *Mission Work*: Bible education is the main thrust of the community work done by Jehovah's Witnesses. During times of local or national disasters, Jehovah's Witnesses have organized relief efforts to help fellow members and others who suffer the effects of calamities.
- *Holidays*: Jehovah's Witnesses commemorate the Memorial of Christ's death, their most important religious event of the year. Throughout the year, Jehovah's Witnesses enjoy parties, picnics, and other events without feeling bound to obligations or to a fixed date. They may also celebrate special events such as weddings and anniversaries. However, they do not celebrate holidays that have non-Christian religious origins (such as Christmas and birthdays) or those that promote nationalism. Jehovah's Witnesses are not opposed to celebrations in general or to the giving of gifts. They respect the right of others to do as they wish.
- Presiding Minister (Elder/Overseer) of local congregation provides pastoral support.

Principles for Clinical Care
Dietary Issues
- Jehovah's Witnesses have no dietary restrictions with respect to religious belief, except one: the eating of blood. It is prohibited.

General Medical Beliefs
- Witnesses believe that God is the ultimate source of all life, health, and healing.
- Witnesses refer to God as the Great Physician.
- Faith Healing: Jehovah's Witnesses do not believe in faith healing as commonly practiced today. They believe that the miraculous healings of Jesus and his apostles were first-century Christianity phenomena and not an ongoing feature of Christianity.
- Witnesses affirm the validity of traditional Western medical procedures in the treatment of illness and disease.
- Jehovah's Witnesses actively seek medical care when needed, and many work in the health care field. They accept the vast majority of treatments available.
- Jehovah's Witnesses avoid the use of tobacco and avoid any form of substance abuse. They do not forbid the use of alcoholic beverages, but they warn against the abuse of alcohol.
- Hospital Liaison Committee (HLC) members are selected elders who provide assistance in resolving spiritual or ethical questions related to medical care, especially nonblood medical management of an illness or medical procedure.

Specific Medical Issues
- **Abortion**: Jehovah's Witnesses believe life begins at conception. Deliberately induced abortion is viewed as the willful taking of human life.

- **Advance Directives**: Most Witnesses have an advance medical directive stating their wishes.
- **Birth Control**: Jehovah's Witnesses believe that birth control is a personal decision, and if married couples do decide on this course, the choice of contraceptive is also a personal matter. "Each one will carry his own load" (Gal. 6:5). However, the method of birth control a couple chooses should be governed by a respect for the sanctity of life. Since the Bible indicates that a person's life begins at conception, Witnesses would avoid contraceptive methods that abort, or end the life of, the developing child. In the case of sterilization, although the decision is one of personal conscience, a Witness couple would not choose voluntary sterilization merely as a convenient means of contraception since the reproductive powers are a gift from the Creator. However, under particular circumstances the couple might reluctantly consider sterilization, such as when there are confirmed medical assurances that the mother or a future child might face a grave medical risk, even a probability of death, with a future pregnancy.
- **Blood Transfusions**: For religious reasons, Jehovah's Witnesses will not accept transfusions of whole blood or any of its primary components – red cells, white cells, platelets, and plasma. Neither will they accept preoperative autologous blood collection and storage for later use.
  ○ Jehovah's Witnesses follow the Bible's command that Christians must "abstain from … blood" (Acts 15:29). Since the Bible makes no clear statement about the use of minor blood fractions or the immediate reinfusion of a patient's own blood during surgery, a medical process known as blood salvaging, the use of such treatments is a personal choice. Jehovah's Witnesses accept reliable nonblood medical alternatives, which are widely recognized and used in the medical field.
  ○ Jehovah's Witnesses will accept most medical treatments, including surgical and anesthetic techniques, various devices, hemostatic or therapeutic agents, and nonblood volume expanders (e.g., dextran, saline, pentastarch).
  ○ Each individual Witness makes a personal decision about whether to accept blood fractions, such as albumin, clotting factors, hemoglobin, hemin, immunoglobulins, interleukins, interferons, and such procedures as autotranfusion, cell salvage, epidural blood patch, labeling or tagging, plasmapheresis (plasma from another person is prohibited), platelet gel, heart-lung machine or heart bypass, hemodialysis and hemodilution (if pumps are primed with nonblood fluids).
- **Circumcision**: Circumcision is not a religious requirement. Male circumcision is a personal choice and, for male infants, a matter for parents to decide. However, in regard to female circumcision, Jehovah's Witnesses view the practice as mutilation. Witnesses living in countries where female circumcision is practiced do not observe this tradition.
- **In Vitro Fertilization**: It is a personal decision if the sperm and the egg came from husband and wife. However, Jehovah's Witnesses avoid surrogate motherhood as well as any procedures that involve the use of *donated* sperm, eggs, or embryos. Also, certain practices sometimes associated with an in vitro

fertilization procedure would be contrary to scriptural indications, such as the disposal of fertilized eggs.

- **Stem Cell Research**: It is a personal decision if adult stem cells are used. However, since Jehovah's Witnesses believe that the life of a human being begins at conception, if embryonic stem cell research involves the destruction of the embryo then that would violate tenets that prohibit the destruction of human life.
- **Vaccinations**: Jehovah's Witnesses have no objection to immunization for the purpose of fighting against disease. Whether a Witness patient allows to be immunized would be a personal decision. Similarly, the taking of a serum injection made from a small fraction of blood is a matter of conscience, too.
- **Withholding/Withdrawing Life Support**: Withholding/withdrawing life support in medically futile cases does not violate teachings of the Jehovah's Witness faith. Jehovah's Witnesses believe that the Bible does not require that extraordinary, complicated, or distressing measures be taken to sustain a person if this would merely prolong the dying process.

Gender and Personal Issues

- Jehovah's Witnesses as a faith tradition have no prescriptions or proscriptions with respect to gender and personal issues.
- Jehovah's Witnesses have no class or racial distinctions, and cultural differences are accepted as long as they do not conflict with Bible teachings.

Principles for Spiritual Care through the Cycles of Life
Concepts of Living and Dying for Spiritual Support

- Life is sacred.
- Death is something all must experience and need not be feared.
- Death is perceived as sleep, a time of total unconsciousness until the time of resurrection.
- Death is called mankind's enemy, and is not a method a God of love uses to populate heaven.
- The hope of the resurrection is a source of comfort. Jehovah's Witnesses have the hope of seeing their loved ones alive again on earth but under very different circumstances – an earth restored to Paradise conditions. At that future time, humans will live on earth under peaceful, righteous conditions while enjoying perfect health, and they will never have to die again (Rev. 21:1–4). God, who started mankind off in a lovely garden, has promised to restore Paradise on this earth under the rule of His heavenly Kingdom in the hands of the now glorified Jesus Christ. Gone, too, will be all hatred, racial prejudice, ethnic violence, and economic oppression. It will be into such a cleansed earth that Jehovah God through Jesus Christ will resurrect the dead and reunite love ones.

During Birth

- The Bible says that children are a blessing from God, an "inheritance" (Ps. 127:3).
- *Birth Control*: As stated earlier, this is a matter of personal choice for Jehovah's Witnesses.
- *Abortion*: As stated earlier, Jehovah's Witnesses believe life begins at conception. Deliberately induced abortion is viewed as the willful taking of human life.

- Although a time of outstanding joy, Jehovah's Witnesses have no religious rituals at time of birth.
- Infant death is a time of great sadness. Comfort comes from reflection on the hope of a resurrection as explained in the section "Concepts of Living and Dying for Spiritual Support."
- During a medical emergency, HLC members visit medical professionals and Witness patients. For more information, see the section "During Illness."

During Illness

- Jehovah's Witnesses have no rituals for the sick.
- Prayer for comfort, strength, and endurance offered on behalf of the ill one is always appropriate. Prayers can be offered by any baptized Witness, especially by local congregation elders during their pastoral visit.
- HLCs and Patient Visitation Groups are made up of selected Jehovah's Witness elders who provide support for Witness patients and can be called upon at any hour of the day or night. HLC members provide services to medical professionals and to Witness patients regarding nonblood medical management at no charge. These services meet current physician demand for readily available information on medical alternatives to blood transfusions. HLC elders also provide personal assistance to Witness patients on resolving spiritual or ethical questions related to medical care.

During End of Life

- Jehovah's Witnesses as a faith tradition have no specific end-of-life rituals.
- Pastoral visits and prayers by congregation elders are customary. Scriptures citing the resurrection hope and the future

Paradise earth may be read. (Jehovah's Witnesses believe that only 144 000 will be resurrected to heaven to become corulers with Jesus Christ in the Kingdom of God. Hence, the vast majority of the dead will be resurrected to an earth restored to Paradise conditions where they will enjoy everlasting life.)

Care of the Body

- Jehovah's Witnesses have no rituals regarding the body or body care.
- Disposition and embalming are personal decisions, based on local legal requirements. Funeral directors may be consulted for assistance.
- Memorial service, which includes a sermon delivered by an elder, can be held by choice at a Kingdom Hall or a funeral home, and a prayer may be said at the gravesite.
- Autopsy and donation of body for medical research are personal decisions.

Organ and Tissue Donation

- Jehovah's Witnesses believe that an organ transplant or organ donation is a personal decision. It may be preferable for a chaplain and/or nurse who are trained designated requesters to be consulted for assistance.

Scriptures, Inspirational Readings, and Prayers

- Prayers are to be performed by only baptized Jehovah's Witnesses, and usually, but not exclusively, by elders.

READINGS DURING ILLNESS

These can be read by family, friends, ministers and health care professionals. (All scripture quotations are from the New World Translation of the Holy Scriptures.)

With that I heard a loud voice from the throne say: "Look! The tent of God is with mankind, and he will reside with them, and they will be his peoples. And God himself will be with them. And he will wipe out every tear from their eyes, and death will be no more, neither will mourning nor outcry nor pain be anymore.

The former things have passed away."

—Rev. 21:3, 4

With that I heard a loud voice from the throne say: "Look! The tent of God is with mankind, and he will reside with them, and they will be his peoples. And God himself will be with them. And he will wipe out every tear from their eyes, and death will be no more, neither will mourning nor outcry nor pain be anymore.

The former things have passed away."

—Rev. 21:3, 4

We are to exercise faith ... Therefore we do not give up, but even if the man we are outside is wasting away, certainly the man we are inside is being renewed from day to day. For though the tribulation is momentary and light, it works out for us a glory that is of more and more surpassing weight and is everlasting; while we keep our eyes, not on the things seen, but on the things unseen. For the things seen are temporary, but the things unseen are everlasting.

—2 Cor. 4:13, 16–18

Jesus said to her: "I am the resurrection and the life. He that exercises faith in me, even though he dies, will come to life; and everyone that is living and exercises faith in me will never die at all."

—John 11:25, 26

He will actually swallow up death forever, and the Sovereign Lord Jehovah will certainly wipe the tears from all faces ... And in that day one will certainly say: "Look! This is our God. We have hoped in him, and he will save us. This is Jehovah. We have hoped in him. Let us be joyful and rejoice in the salvation by him."

—Isa. 25:8

READINGS DURING END-OF-LIFE PROCESS

Scriptural readings can be read by family, friends, ministers and health care professionals. (All scripture quotations are from the New World Translation of the Holy Scriptures.)

Orthodox Christianity

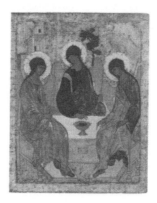

234

Being as Communion[235]

Prepared by:
The Very Reverend Steven Voytovich, DMin, LPC
Director, Orthodox Church in America Department of Institutional Chaplains
Director of Clinical Pastoral Education, Episcopal Health Services
Far Rockaway, NY

History and Facts

A proper understanding of Orthodox (Eastern) Christianity must begin with a discussion of the Christian faith at its inception, following the direct ministry and witness of Jesus Christ Himself. The roots of the Christian faith begin with the Feast of Pentecost, 50 days after Jesus' death, resurrection and ascension. The Holy Spirit descended upon the twelve apostles as "tongues of fire," and these simple fishermen began to bear witness to God in the languages of the people gathered in Jerusalem. Peter, the first among the apostles, preached to those gathered. When Peter "departed to another place" (tradition having that to be Rome), James, the Brother of the Lord, remained in Jerusalem until his death. The early Church was marked by both itinerant preaching and early indwelling leadership

---

234 Ouspensky, L. *The Meaning of Icons.* Crestwood, NY: St. Vladimir's Seminary Press, 1982. The Icon of the Trinity was painted around 1410 by Andrei Rublev. Three angels are depicted visiting Abraham at the Oak of Mamre – but is often interpreted as an icon of the Holy Trinity (Genesis 18). It is sometimes called the icon of the Old Testament Trinity. This icon is full of symbolism – designed to take the viewer into the Mystery of the fullness of communion within the Trinity: Father, Son, and Holy Spirit, embracing all of creation.

235 The quote was provided by V. Rev. Steven Voytovich, the author of this chapter – it is the title of a book by Metropolitan John Zizioulas.

in the local church later known as bishops. Peter is known as the "Apostle of the Circumcised" and Paul as the "Apostle of the Gentiles." Tradition has both Peter and Paul ending their lives in Rome in about 68 CE, at that time the capital of the empire.

The last half of the first century was the period in which many of the gospels and other texts forming the New Testament were written. Also during that time and until the fourth century, Christians were persecuted throughout the empire. To escape persecution, many gathered in secret to celebrate the Eucharist.

With respect to authority within the Church, Saint Ignatius of Antioch bore witness to the local church gathered around its bishop as the fullness of the Church, having the Lord and His Apostles at its head. He was also aware of the concept of "apostolic succession" among the early leaders of the Church. With the peace of Constantine when persecution of Christians ceased, Christianity became the favored religion of the empire and the capital was moved from Rome to Constantinople.

The Ecumenical Councils

The period of the fourth century was a vibrant time in the Christian Church in crystallizing and standardizing its beliefs. Having a clear understanding of the nature of God was paramount. In the East, the Cappadocian Fathers Basil the Great, Gregory the Theologian (Basil's brother) and Saint Gregory Nazianzus developed the term *homooúsios*, found in the Nicene Creed to indicate that "Jesus Christ is of one essence or substance with the Father and yet distinct in *hypostasis* or personhood." Thus, these theologians are credited with developing the Trinitarian understanding of the Father, the Son and the Holy Spirit

as three persons, yet one in essence and undivided, a concept hinted at in several New Testament verses.

This concept of the Godhead is characterized in the Icon of the Holy Trinity (drawing upon Genesis 18, when the three angels visit Abraham under the Oak of Mamre) which depicts the Father sitting on the left side with the Son facing outward toward humanity that he came to save and the Holy Spirit (both inclining their heads toward the Father). Saint Irenaeus of Lyons (second century) speaks of the Son and the Spirit as the two hands of God through which the Father's will is accomplished and perfected. This "mystery" of the Holy Trinity is an important focus in Orthodox spiritual life and contemplation. The relational communion of love among the three persons of the Trinity is the archetype that Christians are called to emulate in their daily lives by receiving this love freely offered, sharing it with one another, and freely offering it back to God. In the East, this relational foundation of faith remains central as represented in the Church as "the gathered community celebrating the Eucharist." This celebration of the Liturgy remains a primary source of unity among the Orthodox to the present day.

Up to the time of the Emperor Justinian (527–565), the political and ecclesial boundaries of the Christian empire were almost synonymous. Five early centers were known: Jerusalem, Rome, Constantinople, Alexandria, and Antioch. Conciliarity was, and remains, a significant pillar for church governance, as was reflected during the period of the seven Ecumenical Councils, with "Catholicity" referring to the universality of the Christian Faith and "Orthodoxy" as right belief or right worship.

1. **The First Council of Nicaea (325)**

condemned Arius and defined the incarnate Son of God as "consubstantial" with the Father. The Nicene Creed was also begun during this council.

2. **The First Council of Constantinople (381)** settled the Arian controversy. Later on, this council was credited with having adopted the present form of the Nicene Creed.

3. **The Council of Ephesus (431)** condemned Nestorianism, declaring there were not two persons existing side by side in Christ – God and a man named Jesus – but that the divinity and humanity were united in one person (hypostatic union), the eternal Word of God incarnate. Consequently, Mary, the Mother of Jesus, is the Mother of God (*Theotókos*).

4. **The Council of Chalcedon (451)** while affirming Jesus Christ's united personhood, also affirmed two natures of Christ: divine and human existing within in one person (*hypostasis*). It should be noted that many of the non-Greek churches in the East (Coptic, Ethiopian, Armenian, and Syro-Jacobite together known as the Miaphysites or Oriental Orthodox today) did not affirm this council, and yet for the same theological beliefs that prompted the acceptance of this council. Movement continues toward the healing of this division.

5. **The Second Council of Constantinople (533)**, lead by the Emperor Justinian, desired to win back the Monophysites by proving that Chalcedon had not fallen into Nestorianism (that Jesus is in fact two distinct persons). Theologians suspected of entertaining Nestorian views were condemned.

6. **The Third Council of Constantinople (680)**, still attempting to restore union, condemned Monothelitism which stated that while Christ has two natures he has only one will, his divine will or "energy." The council maintained that humanity is not an abstract entity in Christ but is manifested by its own will, subject freely and in all things to the divine will. Christ, therefore, has two wills.

7. **The Second Council of Nicaea (787)** defined the largely Orthodox (right worship/praise) doctrine concerning icons representing Christ (icons of saints are known in the Catholic Church as well). While sacred images are to be "venerated" (*proskynesis*), this is not be confused with "true worship" (*latreia*) which is due to God alone. Icons were not returned to the church until 843, known now as the Sunday of Orthodoxy, the first Sunday of Great Lent.

These Councils are still understood by the Catholic and Orthodox Churches as efforts of the early church to remain faithful to the foundation of the faith and the Gospels. Issues of church administration and way of life concerns (through the many canons accepted through these councils) were also results of these councils.

The Great Schism

Unfortunately, the Christian Church became divided between the Latin-speaking West and Greek-speaking East. This separation was exacerbated by the difficulties in communication between Rome and Constantinople. An early political event sparking controversy was the crowning of Charlemagne as Holy Roman Emperor by the pope in Rome in 800, expressing the desire to reestablish Rome as the capital of the empire. Theologically, the *Filioque* clause was added to the Nicene Creed (the Holy Spirit which proceeds from the Father *and* the Son) and celebrated in Rome in the Liturgy/Mass. This strained relations even further between Rome and Constantinople. (Orthodox Christians recite the Nicene Creed without the *Filioque* – *see* Nicene Creed).

These and other events, but mostly poor communication, brought about the Great Schism between the Church of Rome and the Church of Constantinople along with the other three historic centers of the early Christian Church in 1054. Several unsuccessful attempts were made to heal this schism. However, the mutual "anathemas" were lifted in 1969, and though relations are slowly warming, full communion has not yet been restored between what became known as the Roman Catholic Church and the Eastern Orthodox Church representing the other four early centers of Christianity. At present, the Catholic and Orthodox Churches recognize the sacraments of Baptism, Chrismation, and Marriage. What follows is the history of the Orthodox Church representing the Eastern branch of the historic Christian Church.

Eastern Christianity

Developments in the East included the missionary efforts of Saints Cyril and Methodius in developing a form of the Cyrillic alphabet as a written language for the Slavs in order to translate the Liturgy and scripture for that Christian community. This missionary focus of spreading the message of Orthodox Christianity would be repeated through many different cultural contexts, including Russia with the baptism of Vladimir around 988. When Constantinople fell to the Ottoman Empire in 1453, Moscow saw itself as the "Third Rome," with Constantinople being known by those in the East as "new Rome."

Worship styles varied in the differing cultural milieus of Eastern Christianity as well. For example, *Hagia Sophia* (The Church of the Holy Wisdom) featured the richness of the cathedral rite with song services including composed hymns. Monastic communities, on the other hand, offered the less flowery pious chanting of Psalms and services with solemnity. Also, the men and women of the desert built the foundations of monastic life, embraced in its fullness on Mount Athos, but the monks and nuns in Russia lived in the wilderness. Even so, a great school of elders *gerons* (Greek) or *startsy* (Russian), representing those living the depth of the spiritual life, were sought out by the faithful of all traditions for spiritual direction. A series of publications called the *Philokalia* represent the depth of spiritual life from these times. The two traditions of cathedral and monastic worship were combined and are part of the present day liturgical life of the Orthodox Church and lived out in a variety of ways. The beauty and solemnity of liturgical services, most often with responses sung a cappella, is well known in the Orthodox Church.

The Orthodox Church's Arrival in America

The Orthodox Church came to America by way of Alaska. In 1794, a group of monks including Monk Herman, traveled from Valaam Monastery in Finland, through Russia, and across the Bering Strait to the Island of Kodiak where Holy Resurrection Church was later established. The monks were sent by the Russians to support the work of fur trading in this new territory.

However, upon discovering how the native people were exploited, the religious men took a stand for the rights of the indigenous Aleuts. Monk Herman, the last surviving member of that initial group ministered to the needs of the native Aleut people on Spruce Island until his death around 1837. Herman became the first canonized saint in North America in 1970.

A short time before Saint Herman's death, Father John Veniaminov (later becoming Bishop Innocent) was sent to continue the missionary effort begun by those monks. He evangelized the native Aleuts and Tlingits. Through an effort similar to that of Cyril and Methodius, he developed written languages for both peoples in order that they could hear the liturgical services and Scripture in their own languages. To this day, the Orthodox Church is well known among the indigenous people of Alaska. For his dedication and efforts, Bishop Innocent was canonized in 1977.

Approximately a century later, immigration began in earnest to the eastern seaboard of America from various points in Eastern Europe. This was the period when the high point of Orthodox Church life in America occurred (from the 1890s to 1917). Bishop Tikhon, the head of the Russian missionary venture to America, sought to bring together the missionary and immigrant components into one united church. He succeeded in bringing together persons of all ethnic backgrounds to worship, in English, in the Orthodox Church planted in North America. Unfortunately, the Russian Revolution in 1917 caused the American Church to find itself without direction or resources when Bishop (now Saint) Tikhon was recalled to Russia to become the Patriarch of the Church of Russia. The consequences of his leaving were dramatic.

The Greek-speaking Christians looked back to Constantinople for direction, organizing in the 1920s; the Syrian Christians turned to Antioch; and the Slavs simply "toughed it out" locally on their own, awaiting the opportunity to reunite once again with the Russian Orthodox Church.

The Orthodox Church in America

Much of the Eastern Church was captive and had to operate "underground" during the reign of Communism in Eastern Europe. It wasn't until the late 1960s that the functioning remainder of the Russian Mission in America was able to reestablish contact with the Russian Orthodox Church who in 1970 granted autocephaly or self-governance to the Russian Mission in America. This new entity became known as the Orthodox Church in America (OCA). It is ironic that this occurred in the same year that Bishop Herman, the monk who brought Orthodox Christianity to America, was canonized as a saint. Even though there are jurisdictional differences in the American Orthodox Church (i.e., Greek, Russian, Ukrainian, Syrian/Antiochian), these distinctions are largely administrative and have little to do with the faith, which remains one.

Two important points need to be made here concerning the multiple jurisdictions present in the North American Church. The first is that one does not need to be of the ethnic identity of a specific Orthodox Church (Russian, Greek, etc.). This is a worldwide faith, and typically the Orthodox Church in any geographic region is for those living in that region no matter what their ethnic origin. The second point is that how the Orthodox Faith is lived out among the various jurisdictions amount to small "t" traditional differences. The Liturgy and the

Faith are understood as part of the greater Orthodox Christian Faith.

In North America, it is estimated that there are between two and three million Orthodox Christians. Expanding the perspective to worldwide estimation of Orthodox Christians, the estimation is between 200 and 300 million.[236] Such estimation includes divergence on the definition of membership and the reality that for much of the Orthodox Church in captivity, it was impossible to maintain any kind of membership lists.

Basic Teachings

- The Nicene Creed as known in the Orthodox Church is a brief and yet powerful primer concerning the Christian Faith and baptismal affirmation:

Nicene Creed

I believe in one God, the Father Almighty, Maker of heaven and earth, and of all things visible and invisible.

And in one Lord Jesus Christ, the Son of God, the only-begotten, begotten of the Father before all ages. Light of Light; true God of true God; begotten, not made, of one essence with the Father, by whom all things were made;

Who, for us men and for our salvation came down from heaven, and was incarnate of the Holy Spirit and the Virgin Mary, and became man. And was crucified for us under Pontius Pilate, and suffered, and was buried. And the third day He rose again, according to the Scriptures;

and ascended into heaven, and sits at the right hand of the Father; and He shall come again, with glory, to judge the living and the dead; whose Kingdom shall have no end.

And in the Holy Spirit, the Lord, the Giver of Life, who proceeds from the Father; who with the Father and the Son together is worshipped and glorified; who spoke by the prophets.

In one Holy, Catholic, and Apostolic Church; I acknowledge one baptism for the remission of sins; I look for the resurrection of the dead, and the life of the world to come. Amen.[237]

- Human beings were originally created as "good" by God, in God's image and likeness (see Genesis 2–3). The image is planted in people at the moment of conception, and likeness is an ongoing effort to actualize Baptism, as accomplished through the grace of the Holy Spirit, who freely returns the great gift of God's love.
- The Orthodox interpretation of Rom. 5:12 is that the fallen human nature people inherit includes sickness and ultimately physical death. Sin is a dimension of this fallen human nature. As Christ overcame spiritual death (meaning separation from God), physical death becomes a step toward greater communion with Him. Rather than washing away "original sin," baptism is the gift of Jesus Christ's saving death and, God willing, participation in His Resurrection. Infants as well as adults can be baptized.

---

236 These estimates were obtained from the Orthodox Church in America website: www.oca.org.

237 Nicene Creed from the text of *The Divine Liturgy of St. John Chrysostom*, published by the Russian Orthodox Greek Catholic Church of America, New York, 1967, and currently used in the celebration of the Divine Liturgy.

- The Orthodox refer to Holy Tradition as the inheritance they are charged to preserve as a living continuity with the early church. Holy Scripture is central in Holy Tradition. Other dimensions of Holy Tradition include the Nicene Creed, the Ecumenical Councils and their canons; even iconography and hymnography are, in their own ways, vehicles communicating Orthodox theology. The writings of the Patristic Fathers also comprise a portion of Holy Tradition.

- Conciliarity is a significant principle in the Eastern Christian Faith. All bishops are of equal standing, with the head of a particular church being the "first among equals." As such, the church gathers in council praying that God's will be accomplished through inspiration of the assembly by the Holy Spirit.

- The principle of *conciliarity* also guides ethical decision making. The "mind of the church" is prayerfully approached through Holy Tradition, and organically brought to bear on a particular situation. The Orthodox often hold seemingly dichotomous concepts in tension, sometimes known as antinomies, and speak from within these tensions. For example, the local church, gathered around the local bishop in celebration of the Eucharist is constitutive of the fullness of the church, not just one portion of it. This is an expression of unity. The bishops gathered in council represent a unanimity as well as conciliarity expressed from within the Eucharistic assembly.

- The Orthodox continue to hold a circular sense of time within the liturgical year. One is always focused on the Resurrection of Christ: either the Church is approaching **Pascha** (Passover from death to life and used instead of "Easter"), celebrating Pascha, or in the period returning to waiting for the journey to Pascha to begin again. Each Sunday is a little Pascha; Sunday always remembering the Resurrection.

- In continuing the sense of time, Orthodox faithful keep several dimensions of the calendar in unique tension each year. The date of Pascha (computed according to the Julian calendar) leads to Pascha and the journey to and from it is celebrated at distinct times from that of many "Western Christians." Furthermore, each day of the week has its own significance and focus, with a daily cycle of services served in monastic communities and some active parishes. Then the fixed calendar of Feasts and Fasts is "knitted" together with the Pascha determination.

- The Orthodox Christians maintain the prior Jewish practice of beginning each day the night before. Sunday, for example, begins with Vespers Saturday night (for many Orthodox) Matins celebrated prior to the Liturgy (Byzantine practice) and then the Liturgy. Only one Liturgy can be celebrated on a given day.

- Worship in general is a very sensory experience; one lights candles, smells the incense, hears the Word, sees the icons, and tastes of the precious Body and Blood of Christ.

Basic Practices

- The entrance of infants through adults into Orthodox Christianity is through Baptism. This service begins with exorcisms and proceeds through baptism of triple immersion ("the servant of God is baptized in the name of the Father, and the Son, and the Holy Spirit"). Usually, one has at least one sponsor (or witness also in marriage) who must be a practicing Orthodox Christian. As in other traditions, in emergencies such as danger of death, baptism may be performed using this formula.

- In the Orthodox Tradition, Chrismation, being sealed with the gift of the Holy Spirit (known in some traditions as confirmation), is conferred at the time of Baptism. Therefore, the newly baptized and chrismated servant of God is a full member of the Body of Christ from that day forward, able to receive the Eucharist as the fulfillment of Baptism.

- The Eucharist is a sacrifice of thanksgiving offered by the gathered faithful in celebrating the Liturgy (*Leitourgia*, literally the work of God's people). Upward of 95% of the Liturgy is taken directly from scripture. The Liturgy is a journey that begins in the present and leads, through the Gospel, to the Kingdom of Heaven. In the Eucharist, believers taste the precious Body and Blood of Christ of the Kingdom of Heaven mystically transformed from bread and wine.

- The celebration of the Eucharist is also significant to note. Either five loaves or one large loaf of bread stamped with a special seal denoting: "*IC XC NI KA*" or "Jesus Christ conquers all" are prepared for the Liturgy. One loaf (or center portion of large loaf) is cut into a square portion under this seal (the Lamb of God) and placed on the paten. Wine and water are poured into a chalice. Other loaves or portions represent: the Mother of God, the ranks of the Saints, the living, and the departed. Especially for the latter two, portions may be placed for individual names of those sick, departed, and so forth. During the Liturgy, the four portions of the lamb are fractioned. The *IC*

(Body of Christ) is placed in the chalice, the clergy celebrating receive from the *XC* portion, and the *NI KA* portions are cut up and placed in the chalice for the faithful. Warm water is added to the chalice symbolizing the warmth of the Holy Spirit. The faithful receive the Body and Blood together by spoon from the chalice. All remaining portions of the Eucharist are consumed at the end of the Liturgy, though a small amount of reserved sacrament is prepared for communing with those sick or infirm.

- As the Eucharist is constitutive of the Church, only those expressing common belief as Orthodox Christians, are baptized and chrismated, and having prepared through prayer and confession may receive Holy Communion.

- One who is baptized, chrismated, and receives the Eucharist is a full member of the Body of Christ (the priesthood of all believers) and takes his or her place in the assembly to offer the fruits of gifts given unto him or her.

- Depending on the tradition of local parishes, once a child becomes of the age of knowing right from wrong, they begin to participate in the Sacrament of Confession. This sacrament is a reconciliation or *metanoia* (translated "repentance," literally meaning "turning one's journey back toward God" or ongoing spiritual development). From this point onward, the participation in Confession is an integral part of continuing to approach the chalice to receive communion. Because of influences in some cultural settings where penitent and whomever he or she is confessing to were both held accountable for what might be shared, confession was not practiced.

- The practice of confession deserves

some attention here as well. The penitent approaches the priest or confessor, who stands with the person before God as he or she confesses sins. The confessor may offer some comment in terms of understanding or penance, and then pronounces the formula of absolution. This sacrament can be conducted at the bedside as well. The priest holds silent anything brought to him in confession. No one pursues their spiritual life in isolation due to the grave potential for temptation.

- Though the Orthodox Church does not hold sacraments to seven, the Orthodox Church approaches other major steps in the life journey sacramentally. They include but are not limited to: confession, marriage, ordination to holy orders, Holy Unction.

- One is changed through the celebrations of the sacraments. Several have already been explained. In marriage, the bride and groom are two becoming one flesh (Gen. 2:24). One of the two desiring to be married must be an Orthodox Christian, and the other needs to be a practicing Christian who embraces at least baptism using the formula Father, Son, and Spirit.

- In ordination (one remains either celibate or married upon ordination) the ordained is ontologically changed. Ordinations include sub-deacon, deacon, priest, and bishop). Not only discernment and theological studies, but preparation with one's bishop precedes ordination.

- Holy Unction is a special service that in its fullness is celebrated with seven celebrants. A special mixture of wine and oil is prepared, and then each successive celebrant reads assigned scripture readings, prays over the oil, and anoints the person who is ill. The meaning here is anointing unto the health of soul and body, meaning that while physical health may not be the outcome, one is prepared to be in right relationship with God. Those who are communicants are able to receive Holy Unction. It is also the practice in many Orthodox Churches to celebrate the Holy Unction service on Holy Wednesday (of Holy Week) and perhaps at other appointed times according to local tradition when all the faithful may receive this sacrament.

- Besides the real focus and emphasis on community life, Orthodox Christians have prayers morning, evening, and at other times. These are usually developed with one's spiritual father, and may include the *Trisagion* (see "Scriptures, Inspirational Readings, and Prayers" section), daily Epistle and Gospel readings, some written prayers, and quiet or spontaneous dialogue with God. The best possible practice is one who prays regularly, likewise regularly participates in the celebration of the Eucharist and, between times, exercises whatever gifts of ministry one may have.

- Concerning "being saved": one has been saved by Christ, one is being saved in actualizing baptism and one will be saved upon the Second Coming of Christ. An important word for Orthodox Christians concerning salvation is *theosis*. The literal translation is "becoming what God is by nature, through God's grace." Orthodox believe in a life-long actualization of baptism, transformation accomplished through the Grace of the Holy Spirit, to become more fully the image (given at conception) and likeness of God they were created to be.

Principles for Clinical Care
Dietary Issues

- A dimension of the Orthodox Christian that may be helpful in a hospital setting has to do with fasting periods. Particularly during the season of Great Lent – the 6 weeks prior to the celebration of Easter (which may be a different date than that which is popularly celebrated in a given year through the use of the Julian rather than Gregorian calendar) – Orthodox Christians typically fast from meats and from dairy with varying degrees of severity; so dietary sensitivity is appreciated.
- Orthodox in many traditions will fast from meats on Wednesdays and Fridays – Wednesday representing the Betrayal of Christ, and Friday representing the Crucifixion.
- Outside of prescribed fasting periods and weekly observances, there are no real dietary restrictions for Orthodox Christians. Some choose, for example, to eat a vegetarian diet either for personal reasons or for possibly ascetical reasons.

General Medical Beliefs

- The Orthodox Church values life from the moment of conception through end of life, and so has been opposed to any means of shortening that life. At the same time, the Orthodox Church has, in interacting with the medical community, come to appreciate the reality of life-sustaining measures that can prolong the dying process.
- In valuing life from the moment of conception, the Orthodox Church believes from this moment this new life is an "ensouled," personal existence created in the image of God and endowed with a sanctity that destines it for eternal life.
- Jesus' saving death and Resurrection

promises to all the fruits of communion with God as the source of life, communion with our fellow human beings and other creatures of our planet, and the fullness of human nature: light, goodness, truth leading to well-being of mind, soul, and body. This renewed fullness of life is best described as *theosis*.[238]

- A therapeutic, healing approach is at the core of Orthodox Christianity.

> This healing vision of God at work in the world applies primarily to the religious, the spiritual, and the moral dimensions of life, but not exclusively so. It forms a matrix of concern that includes every part of life, restoring and healing the life being transfigured into one fully in communion with God and God's creation. It thus comes naturally to pray to God, "the Physician of our souls and bodies."[239]

- Basil the Great taught that physical and emotional disturbances were equally within the purview of the physician. In the same manner, body and spirit are equally of concern for the church. Both pursue a common goal to cure the whole person using their respective means.
- Suffering, that may come to human life through a variety of means, often uninvited, can, through the understanding of the Orthodox Tradition, be dealt with in a way that transforms us. Intractable pain is beyond the threshold of transformation.

---

238 Notes on general medical beliefs paraphrased from Fr. Stanley Harakas (*Health and Medicine in the Eastern Orthodox Tradition*. [1990]. New York, NY: Crossroad). Please also see *theosis* in glossary at end of chapter.

239 Harakas. *Health and Medicine in the Eastern Orthodox Tradition*, 28.

Specific Medical Issues

- **Abortion**: The Orthodox Church's posture toward abortion as ending the new life ensouled and endowed with personhood remains consistent from biblical times to the present. Abortion has been regarded as the morally condemnable act of destroying an innocent human life. This statement is supported through scripture, early Church writings and canon law. That said, the Church remains pastorally available to those confessing having abortions.

  o While a full articulation the Orthodox Church's posture on this and other bioethical issues can be found in *The Sacred Gift of Life: Orthodox Christianity and Bioethics* by the Very Reverend John Breck,[240] a few points will be included here:

  o Partial-birth abortion is never medically necessary to protect the health of a woman, as stated by a group of physicians known as PHACT, and can pose grave dangers to women.

  o If a woman's life is seriously endangered, she has no real choice. (Fr. John notes that these are the only truly "therapeutic" cases, and account for less than 1% of the nearly 1.4 million abortions performed in North America annually.) In cases of ectopic pregnancy, life-threatening eclampsia, or uterine cancer, the only choice is to work to save the woman's life or else lose both

her and her child.[241] This is not to create a hierarchy of value between mother and child's life, but that the woman has already established relationships and responsibilities with others depending on her. The principle of double effect is present here as the focus is not on ending pregnancy but preserving the mother's life; and the loss of the child's life is both tragic and regrettable.

  o In other cases such as rape and incest, Fr. John notes that procedures in place at hospital emergency departments can "virtually guarantee that fertilization will not occur." This step is primary, preceding the use of miscarriage invoking drugs.

- **Advance Directives**: Orthodox Christians may complete advance directives, and may seek counsel from their parish priest in doing so.

- **Birth Control**: One, not the only, purpose of marriage is the procreation of children. It is also as an expression of the indissoluble bond of love (Gen. 2:24). Entering into marital union implies at least an openness to having a family. Totally excluding procreation from a marital relationship then is not consonant with marriage. It is generally understood, however, that contraceptives utilized toward spacing of children and enhancing the loving unity of the relationship may in fact be helpful in the relationship.[242] Usually such a decision would be arrived at in consultation with one's parish priest and/or in preparation for marriage. Any birth control methods that are abortive in

---

240 Fr. John Breck is a noted ethicist and author on biomedical issues. Please see his books for further reference from which much of this medical/ethical material was presented: *The Sacred Gift of Life: Orthodox Christianity and Bioethics*, SVS Press, 1998; *Stages on Life's Way: Orthodox Thinking on Bioethics*, SVS Press, 2005; and *Longing for God: Orthodox Reflections on Bible, Ethics, and Liturgy*, SVS Press, 2006.

241 Breck, J. *The Sacred Gift of Life: Orthodox Christianity and Bioethics*. SVS Press, 1998, pp. 157–161.

242 Harakas. *Health and Medicine in the Eastern Orthodox Tradition*, 141.

nature are to be rejected (*see* first point in this section, "Abortion").

- **Blood Transfusions**: The Orthodox Church has no resistance to the use of blood and blood products when necessary for treatment of persons.

- **Cell/Gene Manipulation**: In a more general statement then, no manipulation of the human person, on the macro or micro level, can be accepted unless that manipulation is for strictly therapeutic purposes that will best serve the interests of the person concerned.

- **Circumcision**: Circumcision is typically decided on more for medical and hygienic reasons, and is not a requirement in the eyes of the church.

- **In Vitro Fertilization**: Any and all manipulation of human embryos for research purposes is seen as inherently immoral and a violation of human life. Arguments for this position include a post-Holocaust principle, universally accepted by the scientific community, that no experimentation be undertaken on human subjects without informed consent. No one can have proxy rights over the life and well-being of a child in utero or in vitro. The Orthodox Church applauds recent legislation passed in Italy in February 2004 entitled "Rules concerning medically assisted procreation (MAP)" that includes, among other clear and focused guidelines, a limitation of in vitro fertilization to those to be implanted immediately.[243]

- **Prenatal, Neonatal, and Ongoing Care**: Prenatal, neonatal, and ongoing care, including vaccinations, are strongly encouraged.

- **Stem Cell Research**: The scientific community is urged "to devote their time, energy and resources to discovering, harvesting and utilizing non-embryonic stem cells, including those derived from adults, placentas, and umbilical cords."[244]

- **Withholding/Withdrawing Life Support**: Decisions involving withholding/withdrawing life support in medically futile cases typically are worked through with the individual's parish priest in consultation with the health care team. While Orthodox understand medically that artificial respiration, nutrition, and hydration are significant means to prolonging life, they also recognize that there is a boundary to which these measures may simply be prolonging someone's natural departure from this life.

Gender and Personal Issues

- The Orthodox Church upholds the sanctity of marriage as monogamous, heterosexual, blessed, and conjugal, representing the sacrificial love between Christ and the Church. While same gender relationships are not blessed in the Church, legally recognized monogamous civil unions can aid in gaining necessary legal rights.

- Compassionate ministry toward gays and lesbians is a significant pastoral concern that needs more attention in the life of the church.

- In terms of caring for those hospitalized,

---

243 Breck, J. *Longing for God: Orthodox Reflections on Bible, Ethics, and Liturgy.* SVS Press, 2006, pp. 96–97.

244 Statement by the OCA Holy Synod of Bishops, Embryonic Stem Cell Research in the Perspective of Orthodox Christianity, October 17, 2001. Available at: http://oca.org/holy-synod/statements/holy-synod/embryonic-stem-cell-research-in-the-perspective-of-orthodox-christianity (accessed May 2010).

one's gender, sexual orientation, marital status, and age do not preclude being ministered to.

Principles for Spiritual Care through the Cycles of Life

Concepts of Living and Dying for Spiritual Support

- Life is sacred and deserves respect and protection throughout. Sanctity of life resides in the "person," bearing the image and likeness of God, rather than simply in physical existence.
- All human lives are of equal value, from conception to death.
- Suffering (with or without physical pain) is a consequence of fallen human nature (not intended nor sent to us by God) and therefore a reality in our life. Suffering can have redemptive value as we surrender our pain and anguish into the loving hands of God. This redemptive value exists within the bounds of intractable pain that separates us from our ability to pursue life goals within our relationships with God and one another.
- Those who suffer can become beacons of meaning of what life and death are all about for those around them. "Inasmuch as we can turn and direct our lives toward God, through repentance and living His will, He will bear us up and make us whole in a new context. ... Through our active acceptance of suffering, we can be transfigured in radiating God's presence."[245]
- Death is the passage of the soul or life principle into eternity, meaning to dwell in permanent communion with God enduring beyond the limits of earthly existence.

- Resurrection of the physical body (transformed into a spiritual body 1 Cor. 15:44) and reunion of body and soul will happen at the end of time at the Second Coming of Jesus.
- At the Second Coming, God will reveal His presence and will fill all creation with Himself. For those who love Him it will be paradise. For those who hate Him it will be hell. When the Kingdom of God fills all creation, it will once again be that paradise for which it was originally created."[246]

During Birth

- It is a custom in the Orthodox Church to celebrate a service of naming on the eighth day.
- As stated earlier, circumcision is typically decided on more for medical and hygienic reasons, and is not a requirement in the eyes of the church.
- In the case of fetal demise or the death of a baby, many hospitals have developed wonderful ways of ministering to the mother and father. There are prayers in the Orthodox Tradition that are often helpful at this time, and a great deal of follow-up is important on the part of the parish.
- In some institutional settings, it is felt that baptism should be celebrated even if a baby is stillborn. This is not taught in the Orthodox Church. Rather, a service of blessing with the special prayers for the infant and those around him or her are appropriate. Typically, the parish priest will interact with the parents regarding the desire for burial of the infant.
- Miscarriages are a most important time to

---

245 Voytovich, S. (1990). The ministry of those who suffer. Unpublished MDiv thesis, 61–62.

246 Hopko, T. (1981). *The Orthodox Faith*. Vol. 1, *Doctrine*. New York, NY: Department of Religious Education, Orthodox Church in America, 133–134.

support the expectant parents. This devastating loss impacts mother and father but without support can, in some cases, contribute to the ending of the relationship itself. Caring and compassionate counsel are often needed in the days and weeks following a miscarriage.

- It should be noted that in instances where abortion might be favored, it is also known that abortion can often complicate whatever difficulties were present in beginning the pregnancy. Pregnant women favoring abortion need full support and nurture by family and parish alike to overcome feelings of shame and guilt and to continue the journey of bringing new life into the world, with the option of placing the newborn in adoptive care.

During Illness

- The Orthodox Christian faith is a sacramental faith. Thus, sacramental ministry plays a major role in hospital visitation of patients. It is important to realize, however, that this sacramental ministry itself is most fully celebrated within a meaningful pastoral context. Therefore, many patients will anticipate their priest coming to visit. Chaplains should not be put off by that, but rather remain open to offering their pastoral presence.
- Praying with an Orthodox patient, likewise, offers an opportunity to explore prayers in the Orthodox tradition. While the prayer, the "Our Father," is of course well known, it is the practice in any Orthodox service to offer the *Trisagion* prayers (*see* "Scriptures, Inspirational Readings, and Prayers" section). Further, prayers in the Orthodox tradition have a typical characteristic that begins not by calling upon God, but rather calling upon the God who was present with His people.

These prayers recall instances that relate to the present moment whether of hardship or of celebration; and then call upon the God who was present *there* to be present *here*. Thus, there is a connectedness in Orthodox prayers with the generations of God's children in that moment of prayer.

- Sacraments that an Orthodox Christian may receive while hospitalized do need to be offered by their parish priest and they may include **Confession**, **Holy Communion**, and **Holy Unction**.
  - Holy Communion, in and of itself, is a unique experience as Orthodox Christians do not use unleavened bread, but rather an "intincted" portion of a loaf (baked bread from flour, yeast, and water) specially prepared on Holy Thursday in commemoration of the Last Supper – the body and blood of Christ together. The further importance of receiving Communion in the hospital has to do with preparation of **fasting**. It is the tradition of Orthodox Christians when receiving Communion to fast from the time of going to sleep the previous night until receiving Communion. Consequently, it is a challenge for the priest to bring Communion in the morning before the patient has his or her breakfast. This is also a time when many doctors are trying to check in with their patients, and is an area where understanding on the part of caregivers would be received very warmly.
  - Patients also may ask to receive the sacrament of **Holy Unction**, an anointing with a special preparation of wine and oil (see Luke 10:34, James 5:13–16). In its fullness, this service is celebrated with seven celebrants, each reading scripture, praying over the prepared oil

and wine, and anointing the patient. But typically in practice, the priest will offer this to the patient at the bedside. The anointing with the specially blessed mixture of oil and wine as noted in the parable of the Good Samaritan is applied to: the patient's forehead, eyes, mouth, and ears – representing the senses; the base of the throat – representing the body; and on the hands and feet. This is done as completely as possible, given the circumstances of the patient. This sacrament is offered to those who are communicants in the life of the Church.

- Orthodox patients may have icons in their hospital rooms. Icons have a specific meaning and purpose in Orthodox worship. They are an art form representing a two-dimensional window from the temporal world into some portion of the Kingdom. The very first icon, for example, depicts the cloth in which Jesus was buried with features of his face represented in the icon. This icon represents Jesus' humanity as being among his people. Other icons such as of the Mother of God, of the saints, and of various feast days of the Church, likewise, signify the reality of the light of Christ coming into the world. Therefore, simply calling attention to the icon that patients may have with them is a way of valuing their tradition. Since most Orthodox churches are adorned with iconography, this is a meaningful connection for them with the life of the church while hospitalized. Another icon that Orthodox Christians may have is of the patron saints from which they received their names.

During End of Life

- Local clergy of critically ill patients should be contacted to offer the sacraments. It is also important to know that institutional chaplaincy remains a relatively new phenomenon within the Orthodox tradition. Therefore, extra sensitivity may be helpful in interacting with the local parish clergy, who in many cases are willing to be available to minister to the needs of the Orthodox, and yet may appear to be less familiar with the role of institutional chaplains.

- An important point needs to be made here concerning the request for sacraments. It is difficult for the parish priest to be contacted by health care providers to visit someone they do not know who is on their deathbed, with the family requesting sacraments. If a patient's faith tradition is known, and in this case Orthodox, contacting the parish priest as soon as possible offers the best opportunity to prepare the patient and family members for whatever ministry is offered.

- In keeping focus on the whole of life being a sacred gift from God, the Orthodox Church does not support any actions that could be understood as euthanasia or the active taking of one's life. While every effort is made to sustain life toward reasonable quality, there are cases where the moral response is to withhold/withdraw life support in order that a natural death may occur. It is also understood from an Orthodox perspective that suffering can indeed be redemptive up to the point of intractable pain. Offering pain medication is important, even though the law of double effect can be invoked (in offering sufficient pain medication, one's vital functioning of blood flow and respiration can be suppressed, the focus remains on controlling the pain).

- In addition to prayers at end of life, prayers exist to be offered when one is terminally ill, dying, or at the point of death.

- As stated earlier, the Orthodox can certainly exercise advance directives and can be organ donors if they so choose in dialogue with their parish priest.
- Cases of suicide are handled on a case-by-case basis. Suicide represents willfully destroying the temple of God in which the Holy Spirit dwells (1 Corinthians 3), and therefore severing one's relationship with God. In many instances, though, circumstances surrounding the taking of one's life raise serious questions as to this action being of free will. Therefore, these situations need to be dealt with in the most sensitive pastoral manner. The difference here is whether or not services are celebrated and how the family is pastorally supported. In no way, however, is the taking of one's life as avoidance of pain and suffering acceptable.

Care of the Body

- The Orthodox Church currently does not support cremation, unless, for example, in countries where this is required. If remains are cremated, they cannot be brought into the church and no prayers can be said over them. Burial of the body is in keeping with the sacredness of the human body.
- Embalming is regularly practiced today, although there are occasions where someone may indicate they do not want to be embalmed and legally it is not required.
- Autopsies are routinely offered to families. It should be noted that in some cases, when someone dies within 24 hours of arriving at the hospital, an autopsy may be required. Otherwise it is up to the family to make this decision.
- Typically donation of one's body for medical research was not supported for the same reasons of the sacredness of the human body, but recent developments have made this more accessible since bodies are returned for burial and/or families invited to services once research has been completed.
- Typically, if the person is a communicant, services are celebrated in church. If not a communicant, then services are typically celebrated at the funeral home. In some places, it is customary to celebrate the calling hours and services in the church, with the Psalms being read as visitors pay their respects. The casket is most often open for funeral services, no matter what location. The body may be blessed with holy water or anointed with oil during the funeral service. The faithful usually come to give the last kiss to their loved one before the casket is closed. At the cemetery, usually the casket is lowered until it is level with the ground. Following prayers, the priest will sprinkle dirt over the casket and bless the grave.
- Typically beyond the funeral services, memorial services can be celebrated on the 9th day, the 40th day, and annually in remembrance.
- The parish family offers support to bereaved family members in a variety of ways during their journey of grief.

Organ and Tissue Donation

- Orthodox Christians may choose to donate organs and tissue; it is an individual decision made in dialogue with one's parish priest.

Scriptures, Inspirational Readings, and Prayers
TRISAGION PRAYERS

In the Name of the Father, and of the Son, and of the Holy Spirit. Amen.

Prayer to the Holy Spirit

O Heavenly King, the Comforter, the
Spirit of Truth, who art everywhere
and fillest all things; Treasury of
blessings and Giver of life: Come
and abide in us and cleanse us from
every impurity, and save our souls,
O Good One.

Holy God, Holy Mighty, Holy
Immortal: have mercy on us.
(Thrice)

Glory to the Father, and to the Son,
and to the Holy Spirit:

now and ever and unto ages of ages.
Amen.

Prayer to the Holy Trinity

O most-holy Trinity, have mercy on
us. Lord, cleanse us from our sins.
Master, pardon our transgressions.
Holy One, visit and heal our
infirmities for Thy Name's sake.

Lord, have mercy. (Thrice)

Glory to the Father, and to the Son,
and to the Holy Spirit:

now and ever, and unto ages of ages.
Amen.

Our Father, who art in heaven,
hallowed be thy Name; thy kingdom
come; thy will be done on earth,
as it is in heaven. Give us this day
our daily bread; and forgive us our
trespasses, as we forgive those who
trespass against us; and lead us
not into temptation, but deliver us
from evil.

Through the prayers of our holy
Fathers, Lord Jesus Christ our God,
have mercy on us and save us. Amen.

PRAYERS DURING ILLNESS[247]

O Lord our God, Who by Your Word
alone healed all diseases; who cured
the Mother-in-law of Peter of fever;
Who chastises with pity and heals
according to Your goodness; Who
is able to put aside every malady
and infirmity: Do You, the same
Lord, now relieve Your servant(s)
_____, and cure him/her/them
of the sickness which grieve(s) him/
her/them; lift him/her/them up from
his/her/their bed(s) of pain, sending
down upon him/her/them Your
mercy; and if it be Your will, give to
him/her/them health and complete
recovery. For You are the Physician
of our souls and bodies, and to You
we ascribe glory, to the Father, and
to the Son, and to the Holy Spirit,
now and ever and unto ages of ages.
Amen.

When Sickness Increases

O Lord Jesus Christ our Savior: For
our sakes You were born; for our
sakes You were hungry and thirsted;
for our sakes You suffered and gave
Your life over to death. As You have
caused your servant _____, to
share in Your sufferings, so too, cause
him/her to share in Your Grace. May
Your Precious Blood wash away his/
her unrighteousness. Instead, look
upon his/her faith in You, rather
than upon his/her works when he/
she shall stand before You the Judge.
As his/her sickness increases, so also

247 Prayers are taken from *The Book of Needs*
(Abridged), compiled and edited by a Monk of
St. Tikhon's Monastery (South Canaan, PA: St.
Tikhon's Seminary Press; 1987).

let Your plenteous Grace increase on him/her; do not let his/her faith waver, nor his/her hope fail, nor his/her love grow cold; do not let the fear of death cause him/her to cast away his/her trust in You, or to place it anywhere except on You. But looking steadfastly to You to the end, let him/her say: "Into Your hands, O Lord, I commend my spirit," and so enter into Your everlasting Kingdom, of the Father, and of the Son, and of the Holy Spirit, now and ever and unto ages of ages. Amen.

READING DURING ILLNESS OR END OF LIFE

This can be read by family, friends, clergy, and health care professionals. (Scripture cited is from the New Revised Standard Version.)

The Lord is my shepherd I shall not want.
He makes me lie down in green pastures; he restores my soul.
He leads me in right paths for his name's sake.
Even though I walk through the darkest valley, I fear no evil;
for you are with me; your rod and your staff – they comfort me.
You prepare a table before me in the presence of my enemies;
you anoint my head with oil; my cup overflows.
Surely goodness and mercy shall follow me all the days of my life,
and I shall dwell in the house of the Lord my whole life long.

—Psalm 23

(Also Psalm 91, not included here.)

PRAYER AT END OF LIFE

(Prayer said by the priest at the departure of the soul.)

O Master, Lord, Almighty, Father of our Lord Jesus Christ; Who will that all people should be saved and come to the knowledge of the truth; Who desires not the death of a sinner, but that he/she should turn from his way and live, we entreat You and implore You: Absolve the soul of Your servant, _____, from all bonds and free it from every curse. Pardon his/her transgressions, committed from youth, both knowingly and unknowingly, in deed or in word, that which he/she has freely confessed or concealed, either through forgetfulness or through shame. For You alone loose that which is bound and guide the compunctionate. You are the hope of the despairing, mighty to remit the sins of every person who puts his/her trust in You. Yea, O Lord Who loves mankind, command that he/she be released from the bonds of the flesh and sins. Receive in peace the soul of this, Your servant, _____, and grant it rest in the eternal mansions with Your Saints, by the grace of Your Only-begotten Son, our Lord and God and Savior Jesus Christ, with Whom You are blessed, together with Your Most-holy, Good, and Life-creating Spirit, now and ever and unto ages of ages. Amen.

Special Days: Orthodox Christianity

One will notice the parenthetical designations "Eastern" and "Western" in this section. Many Orthodox churches use the Julian Calendar, which is indicated by the use of "Eastern." The majority of Christian Churches use the Gregorian Calendar, which is indicated by the use of "Western." Please also note that the Orthodox Church's Liturgical New Year begins on September 1 each year, and the Catholic Church recognizes November 30 as the beginning of the Church Year.

January 6 *Epiphany* (Western)/*Feast of the Theophany* (Eastern) – Epiphany (usually called Theophany in Eastern churches) celebrates the manifestation of Jesus as Christ. In the Western Church, Epiphany is associated primarily with the journey of the Magi to visit Jesus. The Eastern Church associates Theophany, primarily, with the baptism of Jesus. It is celebrated because, according to tradition, the baptism of Jesus in the Jordan River by John the Baptist marked the only occasion when all three persons of the Holy Trinity manifested their physical presence simultaneously to humanity: God the Father by speaking through the clouds, God the Son being baptized in the river, and God the Holy Spirit in the shape of a dove descending from heaven. Thus, the holy day is considered to be a Trinitarian feast. This date is also Christmas Eve in Eastern churches that follow the Julian calendar instead of the Gregorian calendar.

January 7 *Nativity of Christ, Christmas* (Eastern) – Celebration of the birth of Jesus Christ observed by prayers, exchanging of gifts and family parties; season of the Christian year following Advent and preceding Epiphany. Some Eastern Orthodox churches, such as the Ukrainian, celebrate Christmas according to the Julian calendar.

February 2 *Meeting of the Lord in the Temple* – This feast commemorates Jesus being brought to the Temple 40 days after birth, as was the custom. Simeon and Anna are featured as waiting to see the Messiah as he is brought by Mary and Joseph. Candles are sometimes blessed on this feast as they portray the light of Christ in the Eastern Church.

February 3 *Transfiguration* (Western) – This day celebrates the appearance of Jesus in a transfigured state during his earthly life to three of the disciples. Appearing with him were Moses and Elijah.

February 6 *Ash Wednesday* (Western) – Ash Wednesday is the observance to begin the 40-day period of Lent (excluding Sundays) of prayer, repentance, and self-denial that culminates in Easter. Ashes in the form of a cross are placed on people's foreheads as a sign of penitence.

February 17 *Triodion* – The Easter season in the Eastern and Oriental Orthodox Churches is the cycle of the moveable feasts. This cycle is comprised of approximately 10 weeks before and 7 weeks after Easter. The 10 weeks before Easter are known as the period of the Triodion (referring to the book that contains the services for this liturgical season). This period includes the 3 weeks preceding Great Lent (the "pre-Lenten period"), the 40 days of Lent, and Holy Week.

March 10 *Lent Monday* (Eastern) – Lent is the final 6 weeks of a 10-week period of reflection and preparation for Holy Week and Easter/Pascha. The season is marked by periods of fasting, frequent worship and prayer, and acts of charity.

March 16 *Palm Sunday* (Western) – The Sunday that begins Holy Week commemorates Jesus' entry into Jerusalem riding on a donkey to participate in the Jewish Passover.

March 20 *Maundy Thursday* (Western) – This day commemorates the institution of the Lord's Supper (also referred to as Communion and Eucharist) by Jesus in the upstairs room to his disciples, at which time he also announced his betrayal by Judas and his imminent death.

March 21 *Good Friday* (Western) – This day is the remembrance of the crucifixion of Jesus and related events. Christians observe this sacrificial act typically through somber worship services in dimly lighted settings.

March 23 *Easter* (Western) – The most holy of Christian sacred days celebrates the resurrection of Jesus from the dead. Observances include sunrise worship services with special music, dressing up in special clothes, feasting (including Easter egg hunts for children) and parades. Easter begins the 50-day period culminating on Pentecost Sunday, which commemorates the birth of the Christian Church.

March 25 *Annunciation of the Birth of Christ* – This feast generally occurs during Great Lent, and commemorates the Archangel Gabriel bringing the joyous message of the birth of Jesus Christ. (Eastern: Mary states her well-known Fiat: "Behold I am the handmaid of the Lord; Let it be to me according to your word" (Luke 1:38). This statement is important in underscoring the understanding of Mary in the Orthodox Church [*see Theotókos* in the Glossary of Orthodox Christian Terms]).

April 19 *Lazarus Saturday* (Eastern) – Celebration of the resurrection of Lazarus by Jesus on the eve of Palm Sunday signifies that Jesus is "the resurrection and life" of all mankind. The eve of this 2-day celebration day brings the 40 days fast to an end.

April 20 *Palm Sunday* (Eastern) – The day that begins Holy Week commemorates Jesus' entry into Jerusalem riding on a donkey to participate in the Jewish Passover. Lazarus Saturday and Palm Sunday share John's Gospel, chapters 11–12.

April 24 *Holy Thursday* – This day, called Maundy Thursday in Western Christianity, commemorates the final meal that Jesus shared with his disciples in the upstairs room. It is usually observed with the sacrament of Holy Communion.

April 25 *Holy Friday* (Eastern) – This day, called Good Friday in Western Christianity, is the remembrance of the crucifixion of Jesus and related events. Christians observe this sacrificial act typically through somber worship services in dimly lighted settings.

April 27 *Easter/Pascha* (Eastern) – The most holy of Christian sacred days celebrates the resurrection of Jesus from the dead. Observances include sunrise worship services with special music, dressing up in special clothes, feasting (including Easter egg hunts for children) and parades. Easter begins the 50-day period culminating on Pentecost Sunday, which commemorates the birth of the Christian Church.

May 4 *Ascension* (Western) – This day marks the anniversary of Jesus' ascent into heaven 40 days after Easter.

May 11 *Pentecost* (Western) – Observation of the day when the Holy Spirit came to the disciples in the forms of tongues of fire and rushing wind. It is a traditional day for baptism and confirmation of new Christians.

June 5 *Ascension* (Eastern) – This day marks the anniversary of Jesus' ascent into heaven 40 days after Easter/Pascha.

June 15 *Pentecost* (Eastern) – Observation of the day when the God the Holy Spirit came to the disciples in the forms of tongues of fire and rushing wind. It is a traditional day for baptism and confirmation of new Christians.

June 22 *All Saints Sunday (Sunday after Pentecost)* (Eastern) – On this Sunday following Pentecost, all saints are commemorated as they shine with the light of Christ.

June 29 *All Saints of_____ (Second Sunday after Pentecost)* – On this second Sunday of Pentecost, all saints of the region surrounding the local church are commemorated. For example, all saints of North America in the United States.

June 29 *Feast of Saints Peter and Paul* (Eastern and Western) – Celebration of the pillars of the Apostolic community. Preceeded in the Eastern Church by the Apostles Fast that begins on the Monday following All Saints Sunday (see June 22) when prior to June 29, and continues through the feast. On years when Pascha is celebrated earlier, this fast is longer.

August 6 *Transfiguration* (Eastern and Western) – This day celebrates the appearance of Jesus in a transfigured state during his earthly life to three of the disciples. Appearing with him were Moses and Elijah.

August 15 *Dormition* (Eastern) – This feast day is preceded by a 2-week fast beginning on August 1. This feast is typically celebrated within the context of the church as a mystery. The disciples are gathered from the ends of the earth to witness the falling asleep of the Mother of God. Jesus is depicted as carrying a small child, representing the soul of the Most Holy Mother of God, carrying it to Heaven. There are no scriptural passages representing this feast, so the icon and service texts represent Holy Tradition.

August 15 *Assumption* (Western) – The Western Church celebrates the **Feast of Assumption**, with the difference being the theological assertion here that Mary did not die before being taken to Heaven.

September 8 *Birth of the Theotókos* – The first of the feast days in the Orthodox Liturgical Year, commemorates the birth of Mary to her parents Joachim and Anna. Mary's conception is celebrated on December 9 (1 day less than 9 months, denoting only Jesus being born exactly 9 months after Annunciation (March 25). John the Baptist's conception is celebrated 1 day more than 9 months from his birth.

September 14 *Elevation of the Holy Cross* – One of three times during the year the Cross is commemorated specifically, this feast commemorates the Cross of the Risen Lord, meaning no corpus is typically revealed on the Cross that is placed in solemn procession in the center of the church during the services on the eve of the feast. The faithful, in venerating the cross, typically make two full prostrations, touching one's knees and forehead to the floor, venerating the cross, and again making a third prostration. Flowers and/or basil typically adorn the

Cross. The other two feast days of the Cross include the third Sunday of Great Lent (*see* Great Lent in the Glossary of Orthodox Christian Terms) and on August 1, commemorating the Cross victoriously leading the Greeks and Russians in battle, processed throughout Constantinople for the people to venerate.

November 1 *All Saints' Day* (Western) – Time for honoring saints, known and unknown. In general, saints are persons with reputations for lives of unusual holiness and devotion to God or who were martyred for their faith. It is a Holy Day of Obligation in the Roman Catholic Church where saints have special formal status (Eastern: *see* June 22).

November 15 *Advent* (Eastern) – Time of preparation for observing the birth of Jesus Christ. Advent begins on November 15 and is the beginning of the Christian worship year. Advent is observed with the lighting of advent candles, display of wreaths and special ceremonies. Advent also anticipates the coming again to earth of Jesus Christ. The season continues through December 24.

November 21 *Entrance of the Theotókos into the Temple* – This feast celebrates Mary being brought into the Temple 40 days after birth, as was the practice in those days.

November 30 *Advent* (Western) – Time of preparation for observing the birth of Jesus Christ. Advent begins on the Sunday nearest November 30 and is the beginning of the Christian worship year. Advent is observed with the lighting of advent candles, display of wreaths and special ceremonies. Advent also anticipates the coming again to earth of Jesus Christ. The season continues through December 24.

December 25 *Christmas* (Western) – Celebration of the birth of Jesus Christ observed by prayers, exchanging of gifts, and family parties; season of the Christian year following Advent and preceding Epiphany.

Glossary of Orthodox Christian Terms

Apostles' Creed: An early statement of Christian belief widely used by a number of Christian denominations for both liturgical and catechetical purposes, most visibly by liturgical Churches of Western tradition, including the Latin Rite of the Roman Catholic Church, Lutheranism, the Anglican Communion, and Western Orthodoxy. It is also used by Presbyterians, Methodists, Congregationalists and many Baptists. The theological specifics of the creed appear to have been originally formulated as a refutation of Gnosticism, an early heresy. This can be seen in almost every phrase. For example, the creed states that Christ Jesus was born, suffered and died on the cross. This seems to be a statement directly against the heretical teaching that Christ only appeared to become man and that he did not truly suffer and die, but only appeared to do so. The Apostles' Creed is esteemed as an example of the apostles' teachings and a defense of the Gospel of Christ. The name of the creed comes from the probable fifth-century legend that, under the inspiration of the Holy Spirit after Pentecost, each of the Twelve Apostles dictated part of it. It is still traditionally divided into twelve articles. Because of its early origin, it does not address some Christological issues defined in the later Nicene and other Christian Creeds.

conciliarity: Term referring to the adherence of various Christian communities to the authority of ecumenical councils and to specific church government structure. This term is very significant in outlining how at every level the gathered community comes together to discern the will of God, inspired by the Holy Spirit.

Filioque: Latin term *filius* meaning "and [from] the son" added to the Nicene Creed in 589 causing different views of the Roman Catholic Church and the Eastern Orthodox Church on the relative divinity of the Father compared to the Son. In the place where the original Nicene Creed reads "We believe in the Holy Spirit ... who proceeds from the Father," the amended, Roman Catholic version reads "We believe in the Holy Spirit ... who proceeds from the Father *and the Son*." The addition is accepted by Roman Catholic Christians but rejected by Eastern Orthodox Christians.

40 days of Great Lent: The tone is set for the lenten journey by a special service celebrated during the first week called Great Compline. During this service a portion of the Canon of St. Andrew of Crete is chanted each night, offering a multitude of penitential images drawn from the scriptures. In general, special lenten tones are used for litanies, with churches lit only by candlelight. The faithful stand, kneel, and make prostrations during lenten services. Prayer, fasting, and almsgiving are the three pillars of the lenten effort (Matthew 6), and most Orthodox Christians make a special effort to come to private confession during the course of Great Lent as an important part of the lenten journey. Each Sunday has a special theme or focus during the lenten journey, in addition to the weekly scripture readings. For example, the first Sunday of Great Lent celebrates the return of icons to the Orthodox Church, and the third Sunday (middle of the lenten journey) is the week of the Cross, when the precious Cross is placed in the center of the church to inspire continued efforts during the lenten journey. No liturgies are celebrated during the weekdays of Great Lent, during which time daily readings are drawn from the OT Books of Genesis, Isaiah, and the Proverbs, representing the Pentateuch, the Prophetic writings, and the Wisdom literature streams of the Old Testament. A Presanctified Liturgy is usually celebrated each week. In this service the lamb that has been inticted and sanctified as the precious Body and Blood of Christ on the previous Sunday is distributed to the faithful to strengthen them during the days of the Great Fast. The Akathist Service is celebrated in some Orthodox Churches weekly on Fridays, and in other churches a special celebration is made of the Akathist on the fifth week of Great Lent. Many churches also keep the second through fourth Saturdays of Great Lent that are memorial Saturdays. Memorial services may be celebrated for all the departed of the parish on Friday eveings, followed by Divine Liturgy on Saturday morning. Fasting rules differ according to local tradition. Strict keeping of the fast includes eating no meat or dairy during the course of the fast, and fish is only taken on special days. Not only are certain foods not eaten during Lent, but the amount and number of meals is also reduced. This ascetical fast is also related to fasting in preparation for receiving Holy Communion. Following receiving the precious Body and Blood of the Risen Lord on Pascha, there is often great anticipation of breaking this ascetical fast with the preparation of foods not eaten during the lenten journey.

Great Lent: 40-day period of fasting, penitence and self-denial, traditionally observed by Christians, in preparation for Easter. In Western Christianity, Lent begins on Ash Wednesday; it ends on Holy Saturday, the last day of Holy Week, which immediately precedes Easter Sunday. In the Eastern Christian tradition, Great Lent is known and kept as a very important portion (10%) of the year. This season begins with four Pre-Lenten Sundays, and opens in fullness on the Monday following the fourth of these Sundays. The 40 days of Great Lent are counted during the 6 weekdays of Great Lent. Even though in the midst of Great Lent, an emergence can be perceived through the hymnography of divine services each Saturday and Sunday to celebrate the Resurrection on Sunday as is the case for each Sunday during the year. Vespers on Friday afternoons and Sunday afternoons mark the movement out of and then back into lenten melodies and service structures respectively. The 40 days thus ends on Friday evening of the sixth week. A 2-day celebration then begins of the Raising of Lazarus on Saturday, and the Entrance into Jerusalem on Sunday, connected by a common troparion and readings from John's Gospel (chapter 11 for the Raising of Lazarus and chapter 12 for the Entrance into Jerusalem). Holy Week begins on that Sunday afternoon and culminates in the celebration of Great and Holy Pascha.

Holy Unction: sacrament which provides both physical and spiritual healing with holy oil blessed by the Holy Spirit. It is most commonly celebrated during Holy Week on Holy Wednesday evening, but private services are also common. Everyone in the parish in good ecclesiastical standing may be anointed with the holy oil for the healing of spiritual and bodily ills. The oil carries God's grace both to renew the body and to cleanse the spirit. The service follows the apostolic tradition mentioned in the New Testament: "let him call for the elders of the church, and let them pray over him, anointing him with oil in the name of the Lord; and the prayer of faith will save the sick man, and the Lord will raise him up; and if he has committed sins, he will be forgiven" (James 5:14–15). Holy unction is a sacrament of great comfort to the faithful. It provides uplifting and asks for patience to accept the will of God whatever the physical outcome. When the sacrament is received privately, the full service is often not performed, but simply the anointing itself is done along with a few prayers.

Holy Week: has its own trajectory following the weekend celebration of Lazarus Saturday and the Entrance into Jerusalem. The week begins with Bridegroom Matins (usually celebrated in the afternoon/evening punctuated by the special hymn "Behold the Bridegroom comes at Midnight"). This service speaks of remaining vigilant for the hour when the Bridegroom comes to call us. In the mornings the Presanctified Liturgy is celebrated. On Holy Wednesday the focus shifts to the events of the latter portion of Holy Week. The Matins of Holy Thursday (sung Wednesday evening) may include the washing of the feet from John's Gospel and/or the celebration of Holy Unction, the sacrament of Healing. The Liturgy of Holy Thursday commemorates the Last Supper, during which time reserved communion is prepared for visitation to the sick for the coming year. Thursday evening is the Matins of Holy Friday with the reading of Twelve Gospels recalling the events from the Last Supper to the Crucifixion. On Holy Friday the Royal Hours are celebrated, following a very solemn Vesper service celebrated near 3 p.m. (commemorating the ninth hour) when Jesus gave up the spirit. A special winding sheet is placed in the center of the church where the Golgotha was visible on Holy Thursday, and the faithful come to venerate this special winding sheet while Psalms are read. Matins of Holy Saturday are celebrated later Friday evening where the lamentations are mixed with Resurrectional glimpses, commemorating that even while Jesus is in the tomb He is breaking down the gates of death. On Holy Saturday a special solemn Liturgy is celebrated commemorating the Myrrhbearing Women being the first to witness the Resurrection. This Liturgy was the early celebration of Pascha, and remains a day focused on the Baptism of catechumens who have been preparing for illumination during the lenten journey.

homooúsios: Greek word meaning "of one substance" or "of one essence used as key term of the Christological doctrine formulated at the first ecumenical council at Nicaea in 325 to affirm that God the Son and God the Father are of the same substance. This term is also used in the Nicene Creed.

hypostasis/hypostatic union: Technical term in Christian theology employed in mainstream Christology to describe the presence of both human and divine natures in Jesus Christ. This term captures the reality of both natures being present in their fullness without either confusion or fusion.

latreia: Service of worship directed to God.

Lenten Triodion: Service book of the Orthodox Church that provides the texts for the services for the pre-Lenten weeks of preparation, Great Lent and Holy Week; called *triodion* because the canons for matins celebrated during this period are composed of three odes each.

Liturgy: Term used to mean public worship in general; the Orthodox use the word "Liturgy," especially when preceded by the adjective "Divine" in a more specific sense, to denote the Eucharistic service. The word Liturgy (*Leitourgia*) literally means the work of God's people.

Matins: Term referring to prayers recited in the early part of the day. Matins can be celebrated with Great Vespers, being called then the Vigil, celebrated by some churches on Saturday evenings preparing for the Liturgy on Sunday and/or special feast days. Resurrectional Matins features a cycling of eleven post-Resurrectional pericopes, keeping alive the celebration of the resurrection each Sunday.

Nicene Creed: document written by the early Church and adopted (in a slightly different version) by the Church Council at Nicaea in 325 CE. It is an essential part of the doctrine and liturgy of the Christian Church. It was modified at a later council by the edition of the *Filioque* clause. This altered rendition is the version used by Roman Catholic and many Protestant churches. Orthodox churches, however, use the creed in its original form, without the *Filioque* clause. This Creed was originally a baptismal declaration of faith.

Pascha: Pascha is known as the Feast of Feasts, as the whole liturgical year revolves around this central feast, including pre-lenten and lenten weeks preceding, and the 40-day celebration of the Paschal Feast itself. The meaning of the word Pascha is another expression of passover, in this case from death to life through Jesus' death and Resurrection. The services of Pascha begin with Nocturne, then a procession around the church that culminates in arriving before the doors of the church as at the doors of the tomb. Paschal Matins is begun there, then the faithful and celebrants enter the empty church and there is an explosion of singing, chanting, censing, as the Matins and Liturgy with the general announcement of the Resurrection are celebrated with great joy. As indicated earlier, the breaking of ascetical fast follows the festal services. The day of Pascha continues through the following week called Bright Week, where the Paschal Liturgy can be celebrated daily. The doors of the altar remain open all week. Then on Bright Saturday, with the blessing of the Artos, the special paschal bread that is then distributed to the faithful, the doors are closed once again. Special features of the Paschal Liturgy are then discontinued, though the faithful continue to share the Paschal greeting during the 40 days: "Christ is Risen! Indeed He is Risen!" Each week of Pascha also has a special celebration. The first Sunday of Pascha commemorates Doubting Thomas. The pericope is read on Vespers of Pascha of Jesus seeing the disciples without Thomas, and then 8 days later on this "second Sunday" Thomas is featured as Jesus appears again. The third Sunday commemorates the Myrrhbearing Women. The last day of Pascha is punctuated by again celebrating the fullness of the Paschal Liturgy as on the day of Pascha, followed by the Ascension celebration, and later still the descent of the Holy Spirit on Pentecost.

Pentecost: Commemorates the Descent of the Holy Spirit on the Disciples. Following the Liturgy on this day, a special Vespers is celebrated with "Kneeling Prayers" as there is a dispensation from kneeling during the Paschal season. This service reveals a return to the watchful waiting for the Second Coming of the Lord until again the Great Lenten journey begins again. It should also be noted that the first two Sundays after Pentecost have special meaning. The first Sunday is the Sunday of All Saints (celebrated in the Western Christian Church on November 1), as all saints both reveal the image of Christ and exhibit the Grace of the Holy Spirit. The second Sunday follows this theme by commemorating all the saints of the local land of a particular church. In North America this Sunday commemorates all the Saints of North America.

Pre-Lenten Sundays: In Eastern Christianity, Great Lent is preceded by four preparatory Sundays featuring special Gospel readings: Publican and Pharisee, Prodigal Son, Last Judgment, and Expulsion from Paradise on the Sunday Great Lent begins. Following the Divine Liturgy on the last of these preparatory Sundays, Great Lent in the Orthodox Tradition begins on Monday. In many churches the beginning of Lent is commemorated by Vespers on Sunday followed by the rite of Forgiveness. After Vespers is concluded, each member of the congregation approaches one another and the parish priest asking forgiveness. The community begins the lenten journey having forgiven one another, and ends the journey by exchanging the Paschal kiss (two or three times on the cheek as is the formal greeting of one Orthodox Christian with another).

theosis: In Orthodox and Eastern Catholic theology, *theosis* (meaning *divinization*, or *deification*, or *making divine*) is the call to people to become holy and seek union with God, beginning in this life and later consummated in the resurrection. *Theosis* concerns salvation from sin. It is premised upon apostolic and early Christian understanding of the life of faith. The meaning of this word for Orthodox Christians is: "to become what God is by nature, by God's grace." To say another way, one's baptism is not a static historical event. Rather, one continues to live into the gift of new life through water and the spirit, experiencing renewal and greater depth through repentance and receiving of the sacrament of Holy Communion.

Theotókos: Compound of two Greek words: *theos*, God and *tokos*, parturition, childbirth. Literally, this translates as *God-bearer* or *the one who gives birth to God*; given as title of Mary, the mother of Jesus used especially in the Eastern Orthodox, Oriental Orthodox, and Eastern Catholic Churches. It is important to note that in the Eastern Orthodox Church, Mary is seen as the archetype of the fullness of human nature, an icon of the church. In other words, Mary's humanity is as ours, though she sins not.

Trisagion: standard hymn of the Divine Liturgy in most of the Eastern Orthodox Churches, Oriental Orthodox Churches and Eastern Catholic Churches. In those churches which use the Byzantine Rite, the *Trisagion* is chanted immediately before the Prokeimenon and the Epistle Reading. In the Orthodox Church, it is also included in a set of prayers named for it, called the *Trisagion Prayers*, which forms part of numerous services (the Hours, Vespers, Matins, and as part of the opening prayers for most services). This term is also used in some Orthodox communities to identify a brief memorial service to remember the departed.

Vespers: religious service in the late afternoon or the evening. This service charts the whole of Salvation history in brief. Vespers begins with Psalm 103, the Psalm of Creation. Then with Psalms 140 – following the fall of man is remembered by the phrase, "Lord I Call Upon Thee …" Then the Hymn Gladsome Light reveals the light of Christ entering the world. Later still the Song of Simeon denotes the elder's words indicating that he can depart in peace in having seen Salvation in beholding the Christ child. Vespers contains great teaching potential through the composed hymns that commemorate special feast days (from the Menaion), lives of saints, the progression of the 8-week cycle (called the Octoechos). Vespers also heralds the beginning of the liturgical day. For example, Sunday begins with the celebration of Vespers on Saturday evening.

Protestant Traditions: General Introduction

Prepared by:
Robert E. Johnson, PhD
Professor of Christian Heritage, Central Baptist Theological Seminary
Shawnee, KS

Protestantism connotes a theologically and ecclesiologically diverse amalgam of Church traditions which has evolved from origins in early sixteenth-century Catholicism. The term "Protestant" was originally applied to Lutherans after their leaders "protested" a decision made by Catholic powers at the Second Diet of Speyer in 1529 aimed at limiting the movement's spread. Over time, the term came to be applied to the entire family of Churches derived from the reforming efforts of Martin Luther, Huldrich Zwingli, John Calvin, and related church leaders. Many of these Churches came into being long after the Reformation itself. In general, they hold in common the conviction that the Bible is the sole source of revealed truth, the doctrine of justification by faith alone, and the priesthood of all believers.

In modern times, Protestantism has become such an inclusive term that it often means little more than a faith group that is not Catholic or Orthodox. Consequently, a precise definition is difficult to achieve. Understanding the movement today might be aided by thinking of it in terms of five categories: (1) Anglican Churches, (2) Lutheran Churches, (3) Reformed Churches, (4) Free Churches, and (5) Charismatic Churches. The ways each body applies the previously stated principles in worship and devotion varies enormously. In general, however, each includes some form of participation by the entire congregation, public reading of the Bible in the vernacular, and emphasis on preaching.

(1) The Anglican Communion of Churches

The Anglican Church consists of a global family of autonomous churches united through their communion with the Archbishop of Canterbury. Episcopal in government, England's Archbishop holds the status of president among the heads of the other self-governing Churches of the Anglican communion. The British origins of this communion draw their early sources from both Celtic Christianity and Roman Catholicism. Particularities of the historical context in which the Church developed its independence from Rome during the sixteenth-century resulted in Anglicanism's identity as both Reformed and Catholic. Reformer Thomas Cranmer (1489–1556) guided development of the Church's defining document, *The Book of Common Prayer*, in a fashion that preserved the threefold Catholic ministry of bishops, priests, and deacons together with many other practices of the medieval Catholic Church, while reinterpreting them in a Protestant sense. Today, the Anglican Church includes at least three elements – Anglo-Catholic, Liberal, and Evangelical – leading some to consider it a "bridge" between Protestantism, Roman Catholicism, and Orthodoxy. The Anglican family of churches includes approximately 80 million members worldwide.

(2) The Lutheran Communion of Churches

Lutheran Churches constitute a confessional movement derived from the teachings of Reformer Martin Luther (1483–1564) and the formulae contained in the *Book of Concord*. Central to their confession is the authority of scripture and justification by faith alone. The core tenets of Lutheran doctrine are set forth in the *Augsburg Confession*. In general, Lutherans retained traditional liturgical forms but modified them, giving equal emphasis to preaching and the sacraments. Communion is celebrated every Sunday as well as other festival occasions.

Lutheran churches make up the largest Protestant bodies in Germany and the Scandinavian countries, and also have a significant presence in many other parts of the world – especially in those areas where people of German descent have settled in large numbers. In North America, there are three major Lutheran Churches: (1) the Evangelical Lutheran Church in America (ELCA), (2) the Lutheran Church Missouri Synod, and (3) the Evangelical Lutheran Church in Canada. The Lutheran World Federation is a worldwide communion of Lutheran Churches which includes most, but not all, Lutherans (some churches have not chosen to be members). Globally, Lutherans number about 67 million members.

(3) The Reformed Communion of Churches

Reformed Churches refer to those churches whose origins derive chiefly from the theology of John Calvin, Huldrich Zwingli, and John Knox. These churches generally accepted the basic tenets of Luther's theology, but applied them more thoroughly in reforming their churches and societies. The Bible is held as the supreme authority in Christian life and practice, and preaching the Word is the focal act of liturgy. The Reformed movement includes two major forms of church government – presbyterian and congregational. The presbyterian form organizes local churches into bodies governed by a regional synod made up of ordained presbyters and lay elders. The congregational form recognizes the independence of local churches, each of which is responsible for its own life and order.

(4) The Free Churches

The Free Church movement generally refers to those churches derived from the Reformation, but which refused to conform to the doctrines, polity, or disciplines of either the Anglican, Lutheran, or Reformed churches. For the most part, these Churches emphasize the necessity of a personal experience with God, while relegating such elements as the liturgy, formalism, church organization, and creeds to a secondary position in the life of the faith community. Among the major Church bodies reflective of this movement are Baptist Churches, Methodist Churches, the Salvation Army, and the Pentecostal Churches. Collectively these Churches number about 150 million members worldwide.

(5) The Charismatic Churches

The Charismatic movement has influenced many, if not most, Christian communions. However, several Church bodies that cannot historically fit into the previous categories, yet which possess some theological lineage to Churches of the Reformation tradition, might be classified under this rubric. Among them are some of the African Independent Churches and many of the House Churches. The African Independent Churches constitute a rapidly growing body of Churches for whom the black African experience is pivotal to their self-understanding. These churches differ greatly, but are generally characterized by combinations of charismatic practices (gifts of the Spirit, ecstatic experiences, miraculous healings, and speaking in tongues), indigenous religious practices and beliefs, and liberation theology. House Churches vary widely in beliefs and practices, and are of two major origins: the Chinese House Churches and those derived from conservative evangelical sources. In both cases, these Churches are distinguished by rejection of the institutional church and an ordained ministry, informal worship, efforts to recapture what they consider to be a New Testament pattern, and often emphasize charismatic practices.

Several Other Faith Groups

Several other faith groups are popularly thought of as being Protestant, but should not be included in this general category because they do not share the essential doctrinal core common to that designation: conviction that the Bible is the sole source of revealed truth, the doctrine of justification by faith alone, and the priesthood of all believers. Among these bodies would be The Church of Jesus Christ of Latter-Day Saints (Mormons) and Jehovah's Witnesses. While often sharing some historical connection, certain dimensions of belief, and other elements, these well-known faith groups differ from Protestant theology and practice in important ways.

The Ecumenical Movement

Many Protestant and other Christian bodies are committed to promoting better understanding and cooperation between Christians. While not organically united, churches supportive of the Ecumenical Movement, often through efforts associated with the World Council of Churches, seek to achieve greater harmony among this plethora of divided communions.

African American Baptist/Protestantism

*Continuing the quest and meeting the challenge of linking
a hurting community with healing God*

Prepared by:
The Reverend L. Henderson Bell
Former President at Large, Progressive National Baptist Convention, Mid-West Region
Pastor, Mt. Pleasant Missionary Baptist Church
Kansas City, MO

History and Facts

The African American Protestant community emerged as the result of European missionary efforts to proselytize the inhabitants of an indentured, enslaved population with the intent to assimilate them into an organized assembly being tutored by and tied to the Southern Baptist church population. This relationship between the Christian slave and the Christian slave master eroded over time to the degree that African American Protestants sought a means to develop their own identity as a Christian community by embracing the tenets of Christianity and exercising freedom of its belief in the salvation message brought by the missionaries. This new identity of African American Protestants became a reality, at least in part, by the establishment of National Baptists church organizations along the Eastern and Southern seaboards; in the year of 1962 the religious movements among African Americans witnessed an amoebic generation with the development of the Progressive National Baptist Convention. The Progressive National Baptist Convention (PNBC) was founded by the Reverend L. Venchel Booth and organized in the city of Cincinnati, Ohio. PNBC headquarters is presently located in Washington, DC.

The ministry and vision of National Baptist/Protestant church community was to unite persons of African descent and heritage in a religious and Christian configuration that reflect the tenets of the New Testament Christian scriptures.

Fortunately, the National Baptist/Protestant church communities did embrace the teachings of the gospel of the New Testament and blended the teachings of the gospel into their historical fabric for freedom of body and mind. It is against this canvas of the gospel that the National Baptist/Protestant church community has developed its theology and the religious principles by which it lives and exercises its religious being.

The Progressive (National) Baptist Convention is a branch and continuation in kind of all the National Baptist Conventions of America USA, Inc. The National Baptist Convention is the identifying label that characterizes the African American Baptist/

Protestant denomination. The African American Baptist/Protestant denomination embraces the protestant ideology and holds to the theological tenets and doctrine of Baptist universal; it too, is Christian in its principle and practice. It holds and promotes the belief that all Christians are able to communicate with God without the mediation of clergy.

Basic Teachings

National Baptists/Protestants affirm the content of the ancient *Apostle's Creed*, which is a brief statement of faith attributed to the early church.

The Apostle's Creed

I believe in God, the Father almighty, creator of heaven and earth,
I believe in Jesus Christ, His only Son, our Lord.
Who was conceived by the power of the Holy Spirit;
Born of the Virgin Mary;
Suffered under Pontius Pilate;
Was crucified, died, and buried.
He descended into hell (or the realm of the dead).
On the third day he rose again.
He ascended into heaven and is seated at the right hand of the Father.
He will come again to judge the living and the dead.
I believe in the Holy Spirit,
The holy catholic (universal) church,
The communion of saints,
The forgiveness of sins,
The resurrection of the body and the life everlasting. Amen.

- All humans are fallen from an original state of innocence and are bent toward actions (i.e., sins) that disconnect them from God and others.
- All humans are experiencing consequences and punishment for continued misdeeds.
- Salvation and heavenly hope are the result of one's faith rather than through one's actions, although Christian practices issue forth from an experience of grace.
- The final destination for those who have been saved from the consequences of their misdeeds is an eternal state of existence often referred to as heaven; this concept suggests communion with God and all the redeemed in a state of peace, justice, and perfect love.
- The final destination of those who are not saved is hell, a state of present confusion, fear, and experiential punishment that is associated with disconnected-ness from God and the saved. Opinions differ as to whether or not hell is eternal, but the teachings of the National Baptists/Protestants suggest that all mankind will live in an eternal state of happiness or punishment according to scripture.
- Scripture is more central to the faith than the traditions of the church. National Baptist/Protestant Christians affirm the Bible, or Holy Scriptures, which is a compilation of 66 different books written over a 1000-year period.
- The National Baptist/Protestant community believes that the New Testament scriptures are the interpretative results of the teachings of Jesus Christ. The scriptures have universal application and are beneficial for the orderly function of the Christian community and the source of strength and inspiration for the inner person.

Basic Practices

- National Baptist/Protestant Christians value communal worship, and will gather on Sundays and at other times to hear preaching, study scripture, sing hymns, give personal testimonies, and pray.
- The sharing of one's faith (evangelism) is of great importance to the National Baptist/Protestant community. Some of the ways it is communicated is through loving actions, talking about personal spiritual experiences, reading scriptures, distributing informational tracts and discussions of doctrinal positions.
- The Lord's Supper (also called Holy Communion or Eucharist, which means "thanksgiving") is a powerful ordinance (sacrament or ritual). It is a liturgical reenactment of the crucifixion, death, burial, and resurrection of Jesus, in which Christians eat bread (to commemorate the broken body of Jesus) and drink grape juice (to symbolize Jesus' shed blood). This can be done during communal worship or in other settings and is usually administered by ordained clergy or other ordained persons.
- Prayer and scripture study are the fundamental spiritual practices for National Baptists/Protestants. The many forms of these practices include reading and/or silent contemplation upon scripture or doctrinal beliefs and prayers of various kinds – petition, healing, repentance for unethical thoughts and actions, praise, worship, and thanksgiving to God.
- Mission work is important to National Baptists/Protestants. These acts of service take the forms of – working for social justice with marginalized peoples, charitable giving to provide food, building, and educational programs for the poor, volunteerism, and so forth. Mission work

is also an intentional witness to one's faith through proclamation and teaching.
- Believer's baptism is the practice of the National Baptists/Protestants. However, the National Baptist/Protestant tradition also practices infant dedication, which includes the church community as an integral part of the faith-journey of the child. The infant is presented to the church congregation when he or she is 3 months of age for the purpose of dedication to God. This ceremony is usually presided over by the pastor of the church or other ordained ministers as appointed by the pastor. This tradition places a great responsibility upon the church community to raise the child to make responsible ethical and spiritual decisions and to influence the child to choose to follow God.

Principles for Clinical Care
Dietary Issues

- The National Baptist/Protestant congregations align with most Christians and do not have any dietary restrictions with respect to their religious beliefs. However each individual congregation is encouraged to inform their parishioners to practice healthy dietary habits, which includes abstaining from the consumption of alcoholic beverages.

General Medical Beliefs

- National Baptist/Protestant Christians believe that God is the ultimate source of all life, health and healing. Therefore if people are to have health and longevity of life, they must be properly aligned with the will of God for daily living.
- The doctrine of the "New Birth" is central in the teaching of the Bible and the

National Baptist/Protestant church community; it is this belief that energizes the parishioners of the National Baptist/Protestant church community to believe that the "Word of God" has healing qualities for both the body and the mind of the believer.

- The Bible is the foundation of the National Baptist/Protestant churches giving them the encouragement to trust God for all its many challenging trials for a healthy life. It further holds that the will of God is discovered through the study and implementation of the scriptures, which teach that God is the source of life for the human family and for anyone to be separated from Him is to be exposed to the dangers that bring death through disease of body and mind.

- National Baptist/Protestant Christians refer to God as the Great Physician. Therefore, prayers are made to God for the overall protection, restoration, and eradication of various sicknesses and disease that may manifest themselves in the lives of believers; prayer is also made for the physicians, who are viewed as the medical ministers to the physical bodies that are under the dominance of sickness and often paralyzed by disease, that they might receive revelations as to how to treat, comfort, and dispel sickness in the individual persons.

- It is important that medical professionals attribute the healing procedure to "God" and not to medications. Many National Baptist/Protestant Christians have the assurance that if they are healed it is God's will.

- National Baptist/Protestant Christians affirm the validity of traditional Western medical procedures in the treatment of illness and disease.

Specific Medical Issues

Some National Baptists/Protestants have serious reservations about certain medical procedures and practices such as abortion, in vitro fertilization, and blood transfusions. The reason for this is the limited knowledge circulated through the majority of National Baptist/Protestant churches concerning the particulars surrounding certain medical procedures. However, when information is provided in lay-friendly terminology about these and other controversial matters, the invaluable insight and understanding enables them to make informed decisions. The following bullets convey the informed viewpoint of the majority of National Baptist/Protestant communities on some of the issues mentioned.

- **Abortion**: The National Baptist/Protestant community does not endorse abortion as a general rule; if the circumstances of the pregnancy warrant medical procedures that might ensure the continued health and longevity of the mother, the families are given the latitude to follow medically devised procedures as determined by a physician.

- **Advance Directives**: The National Baptist/Protestant community is encouraging its members to begin to plan for the continued care in the event of illness through the use of advance directives; caregivers for dependent children and aged parents are encouraged to document information concerning the continued care of those for whom they are responsible.

- **Birth Control**: The National Baptist/Protestant community allows the practice of birth control, as this practice may deter unwanted pregnancies that might impose hardship on families that are unable to care for or maintain children in the existing family structure. Baptists believe that birth control may be used to regulate the number and spacing of children. It is a moral decision for each couple. However, Baptists specify that the form of contraception prevents conception.

- **Blood Transfusions**: The National Baptist/Protestant community has no restrictions as it relates to blood transfusions. It is left to the individual patient to receive or refuse the procedure.
- **Circumcision**: National Baptists/Protestants view circumcision for male infants as a cultural decision and not for religious reasons.
- **In Vitro Fertilization**: The National Baptist/Protestant community does not in a general sense support the procedure of in vitro fertilization; it is believed that life is under the direct superintendence of Almighty God, who has designed and designated the medium through which life is processed and any other means is a breach of Divine authority.
- **Stem Cell Research**: The National Baptist/Protestant community supports the research involving stem cells because of the promise to minimize the effects of terminal illness and disease. The National Baptist/Protestant community does not subscribe to nor endorse the practice of human cloning. This practice is a breach of Divine order and authority for life.
- **Vaccinations**: The National Baptist/Protestant community has issued no official statement on vaccinations but encourages their utilization as contributing to community health; it is an individual decision.
- **Withholding/Withdrawing Life Support**: National Baptists/Protestants are of the opinion that withholding/withdrawing life support in medically futile cases does not violate teachings of Christian faith. It is an individual decision.

Gender and Personal Issues
- National Baptists/Protestants as a faith community have no prescriptions or proscriptions with respect to gender and personal issues.

Principles for Spiritual Care through the Cycles of Life
Concepts of Living and Dying for Spiritual Support
- National Baptists/Protestants believe that life is sacred. They also believe that the physical existence is an altered state of the original creation of life and that life is secured through the spiritual relationship with God Almighty.
- National Baptists/Protestants believe that death is something all must experience and should not be feared. It is the means by which God gathers the souls of people to Himself in an eternal state of blissful existence.
- Death is perceived by National Baptists/Protestants Christians as sleep, a time of peaceful comfort until the Second Coming of Jesus.
- National Baptists/Protestants believe that the spirit of the deceased ascends to heaven at the moment of death, and will remain in that state until the Second Coming of Christ.
- Resurrection of the physical body and the reunion of spirit, soul, and body in some form will happen at the Second Coming of Jesus Christ. Humanity, all living creatures, and the entire cosmos will be healed and restored to a state of original perfection.

During Birth

- The National Baptist/Protestant community does not practice the christening of a baby or a child, living or deceased. In the event of birth complications where death results, National Baptist ministers will perform the normal duties as administered during times of death.
- As stated earlier, National Baptists/Protestants view circumcision for male infants as a cultural decision and not for religious reasons.

During Illness

- Patients may receive comfort from the reading of scriptures or other devotional material, listening to religious music, watching televised worship services of their own or a similar tradition. Patients may request Holy Communion. The chaplain or clergy should be consulted for assistance.
- National Baptist Christian/Protestant patients may receive comfort from healing prayers. These can be offered by health care professionals.
- Patients may request baptism. In the clinical setting, sprinkling is an acceptable mode of baptism, even for National Baptists/Protestants who practice immersion. The chaplain or clergy should be consulted for assistance.
- Health care professionals can ask patients if they would like to have a visit from the chaplain or contact the minister of their church for a visit during difficult, complex or dangerous procedures. This display of concern may change the attitude and enhance the emotional participation of patients in their recovery.

During End of Life

- Patient or the family may request baptism. The chaplain or clergy should be consulted for assistance.
- Patient or the family may request Holy Communion. The chaplain or clergy should be consulted for assistance.
- In situations where medical futility becomes the subject for discussion, the minister can help family members understand that withholding/withdrawing life support in such cases does not violate teachings of their Christian faith. Even so, some in the National Baptist/Protestant community would be resistant to that notion, choosing to believe that the death of loved ones is accomplished according to the will of God, not members of the medical profession; the belief in the will of God being performed in the life of an individual is active as long as the individual is designated as alive by medical professionals. In these situations, the presence of the minister is crucial in helping the family accept the reality of their loved one's medical condition.
- The dying process and death of loved ones is a difficult time for the National Baptist/Protestant community; during such times, there will most probably be emotional outbursts.
- Some National Baptists/Protestants family members may assign cause and blame for their loved one's death and this may be directed toward the medical professional; the earlier the minister of the family arrives, the better the chances are that this attitude resulting in accusations will be dispelled.
- Family may request prayers for the deceased. These can be offered by chaplains, clergy, family, friends, and health care professionals.

Care of the Body

- Family may wish to view the body of the deceased in the hospital room or the chapel. Nurse and chaplain should be consulted for assistance.
- Disposition and embalming are individual decisions. Cremation is now the choice of many Christians. The National Baptist/Protestant community has no restrictions as to the process of burial or disposition of the body of deceased persons; the family of the deceased person has the responsibility to administer the wishes of the deceased relative. The pastor and the funeral home director should be consulted for assistance.
- Autopsy is an individual decision unless required by law. The chaplain and/or nurse should be consulted for assistance.
- Donation for medical research is an individual decision. The National Baptist/Protestant community endorses the right of individuals to donate their remains for the purpose of medical research; this donation is an individual decision; most often the pastor of the individual has been consulted and has given spiritual counsel to the individual who wishes to donate their bodies. Advance planning for such donations is required by most receiving organizations. Last-minute donations are usually not possible.

Organ and Tissue Donation

- Organ and tissue donation is permitted and is an individual decision. The National Baptist/Protestant community endorses the right of individuals to donate organ and tissue for the purpose of assisting in the prolongation of the health of others. National Baptist/Protestant pastors and ministers are attempting to alert their individual congregations about the process and viability of organ donation. Pastors are encouraged to get assistance from hospital chaplains and/or nurses who are trained designated requesters for assistance.

Scriptures, Inspirational Readings, and Prayers

READINGS DURING ILLNESS

These can be read by family, friends, clergy, and health care professionals. (All scripture quotations are from the New Revised Standard Version.)

The Lord is my shepherd I shall not want.
He makes me lie down in green pastures; he restores my soul.
He leads me in right paths for his name's sake.
Even though I walk through the darkest valley, I fear no evil;
for you are with me; your rod and your staff – they comfort me.
You prepare a table before me in the presence of my enemies;
you anoint my head with oil; my cup overflows.
Surely goodness and mercy shall follow me all the days of my life,
and I shall dwell in the house of the Lord my whole life long.

—Psalm 23

Lord, You have been our dwelling place in all generations.
Before the mountains were brought forth, Or ever You had formed the earth and the world, Even from everlasting to everlasting, You are God.

You turn man to destruction, And say,
"Return, O children of men."
For a thousand years in Your sight
Are like yesterday when it is past,
And like a watch in the night.
You carry them away like a flood;
They are like a sleep. In the
morning they are like grass which
grows up:
In the morning it flourishes and
grows up; In the evening it is cut
down and withers.
For we have been consumed by Your
anger, And by Your wrath we are
terrified.
You have set our iniquities before
You, Our secret sins in the light of
Your countenance.
For all our days have passed away in
Your wrath; We finish our years like
a sigh.
The days of our lives are seventy
years; And if by reason of strength
they are eighty years,
Yet their boast is only labor and
sorrow; For it is soon cut off, and
we fly away.

— Ps. 90:1–10

Man who is born of woman Is of few
days and full of trouble.
He comes forth like a flower and
fades away; He flees like a shadow
and does not continue.
And do You open Your eyes on such a
one, And bring me to judgment with
Yourself?
Who can bring a clean thing out of an
unclean? No one!
Since his days are determined, The
number of his months is with You;

You have appointed his limits, so
that he cannot pass.
Look away from him that he may rest,
Till like a hired man he finishes his
day.
"For there is hope for a tree, If it is
cut down, that it will sprout again,
And that its tender shoots will not
cease.
Though its root may grow old in the
earth, And its stump may die in the
ground,
Yet at the scent of water it will bud
and bring forth branches like a
plant.
But man dies and is laid away; Indeed
he breathes his last And where is
he?
As water disappears from the sea,
And a river becomes parched and
dries up,
So man lies down and does not rise.
Till the heavens are no more, They
will not awake nor be roused from
their sleep.
Oh, that You would hide me in the
grave, That You would conceal me
until Your wrath is past, that You
would appoint me a set time, and
remember me!
If a man dies, shall he live again? All
the days of my hard service I will
wait, till my change comes.
You shall call, and I will answer You;
You shall desire the work of Your
hands.

— Job 14:1–15

We know that all things work
together for good …
For I am convinced that neither

death, nor life, nor angels, nor rulers, nor things present, nor things to come, nor powers, nor height, nor depth, nor anything else in all creation, will be able to separate us from the love of God in Christ Jesus our Lord.

—Rom. 8:28a, 38–39

READINGS DURING END-OF-LIFE PROCESS

These can be read by family, friends, clergy, and health care professionals. (All scripture quotations are from the New Revised Standard Version, unless specified differently.)

I am the resurrection and the life. Those who believe in me, even though they die, will live, and everyone who lives and believes in me will never die.

—John 11:25–26

Let not your heart be troubled; you believe in God, believe also in Me. In My Father's house are many mansions; if it were not so, I would have told you. I go to prepare a place for you. And if I go and prepare a place for you, I will come again and receive you to Myself; that where I am, there you may be also.

—John 14:1–3 (NKJV)[248]

For we know that if our earthly house, this tent, is destroyed, we have a building from God, a house not made with hands, eternal in the heavens. For in this we groan, earnestly desiring to be clothed with our habitation which is from heaven, if indeed, having been clothed, we shall not be found naked. For we who are in this tent groan, being burdened, not because we want to be unclothed, but further clothed, that mortality may be swallowed up by life. Now He who has prepared us for this very thing is God, who also has given us the Spirit as a guarantee. So we are always confident, knowing that while we are at home in the body we are absent from the Lord. For we walk by faith, not by sight. We are confident, yes, well pleased rather to be absent from the body and to be present with the Lord.

—2 Cor. 5:1–7 (NKJV)

PRAYERS DURING END-OF-LIFE PROCESS

These prayers can be offered by family, friends, clergy, and health care professionals.

Holy and Merciful Father,
We thank you for the gift of your Son, Jesus, whom you sent to die that we might live. We thank you also that you raised Him from the dead, and that He is seated with you in heaven. We acknowledge that you are the Lord of Life and the Lord of Death. We ask that you send your holy angels to escort our brother/ sister _____ through death into your presence. Give our brother/sister _____ peace and comfort the

---

248 NKJV refers to New King James Version.

family who will be saddened by the loss.

In Jesus' precious name, we pray. Amen.

Eternal God our Father and creator of all things, we come in the knowledge that you have made all things and persons for your Divine pleasure; we thank you for all of your considerations and blessings to us and even now during this time of sorrow and mixed emotions, we thank you for the earthly tenure of our deceased brother/sister; we ask that you be merciful unto us as you bring them into your eternal presence, we ask that you will allow us to continue in faith and to lift and applaud your call of our loved one unto yourself; now bless us with all spiritual graces that we may be empowered to receive and accept your divine will for this hour. In the authority of the name of Jesus Christ we ask these things. Amen.

African Methodist Episcopal Church (AME)

God our Father, Christ our Redeemer, and Man our Brother [249]

Prepared by:
The Reverend Natalie Mitchem, MDiv, RD
Itinerant Elder, First Episcopal District Health
  Commission Coordinator
Philadelphia, PA

Reviewed and approved by:
The Right Reverend Richard F. Norris
Presiding Prelate of the First Episcopal District
Philadelphia, PA

History and Facts

Prior to a discussion of the history of the African Methodist Episcopal Church (AME Church), it will be helpful to the reader to understand the rationale behind the church's name. African is in the title because the majority of its membership is of African descent. However, this does not mean the church is only for people of Africa. Methodist is in the title because Methodism presents an orderly "method" of worship, rules, and regulations, with a focus on a simple and plain gospel. Episcopal is in the title because it indicates the form of government under which the church operates; the church is lead by a Council of Bishops.

The following historical overview of the African Methodist Episcopal Church is taken from the "historical statement" as recorded in the church's *Book of Doctrine and Discipline*.[250]

In November, 1781, the colored people belonging to the Methodist Society of Philadelphia convened together in order to take into consideration the evils under which they labored, arising from the unkind treatment by their white brethren, who considered them a nuisance in the house of worship, and even pulled them off their knees while in the act of prayer and ordered them to the back seats. Because of this unchristian conduct, they considered it their duty to devise a plan to build a house of their own in which they could worship God under their own vine and fig tree.

Being now as outcasts, they had to seek for friends where they could. The Lord put it into the hearts of Dr. Benjamin Rush, Mr. R. Raltson, and other respectable citizens to interpose for them, both by advice and assistance, in getting their building finished. Bishop White also aided them, and ordained one from among themselves, after the order of the Protestant Episcopal Church, to be their Pastor. In 1793, the number of serious people of color had increased and there were different opinions with respect to the mode of religious worship. Inasmuch as many felt a strong partiality for the order adopted by the Methodists, Richard Allen, with the advice of some of his brethren, proposed erecting a place of worship on his

---

249 Quote provided by Rev. Natalie Mitchem, author of this chapter, as the motto of the AME Church.

250 *The Doctrine and Discipline of the African Methodist Episcopal Church 2004–2008.* (2005). Nashville, TN: AMEC Publishing House, 5–9.

own ground and at his own expense as an African Methodist meetinghouse.

Francis Asbury, then bishop of the Methodist Episcopal Church, was invited to open the house for divine service. The invitation was accepted and the house was named Bethel (see Gen. 28:19).

The colored people at Baltimore and other places were treated in a similar manner as those in Philadelphia, and they were compelled to seek places of worship for themselves, rather than go to the law. This induced the people to call General Conference in April, 1816, to form a Connection. Delegates appointed to represent different churches met those of Philadelphia and taking into consideration their grievances, and in order to secure their privilege and promote union among themselves, it was resolved: "That the people of Philadelphia, Baltimore and all other places who should unite with them, should become one body under the name and style of the African Methodist Church."

We believe that it was the design of a gracious Providence in thus uniting to mark out a way by which the despised African race might have an opportunity to receive from their own brethren that religious instruction from which they had been kept by persons claiming to be their superiors, and thereby privileged to sit under their own vine and fig tree. The work of God has spread, through our instrumentality, for Philadelphia throughout the entire United States and into Canada, the West Indies, South America, and Africa. Richard Allen became the first consecrated Bishop of the African Methodist Episcopal church in Philadelphia, Pennsylvania, in 1816 and he served for 15 years.

The AME Church is the first major religious denomination in the Western world that had its origin over sociological rather than theological beliefs and differences. Today, the denomination consists of 20 Episcopal Districts with over 4500 churches around the world. The current church structure includes the AMEC Connectional Health Commission. The commission serves, among other tasks, to help the denomination understand health as an integral part of the faith of the Christian Church, to seek to make our denomination a healing faith community, and to promote the health concerns of its members. In order to accomplish these directives, each region and sub-region (Episcopal District and Annual Conference, respectively) is responsible for appointing a District/Conference Director of Health. Within each Annual Conference, there is to be a coordinating committee of 3–5 persons who help to inform and train each local congregation's committee.[251]

Basic Teachings

The Mission of the AME Church is to minister to the spiritual, intellectual, physical, emotional, and environmental needs of all people by spreading Christ's liberating gospel through word and deed. At the every level of the Connection and in every local church, the African Methodist Episcopal Church shall engage in carrying out the spirit of the original Free African Society, out of which the AME Church evolved, to seek out and save the lost, and serve the needy through a continuing program of:

• preaching the gospel
• feeding the hungry
• clothing the naked

---

251 African Methodist Episcopal Church Connectional Health Commission website www.AMECHealth.org (accessed 15 Sept 2012).

- housing the homeless
- cheering the fallen
- providing jobs for the jobless
- administering to the needs of those in prisons, hospitals, nursing homes, asylums and mental institutions, senior citizens' homes; caring for the sick, the shut-in, the mentally and socially disturbed
- encouraging thrift and economic advancement.[252]

The African Methodist Episcopal Church has 25 Articles of Religion, found on pages 15–20 of its book of *Doctrine and Discipline*. These 25 articles are statements of the church's basic teachings. Four of them are mentioned here.

- **Article One**: Of Faith in the Holy Trinity – There is but one living and true God, everlasting, without body or parts, of infinite power, wisdom, and goodness; the Maker and Preserver of all things, both visible and invisible. In unity of this Godhead, there are three persons, of one substance, power, and eternity – the Father, the Son, and the Holy Ghost.
- **Article Two**: Of the Word, or Son of God, Who Was Made Very Man – The Son, who is the Word of the Father, the very and eternal God, of one substance with the Father, took man's nature in the womb of the blessed Virgin; so that two whole and perfect natures, that is to say, the Godhead and manhood, were joined together in one person, never to be divided; whereof is one Christ, very God and very Man, who truly suffered, was crucified, dead, and buried, to reconcile his Father to us and to be a sacrifice, not

only for original guilt, but also for the actual sins of men.
- **Article Three**: Of the Resurrection of Christ – Christ did truly rise again from the dead, and took again his body with all things appertaining to the perfection of man's nature, wherewith he ascended into heaven, and there sitteth until he returns to judge all men at the last day.
- **Article Four**: Of the Holy Ghost – The Holy Ghost, proceeding from the Father and the Son, is of one substance, majesty, and glory with the Father and the Son, very and eternal God.

Additional doctrinal beliefs include:[253]
- The Affirmation of Faith or the *Apostles' Creed*: I believe in God, the Father Almighty, Maker of heaven and earth, and in Jesus Christ his only son our Lord, who was conceived by the Holy Spirit, born of the Virgin Mary, suffered under Pontius Pilate, was crucified, dead, and buried. The third day he arose from the dead; he ascended into heaven and sits at the right hand of God the Father Almighty; from thence he shall come to judge the quick and the dead. I believe in the Holy Spirit, the Church universal, the communion of saints, the forgiveness of sins, the resurrection of the body and the life everlasting. Amen. (480)
- The Sacrament of the Lord's Supper or Holy Communion – the elements for our communion consist of unleavened bread and the unfermented juice of the vine. The table used for the service should be covered with a clean, white, linen cloth. (487)

---

252 *The Doctrine and Discipline of the African Methodist Episcopal Church 2004–2008*, 15.

253 *The Doctrine and Discipline of the African Methodist Episcopal Church 2004–2008*. The page numbers for the statements following "additional doctrinal beliefs include" are cited in the text at the end of each of the bulleted statements.

- The Sacrament of Baptism – every adult person and parents of every child to be baptized have their choice of either the three modes of baptism, immersion, sprinkling or pouring. But in no case shall our ministers re-baptize any person. (493)
- The Holy Scriptures contain every thing necessary for salvation and to understand salvation as stated in Article Five. (16)
- There are two Sacraments set forth by and ordained by Christ our Lord: Baptism and the Holy Communion as stated in Article Sixteen. (18)
- The lay persons and ordained persons take part in Holy Communion, drinking the juice and eating the bread as stated in Article Nineteen. (19)
- Ministers are permitted to marry as stated in Article Twenty-One. (19)

Basic Practices

- The Decalogue (also known as the Ten Commandments) is recited every Sunday either in full or in abridged version reverently and as a part of the worship service.
- The purpose and practices of The Health Commission as recorded in *Doctrine and Discipline* are:[254]
  - To help the denomination understand health as an integral part of the faith of the Christian Church.
  - To promote the health issues of its members.
  - To advocate access to health care as a right and not a privilege.
  - To challenge and work to reform the unjust structure of the health delivery systems.
  - To seek to make our denomination a healing faith community.
  - To collaborate with community organizations to improve the health care system.
  - To encourage each connectional organization to include a health component in its life and work.
- Christians value communal worship, and will gather on Sundays and at other times to hear preaching, study scripture, sing hymns, and pray.
- The sharing of one's faith (evangelism) is of great importance in many denominations. Some of the ways it is communicated is through loving actions, talking about personal spiritual experiences, reading scriptures, distributing informational tracts, and discussions of doctrinal positions.
- The Lord's Supper, also called Holy Communion, is a powerful sacrament. Christians eat bread (to commemorate the broken body of Jesus) and drink wine or grape juice (to symbolize Jesus' shed blood). This can be done during communal worship or in other settings and is administered by ordained clergy.
- Prayer, meditation, and scripture are the fundamental spiritual practices for many Christians. The many forms of these practices include reading and/or silent contemplation upon scripture or doctrinal beliefs and prayers of various kinds – petition, healing, repentance for unethical thoughts and actions, praise, worship, and thanksgiving to God.
- Mission work is important to Christians. These acts of service take the forms of working for social justice with marginalized peoples, charitable giving to provide food, building, and educational programs for the poor, volunteerism, and so forth.

---

254 *The Doctrine and Discipline of the African Methodist Episcopal Church 2004–2008*, 459.

Mission work is also an intentional witness to one's faith through proclamation and teaching.

Principles of Clinical Care
Dietary Issues
- The African Methodist Episcopal Church has no dietary restrictions with respect to religious beliefs.

General Medical Beliefs
- The Health Commission publishes occasional newsletters, educational information, hosts workshops, lectures, seminars, health screenings, health fairs, and other preventive practices that address critical health issues, including HIV/AIDS.[255]
- The Connectional Health Commission has developed forms, screening guidelines, First Aid care guidelines and protocol in line with HIPPA guidelines for all local churches. This information is available on the Connectional Health Commission website (www.AMECHealth.org).
- The church teaches that God is the ultimate source of all life, health, and healing.
- The church refers to God as the Great Physician.
- The church affirms the validity of traditional Western medical procedures in the treatment of illness and disease.

Specific Medical Issues
- **Abortion**: The Church has no official statement on abortion; it is an individual decision.
- **Advance Directives**: The Church supports the use of advance directives in health care preplanning.
- **Birth Control**: The African Methodist Episcopal Church does not have a birth control statement in the book of Discipline nor any other official documents for the church.
- **Blood Transfusions**: The church is not opposed to blood transfusions.
- **Circumcision**: AME Christians in Western societies have requested circumcision of male infants for cultural and health reasons and not religious reasons.
- **In Vitro Fertilization**: The Church has no official statement on in vitro fertilization; it is an individual decision.
- **Stem Cell Rersearch**: The Church has no official statement on stem cell research; it is an individual decision.
- **Vaccinations**: The Church does not have an official statement or doctrine addressing vaccinations. Parents should seek the advice of their child's physician regarding vaccinations.
- **Withholding/Withdrawing Life Support**: Withholding/withdrawing life support in medically futile cases does not violate the teachings of the church. It is an individual decision.

Gender and Personal Issues
- The church has no prescriptions or proscriptions with respect to gender and personal issues.

Principles for Spiritual Care through the Cycles of Life
Concepts of Living and Dying for Spiritual Support
- Life is sacred.
- Death is something all must experience and should not be feared.

---

255 *The Doctrine and Discipline of the African Methodist Episcopal Church 2004–2008*, 461.

- Death is perceived as sleep, a time of peaceful comfort until the Second Coming of Jesus. Others perceive that Christians are "with Christ," though not in the final resurrection state.
- The soul and spirit of the deceased ascend to heaven at the moment of death.
- Resurrection of the physical body and the reunion of spirit, soul, and body will happen at the Second Coming of Jesus. Humanity, all living creatures, and the entire cosmos will be healed and restored to a state of perfection.

During Birth

- Baptism may be requested by family for a baby, living or deceased. The chaplain or clergy should be consulted for assistance.
- As stated earlier, AME Christians in Western societies have requested circumcision of male infants for cultural and health reasons and not religious reasons.

During Illness

- African Methodist Episcopal clergy, laypersons, and the Missionary Society are encouraged to visit the sick and address their physical and spiritual needs.
- The local Health Commission is available to act as a resource and advocate for the sick.
- Patients may receive comfort from the reading of scriptures or other devotional material, listening to religious music, watching televised worship services of their own or a similar tradition. Patients may request Holy Communion. The chaplain or clergy should be consulted for assistance.
- Patients may receive comfort from healing prayers. These can be offered by health care professionals. Some patients may ask for healing prayer to be connected with "anointing with oil" or the "the laying on of hands." The chaplain or clergy should be consulted for assistance for these requests.
- Patients may request baptism. The chaplain or clergy should be consulted for assistance.

During End of Life

- Ordained African Methodist Episcopal clergy are to minister to the dying person and the family.
- The Health Commission is available to act as a resource for the dying person and the family and clergy.
- Patient or the family may request baptism. The chaplain or clergy should be consulted for assistance.
- Patient or the family may request Holy Communion. The chaplain or clergy should be consulted for assistance.
- Family may wish to view the body of the deceased in the hospital room or the chapel. A nurse and chaplain should be consulted for assistance.

Care of the Body

- Disposition and embalming are individual decisions. The chaplain and the funeral home director should be consulted for assistance.
- Autopsy is an individual decision unless required by law. The chaplain and/or nurse should be consulted for assistance.
- Donation for medical research is an individual decision. The chaplain and/or nurse should be consulted for assistance. Advance planning for such donations is required by most receiving organizations. Last-minute donations are usually not possible.
- The body is cared for by the funeral home.
- The casket should be closed before

the service begins and remain closed throughout the service after the family has viewed the body. Concerning the processional, "the clergy shall lead, followed by the body and family."[256]

Organ and Tissue Donation

• Organ and tissue donation is permitted and is an individual decision. It may be preferable for a chaplain and/or nurse who are trained designated requesters to be consulted for assistance.

Scriptures, Inspirational Readings, and Prayers

• The Book of Worship contains hymns, scriptures, and prayers. Scriptures, inspirational readings, and prayers may also be selected by the family with consultation from the Ordained Elder in charge.

READING DURING ILLNESS

This can be read by family, friends, clergy, and health care professionals.

The Lord is my shepherd I shall not want.
He makes me lie down in green pastures; he restores my soul.
He leads me in right paths for his name's sake.
Even though I walk through the darkest valley, I fear no evil;
for you are with me; your rod and your staff – they comfort me.
You prepare a table before me in the presence of my enemies;

you anoint my head with oil; my cup overflows.
Surely goodness and mercy shall follow me all the days of my life,
and I shall dwell in the house of the Lord my whole life long.

— Psalm 23 (New Revised Standard Version)

PRAYER DURING ILLNESS

This prayer can be offered by family, friends, clergy, and health care professionals.

Our Father which art in heaven,
Hallowed be thy name.
Thy kingdom come.
Thy will be done in earth, as it is in heaven.
Give us this day our daily bread.
And forgive us our debts, as we forgive our debtors.
And lead us not into temptation, but deliver us from evil:
For thine is the kingdom, and the power, and the glory, forever. Amen.

— Matt. 6:9–13 (Authorized [King James] Version)

READINGS DURING END-OF-LIFE PROCESS

These can be read by family, friends, clergy, and health care professionals.[257]

Jesus said to her, I am the resurrection and the life; he who believes in me, though he die, yet

---

256 *African Methodist Episcopal Church Book of Worship.* (1984). Nashville, TN: AME Sunday School Union, 71.

257 *African Methodist Episcopal Church Book of Worship.*

shall he live and whoever lives and believes in me shall never die.

Do you believe this?

—John 11:25–26

For I know that my Redeemer lives and at last he will stand upon the earth; and after my skin has been thus destroyed, then from my flesh I shall

see God, who I shall see on my side, and my eyes shall behold, and not another. My heart faints within me.

—Job 19:25–27

For we brought nothing into the world and we cannot take anything out of the world.

—1 Tim. 6:7

Assemblies of God

We believe in the God of the Bible and have embraced the salvation
provided through His Son, Jesus Christ. We believe God is at
work today through the power of His Holy Spirit.[258]

Prepared by:
Emanuel Williams, MDiv, BCC
Healthcare Chaplaincy Representative;
Keith Surface
Representative, Office of Public Relations;

Alvin F. Worthley, MDiv
Director of Chaplaincy,
All affiliated with the Assemblies of God World
  Headquarters
Springfield, MO

History and Facts

The Assemblies of God has its roots in a religious revival that began in the late 1800s and swept into the twentieth century with widespread repetition of biblical spiritual experiences. In the United States, the revival is generally traced to a prayer meeting in Topeka, Kansas, on January 1, 1901, that subsequently spread to Missouri, Texas, and California. A 3-year revival meeting at Azusa Street Mission in Los Angeles attracted believers from across the nation and overseas and served as a springboard to send the Pentecostal message around the world. The Pentecostal aspects of the revival were not generally welcomed by the established churches, and participants in the movement soon found themselves outside existing religious bodies and forced to seek their own places of worship.

By 1914, many ministers and laymen alike had begun to realize the rapid spread of the revival, and the many evangelistic outreaches it spawned had created a number of practical problems. These concerned leaders realized that to protect and preserve the results of the revival the thousands of newly Spirit-baptized believers should be united in a cooperative fellowship. In 1914 about 300 preachers and laymen gathered from 20 states and several foreign countries for a "general council" in Hot Springs, Arkansas, to discuss and take action on the growing need.

A cooperative fellowship emerged from the meeting and was incorporated under the name "The General Council of the Assemblies of God." The new organization was structured to unite the assemblies in ministry and legal identity while leaving each congregation self-governing and self-supporting.

Assemblies of God ministries have focused on evangelism and missions and have resulted in a continuing growth at home and abroad. The constituency has climbed from the founding convention attendance of 300 to more than 2.6 million

---

258 Quote provided by Alvin Worthley from the General Council of the Assemblies of God, Springfield, Missouri.

in the United States and over 48 million overseas. Today, Assemblies of God people worship in over 12 100 churches in the United States and in 236 022 churches and outstations in 191 other nations. The Assemblies of God has 19 endorsed Bible colleges, liberal arts colleges, and a seminary in the United States.

Basic Teachings

In 1916 the General Council approved a Statement of Fundamental Truths that remains virtually unchanged and continues to provide a sound basis for the Fellowship, giving a firm position on vital doctrines. These truths are:

- **The Scriptures Inspired**: The scriptures, both the Old and New Testaments, are verbally inspired of God, the revelation of God to man and the infallible, authoritative rule of faith and conduct.
- **The One True God**: The one true God has revealed Himself as the eternally self-existent "I AM," the Creator of heaven and earth and the Redeemer of mankind. He has further revealed Himself as embodying the principles of relationship and association as Father, Son, and Holy Ghost.
- **The Deity of the Lord Jesus Christ**: The Lord Jesus Christ is the eternal Son of God. Jesus was both human and divine.
- **The Fall of Man**: Man was created good and upright; for God said, "Let us make man in our own image, after our likeness." However, man by voluntary transgression fell and thereby incurred not only physical death but also spiritual death, which is separation from God.
- **The Salvation of Man**: Man's only hope of redemption is through the shed blood of Jesus Christ the Son of God.
- **The Ordinances of the Church**: Baptism

by immersion in water and Holy Communion

- **The Baptism in the Holy Ghost**: All believers are entitled to and should ardently expect and earnestly seek the promise of the Father, the baptism in the Holy Ghost and fire, according to the command of the Lord Jesus Christ. This was the normal experience of all in the early Christian Church. With it comes the empowerment for life and service, the bestowment of the gifts and their uses in the work of the ministry.
- **The Initial Physical Evidence of the Baptism in the Holy Ghost**: The baptism of believers in the Holy Ghost is witnessed by the initial physical sign of speaking with other tongues as the Spirit of God gives them utterance.
- **Sanctification**: Sanctification is an act of separation from that which is evil, and of dedication unto God.
- **The Church and its Mission**: The Church is the Body of Christ, the habitation of God through the Spirit, with divine appointments for the fulfillment of the great commission. Each believer, born of the Spirit, is an integral part of the General Assembly and Church of the Firstborn, which are written in heaven.
- **The Ministry**: A divinely called and scripturally ordained ministry has been provided by the Lord for the threefold purpose of leading the Church in:
  o *Evangelization of the world* (Mark 16:15–20)
  o *Worship of God* (John 4:23–24)
  o *Building body of saints being perfected in image of God's Son* (Eph. 4:11, 16).
- **Divine Healing**: Divine healing is an integral part of the gospel. Deliverance from sickness is provided for in the atonement, and is the privilege of all believers.

- **The Blessed Hope**: The resurrection of those who have "fallen asleep" (i.e., experienced physical death) in Christ and their translation (i.e., union with Christ) together with those who are alive and remain unto the coming of the Lord is the imminent and blessed hope of the church.
- **The Millennial Reign of Christ**: The Second Coming of Christ includes the rapture of the saints, which is the blessed hope, followed by the visible return of Christ with His saints to reign on earth for 1000 years.
- **The Final Judgment**: There will be a final judgment in which the wicked dead will be raised and judged according to their works. Whosoever is not found written in the Book of Life, together with the devil and his angels, the beast and the false prophet, will be consigned to the everlasting punishment in the lake which burns with fire and brimstone, which is the second death.
- **The New Heavens and the New Earth**: "We, according to His promise, look for new heavens and a new earth wherein dwelleth righteousness."

Basic Practices

- Church members value communal worship, and will gather on Sundays and at other times to study scripture, worship God through the singing of songs, pray, and hear preaching from the Bible.
- The sharing of one's faith (evangelism) is of great importance. Some of the ways it is communicated is through loving actions, talking about personal spiritual experiences, reading scriptures, distributing informational tracts and discussions of doctrinal positions.

- The Lord's Supper, also called Holy Communion, is a powerful ordinance. It is a symbolic memorial of the suffering and death of Jesus, in which Christians eat bread (to commemorate the broken body of Jesus) and drink grape juice (to symbolize Jesus' shed blood). This can be done during communal worship or in other settings and is usually administered by ordained clergy.
- Prayer, meditation, and scripture are the fundamental spiritual practices for many Christians. The many forms of these practices include: reading and/or silent contemplation on scripture or doctrinal beliefs and prayers of various kinds – petition, healing, repentance for unethical thoughts and actions, praise, worship, and thanksgiving to God.
- Mission work is important to the Church. This is accomplished through intentional witness to one's faith through proclamation and teaching. Mission work is also accomplished through acts of service in the form of working for social justice with marginalized peoples, charitable giving to provide food, building, and educational programs for the poor, volunteerism, and so forth.
- Ordinance of baptism is by immersion of an individual at the age of responsibility and understanding. This emphasizes waiting until a child is old enough to make an informed decision with respect to his or her relationship to God. Through baptism, believers symbolically declare to the world that they have died with Christ and that they also have been raised with Him to walk in newness of life.
- Clergy are required to officiate at the table of Holy Communion and in baptism.

Principles for Clinical Care
Dietary Issues

- The General Council of the Assemblies of God has no dietary restrictions with respect to religious beliefs. However, fasting is encouraged for spiritual growth.

General Medical Beliefs

The General Council of the Assemblies of God:

- Refers to God as the Great Physician.
- Affirms the validity of traditional Western medical procedures in the treatment of illness and disease.
- Does not take an official stand on the appropriateness of contraception within a heterosexual marriage for purposes of regulating the number of children, determining the time of their birth, or safeguarding the health of the mother. This is an individual decision.

Specific Medical Issues

- **Abortion**: The Church views abortion as evil and an unacceptable alternative for birth control. This concept is based upon the scriptures that regularly treat the unborn as a person under the care of God. A potentially legitimate exception would be in the infrequent cases where responsible diagnoses confirm that childbirth is likely to result in the death of the mother. The Church strongly encourages couples faced with this dilemma to prayerfully evaluate the medical diagnoses with the assistance of humane physicians and godly leaders prior to making their decision.
- **Advance Directives**: A health care directive (also called "living will") which clearly states a person's wishes for end-of-life care can help to alleviate painful decisions for family and loved ones and is therefore encouraged.

- **Birth Control**: The Assemblies of God acknowledges that the first command of God in the Bible (Gen. 1:28) is "Be fruitful and multiply, and fill the earth and subdue it." Therefore, the common expectation is that most Christians will marry and bring children into this world to be raised in the love and admonition of the Lord. However, the Assemblies of God also believes there may be valid reasons for delaying, limiting, or not having children which should be prayerfully taken into consideration. Generally speaking, the Assemblies of God leaves the decisions regarding birth control up to the couples concerned except as noted here.

Specific prohibitions regarding birth control practices

1. **The use of chemically induced or surgical abortion.**
2. **Any birth control method that functions to destroy a fertilized egg, rather than actually preventing conception.**

Additional information may be found on the Assemblies of God website (www.ag.org) under "Beliefs."

- **Blood Transfusions**: The Church has no official position and no reservations regarding blood transfusions.
- **Circumcision**: The Assemblies of God has no official position on circumcision. However, church members in Western societies have requested circumcision of male infants for cultural, not religious, reasons.
- **In Vitro Fertilization**: Infertile heterosexual couples (who have pursued all viable treatments without success) considering in vitro fertilization, should give careful and prayerful attention with knowledgeable and godly counsel regarding all

pertinent issues and make decisions in good conscience with the guidance of the Spirit of God. The church disapproves of any procedure that results in the destruction of unimplanted embryos.

- **Stem Cell Research**: The Church believes Somatic Gene Transfer for therapeutic purposes is morally acceptable. However, it believes that reproductive cloning is immoral and not permissible.
- **Vaccinations**: The Assemblies of God has no official position on immunization. However, most church members would view immunization as an effective medical treatment that has the potential for both individual and societal prevention of substantial harm, suffering, or death and therefore accepts safe and properly administered immunization. The right of individuals to make these kinds of decisions would be respected so that those individuals who hold genuine and sincere religious beliefs contrary to immunization would not be precluded from choosing to decline immunization.
- **Withholding/Withdrawing Life Support**: The Church does not view the withholding/withdrawing of life support in medically futile cases as a violation of teachings of the Assemblies of God. It is an individual decision that should be made by the patient whenever possible, after prayerful consultation with a Christian doctor and a respected spiritual leader. It is wise for believers to consider and decide these matters before the moment of crisis.

Gender and Personal Issues

- Within the context of clinical care, the General Council of the Assemblies of God as a faith tradition has no prescriptions or proscriptions with respect to gender and personal issues.

- There are no cultural differences from a denominational standpoint that impact the provision of spiritual care. However, there are numerous ethnic groups represented in the denomination, and members of these groups may express preferences for specific kinds of pastoral care.

Principles for Spiritual Care through the Cycles of Life

Concepts of Living and Dying for Spiritual Support

- Every human life, from conception through death is to be valued, respected, nurtured, and protected.
- God is the ultimate source of all life, health, and healing.
- Divine healing is an integral part of the gospel. Deliverance from sickness is provided for in the Atonement, and is the privilege of all believers.
- Death is the result of human sin and comes eventually to all, except those believers alive at the coming of Christ.
- Following the death of a believer, the spirit of the deceased ascend to heaven at the moment of death and will be with the Lord forever (2 Cor. 5:6–9; Phil. 1:23).
- Resurrection of the physical body and the reunion of spirit and body in some form will happen at the Second Coming of Jesus.

During Birth

- As stated earlier, church members in Western societies have requested circumcision of male infants for cultural, not religious, reasons.

During Illness

- Patients may receive comfort from the reading of scriptures or other devotional material, listening to religious music, or watching televised worship services of their own or a similar tradition. Patients may request Holy Communion. The chaplain or clergy should be consulted for assistance.

- Patients may receive comfort from healing prayers. These can be offered by health care professionals; however, patients may ask for healing prayer to be connected with "anointing with oil" or the "the laying on of hands." The chaplain or clergy should be consulted for assistance for these requests.
- Patients may request baptism. In the clinical setting, sprinkling is an acceptable mode of baptism, even though the Assemblies of God practices immersion. The chaplain or clergy should be consulted for assistance.
- Pastors are the primary spiritual leaders for the members of their congregations and are normally the clergy person who will make hospital visits.
- Deacons and church elders may also make hospital calls on the sick.
- Prayer for the healing of the sick is a normative practice and may be performed by clergy and/or laypersons. James 5:14, 15 instruct the sick to call the elders of the church to anoint them with oil in the name of the Lord. Appropriate scriptures may also be read in conjunction with the prayers.

During End of Life

- Patient or the family may request that clergy and/or the chaplain offer prayer.
- Family members who wish to view the body of the deceased should consult with the chaplain and/or hospital staff to arrange an appropriate setting in the hospital.

- Family members may request that the chaplain and/or clergy offer prayers and read scripture for those near death.

Care of the Body

- There are no specific protocols regarding the handling of the body except for treating the body with the utmost respect.
- Disposition and embalming are individual decisions. Cremation is also a choice of some Christians. The Assemblies of God has no restrictions on method of burial, believing that one's commitment to Christ in life and not the manner of burial after death affects one's eternal reward.
- Autopsy is an individual decision unless required by law. The chaplain and/or nurse should be consulted for assistance.
- Donation for medical research is an individual decision. The chaplain and/or nurse should be consulted for assistance. Advance planning for such donations is required by most receiving organizations. Last-minute donations are usually not possible.

Organ and Tissue Donation

- The denomination has taken no doctrinal position on organ donation. It is an individual decision. However, organ and tissue donation is permitted as an individual decision. It may be preferable for a chaplain and/or nurse who are trained designated requesters to be consulted for assistance.

Scriptures, Inspirational Readings, and Prayers

READINGS DURING ILLNESS

These can be read by family, friends, clergy, and health care professionals. (All scripture quotations are from the New International Version.)

The Lord is my shepherd, I shall not
be in want.
He makes me lie down in green
pastures;
He leads me beside quiet waters,
He restores my soul.
He guides me in paths of
righteousness for his name's sake.
Even though I walk through the
valley of the shadow of death, I will
fear no evil;
for you are with me; your rod and
your staff – they comfort me.
You prepare a table before me in the
presence of my enemies;
You anoint my head with oil; my cup
overflows.
Surely goodness and love will follow
me all the days of my life,
and I will dwell in the house of the
Lord forever.

—Psalm 23

Fear not, for I have redeemed you; I
have summoned you be name; you
are mine.
When you pass through the waters,
I will be with you; and when you
pass through the rivers, they will
not sweep over you. When you walk
through the fire, you will not be
burned; the flames will not set you
ablaze.
For I am the Lord, your God.

—Isa. 43:1–3

And we know that in all things God
works for the good of those who
love him, who have been called
according to his purpose.
For I am convinced that neither
death, nor life, neither angel nor
demons, neither the present, nor
the future, nor any powers, neither
height nor depth, not anything
else in all creation, will be able to
separate us from the love of God
that is in Christ Jesus our Lord.

—Rom. 8:28, 38–39

READINGS DURING END-OF-LIFE PROCESS

These can be read by family, friends, clergy, and health care professionals. (All scripture quotations are from the New International Version.)

I am the resurrection and the life.
He who believes in me will live, even
though he dies; and whoever lives and
believes in me will never die.

—John 11:25–26

Do not let your hearts be troubled.
Trust in God, trust also in me.
In my Father's house there are many
rooms. If it were not so, I would
have told you.
I am going there to prepare a place
for you. And if I go and prepare a
place for you, I will come back and
take you to be with me that you also
may be where I am.

—John 14:1–3

PRAYER DURING END-OF-LIFE PROCESS
This prayer can be offered by family, friends, clergy, and health care professionals.

Our heavenly Father,
We praise you for your faithfulness
through life and through death. And
as we sense the nearness of death
the significance of your faithfulness
deepens.
Entering the unknown is frightening
and leaving our loved ones is hard.

Wondering just how and when
death will come is tedious.
Give us courage to face the
challenges. Give us patience to
endure the trials. Give us faith
to overcome our fears. Give us
guidance to reach the promised rest.
We ask these things in the name of
Jesus.

Baptist Church

A free church in a free state, reflecting the Baptist ideal of religious liberty.[259]

Prepared by:
C. Michael Fuhrman, PhD
Professor of Christian Studies, Southwest Baptist University
Bolivar, MO

History and Facts

Some Baptist historians trace Baptist origins in the English-speaking world to the Anabaptist groups of the Reformation Era, but evidence of such influences has proven difficult to document. Other Baptists, particularly some in the south-central United States, maintain the belief (on a popular level) that the Baptist church has existed from the New Testament Era until the present time. This view, called the Landmark Theory, holds that a wide number of dissenting groups in Christian history, such as the Cathari or the Bogomiles, in actuality were "Baptists by another name," and that they existed in an unbroken line of succession back to the time of Jesus and the apostles. While this view has never found acceptance by Baptist historians, in some regions of North America, it has enjoyed considerable popularity among Baptist laity.

The predominant view of Baptist origins holds that Baptists began as a persecuted minority in Elizabethan England, with their roots in English Separatism. The Puritans of the time wanted to remain in the Church of England and purify it from within. Separatists considered the Church of England of that time as too corrupt to preserve and hence advocated establishing a new church altogether. In 1607, under the leadership of John Smyth and Thomas Helwys, a group of Separatists from the English town of Gainsborough fled from persecution under James I and took up temporary refuge in Holland. There, Smyth led the group to embrace believer's baptism. Historians date the establishment of the first Baptist church in the world to this event, which occurred about 1609. Sometime during the winter of 1611/1612 CE, Helwys led a small number of this congregation to return to England, where they established the first Baptist congregation on English soil. From this beginning Baptists have grown to become a major faith group within Protestant Christianity.

Within a generation of their origins in England, Roger Williams planted the first Baptist congregation in North America: the First Baptist Church of Providence, Rhode Island, in 1638. Baptists, both in England and in colonial America, suffered greatly from being persecuted as a dissenting group. Indeed, Baptists have spent much of

---

259 Quote provided by C. Michael Fuhrman, author of this chapter.

their four centuries of existence as a persecuted minority, with the persecution often coming at the hands of a state church. This heritage of persecution has shaped Baptist views on both religious liberty and matters relating to liberty of conscience. For example, Baptists in Virginia and Massachusetts championed the cause of religious liberty in the years of the Revolutionary War Era, and, partly as a result of their dissent, the First Amendment (which guaranteed religious liberty for all) was added to the United States' Constitution. Similarly, because Baptists remember those times when their own liberty of conscience was threatened by the creed of the state church, they have historically shown an aversion to creeds. While Baptists would broadly agree with the doctrinal positions of the historic creeds of the church, Baptists historically have resisted the use of such doctrinal statements as tools to compel belief. For this reason, Baptists prefer to compose confessions of faith, statements declaring what a group of Baptists at a certain time and place do believe, rather than creeds or statements of faith declaring what a Christian must believe.

Baptists grew exponentially as a result of the First and Second Great Awakenings on the American frontier, and they have continued to grow vigorously since. At last count, some fifty-two different Baptist groups exist in the United States alone, not counting many "independent" or nondenominational Baptist congregations scattered all across the country. There are a variety of reasons Baptists have fragmented into the many different groups, including, but certainly not limited to (1) ethnicity; (2) the Baptist ideal regarding the autonomy of the local church, or its right to self-governance; and (3) the Baptist core value regarding the priesthood of the believer, or the right

of each individual to interpret the Bible, approach God, and decide for themselves regarding theological and ethical concerns. Furthermore, in the Baptist world, one will find widely varying positions on such matters as the ordination of women for the pastoral ministry or ecumenism. On certain matters of theology (such as the Second Coming of Christ), one will find Baptists "all over the map."

As one would expect, this diversity renders generalizing about Baptists difficult. Moreover, because of this diversity and lack of a single denominational structure, accurate membership statistics are rendered somewhat difficult to calculate. With that qualification in mind, by the year 2000, Baptists collectively had grown to number in excess of 30 million members in the United States and 45 million members worldwide. Baptists, thus represent the largest Protestant group in the United States, with the largest single Baptist group being the Southern Baptist Convention, with over 16 million members.

Basic Teachings

- Baptists affirm the teachings of historic Protestant orthodoxy.
- The inspired scriptures provide the guide and norm for the Christian life.
- Every believer is a priest before God who can approach God in prayer and interpret the Bible without any mediator except for Jesus Christ.
- Each local congregation is self-governing or autonomous. The local church represents denominational headquarters in Baptist life.
- Baptism is of believers and by immersion. An experience of Christian conversion must precede baptism.

- Religious liberty is the right of all. Historically, Baptists have championed the ideal of a free church in a free state.

Basic Practices

- Baptists value regular times of worship, prayer, and Bible study as a community of faith.
- Baptists do not typically call baptism and the Lord's Supper "sacraments," preferring to view them as symbolic "ordinances" instead.
- The Lord's Supper is typically observed regularly, but not weekly.
- Baptists believe that sharing their faith with unbelievers is every Christian's responsibility.
- God has commissioned the followers of Christ to conduct mission work throughout the world.
- Infants and their parents may participate in dedication services, but because they are not old enough to understand the Christian Gospel and respond to it, infants are not baptized.

Principles for Clinical Care
Dietary Issues

- Baptists have no dietary restrictions with regard to religious beliefs.

General Medical Beliefs

- Baptists believe that God is the ultimate source of all life, health, and healing.
- Baptists refer to Christ as the Great Physician.
- Baptists affirm the validity of traditional Western medical procedures in the treatment of illness and disease.

Specific Medical Issues

- **Abortion**: Baptists generally oppose abortion.
- **Advance Directives**: Baptists have generally not taken a position on advance directives for health care preplanning, leaving this as an individual decision.
- **Birth Control**: Baptists believe that birth control may be used to regulate the number and spacing of children. It is a moral decision for each couple. However, Baptists specify that the form of contraception prevents conception.
- **Blood Transfusions**: Baptists have no reservations regarding blood transfusions.
- **Circumcision**: Circumcision for male infants is widely followed for cultural, not religious, reasons.
- **In Vitro Ferilization**: Opinions with regard to in vitro fertilization vary widely among the various Baptist groups. Generally speaking, it is probably fair to say that in vitro fertilization is discouraged, while realizing that it ultimately represents an individual decision.
- **Stem Cell Research**: Some Baptist groups, but not all, have taken an official position in opposition to embryonic stem cell research, although the use of adult stem cells for therapeutic purposes enjoys much wider support. Baptists generally oppose human cloning.
- **Vaccinations**: The Baptist tradition embraces the value of vaccinations, given at appropriate times and to appropriate subjects, as a disease preventive.
- **Withholding/Withdrawing Life Support**: Withholding/withdrawing life support in medically futile cases does not violate Baptist teachings; it is an individual decision.

Gender and Personal Issues

- Baptists have no prescriptions or pro-scriptions with respect to gender and personal issues concerning the delivery of health care in a clinical setting.

Principles for Spiritual Care through the Cycles of Life

Concepts of Living and Dying for Spiritual Support

- Life is sacred.
- Death is something all must experience.
- Christians experience the immediate presence of God in heaven upon their death.
- Believers receive a resurrection body after they die.

During Birth

- Babies may be dedicated to God but are not baptized.
- As stated earlier, circumcision for male infants is widely followed for cultural, not religious, reasons.

During Illness

- Patients may receive comfort from the reading of scriptures or other devotional material, listening to Christian music, watching televised worship services of their own or of a similar faith tradition.
- Patients may receive the Lord's Supper from chaplains, clergy, or deacons upon their request (although this is not widely practiced).
- Patients may receive comfort from healing prayers. While Baptists do not widely practice "anointing with oil" or "the laying on of hands," there is nothing in the Baptist heritage that would oppose these practices.

- Christian patients may receive assurance from their faith-relationship with God through Jesus Christ.

During End of Life

- The patient or family may request Christian conversion. The chaplain or clergy should be consulted for assistance.
- The patient or family may request the Lord's Supper from chaplains, clergy, or deacons.
- The patient or family may request prayer for the dying and the reading of appropriate scripture texts.
- The family may wish to view the body of the deceased in the hospital room. The nursing staff and chaplain should be consulted for assistance.
- The grieving family members may request prayer for themselves, which can be offered by the chaplain, clergy, friends, or health care professionals.

Care of the Body

- Disposition and embalming are individual decisions. The chaplain and the funeral home director should be consulted for assistance.
- Autopsy is an individual decision unless required by law. The chaplain and/or nurse should be consulted for assistance.
- Donation for medical research is an individual decision. The chaplain or nursing staff should be consulted for assistance. Advance planning for such donations is required by most receiving organizations. Last-minute donations are usually not possible.

Organ and Tissue Donation

- Organ and tissue donation is permitted and is an individual decision. It may be preferable for a chaplain and/or nurse who are trained designated requesters to be consulted for assistance.

Scriptures, Inspirational Readings, and Prayers

READINGS DURING ILLNESS

These can be read by family, friends, clergy, and health care professionals. (All scripture quotations are from the New Revised Standard translation.)

The Lord is my shepherd I shall not want.
He makes me like down in green pastures: he restores my soul.
He leads me in right paths for his name's sake.
Even though I walk through the darkest valley, I fear no evil;
For you are with me; your rod and your staff – they comfort me.
You prepare a table before me in the presence of my enemies;
You anoint my head with oil; my cup overflows.
Surely goodness and mercy shall follow me all the days of my life,
and I shall dwell in the house of the Lord my whole life long.

— Psalm 23

We know that all things work together for good ...
For I am convinced that neither death, nor life, nor angels, nor rulers, nor things present, nor things to come, nor powers, nor height, nor depth, nor anything else in all creation, will be able to separate us from the love of God in Christ Jesus our Lord.

— Rom. 8:28a, 38–39

READINGS DURING END-OF-LIFE PROCESS

These can be ready by family, friends, clergy, and health care professionals. (All scripture quotations are from the New Revised Standard Version.)

I am the resurrection and the life. Those who believe in me, even though they die, will live, and everyone who lives and believes in me will never die."

— John 11:25–26

Do not let your hearts be troubled. Believe in God, believe also in me.
In my Father's house there are many dwelling places. If it were not so, would I have told you that I go to prepare a place for you?
And if I go and prepare a place for you, I will come again and will take you to myself, so that were I am, there you may be also.

— John 14:1–3

PRAYER DURING END-OF-LIFE PROCESS

This prayer can be offered by family, friends, clergy, and health care professionals.

Holy and Merciful Father,
We thank you for the gift of your Son, Jesus, whom you sent to die that we might live. We thank you

also that you raised Him from the dead, and that He is seated with you in heaven. We acknowledge that you are the Lord of Life and the Lord of Death. We ask that you send your holy angels to escort our brother/sister _____ through death into your presence. Give our brother/sister _____ peace and comfort the family who will be saddened by the loss.

In Jesus' precious name, we pray. Amen.

Christian Church (Disciples of Christ)

Seeking unity in the diversity[260]

Prepared by:
The Reverend Quentin B. Jones, MDiv, BCC
Chaplain, Lakeview Village
Lenexa, KS

Reviewed and approved by:
The Reverend Dr. Paul J. Diehl
Regional Minister/President, Christian Church
(Disciples of Christ) of Greater Kansas City
Overland Park, KS

History and Facts

The Christian Church (Disciples of Christ) began in the early 1800s as a result of the increasing concern shared by three Protestant clergymen of the division among the Christian community caused by denominational exclusivity. Barton Stone, Thomas Campbell, and his son Alexander Campbell set out to dissolve these denominational differences and restore unity following, what they believed to be, the model of the early church of the New Testament period. Their ultimate goal in this effort was that all Christians could gather at the table of Holy Communion and worship together. This initiative of seeking unity among Christians became known as the Restoration Movement.

However, these three men were not initially together with respect to their common goal. Barton Stone was the leader of one group of people who called themselves "Christians." Thomas and Alexander Campbell were the leaders of the other group called "Disciples." By the middle of

the nineteenth century, the Stone-Campbell groups united and became known as the Disciples of Christ. This church movement which had earlier sought to break the bonds of denominationalism within Christianity became identified as a denomination themselves in the early twentieth century. Today, the Christian Church (Disciples of Christ) is the first and one of the largest Christian faith groups founded on US soil, with over 800 000 members in the United States and Canada.

Basic Teachings

Many Disciples will affirm the content of the ancient *Apostles' Creed*, which is a brief statement of faith attributed to the early church.

The Apostles' Creed

I believe in God, the Father almighty,
    creator of heaven and earth,
I believe in Jesus Christ, His only
    Son, our Lord.
Who was conceived by the power of
    the Holy Spirit;
Born of the virgin Mary;
Suffered under Pontius Pilate;

---

260 Quote provided by Rev. Quentin Jones, author of this chapter.

Was crucified, died, and buried.
He descended into hell (or the realm
   of the dead).
On the third day he rose again.
He ascended into heaven and is
   seated at the right hand of the
   Father.
He will come again to judge the living
   and the dead.
I believe in the Holy Spirit,
The holy catholic (universal) church,
The communion of saints,
The forgiveness of sins,
The resurrection of the body and the
   life everlasting. Amen.

- All humans are fallen from an original state of innocence and are bent toward actions (i.e., sins) that disconnect them from God and others.
- All humans deserve just punishment for misdeeds.
- Humans can be rescued (i.e., saved) from just punishment through faith in the death, burial, and resurrection of Jesus.
- The final destination for those who have been saved from the consequences of their misdeeds is heaven, which is communion with God and all the redeemed in a state of peace, justice, and perfect love.
- The final destination of those who are not saved is hell, a state of punishment and disconnected-ness from God and the saved. Opinions differ as to whether or not hell is eternal.
- Disciples affirm the Bible, or Holy Scriptures, which is a compilation of 66 different books written over a thousand-year period. These writings contain wisdom sayings, history, poetry, social commentary, and devotional literature from ancient Semitic Jewish, Hellenistic Jewish, and early Christian authors. Some

Christians also include additional books from Hellenistic Jewish culture called the Apocrypha. The number of these books varies according to the different traditions.
- All baptized persons are called to ministry.
- All Disciples are capable of study and interpretation of scripture.
- No requirement for subscription to any creed for membership in the Christian Church. Creeds are viewed as helpful statements in articulating the tenets of the faith. A common phrase is "No creed but Christ; no book but the Bible."
- Two sacraments are recognized: baptism and Holy Communion.

Basic Practices
- Disciples value communal worship, and will gather on Sundays and at other times to hear preaching, study scripture, sing hymns, and pray.
- The sharing of one's faith (evangelism) is of great importance to Disciples. Some of the ways it is communicated is through loving actions, talking about personal spiritual experiences, reading scriptures, distributing informational tracts and discussions of doctrinal positions.
- The Lord's Supper, also called Holy Communion or Eucharist (meaning "thanksgiving"), is a powerful ordinance (sacrament or ritual). It is a liturgical reenactment of the crucifixion, death, burial and resurrection of Jesus, in which Christians eat bread (to commemorate the broken body of Jesus) and drink wine or grape juice (to symbolize Jesus' shed blood). Holy Communion is an integral part of weekly worship.
- Prayer, meditation, and scripture are the fundamental spiritual practices for many

Christians. The many forms of these practices include reading and/or silent contemplation upon scripture or doctrinal beliefs and prayers of various kinds – petition, healing, repentance for unethical thoughts and actions, praise, worship, and thanksgiving to God.

- Mission work is important to Disciples. These acts of service take the forms of working for social justice with marginalized peoples, charitable giving to provide food, building, and educational programs for the poor, volunteerism, and so forth. Mission work is also an intentional witness to one's faith through proclamation and teaching.
- Christening is the ceremonial act which includes naming of the child. It can be an official part of the ceremony of baptism or combined with infant dedication.
- Clergy and non-ordained laypersons have equal standing at the table of Holy Communion and in baptism.
- Sacrament of baptism is usually by immersion of an individual at the age of responsibility and understanding. However, infant baptism and "sprinkling" are also generally recognized and accepted.
- Social action and pursuit of justice for all people are strongly encouraged.

Principles for Clinical Care
Dietary Issues
- Christian Church has no dietary restrictions with respect to religious beliefs.

General Medical Beliefs
- Christians believe that God is the ultimate source of all life, health, and healing.
- Christians refer to God as the Great Physician.

- Christians affirm the validity of traditional Western medical procedures in the treatment of illness and disease.

Specific Medical Issues
- **Abortion**: Abortion is acceptable only in certain circumstances. Generally, there is some concession to abortion to save the life of the mother and in cases of rape or incest.
- **Advance Directives**: Christian Church has no reservations about and supports the use of advance directives for health care preplanning.
- **Birth Control**: The Christian Church (Disciples of Christ) has no pronouncement about birth control. As far as the church is concerned, it is a matter of personal conscience and prayerful consideration.
- **Blood Transfusions**: Christian Church has no reservations about blood transfusions.
- **Circumcision**: Christians in Western societies have requested circumcision of male infants for cultural, not religious, reasons.
- **In Vitro Fertilization**: Christian Church has no reservations about in vitro fertilization and birth control.
- **Stem Cell Research**: Christian Church has made no declaration regarding stem cell research. Thus, it is assumed to be a matter of individual conscience. Human cloning is not an endorsed practice of the Christian Church.
- **Vaccinations**: Christian Church has issued no statement on vaccinations. Thus, it is a matter of personal conscience. The church does promote wellness and health, however.
- **Withholding/Withdrawing Life Support**: Withholding/withdrawing life

support in medically futile cases does not violate teachings of the Christian Church. It is an individual decision.

Gender and Personal Issues

- Christian Church as a faith tradition has no prescriptions or proscriptions with respect to gender and personal issues.

Principles for Spiritual Care through the Cycles of Life

Concepts of Living and Dying for Spiritual Support

- Life is sacred.
- Death is something all must experience and should not be feared.
- Death is not perceived as sleep. People can be traumatized by the connection between death and sleep and, thus, afraid to go to sleep. This is especially true with children.
- The soul and spirit of the deceased ascend to heaven at the moment of death.
- Resurrection of the physical body and the reunion of spirit, soul, and body in some form will happen at the Second Coming of Jesus. Humanity, all living creatures, and the entire cosmos will be healed and restored to a state of perfection.

During Birth

- Christening or baptism may be requested by family for a baby, living or deceased. The chaplain or clergy should be consulted for assistance.
- As stated earlier, Christians in Western societies have requested circumcision of male infants for cultural, not religious, reasons.

During Illness

- Patients may receive comfort from the reading of scriptures or other devotional material, listening to religious music, or watching televised worship services of their own or a similar tradition. Patients may request Holy Communion. The chaplain or clergy should be consulted for assistance.
- Patients may receive comfort from healing prayers. These can be offered by health care professionals. Patients from some traditions, however, may ask for healing prayer to be connected with "anointing with oil" or the "the laying on of hands." The chaplain or clergy should be consulted for assistance for these requests.
- Patients may request baptism. In the clinical setting, sprinkling is an acceptable mode of baptism, even for traditions that practice immersion. The chaplain or clergy should be consulted for assistance.

During End of Life

- Patient or the family may request baptism. The chaplain or clergy should be consulted for assistance.
- Patient or the family may request Holy Communion. The chaplain or clergy should be consulted for assistance.
- Family may wish to view the body of the deceased in the hospital room or the chapel. The nurse and chaplain should be consulted for assistance.
- Family may request prayers for the deceased. These can be offered by the chaplain, clergy, family, friends, and health care professionals.

Care of the Body

- Disposition and embalming are individual decisions. Cremation is now the choice of many Christians. The chaplain and the funeral home director should be consulted for assistance.

- Autopsy is an individual decision unless required by law. The chaplain and/or nurse should be consulted for assistance.
- Donation for medical research is an individual decision. The chaplain and/or nurse should be consulted for assistance. Advance planning for such donations is required by most receiving organizations. Last-minute donations are usually not possible.

Organ and Tissue Donation

- Organ and tissue donation is permitted and is an individual decision. It may be preferable for a chaplain and/or nurse who are trained designated requesters to be consulted for assistance.

Scriptures, Inspirational Readings, and Prayers

- Ask the patient and/or family if there are favorite texts of scripture or devotional readings.
- All those of "Christianity" apply.
- Many Christian Church individuals will have developed a "list" of favorite passages from which they draw comfort, encouragement, hope, and/or vision for the future as the disease process is treated or as the end of life draws closer. In addition to the ones provided in the general Christianity section are Psalms 46 and 91 and Revelation 21.

READINGS DURING ILLNESS

These can be read by family, friends, clergy, and health care professionals. (All scripture quotations are from the Revised Standard Version.)

God is our refuge and strength, a very present help in trouble.

Therefore we will not fear though the earth should change, though the mountains shake in the heart of the sea, though its waters roar and foam, though the mountains tremble with its tumult. Selah.

There is a river whose streams make glad the city of God, the holy habitation of the Most High.

God is in the midst of her, she shall not be moved; God will help her right early.

The nations rage, the kingdoms totter; he utters his voice, the earth melts.

The LORD of hosts is with us; the God of Jacob is our refuge. Selah.

Come, behold the works of the LORD, how he has wrought desolations in the earth.

He makes wars cease to the end of the earth; he breaks the bow, and shatters the spear, he burns the chariots with fire!

"Be still, and know that I am God. I am exalted among the nations. I am exalted in the earth!"

The LORD of hosts is with us; the God of Jacob is our refuge.

— Psalm 46

He who dwells in the shelter of the Most High, who abides in the shadow of the Almighty, will say to the Lord, "My refuge and my fortress; my God, in whom I trust."

For he will deliver you from the snare of the fowler and from the deadly pestilence; he will cover you with his pinions, and under his wings you will find refuge; his faithfulness is a shield and buckler. You will not fear the terror of the night, nor the arrow that flies by day, nor the pestilence that stalks in darkness, nor the destruction that wastes at noonday.

A thousand may fall at your side, ten thousand at your right hand; but it will not come near you. You will only look with your eyes and see the recompense of the wicked.

Because you have made the Lord your refuge, the Most High your habitation, no evil shall befall you, no scourge come near your tent:

for he will give his angels charge of you to guard you in all your ways. On their hands they will bear you up, lest you dash your foot against a stone. You will tread on the lion and the adder, the young lion and the serpent you will trample under foot.

Because he cleaves to me in love, I will deliver him; I will protect him, because he knows my name. When he calls to me, I will answer him; I will be with him in trouble, I will rescue him and honor him. With long life I will satisfy him, and show him my salvation.

—Psalm 91

READING DURING END-OF-LIFE PROCESS
This can be read by family, friends, clergy, and health care professionals. (This scripture quotation is from the Revised Standard Version.)

Then I saw a new heaven and a new earth; for the first heaven and the first earth had passed away, and the sea was no more. And I saw the holy city, New Jerusalem, coming down out of heaven from God, prepared as a bride adorned for her husband; and I heard a loud voice from the throne saying, "Behold, the dwelling of God is with men. He will dwell with them, and they shall be his people, and God himself will be with them; he will wipe away every tear from their eyes, and death shall be no more, neither shall there be mourning nor crying nor pain any more, for the former things have passed away."

And he who sat upon the throne said, "Behold, I make all things new." Also he said, "Write this, for these words are trustworthy and true." And he said to me, "It is done! I am the Alpha and the Omega, the beginning and the end."

—Rev. 21:1–6a

Christian Science

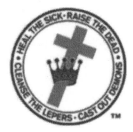

Divine Love always has met and always will meet every human need.[261]

Prepared by:
Committee on Publication
The First Church of Christ, Scientist
Boston, MA

History and Facts

Christian Science is based on the teachings of Jesus. It presents God as all-powerful, ever-present, and all-good, and it presents each individual, therefore, as inseparable from God and God's love. In Christian Science, it is the unfolding understanding of this reality that brings about healing. The most complete explanation of Christian Science can be found in *Science and Health with Key to the Scriptures* by Mary Baker Eddy, which is read along with the Holy Bible at church services and in individual study and prayer.

Mary Baker Eddy (1821–1910)

discovered Christian Science in 1866 and, later, founded The Church of Christ, Scientist, which today has members and branches throughout the world. Although the church is frequently referred to as the "Christian Science Church," the teachings of Christian Science are studied and practiced by people throughout the world, irrespective of cultural, ethnic or religious background.

Eddy spent much of the first half of her life searching for an effective means of relief from the severe chronic health problems that plagued her. A deeply spiritual woman, she was convinced that the teachings contained in the Bible, particularly those of Jesus, were somehow applicable to the present-day cure of disease. She also became increasingly convinced of the power of thought; that it played a primary role in both the cause and cure of disease. In several instances, she healed other people through her prayers,

---

261 Eddy, M. *Science and Health with Key to the Scriptures.* (1971). Boston, MA: Christian Science Publishing Society/Christian Science Board of Directors, 494. With respect to the logo, the Cross and Crown design is a trademark of the Christian Science Board of Directors and is used by permission.

although she was unable to explain just how the healing work was accomplished.

The restoration of her health, though, remained elusive.

In February 1866, Eddy fell on an icy sidewalk and sustained serious injuries. After several days of intense suffering, Eddy then asked for her Bible and, while reading an account of Jesus' healing, had what she later characterized as a deeply transforming spiritual experience. She became keenly aware of God's presence, so much so that she experienced an immediate recovery. She got up, dressed, and, to the reported surprise of those present, walked into the next room. Years later, she wrote, "That short experience included a glimpse of the great fact that I have since tried to make plain to others, namely, Life in and of Spirit; this Life being the sole reality of existence."[262] The "Christian Science" concept was beginning to evolve.

The next several years were characterized by intensive study of the Bible, wrestling with old and new theological concepts and significant healing work. Eddy's newfound discovery, which she later named Christian Science, was coming into clearer and clearer focus.

Mary Baker Eddy also taught others how to heal. Hundreds of her students, both past and present, and both male and female, established successful healing practices across the United States and abroad. Some of these practitioners later became teachers of Christian Science, meaning that they've been qualified to teach an intensive course, called Primary Class, to individuals interested in learning more about how to heal

themselves and others using the method of Christian Science healing. Teachers also continue to act as mentors to these pupils for their spiritual growth. Both Christian Science practitioners and teachers continue to be available worldwide today to assist, through prayer, individuals struggling with physical, mental, emotional, relationship, and other difficulties.

Later, Eddy also instituted a program of Christian Science nursing care for those relying exclusively on Christian Science for physical healing, but who required skilled assistance.

Science and Health with Key to the Scriptures

Eddy wrote and circulated short essays on her discovery, but the need for a more comprehensive treatment had become apparent. *Science and Health with Key to the Scriptures* was first published in 1875 and has remained in continuous publication since that time. Over her lifetime, Eddy revised this book many times, continually refining and clarifying its message and scriptural exegeses.

Establishing the Church of Christ, Scientist

Mary Baker Eddy's initial hope was that existing Christian churches would embrace her discovery. It soon became clear that this was not to be, and so she founded her own church in 1879, later naming it the Church of Christ, Scientist. It was established, she wrote, "to commemorate the word and works of our Master, which should reinstate primitive Christianity and its lost element of healing."[263] Eddy's purpose in founding the church was to make the system

---

262 Eddy, M. *Miscellaneous Writings 1883–1896.* (1953). Boston, MA: Christian Science Publishing Society/Christian Science Board of Directors, 24.

263 www.marybakereddylibrary.org/mary-baker-eddy/life (accessed 8 Sept 2012).

of spiritual healing she discovered more widely available and accessible. Today, as then, individuals need not be members of the church in order to practice Christian Science healing. Individuals of various faith traditions regularly study *Science and Health*, and rely on and practice the healing system it explains.

The Church of Christ, Scientist is a "lay" church without ordained clergy or ecclesiastical body of any kind. It does not dictate members' practice of Christian Science, reflecting a conviction that personal matters are best decided by the individual with the Bible and the writings of Mary Baker Eddy as the guide. Telling, perhaps, is a convention among church members – be they Sunday School pupils or senior church officials – to refer to themselves as "students" of Christian Science, implying that no one individual has all the answers.

The Church of Christ, Scientist is also an international body consisting of The First Church of Christ, Scientist in Boston, Massachusetts – also known as The Mother Church – and its branches around the world. Branch churches are democratic, self-governing bodies. Today, there are over 1700 branch churches in 70 countries (see www.churchofchristscientist.org).

Basic Teachings

Foundational to the theology of Christian Science is the fact of each individual's inseparability from God. This belief, which suggests that no one has the ability, much less the authority, to interfere with or mediate in this relationship, was a major point in the early theological tenets of Christian Science thought. Those tenets are:

• God is infinite Father-Mother. God, Spirit, is all and wholly good.

• God created everything, and everything created reflects God's goodness.

• Individuals are made in the "image and likeness" of God as the Bible teaches. Each individual is spiritual and reflects God's goodness.

• The relationship of God and His/Her creation is indestructible and eternal. The Supreme Being is forever governing His/Her children in perfect harmony.

Mary Baker Eddy believed that these and related concepts were not just theological ideas, but actual spiritual laws – laws that govern the entire being and function of creation, including men and women. She felt it was Jesus' pure, unparalleled faith in these divine laws of goodness that explained his remarkable healing work. She was convinced that these universal, spiritual laws, prayerfully understood and applied in daily life, would allow anyone to heal the sick, and thus confirm Jesus' own statement that "these signs shall follow them that believe" (Mark 16:17).

In *Science and Health*, Eddy further expanded her thought by stating the basic principles of Christian Science as follows:

1. As adherents of Truth, we take the inspired Word of the Bible as our sufficient guide to eternal Life.
2. We acknowledge and adore one supreme and infinite God. We acknowledge His Son, one Christ; the Holy Ghost or divine Comforter; and man in God's image and likeness.
3. We acknowledge God's forgiveness of sin in the destruction of sin and the spiritual understanding that casts out evil as unreal. But the belief in sin is punished so long as the belief lasts.
4. We acknowledge Jesus' atonement as the evidence of divine, efficacious

Love, unfolding man's unity with God through Christ Jesus the Way-shower; and we acknowledge that man is saved through Christ, through Truth, Life, and Love as demonstrated by the Galilean Prophet in healing the sick and overcoming sin and death.

5. We acknowledge that the crucifixion of Jesus and his resurrection served to uplift faith to understand eternal Life, even the allness of Soul, Spirit, and the nothingness of matter.

6. And we solemnly promise to watch, and pray for that Mind to be in us which was also in Christ Jesus; to do unto others as we would have them do unto us; and to be merciful, just, and pure.[264]

Also from *Science and Health*, the "Scientific Statement of Being" is read each week in Churches of Christ, Scientist, throughout the world:

> "There is no life, truth, intelligence, nor substance in matter. All is infinite Mind and its infinite manifestation, for God is All-in-all. Spirit is immortal Truth, matter is mortal error. Spirit is the real and eternal. Matter is the unreal and temporal. Spirit is God, and man is His image and likeness. Therefore, man is not material, he is spiritual."[265]

In addition to *Science and Health*, the Christian Science Publishing Society publishes several magazines, each of which contains verified accounts of healing through the application of the teachings of Christian Science. While many of these healings involve healings of diseases and

---

264 Eddy. *Science and Health with Key to the Scriptures*, 497.
265 Eddy. *Science and Health with Key to the Scriptures*, 468.

other physical conditions, others involve the resolution of various life challenges.

Basic Practices

Fundamental to the practice of Christian Science is an appreciation of every individual's unique relationship with God, and an acknowledgement of the uniqueness of each person's spiritual journey. Nothing in Christian Science teaching or practice supports or justifies interference with an individual's prerogative to make decisions about his or her health care or any other aspect of daily life.

- Sunday worship services include music, singing, prayer, and readings from the Bible and *Science and Health*.
- Wednesday testimony meetings are similar to the Sunday services but also include people sharing their own experiences and practical "how to's" of healing.
- Christian Scientists provide Reading Rooms, which serve as bookstores and libraries, in communities throughout the world.

Principles for Clinical Care
Dietary Issues

- Christian Science teaching has no dietary prescriptions or proscriptions. Diet is a matter of individual choice.

General Medical Beliefs

- The importance of individual choice is a hallmark of the practice of Christian Science. Each individual has his or her own relationship to God, and each individual will make his or her own decision as to what best meets the need at the moment, based on prayer and, perhaps, consultation with loved ones.

- Many, if not most, Christian Scientists have come to rely on prayer as a curative measure.
- Consider the possibility of retesting the patient or reevaluating an impending procedure after the patient has had time to pray for healing.
- Questions relating to diagnosis, treatment, birth, death, or any other issue arising in the health care setting are always an individual or family decision.
- A Christian Scientist who enters a medical care facility voluntarily will likely accept conventional medical treatment.
- A Christian Scientist seeking conventional medical treatment may ask that drugs/therapy be kept to a minimum.
- A Christian Scientist request to decline some aspects of medical care should be honored.
- Therapeutic choices are always left to the individual, in accord with applicable law.
- Christian Science practitioners can be consulted on spiritual/theological topics and Christian Science nurses can be consulted for nonmedical physical care (*see* information in Christian Science Practitioners and Nurses).

CHRISTIAN SCIENCE PRACTITIONERS AND NURSES

Eddy established a professional infrastructure to support the practice of Christian Science healing. Christian Science practitioners heal through the prayer-based approach taught in Christian Science. Christian Science nurses offer skilled physical (nonmedical) care to those requiring assistance while they seek healing through Christian Science treatment. A worldwide directory of Christian Science nurses and practitioners can be found in the church's monthly magazine,

the *Christian Science Journal*, or online (http://christianscience.com/prayer-and-health/talk-with-someone-or-get-help/christian-science-practitioners).

Specific Medical Issues

- **Abortion**: Issues such as abortion are individual and/or family decisions.
- **Advance Directives**: In a case of incapacity, it should be explored whether or not a Christian Scientist has legally empowered another individual to make health care decisions on his or her behalf. Many Christian Scientists are likely to have taken such a step, but without first consulting a medical professional.
- **Birth Control**: Issues such as birth control are individual and/or family decisions.
- **Blood Transfusions**: Issues such as blood transfusions are individual and/or family decisions.
- **Circumcision**: Circumcision is an individual and/or family decision.
- **In Vitro Fertilization**: The Church does not have an official position on in vitro fertilization. This issue is an individual and/or family decision.
- **Stem Cell Research**: The Church does not have an official position on stem cell research for therapeutic purposes. This issue is an individual and/or family decision.
- **Vaccinations**: For more than 100 years, Christian Science prayer has been effective in both preventing and healing infectious diseases. Communicable disease is a serious issue that is not taken lightly by Christian Scientists. For decades, Christian Scientists have a long record of notifiying and staying in close touch with public health authorities when there are cases of infectious disease. Their diligence in this matter is not simply a

matter of obeying the law, but out of Christian concern for their neighbor. Where there is an accommodation in the law regarding vaccinations for those with sincerely held religious beliefs, the choice to utilize that accommodation is an individual and/or family decision.

- **Withholding/Withdrawing Life Support**: Issues such as last wishes (e.g., withholding/withdrawing life support) are individual and/or family decisions.

Gender and Personal Issues

- Christian Scientists and their families make their own decisions concerning gender and personal issues.

Principles for Spiritual Care through the Cycles of Life
Concepts of Living and Dying for Spiritual Support

- The human condition is understood to be the outgrowth of thought. When through prayer an individual gains a clearer understanding of his or her identity as the "image and likeness" of an all-loving God with whom there is an unbroken relationship, healing occurs.
- Death is a transitional stage of experience; a person's life and identity continue beyond this transition.
- God is always governing His/Her children in perfect harmony.
- God is only good and never sends or sanctions disease or death.
- Each individual is spiritual and reflects the goodness of God.
- God and His/Her creation are inseparable and coexist eternally.

During Birth

- Christian Scientists do not see birth as a medical condition but, rather, as a natural event.
- There are no prescribed religious rituals surrounding the birth event.
- Christian Scientists can and do choose different forms of child birthing, such as home birth and/or state certified midwives, but are known for staying within the bounds of what is required by law.

During Illness

Physicians, nurses, mental health professionals, chaplains, and other providers will find that there are numerous, meaningful ways that they can show support for their Christian Scientist patients. Of course, the best way to ascertain what would be most helpful in any circumstance is to ask the individual patient. Some of the following might be requested by a patient, or could be offered by the health care professional:

- Providing the patient time and a quiet space to pray in the various stages of diagnosis and treatment.
- Facilitating the patient's contact with a Christian Science practitioner. A worldwide directory of Christian Science practitioners can be found online (http://christianscience.com/prayer-and-health/talk-with-someone-or-get-help/christian-science-practitioners).
- Making sure that the patient has access to the Bible and *Science and Health with Key to the Scriptures* by Mary Baker Eddy.
- Reading aloud requested passages from these books (or other Christian Science literature) to the patient.

During End of Life

- In Christian Science, there are no specified "last rites."

- Ask patient and/or family how you can best support them during this time.
- In a case of incapacity, it should be explored whether or not a Christian Scientist has legally empowered another individual to make health care decisions on his or her behalf. Many Christian Scientists are likely to have taken such a step, but without first consulting a medical professional.

Care of the Body
- Disposition of the body and/or autopsy is an individual and/or family decision.
- Donation for medical research is an individual and/or family decision.

Organ and Tissue Donation
- Organ and/or tissue donation is an individual and/or family decision. It may be preferable for a chaplain and/or nurse who are trained designated requesters to be consulted for assistance.

Scriptures, Inspirational Readings, and Prayers
In *Science and Health*, Mary Baker Eddy gave what she called the "spiritual sense" of the Lord's Prayer, which is read during the Sunday service in Churches of Christ, Scientist, throughout the world; and is a source of comfort and healing.[266]

Our Father which art in heaven,
Our Father-Mother God, all-harmonious,
Hallowed be Thy name.
Adorable One.
Thy kingdom come.
*Thy kingdom is come; Thou art
ever-present.*
Thy will be done in earth, as it is in heaven.
*Enable us to know, – as in heaven, so on
earth, – God is omnipotent, supreme.*
Give us this day our daily bread;
*Give us grace for to-day; feed the famished
affections;*
And forgive us our debts, as we forgive our debtors.
And Love is reflected in love;
And lead us not into temptation, but deliver us from evil;
*And God leadeth us not into temptation,
but delivereth us from sin, disease, and
death.*
For Thine is the kingdom, and the power, and the glory, forever.
*For God is infinite, all-power, all Life,
Truth, Love, over all, and All.*

For more inspirational readings from the Bible, *Science and Health with Key to the Scriptures*, and articles from the Christian Science periodicals, *see* www.spirituality.com.

---

266 Eddy. *Science and Health with Key to the Scriptures*, 16–17.

Church of God Movement (Anderson, IN)

A united church for a divided world, where Christian experience makes you a member.[267]

Prepared by:
Barry L. Callen
Special Assistant to the General Director, Church of God Ministries, Inc.
Anderson, IN

History and Facts

Following the Civil War in the United States, the religious scene was dominated by a neglect and even denial of much that had previously been held as basic within the Christian community. The Church of God movement (Anderson) emerged at this time as part of the larger Holiness Movement. It was a "reformation movement" seeking to "come out" of the competitive and compromising chaos of divisive denominationalism. A primary pioneer leader was Daniel S. Warner (1842–1895). His biography is titled *It's God's Church!* (by Barry L. Callen, Warner Press, 1995).

The reforming Christians of the early Church of God movement intended to pioneer a better way for the church. They spoke of the "early morning light" shining again in the "evening time" of the church's troubled history. These "early" and "evening" references were to the original apostolic church, now being recovered prior to the assumed nearness of Christ's return. These early Church of God Christians sensed a divine commission to accept fully the apostolic faith as defined by the New Testament and to fulfill the church's mission by reemphasizing an open and free fellowship of sanctified and unified believers. They spoke of the Bible being their only creed and the church being the family of all the redeemed. They reached their hands "to every blood-washed one," that is, they wished to be in fellowship with all Christians (those who have accepted their forgiveness through the blood of Jesus) regardless of church affiliations.

Today, the Church of God movement is a fellowship of about 625 000 persons worshipping in more than 5000 congregations located in 85 countries. Administrative offices in North America are in Anderson, Indiana. They exist to serve local congregations, not act as an authoritarian denominational headquarters. The movement recently published a book summarizing its basic teachings and practices (Barry L. Callen, *Following Our Lord*, Warner Press, 2008).

---

267 Quote provided by Barry L. Callen, author of this chapter.

Basic Teachings

One historian of the Church of God movement, John W. V. Smith,[268] summarized the core teaching of the movement's earliest leaders. They affirmed:

- The Protestant precept that the Bible is the sole foundation of the Christian faith.
- The basic conviction that religion, for the Christian, is essentially experiential.
- That God was calling them to proclaim and to model the visible earthly expression of God's one, holy, catholic church.
- That the church could not be equated with any existing denomination. They had received "light on the church." The light was that the church is to be holy, unified, and not controlled by any creed, structure, or tradition.
- That they were participants in the fulfillment of a segment of divine destiny for all humanity. They understood their role as being the heralds of God's ultimate will for the church.

The Church of God movement has not developed denominational distinctives framed in official and mandatory creedal statements – typical denominational actions that tend to divide Christians unnecessarily. It claims no special revelations beyond the Bible and affirms all major elements of what would be called "orthodox" Christianity as stated, for instance, in the *Apostles' Creed*.

I believe in God, the Father almighty, creator of heaven and earth,
I believe in Jesus Christ, His only Son, our Lord.
Who was conceived by the power of the Holy Spirit;
Born of the virgin Mary;
Suffered under Pontius Pilate;
Was crucified, died, and buried.
He descended into hell (or the realm of the dead).
On the third day he rose again.
He ascended into heaven and is seated at the right hand of the Father.
He will come again to judge the living and the dead.
I believe in the Holy Spirit,
The holy catholic (universal) church,
The communion of saints,
The forgiveness of sins,
The resurrection of the body and the life everlasting. Amen.

The booklet titled "We Believe" authored by the faculty of Anderson School of Theology (seminary of the Church of God), concludes with the following – a fitting summary of the believing tradition of the Church of God movement:[269]

In devotion to Christ as the head of the church, we desire to be a biblical people, a people who worship the triune God, a people transformed by the grace of God, a people of the kingdom of God, a people committed to building up the one, universal church of God, and a people who, in God's love, care for the whole world.

The goals of the movement are still serious discipleship, a unified church, and sharing the good news of Jesus Christ with the

---

268 Smith, J. (1980). *The Quest for Holiness and Unity.* Anderson, IN: Warner Press, 81–100.

269 Faculty of Anderson University School of Theology. (1979). *We Believe: A Statement of Conviction on the Occasion of the Centennial of the Church of God Reformation Movement.* Anderson, IN: Anderson University School of Theology. No page numbers in booklet.

whole world. Rather than speculating about some "millennium" of Christ's future reign on earth, the emphasis is on faithful life now, in the power and on behalf of the Spirit of God.

Basic Practices

Merle D. Strege, current church historian of the Church of God movement, speaks of the church's practices as the elements of the church's social and public life that are pursued because of the ends for which the church exists.[270] The basic practices of congregations of the Church of God movement include especially:

- Regular corporate and private worship of God.
- The acts of baptism (the immersing of non-infant believers), the Lord's Supper, and foot washing. These sacramental practices tell the stories of individual incorporation into the church, the basis of the faith itself (the life, death, and resurrection of Jesus) and the resulting life of humble service.
- Acts of love to church members, neighbors, and "enemies" alike. Compassion and justice are essential components of Christlike love.
- Programs of Christian education that assist believers to be mature disciples.
- Stewardship of time, talents, and resources that reflects life priorities.
- Focus on telling the good news of Jesus Christ to the world – programs of evangelism and world mission.

---

270 Strege, M. (1993). *Tell Me Another Tale*. Anderson, IN: Warner Press, 3. The bulleted list which follows is not taken specifically from this reference; it is the author of this chapter's general overview of practices.

Principles for Clinical Care
Dietary Issues

- The Church of God does not have specific teachings regarding eating habits and religious beliefs. Moderation in all things is the typical rule.
- Fasting is practiced on occasion for spiritual and/or bodily health.
- The use of alcoholic beverages is avoided typically, with high sensitivity to the personal and social damage caused by their abuse.
- The general goal is to respect and care for the body, which is understood to be the temple of the Holy Spirit.

General Medical Beliefs

- There is a strong tradition of divine healing, but also an appreciation of modern medical technology that is encouraged whenever the quality of life can be preserved and enhanced. Such technology is a gift of God. God is the Great Physician; human health care providers are instruments of God.
- The use of tobacco in any form is opposed because of its harmful effects on the body.

Specific Medical Issues

- **Abortion**: There is opposition to abortion on demand, recognizing that the unborn fetus is a living human being and thus should be protected. Christian compassion should be extended both to life before birth and to the lives thus preserved.
- **Advance Directives**: Persons are encouraged to express their desires for end-of-life decisions in the form of "advance directives."
- **Birth Control**: In the name of radical faith in the power and faithfulness of God, the earliest phase of the tradition of the Church of God found many believers

resisting the use of medicine altogether, preferring instead faith in the Great Physician. A more wholesome balance of faith and medicine soon evolved. The general result of the theological perspectives of this movement in recent decades evidences few if any special prohibitions regarding the use of medicine. This issue is left as a matter of personal conscience and preference.

- **Blood Transfusions**: There are no religious reservations regarding blood transfusions.
- **Circumcision**: Circumcision of newborn males is often chosen by parents, but for reasons other than religious ones.
- **In Vitro Fertilization**: The Church has issued no statement on in vitro fertilization. It is an individual decision.
- **Stem Cell Research**: The Church has issued no statement on stem cell research for therapeutic purposes. It is an individual decision.
- **Vaccinations**: The Church has issued no specific statement on vaccinations; it is an individual decision.
- **Withholding/Withdrawing Life Support**: Christians are to exercise freedom of conscience concerning the use of life support systems.

Gender and Personal Issues
- There is active encouragement of personal modesty in dress and behavior as a wise means of expressing Christian holiness.
- Affirmed is the equal worth of women and men and rejection of practices that support superiority of one over the other.
- Christians are called to demonstrate love, compassion, and counsel to assist disabled persons and their families, avoiding any implication that the disabled person is a second-class citizen.

- Sexuality is a gift from God that is to be affirmed and celebrated, although practiced lovingly only within the sacred bounds of marriage.
- Persons practicing homosexuality are viewed as persons of worth who should be treated with care and respect. Even so, it is assumed that the practice of homosexuality is incompatible with Church of God teaching and Christlike living.

Principles for Spiritual Care through the Cycles of Life
Concepts of Living and Dying for Spiritual Support
- Human life is God's good creation and thus sacred. All human beings are created in the image of God. The body is a gift of God.
- God is the ultimate source of all life, health, and healing.
- All people are called to faithful living in this earthly life, including care of the body as part of God's creation.
- The rites of passage – birth, baptism, marriage and death – are to be celebrated within the context of the church. As individuals make covenantal commitments, for instance marriage and baptism, the church enters into covenantal commitment with the individuals or couple to pray for them, love them, and support them.
- Knowing that life in this world is limited should motivate Christians to "redeem the time." Every moment should be made to count for the glory of God, even the moments of sickness and death.
- Death is a sign of one's mortal life and human finitude. While individuals may seek to prolong meaningful life, death should not be feared. It is something that

all must experience. Through the death and resurrection of Jesus Christ, we are assured of eternal life.

During Birth

- As stated earlier, circumcision of newborn males is often chosen by parents, but for reasons other than religious ones.
- The Church of God dedicates infants, offering them back to God. The family and congregation dedicate themselves to nurturing and educating the child in the faith.

During Illness

- Illness is not to be understood as the punishment of God for sin. It is part of one's mortal existence and comes to believers and nonbelievers alike.
- "Laying on of hands" and anointing with oil is practiced because it is biblically recommended. Typically, this is done by the patient's pastor, but others may do it when the pastor is not available – including chaplains or health care professionals. Often family and close friends share in this act of prayer and faith.
- Physical healing can come through the exercise of faith and prayer, especially when supported by the community of believers. Whether physical healing occurs in this life or ultimate healing occurs in the life to come is within the provision of sovereign grace according to the wisdom of God.
- Patients may receive comfort from the reading of scriptures or other devotional material, listening to religious music, watching televised worship services of their own or a similar tradition.

During End of Life

- All efforts are made to ensure the comfort and dignity of the dying and the provision of pastoral care for the dying and their families.
- Persons are encouraged to express their desires for end-of-life decisions in the form of "advance directives."
- Dying persons and their families should avail themselves of all medical technology, but are under no religious or moral obligation to continue life-sustaining treatments when they cease to be beneficial or are being used merely to prolong the process of dying.
- The use of palliative care and hospice services, when appropriate, is encouraged.
- Christians are called to live in constant readiness because the timing and circumstances of death are not theirs to know or determine. A consistent life of faithfulness and obedience to God, rather than deathbed conversion, is the best way to prepare for death and the life to come.
- Baptism is the expected act of public witness of a believer's conversion to Jesus Christ. Should such conversion occur near the time of death, however, baptism is not essential for salvation to be assured.
- Often a dying person will find comfort in having planned his or her own funeral with the pastor and/or family members. Such planning should be honored as much as is feasible.
- Customs related to dying vary by region and/or culture. There are no required sacramental rites for the dying, although persons or families may request Holy Communion, sacred music, and so forth.

Care of the Body

- The Church of God has no specific rituals or beliefs regarding care of the deceased's body. Whatever is done should always show respect.

- Decisions regarding disposition of the body should be made according to the preferences of the family, in consideration of the wishes of the deceased. Both burial and cremation are acceptable Christian choices.
- Donation of the body for medical research is an individual/family decision.

Organ and Tissue Donation

- While having no specific policy, the Church of God respects the practice of organ and tissue donation as an act of self-sacrificing love. It may be preferable for a chaplain and/or nurse who are trained designated requesters to be consulted for assistance.

Scriptures, Inspirational Readings, and Prayers

THE USE OF SCRIPTURES, HYMNS, AND PRAYERS

Church of God people are a Bible-reading, praying, and singing people. Often, the dying person will be comforted by hearing particular biblical passages read, such as those glorifying God (Psalm 24), assuring guidance and protection (Psalm 23), and speaking of an eternal home with God (John 14:1–4).

READINGS DURING ILLNESS OR END-OF-LIFE PROCESS

The following can be read by family, friends, clergy, and health care professionals. (All scripture quotations are from the New Revised Standard Version.)

The earth is the Lord's and all that is in it, the world and those who live in it; for he has founded it on the seas,

and established it on the rivers. Who shall ascend the hill of the Lord? And who shall stand in his holy place? Those who have clean hands and pure hearts, who do not lift up their souls to what is false, and do not swear deceitfully. They will receive blessing from the Lord, and vindication from the God of their salvation. Such is the company of those who seek him, who seek the face of the God of Jacob.

Lift up your heads, O gates! And be lifted up O ancient doors! That the king of glory may come in. Who is the King of glory? The Lord, strong and mighty, the Lord, mighty in battle. Lift up your heads, O gates! And be lifted up, O ancient doors! That the King of glory may come in. Who is this King of glory? The Lord of hosts, he is the King of glory.

—Psalm 24

READINGS DURING END-OF-LIFE PROCESS

The following can be read by family, friends, clergy, and health care professionals. (All scripture quotations are from the New Revised Standard Version.)

The Lord is my shepherd, I shall not want.
He makes me lie down in green pastures; he restores my soul.
He leads me in right paths for his name's sake.
Even though I walk through the darkest valley, I fear no evil;
for you are with me; your rod and your staff – they comfort me.
You prepare a table before me in the presence of my enemies;

you anoint my head with oil; my cup
overflows.
Surely goodness and mercy shall
follow me all the days of my life,
and I shall dwell in the house of the
Lord my whole life long.

—Psalm 23

Do not let your hearts be troubled.
Believe in God, believe also in me.
In my Father's house there are many
dwelling places. If it were not so,
would I have told you that I go to
prepare a place for you?
And if I go and prepare a place for
you, I will come again and will take
you to myself, so that where I am,
there you may be also.
And you know the way to the place
where I am going.

—John 14:1–4

Prayer is always central. Common is the
prayer of faith for physical healing, or at
least for comfort and even joy until final
healing is experienced beyond this mortal
life. Always appropriate is the Lord's Prayer
found in Matt. 6: 9–14.

PRAYER DURING ILLNESS OR END-OF-LIFE PROCESS
This prayer can be offered by family, friends,
clergy, and health care professionals.

The Lord's Prayer
Our Father in heaven, hallowed be
your name.

Your kingdom come, Your will be
done,
On earth as it is in heaven.
Give us this day our daily bread.
And forgive us our debts,
As we also have forgiven our debtors.
And do not bring us to the time of
trial,
But rescue us from the evil one.
For Thine is the kingdom, and the
power, and the glory, forever!
Amen.

HYMN FOR END OF LIFE
Mature believers usually have favorite
hymns that bring comfort and assurance.
Singing or hearing these sung by others is
common practice, both during the dying
process and later for the sake of family and
friends during the funeral service. The hymnal of the church is the key source (*Worship
the Lord: Hymnal of the Church of God*,
Warner Press, 1989). One example is the
hymn by Charles Wesley titled "Christ the
Lord is Risen Today" (p. 203). The words
from verses two and three rejoice in the victory over death and the hope of life eternal.

Christ the Lord is Risen Today
Lives again our glorious King.
Where, O death, is now thy sting?
Dying once, He all doth save,
Where thy victory, O grave?
Love's redeeming work is done,
Fought the fight, the battle won,
Death in vain forbids Him rise,
Christ has opened paradise.

Episcopal Church

O God of unchangeable power and eternal light: Look favorably on your
whole Church, that wonderful and sacred mystery; by the effectual working
of your providence, carry out in tranquility the plan of salvation; let the
whole world see and know that things which were cast down are being
raised up, and things which had grown old are being made new, and that
all things are being brought to their perfection by him through whom
all things were made, your Son Jesus Christ our Lord. Amen.[271]

Prepared by:
Marshall S. Scott, MDiv, BCC
Episcopal Priest and Chaplain, Saint Luke's South
  Hospital
Overland Park, KS

Reviewed and approved by:
The Right Reverend Barry Howe
Bishop of the Diocese of West Missouri
Kansas City, MO

History and Facts

The Episcopal Church in the United States of America is the American daughter church of the Church of England. With the Church of England and other daughter churches around the world the Episcopal Church participates in the worldwide Anglican Communion. Although considered comparable in many ways with the Roman Catholic communion, the Anglican Communion has no central figure or institution of jurisdictional authority.

Rather, the Anglican churches are united in a "communion of love." Asked what held the Anglican Communion together, Archbishop Desmond Tutu of South Africa said, "We meet." Joint efforts among Anglicans are facilitated by the office of the Archbishop of Canterbury, and by meetings of the Lambeth Conference, the Anglican Consultative Council, and the Primates' Meeting.

The Episcopal Church is rooted in the Church of the English Reformation. The Church in England separated politically from the Roman Catholic Church under Henry VIII, and became the Church of England under Edward VI. The Church of England was brought to North America with the foundation of the thirteen colonies, and eventually it became the established church. With the American Revolution the Church in America separated from the Church of England, and reestablished

---

271 Guilbert, C. (Custodian of the *Standard Book of Common Prayer*). (1990). *The Book of Common Prayer*. New York, NY: Oxford University Press, 291. This prayer is the final Collect of the Great Vigil of Easter. It is also the final Solemn Collect of the Proper Liturgy for Good Friday, and is the central collect for all ordinations in the Episcopal Church (bishops, priests, and deacons). This prayer is both central in the life of the Church and as representative of the Episcopal Church in many ways as anything else.

itself as the Protestant Episcopal Church in the USA. For most of its history it has been known more commonly simply as the Episcopal Church.

The Episcopal Church grew as the nation grew, spreading into new territories as they were opened to settlement. While not noted as a "missionary church," the church was especially successful in ministering among the Native American tribes in northern states. While other church bodies divided during the Civil War, the Episcopal Church did not. Efforts were made to form a separate body for the Confederacy, and several Episcopal bishops served as both chaplains and officers in the Confederate Army. However, that effort was abandoned with the fall of the Confederacy.

Basic Teachings

In 1886, bishops of the Episcopal Church accepted four principles as describing "inherent parts" of "principles we believe to be the substantial deposit of Christian Faith and Order committed by Christ and his Apostles to the Church unto the end of the world." These principles, with slight changes, were adopted by the 1888 Lambeth Conference, the gathering each decade of all the bishops of the Anglican Communion, as a basis for all ecumenical conversation. These principles taken from the *Book of Common Prayer*[272] were:

- The Holy Scriptures of the Old and New Testaments, as "containing all things necessary to salvation," and as being the rule and ultimate standard of faith.
- The Apostles' Creed, as the Baptismal Symbol; and the Nicene Creed, as the sufficient statement of the Christian faith.

---

272 Guilbert. *The Book of Common Prayer*, 877–878.

- The two Sacraments ordained by Christ Himself – Baptism and the Supper of the Lord – ministered with unfailing use of Christ's words of Institution, and of the elements ordained by Him.
- The Historic Episcopate, locally adapted in the methods of its administration to the varying needs of the nations and peoples called of God into the Unity of His Church.

These principles are called collectively "The Chicago-Lambeth Quadrilateral." Most Episcopalians would acknowledge that these principles are essential, if not sufficient, for understanding the Episcopal expression of the Christian faith.

As expressions of these principles, Episcopalians would affirm the following.
- The doctrine of the Trinity: one God known in three Persons of Father, Son, and Holy Spirit.
- The doctrine of Incarnation: that Jesus is God made flesh, both fully human and fully divine.
- From baptism the Holy Spirit dwells in the Christian, empowering the person for ministry and growth in Christ.
- The Episcopal Church is a part of the whole Body of Christ, which consists of all the baptized.
- Two sacraments are commanded by Christ for all Christians: Baptism with water in the name of the Trinity; and Holy Eucharist (Communion) with the elements of bread and wine.
- Baptism is appropriate for infants as well as adults.
- Holy Eucharist is appropriate for all baptized members, and in some congregations children may be admitted to communion.
- The ministry of the Church is carried

out by ministers in four orders: bishops, priests, deacons, and laypersons.

Basic Practices

- Episcopalians value communal worship, and will gather on Sundays and at other times to hear preaching, study scripture, receive communion, sing hymns, and pray.
- The sharing of one's faith (evangelism) is of great importance as in many denominations. In the Episcopal Church, it is communicated through loving actions, talking about personal spiritual experiences, reading scriptures, and invitations to share in worship.
- The Eucharist (meaning "thanksgiving"), also called Holy Communion or the Lord's Supper, is considered a sacrament and an integral part of weekly worship. It is a liturgical reenactment of the crucifixion, death, burial, and resurrection of Jesus, in which Christians eat bread (to commemorate the broken body of Jesus) and drink wine (to symbolize Jesus' shed blood). This can be done during communal worship or in other settings and is celebrated and usually administered by ordained clergy.
- Baptism is the ceremonial act which includes naming of the child. It commonly includes christening, which is anointing with oil blessed for the purpose by the bishop.
- Sacrament of baptism is usually by pouring water over the head of the person to be baptized, although immersion is acceptable.
- Baptism and Eucharist are celebrated by ordained clergy, who may be assisted by laypersons.
- Prayer, meditation, and scripture are the

fundamental spiritual practices for many Episcopalians. The many forms of these practices include: reading and/or silent contemplation upon scripture or doctrinal beliefs and prayers of various kinds – petition, healing, repentance for unethical thoughts and actions, praise, worship, and thanksgiving to God.
- Mission work is important to Episcopalians. These acts of service take the forms of working for social justice with marginalized peoples, charitable giving to provide food, building, and educational programs for the poor, volunteerism, and so forth. Mission work is also an intentional witness to one's faith through proclamation and teaching.
- Social action and pursuit of justice for all people are strongly encouraged.

Principles for Clinical Care
Dietary Issues

- The Episcopal Church has no dietary restrictions with respect to religious beliefs. Some Episcopalians may choose to fast before receiving the Holy Eucharist.

General Medical Beliefs

- Episcopalians believe that God is the ultimate source of all life, health, and healing.
- Episcopalians refer to God as the Great Physician.
- Episcopalians affirm the validity of traditional Western medical procedures in the treatment of illness and disease.

Specific Medical Issues

- **Abortion**: Abortion is primarily a decision between woman and physician. While it is always regrettable, it is acceptable to protect the physical and mental health of the mother. It is not acceptable for birth control, sex selection, or convenience.

- **Advance Directives**: The 70th General Convention of the Episcopal Church (1991), Resolution A093, states that advance written directives (so-called "living wills," "declarations concerning medical treatment" and "durable powers of attorney setting forth medical declarations") that make a person's wishes concerning the continuation or withholding or removing of life-sustaining systems should be encouraged, and this Church's members are encouraged to execute such advance written directives during good health and competence and that the execution of such advance written directives constitutes loving and moral acts.

- **Birth Control**: The Episcopal Church recognizes the right of individuals to use any natural or safe artificial means of conception control, and to the full range of affordable, acceptable, safe, and noncoercive contraceptive and reproductive health care services.

- **Blood Transfusions**: The Episcopal Church has no reservations about blood transfusions.

- **Circumcision**: Episcopalians in Western societies have requested circumcision of male infants for cultural, not religious, reasons.

- **In Vitro Ferilization**: The Episcopal Church has no reservations about in vitro fertilization and birth control.

- **Stem Cell Research**: Reproductive cloning is not morally permissible. Somatic Gene Transfer for therapeutic purposes is morally acceptable.

- **Vaccinations**: The General Convention has not made a specific statement, but based on statements regarding the importance of health care for children, and especially preventive care, the General Convention would support vaccination for all children. The Episcopal Church considers as valid "for example and instruction, but not to establish doctrine." Eccles. 38:4: "The Lord created medicines out of the earth, and the sensible will not despise them."

- **Withholding/Withdrawing Life Support**: Withholding/withdrawing life support in medically futile cases does not violate teachings of the Episcopal Church. It is an individual decision.

Gender and Personal Issues

- The Episcopal Church as a faith tradition has no prescriptions or proscriptions with respect to gender and personal issues.

Principles for Spiritual Care through the Cycles of Life

Concepts of Living and Dying for Spiritual Support

- Life is sacred.
- Death is something all must experience and should not be feared.
- Death is not perceived as sleep. People can be traumatized by the connection between death and sleep and, thus, afraid to go to sleep. This is especially true with children.
- The soul and spirit of the deceased ascend to heaven at the moment of death, according to most traditions.
- Resurrection of the physical body and the reunion of spirit, soul and body in some form will happen at the Second Coming of Jesus. Humanity, all living creatures and the entire cosmos will be healed and restored to a state of perfection.

During Birth

- Baptism or christening may be requested by family for a living baby. The chaplain or clergy should be consulted for assistance.
- As stated earlier, Episcopalians in Western societies have requested circumcision of male infants for cultural, not religious, reasons.

During Illness

- Patients may receive comfort from the reading of scriptures or other devotional material, listening to religious music, watching televised worship services of their own or a similar tradition. Patients may request Holy Communion. The chaplain or clergy should be consulted for assistance.
- Patients may receive comfort from healing prayers. These can be offered by health care professionals. Patients from some traditions, however, may ask for healing prayer to be connected with "anointing with oil" or the "the laying on of hands." The chaplain or clergy should be consulted for assistance for these requests.
- Patients may request baptism. In the clinical setting, sprinkling is an acceptable mode of baptism for Episcopalians. The chaplain or clergy should be consulted for assistance.

During End of Life

- The patient or the family may request baptism. The chaplain or clergy should be consulted for assistance.
- The patient or the family may request Holy Communion. The chaplain or clergy should be consulted for assistance.
- Family may wish to view the body of the deceased in the hospital room or the chapel. Nurse and chaplain should be consulted for assistance.

- Family may request prayers for the deceased. These can be offered by the chaplain, clergy, family, friends, and health care professionals.

Care of the Body

- Disposition and embalming are individual decisions. Cremation is now the choice of many Episcopalians. The chaplain and the funeral home director should be consulted for assistance.
- Autopsy is an individual decision unless required by law. The chaplain and/or nurse should be consulted for assistance.
- Donation for medical research is an individual decision. The chaplain and/or nurse should be consulted for assistance. Advance planning for such donations is required by most receiving organizations. Last-minute donations are usually not possible.

Organ and Tissue Donation

- Organ and tissue donation is permitted and is an individual decision. It may be preferable for a chaplain and/or nurse who are trained designated requesters to be consulted for assistance.

Scriptures, Inspirational Readings, and Prayers

READINGS DURING ILLNESS

These can be read by family, friends, clergy, and health care professionals. (All scripture quotations are from the New Revised Standard Version.)

The Lord is my shepherd I shall not want.
He makes me lie down in green pastures; he restores my soul.
He leads me in right paths for his name's sake.

Even though I walk through the
darkest valley, I fear no evil;
for you are with me; your rod and
your staff – they comfort me.
You prepare a table before me in the
presence of my enemies;
you anoint my head with oil; my cup
overflows.
Surely goodness and mercy shall
follow me all the days of my life,
and I shall dwell in the house of the
Lord my whole life long.

—Psalm 23

We know that all things work
together for good …
For I am convinced that neither
death, nor life, nor angels, nor
rulers, nor things present, nor things
to come, nor powers, nor height,
nor depth, nor anything else in all
creation, will be able to separate
us from the love of God in Christ
Jesus our Lord.

—Rom. 8:28a, 38–39

READINGS DURING END-OF-LIFE PROCESS

These can be read by family, friends, clergy,
and health care professionals. (All scripture quotations are from the New Revised
Standard Version.)

I am the resurrection and the life.
Those who believe in me, even though
they die, will live, and everyone who
lives and believes in me will never die.

—John 11:25–26

Do not let your hearts be troubled.
Believe in God, believe also in me.
In my Father's house there are many
dwelling places. If it were not so,
would I have told you that I go to
prepare a place for you?
And if I go and prepare a place for
you, I will come again and will take
you to myself, so that where I am,
there you may be also.

—John 14:1–3

PRAYER DURING END-OF-LIFE PROCESS

These prayers can be offered by family,
friends, clergy, and health care professionals.
For the patient:

Into your hands, O merciful
Savior, we commend your servant
_____. Acknowledge, we
humbly beseech you, a sheep of your
own fold, a lamb of your own flock,
a sinner of your own redeeming.
Receive (him or her) into the arms
of your mercy, into the blessed rest
of everlasting peace, and into the
glorious company of the saints in
light. Amen.

For the family:

Almighty God, look with pity upon
the sorrows of your servants for
whom we pray. Remember them,
Lord, in mercy; nourish them with
patience; comfort them with a
sense of your goodness; lift up your
countenance upon them; and give
them peace; through Jesus Christ our
Lord. Amen.

Evangelical Covenant Church

A communion of congregations gathered by God, united in Christ, and empowered by the Holy Spirit to obey the great commandment and the great commission.[273]

Prepared by:
Thomas B. Anderson
Pastor, Community Covenant Church
Lenexa, KS

Reviewed and approved by:
Ken Carlson
Superintendent, Midwest Covenant Conference
Omaha, NE

History and Facts

The Evangelical Covenant Church was founded in 1885. Its roots are anchored in historical Christianity, the Protestant Reformation, the biblical instruction of the Lutheran Church of Sweden, the great spiritual awakenings of the eighteenth and nineteenth centuries, and the more recent renewal movements in North America. Historically the church has emphasized missions, youth ministry, Christian education and evangelism. The Evangelical Covenant Church is committed to reaching across boundaries of race, ethnicity, culture, gender, age, and status in the cultivation of communities of faith and service.

The Evangelical Covenant Church adheres to the affirmation of the Protestant Reformation regarding the Bible. It confesses that the Holy Scripture, the Old and the New Testaments, is the Word of God and the only perfect rule for faith, doctrine, and conduct. It affirms the historic confessions of the Christian Church, particularly the *Apostles' Creed* and the *Nicene Creed*, while emphasizing the sovereignty of the Word of God over all creedal interpretations.

In continuity with the renewal movements of historic Pietism, the Evangelical Covenant Church especially cherishes the dual emphasis on the new birth and new life in Christ, believing that personal faith in Jesus Christ as Savior and Lord is the foundation for the mission of evangelism and Christian nurture. The common experience of God's grace and love in Jesus Christ continues to sustain the Evangelical Covenant Church as an interdependent body of believers that recognizes but transcends theological differences.

The Evangelical Covenant Church celebrates two divinely ordained sacraments, baptism and the Lord's Supper. Recognizing the reality of freedom in Christ, and in conscious dependence on the work of the Holy Spirit, the Church practices both the baptism of infants and believer baptism. The Evangelical Covenant Church embraces this freedom in Christ as a gift that preserves personal conviction, yet guards against an individualism that disregards the centrality of the Word of God and the mutual respon-

---

273 Quote provided by Rev. Tom Anderson, author of this chapter.

sibilities and disciplines of the spiritual community.

United States membership in the Evangelical Covenant Church stands at 116 000, with an average attendance of 161 000. Ethnic and multiethnic congregations comprise more than 21% of all Covenant Churches. Worldwide, there are 277 814 members in 2624 churches. Denominational headquarters are in Chicago, Illinois.

- The church is "Trinitarian" (belief in God the Father, God the Son, and God the Holy Spirit) and affirms a conscious dependence on the Holy Spirit.
- The church is devotional, meaning that personal scripture reading and prayer are critical to one's common life.
- It is congregational, meaning that the congregation is the highest constituted authority of the church.
- The church is pro-life.

Basic Teachings

- The Covenant Church is non-creedal, but adheres to the *Apostles' Creed*.
- It is an evangelical church, believing that "all have sinned and fallen short of the glory of God." Since people cannot save themselves, salvation must come from God. The church believes that Jesus Christ is Savior and salvation is anchored in a "Saving Event," which is the cross and resurrection of Jesus Christ. This is to be believed and received.
- The church believes the Bible (the Old and New Testaments) is the inspired Word of God, and the only perfect rule for faith, doctrine, and conduct.
- It is a reformation church, with particular emphasis on the doctrine of justification by faith through grace.
- It is committed to the whole mission of the church. The early name given to Covenanters was "Mission Friends," people who gathered together for the purpose of common mission both near and far.
- The church understands mission to include evangelism, Christian formation, and benevolent ministries of compassion and justice.
- It believes the church is the "fellowship of believers."

Basic Practices

- Christians value communal worship, and will gather on Sundays and at other times to hear preaching, study scripture, sing hymns, and pray. A variety of worship styles is offered.
- Ministries of evangelism, compassion and justice together comprise the Church's outreach. Some of the ways evangelism is communicated is through loving actions, talking about personal spiritual experiences, reading scriptures, distributing informational tracts, and discussions of doctrinal positions.
- The Lord's Supper, also called Holy Communion or Eucharist (meaning "thanksgiving"), is a powerful ordinance (sacrament or ritual). It is a liturgical reenactment of the crucifixion, death, burial, and resurrection of Jesus, in which Christians eat bread (to commemorate the broken body of Jesus) and drink wine or grape juice (to symbolize Jesus' shed blood). This can be done during communal worship or in other settings and is usually administered by ordained clergy. Communion is practiced monthly.
- Prayer, meditation, and scripture are the fundamental spiritual practices for many Christians. The many forms of these

practices include: reading and/or silent contemplation upon scripture or doctrinal beliefs and prayers of various kinds – petition, healing, repentance for unethical thoughts and actions, praise, worship, and thanksgiving to God.

- Mission work is important to Christians. These acts of service take the forms of working for social justice with marginalized peoples, charitable giving to provide food, building, and educational programs for the poor, volunteerism, and so forth. Mission work is also an intentional witness to one's faith through proclamation and teaching.
- The Great Commandment and the Great Commission are the marching orders of the church.
- The establishment of ethnic churches is a priority.
- Church growth through the planting of new churches is a priority.
- Infant baptism, infant dedication, and believers' baptism by immersion are practiced. The pastor is the servant of the church in these matters.
- Christening is the ceremonial act which includes naming of the child. It can be an official part of the ceremony of baptism or combined with infant dedication.
- Whole-life stewardship is practiced, with the emphasis on the "tithe" or 10% given to the Lord's work.
- The church understands itself as a "Fellowship of Believers" and sees itself as simply a small part of whole family of God. Words like "independent and separate" are not in the church's vocabulary.

Principles for Clinical Care
Dietary Issues
- The Covenant Church offers no dietary rules.
- Fasting is encouraged on occasion to sharpen one's prayer life.
- Self-care is encouraged; this is understood to mean physical, spiritual, and emotional care.

General Medical Beliefs
- The church believes that all healing comes from God.
- The church believes that Jesus Christ is the "Divine Physician" and that the source of healing flows from the cross and resurrection.
- The church believes in practicing the best that Western medicine has to offer.
- The church opposes any legislation that legalizes assisted suicide.

Specific Medical Issues
The Covenant Church has not created a generalized statement about its medical beliefs. However, the following statements reflect what it believes.

- **Abortion**: The church believes abortion to be wrong and grieve whenever an abortion takes place. However, it recognizes that in some tragic instances, abortion may need to be considered to safeguard the life of the mother.
- **Advance Directives**: The church encourages people to plan for "end of life issues": this means health care directives, durable power of attorney for health care decisions, and estate planning.
- **Birth Control**: The Evangelical Covenant Church holds no position on birth control. It allows individuals or couples the freedom to decide whether or not to use

birth control, the circumstances for its use, and the type of birth control to use.

- **Blood Transfusions**: The church encourages blood transfusions and the use of other blood products when the health needs of the patient require them.
- **Circumcision**: Circumcism is a matter of personal preference and the Evangelical Covenant Church takes no position on the issue. Most Covenant families choose to circumcise their boys, primarily for health and hygiene reasons.
- **In Vitro Fertilization**: The church has no specific teaching on in vitro fertilization. Any decisions related to that issue are left to individual discretion.
- **Stem Cell Research**: Regarding stem cell research, the church opposes the research for therapeutic use of human embryos, or cell lines derived from the destruction of human embryos. However, the church strongly encourages biomedical research (such as using adult stem cells for therapeutic use) that does not result in destruction of human life.
- **Vaccinations**: The church supports all vaccinations, immunizations, and flu shots. Anything that can function to prevent disease is consistent with the church's ethical practice.
- **Withholding/Withdrawing Life Support**: Concerning withholding or withdrawing life support, the church makes a distinction between assisted suicide and removing life support. When sound clinical judgment in terminal cases indicates that continued life without life support is impossible, the church supports the "Do not resuscitate order."

Gender and Personal Issues
- The dignity of every person must be honored.

- The Covenant Church ordains women and sees them as gifted and called by God.
- There is freedom in personal issues, but they are circumscribed by the teaching of scripture, the conviction of the Holy Spirit, and the greater good of the church.

Principles for Spiritual Care through the Cycles of Life
Concepts of Living and Dying for Spiritual Support
- Human life is sacred.
- Death for a believer is a graduation exercise into heaven. It is not to be feared.

During Birth
- Life begins at conception.
- Every birth is celebrated with a rose, a bulletin announcement, a CD of lullabies, and a pastoral visit.
- Miscarriages are noted and mourned and pastoral care is provided.
- The death of a baby is especially tragic and is handled with tenderness, dignity, and much care for the family.

During Illness
- The church offers the services of a parish nurse to its congregation.
- The church offers services of healing, including anointing with oil and the "laying on of hands."
- The church provides visits to patients prior to surgery or major procedures and then follow-ups after the surgery.
- Meals are brought in.
- Chaplains and counselors are valued for the role they play in providing comfort and hope.

During End of Life

- The church brings communion upon request or suggestion.
- The wishes of the dying person take precedence over the wishes of the family.
- The church encourages patients to complete "advance directives."
- The church encourages a bedside service when a decision has been made to terminate life support.
- The church affirms the importance of hospice ministry.
- Viewing of the body is a personal or family decision. The church honors the choice of the family.
- Chaplains and counselors are valued for the role they play in providing comfort and hope.
- The church assists the family in planning the service, providing a family meal, in printing the bulletin, and extending support both prior to and after the funeral.
- The church encourages funerals to be held in church.
- The church has a Stephen Ministry (a lay ministry) to care for people who suffer loss or grief.

Care of the Body

- The church encourages funerals to be held in church.
- The church has a Stephen Ministry to care for people who suffer loss or grief.
- The body is honored, treated reverently, and with great care.
- The church honors the preference of cremation or burial.
- Autopsy is an individual decision unless required by law. The chaplain and/or nurse should be consulted for assistance.
- Donation for medical research is an individual decision. The chaplain and/or nurse should be consulted for assistance.

Advance planning for such donations is required by most receiving organizations. Last-minute donations are usually not possible.

- The memory of the deceased is also treated reverently and with care.

Organ and Tissue Donation

- The church honors the choice of individuals in this matter.
- When asked, however, the church would encourage organ donation and see it as part of whole-life stewardship. It may be preferable for a chaplain and/or nurse who are trained designated requesters to be consulted for assistance.

Scriptures, Inspirational Readings, and Prayers

READINGS DURING ILLNESS

These can be read by family, friends, clergy, and health care professionals. (All scripture quotations are from the Revised Standard Version Version.)

"Cast all your cares on Him, for he cares for you."

—1 Pet. 5:7

"We are protected by the power of God through faith for a salvation ready to be revealed in the last time."

—1 Pet. 1:5

"Wait for the Lord; be strong and take heart and wait for the Lord."

—Ps. 27:14

"For I know the plans I have for you," declares the Lord, "plans to prosper you and not to harm you, plans to give you hope and a future."

—Jer. 29:11

"How precious also are your thoughts to me, O God! How great is the sum of them!
If I should count them, they would be more in number than the sand; when I awake, I am still with you."

—Ps. 139:17–18

"Look at the birds of the air; they do not sow or reap or store away in barns, and yet your heavenly Father feeds them. Are you not much more valuable than they?"

—Matt. 6:26

"For once you were not a people, but now you are the people of God. Once you had not received mercy, but now you have received mercy."

—1 Pet. 2:10

READINGS DURING END-OF-LIFE PROCESS

These can be read by family, friends, clergy, and health care professionals. (All scripture quotations are from the Revised Standard Version.)

"He will swallow up death forever. The Sovereign LORD will wipe away the tears from all faces; he will remove the disgrace of his people from all the earth. The LORD has spoken."

—Isa. 25:7b–8

"I am still confident of this: I will see the goodness of the LORD in the land of the living."

—Ps. 27:13

"For he has rescued us from the dominion of darkness and brought us into the kingdom of the Son he loves."

—Col. 1:13

"So do not fear, for I am with you; do not be dismayed, for I am your God. I will strengthen you and help you; I will uphold you with my righteous right hand."

—Isa. 41:10

"Thanks be to God who gives us the victory through Jesus Christ our Lord."

—1 Cor. 15:57

"But now, this is what the Lord says,
'he who created you, O Jacob,
he who formed you, O Israel: Fear
not, for I have redeemed you;
I have summoned you by name; you
are mine.'"

—Isa. 43:1

"What, then, shall we say in response
to this? If God is for us, who can be
against us? He who did not spare
his own Son, but gave him up for
us all;
how will he not also, along with him,
graciously give us all things?"

—Rom. 8:31–32

"For we are more than conquerors
through him who loved us and gave
his life for us."

—Rom. 8:37

"Naked I came from my mother's
womb, and naked shall I return there;
the Lord gives and the Lord takes
away, blessed be the name of the
Lord."

—Job 1:21

"Weeping may last for the night, but a
shout of joy comes in the morning."

—Ps. 30:5b

"We are hard pressed on every side,
but not crushed; perplexed, but
not in despair; persecuted, but not
abandoned; struck down, but not
destroyed. Therefore, we do not lose
heart. Though outwardly we are
wasting away, yet inwardly we are
being renewed day by day."

—2 Cor. 4:8, 9, 16

Lutheran Church

Justification is by God's grace alone (Sola Gratia), through faith alone (Sola Fide), revealed through scripture alone (Sola Scriptura)[274]

Prepared by:
The Reverend John D. Kreidler
Bishop's Associate, Central States Synod of the Evangelical Lutheran Church in America
Kansas City, MO

History and Facts

Lutheranism is a Christian faith tradition originating in the sixteenth-century Protestant Reformation based largely on the writings and action of Martin Luther and those of his immediate adherents. Lutheranism in various forms came to the United States during the European immigrations of the eighteenth, nineteenth, and twentieth centuries. Initially, Lutherans from Europe settled in the northeast, the Atlantic coast of Virginia and the Carolinas and in the Midwest. Since the arrival of the Lutheran immigrant populations, Lutheranism has spread throughout the United States.

Over the years, American Lutheranism has been represented by numerous organizational formations often referred to as *synods*, which represent either national or geographical combinations of congregations (e.g., *Wisconsin Synod* and *Missouri Synod* are commonly used abbreviated names for national churches while the national body of the *Evangelical Lutheran Church in*

America is divided into 65 synods). These organizational formations of Lutheranism have periodically broken apart based on disputes regarding doctrine and polity. On the other hand, they have come together in new organizational formations based on ministry and mission. Currently, the three largest Lutheran bodies in the United States are the *Evangelical Lutheran Church in America*, the *Lutheran Church–Missouri Synod*, and the *Wisconsin Evangelical Lutheran Synod*. Because of the nature of the separations within Lutheranism, it may be possible for some of the Lutheran bodies to relate to other Christian traditions more fully than with other Lutheran bodies (e.g., at the time of this writing, the *Evangelical Lutheran Church in America* has full communion relationships with six other Christian bodies but not with the *Lutheran Church–Missouri Synod* or the *Wisconsin Evangelical Lutheran Synod*). For most Lutherans, the local congregation is their primary reference both for teaching and practice. Therefore, the individual's personal practice may include or exclude items that are not accounted for by general Lutheran teaching and practice.

Membership in Lutheran churches is

---

274 Quote provided by Rev. John D. Kreidler, author of this section.

almost 70 million worldwide. As of 2005, there are 8 million Lutherans who are members of 28 Lutheran bodies in North America. In the United States, the distribution of these Lutheran bodies ranges from the Evangelical Lutheran Church in America which has 10 585 congregations in 47 states to bodies such as the Conservative Lutheran Association which has three congregations according to the *2006 Yearbook of American & Canadian Churches*.

Basic Teachings

The pastors and writings of the various Lutheran churches should be consulted regarding specific teachings and practices. However, what follows is generally applicable to Lutheran faith and practice.

- Lutheranism is "Trinitarian" in its belief.
- Lutheranism regards the Bible as the Word of God and, as such, is the sole rule and norm of faith. The Bible includes 66 different books divided into the old and new testaments. These writings include wisdom literature and poetry, historical writings, the books of the law as well as the four gospels, letters to the early Christian churches, and apocalyptic literature.
- The understanding of the Word of God that forms the basis of Lutheran teaching is gathered together in the *Book of Concord*, also referred to as the Lutheran Confessions. This book includes the *Apostles, Nicene and Athanasian Creeds* together with confessional documents written in the sixteenth century at the time of the separation of what would become the Lutheran Church from the Roman Catholicism.
- According to Lutheran teaching, humanity is by nature sinful. This sinfulness separates humanity from God who is the creator of all things and who continues to have unconditional love for sinful humanity. This unconditional love is fully expressed in Jesus Christ.
- Jesus Christ upon his birth, was fully and completely a human being and fully and completely God.
- Through the life, suffering, and death on the cross, and resurrection on Easter of Jesus Christ, humanity can be reconciled to God. This reconciliation is realized in a person's life by the grace of God through faith. Though through faith a person has received salvation, the person still struggles with sinfulness. This is expressed in the expression that a Christian is at once a saint and a sinner.
- Each person is by nature sinful and eternally separated from God, yet through faith in Jesus Christ, the believer is assured of eternal life.
- Lutherans teach that the Holy Spirit gathers the church together in order that forgiveness may be given and received, that the Word of God may be proclaimed, and the sacraments administered. This is done both for the sake of Christians and also in order that Christians may live by faith in their everyday lives so that others may realize the presence of Jesus Christ in the world.
- There is an ordained ministry of Word and Sacrament in each of the Lutheran bodies. The ordained pastor fully acts on behalf of the church regarding the proclamation of the Word and administration of the Sacraments though in some cases, the church's ministry of Word and Sacrament is extended by granting to laypersons authority to perform certain functions. The ordained person is usually addressed with the title of "pastor" or

"reverend." Some Lutherans ordain both men and women (e.g., the *Evangelical Lutheran Church in America*) and others only ordain men (e.g., the *Lutheran Church–Missouri Synod* and the *Wisconsin Evangelical Lutheran Synod*).

- The Lutheran church recognizes two sacraments. In a sacrament, the Word of God joins with the physical elements as a means of God's grace for the recipient.
  - Baptism joins the Word of God with water. Sprinkling, pouring, and immersion are all acceptable modes of baptism with the general rule that the water should be applied in sufficient quantity that it "runs." Lutherans teach and practice infant baptism.
  - Holy Communion or the Eucharist joins the Word of God with bread and wine. For some Lutherans, grape juice may be substituted for wine especially due to health issues. Also, for some, substitution of non-wheat bread is approved, especially where there are health concerns related to traditional forms of bread.

Basic Practices

All of Lutheranism shares: in being Trinitarian; use of the *Book of Concord* as the basis of its teaching; belief that justification is by grace through faith in Jesus Christ; understanding of the Word of God as the sole rule and norm of the faith. However, the practices which result from these beliefs are not uniform and may be sources of division within Lutheranism. Therefore, it is important to not only know that a person is Lutheran as opposed to another Christian tradition, but also to know with which specific Lutheran body the person is affiliated. Following are some points of practice that

may be considered in providing pastoral care.

- Lutheranism recognizes that the church extends beyond the local congregation. It also recognizes that ordained persons are ordained for the whole church and so may provide Word and Sacrament ministry to people who are not members of the congregation to which they are immediately called. However, for the individual there is often a very close identification with and high expectation of his or her congregation of membership and the pastor of that congregation. Therefore, it is important to seek the individual's permission to notify his or her pastor and include that pastor in providing pastoral care. It should be expected that in some cases, the individual will not approve this notification or the involvement of the local pastor.
- Worship in the Lutheran tradition is ordinarily liturgical in nature because worship is a confession of faith and because the church extends beyond the local congregation. This liturgical form is reflected in the administration of the sacraments, the proclamation of the Word, prayer, and other rites that may be provided outside of communal worship. Lutheran churches publish some form of pastoral aid or handbook to provide models for pastoral care in a variety of settings including hospitals, nursing facilities, and homes. The models provided by these books are useful, but in the end what is most important is that the individual have access to the sacraments, the Word, and prayer.
- There is an expectation of communal worship at least once each week.
- Lutherans may choose to participate

in worship, devotional, or educational activities with other Christians.

- Study and meditation based on the Bible; spoken and silent prayer; singing of hymns; regular use of the Lord's Prayer, the Apostles' Creed, and the Psalms are all practices that may be included in a Lutheran's life in formal communal worship, individual or small group devotional activities, and during informal interaction with others.
- There are practices which are within the Lutheran tradition, but that may be unfamiliar to the individual Lutheran church member (e.g., individual private confession). The individual's personal experience may not lead that person to be aware of or to ask for a certain pastoral act suggested by particular circumstances.
- Baptism is ordinarily administered by an ordained person. In an emergency situation, Baptism may be administered using a Trinitarian formula by any Christian. When this occurs, permission should be sought to notify the congregation and pastor where the person [or, in the case of a child, the child's parent(s) or guardian(s)], is a member or would desire to be a member.
- Holy Communion should be offered to individuals on a regular basis when they are in circumstances that keep them from participating in communal worship. Given the opportunity, an individual may choose to receive communion from a non-Lutheran pastor, priest, or other communion minister.
- Lutherans have the responsibility and privilege to share their faith in their words and action in all of life's settings.

Historically, the bench mark for Lutheran practice in the United States has been established based on the northern European immigrants' cultural and spiritual experience, which in turn has been passed on, though sometimes imperfectly, to subsequent generations. However, there are some communities of Lutheranism that have been influenced by Hispanic, African American, or other racial or ethnic cultures and spiritual experiences. These are not so common as to be able to provide any general guidance regarding modification of practice. The pastoral care provider and the local pastor may and will need to be flexible in form and style in meeting the spiritual needs of culturally diverse Lutherans.

Principles for Clinical Care
Dietary Issues
- There are no specific dietary restrictions or practices proscribed by Lutheran teaching. Individuals may choose to fast or practice other dietary disciplines as a personal choice.

General Medical Beliefs
- The various Lutheran bodies have published statements of the church regarding various social issues. Some of these may relate to medical concerns (e.g., abortion). In general, however, there are no statements that would preclude ordinarily accepted medical practice.
- Consulting with a Lutheran pastor is advised whenever a socially sensitive condition is involved or when the individual seems to have personal questions of conscience.
- The local Lutheran pastor is the best resource for assisting the health care personnel in identifying and understanding the full breadth of possible options

in providing pastoral care to a specific individual.

- Generally, Lutheran teaching recognizes life as a gift from God. As such, medical decisions regarding initiation or termination of human life, at whatever stage and for whatever reason, must include: willingness to humbly discern God's will; willingness to accept our sinfulness and to seek God's mercy and grace; and compassion for those most immediately affected by the necessary medical decisions.

Specific Medical Issues

- **Abortion**: Induced abortion is one of the issues about which Lutherans have serious differences. These differences are reflected in the social teaching statements of the various Lutheran bodies. Medical decisions regarding abortion are finally individual decisions. A discussion regarding these medical options is best pursued with the inclusion of an appropriate Lutheran pastor.

- **Advance Directives**: Use of advance directives in health care preplanning does not violate teachings of Lutheran faith. It is an individual decision.

- **Birth Control**: There is no categorical proscription regarding birth control in Lutheran teaching. However, within the various Lutheran groups or as a matter of faith and conscience for individual Lutherans, there may be concerns regarding specific birth control procedures or the circumstances surrounding birth control decisions. A full discussion of these procedures is best pursued with inclusion of an appropriate Lutheran pastor.

- **Blood Transfusions**: The use of blood products (e.g., blood transfusions) does not violate teachings of Lutheran faith. It is an individual decision.

- **Circumcsion**: Circumcision for male infants is a personal decision rather than a religious one.

- **In Vitro Fertilization**: While in vitro fertilization may not violate teachings of the Lutheran faith per se, prayerful discussion continues regarding this subject in many Lutheran bodies. Therefore, while these are finally individual decisions, a discussion regarding these medical options is best pursued with the inclusion of an appropriate Lutheran pastor.

- **Stem Cell Research**: While stem cell research for therapeutic purposes may not violate teachings of the Lutheran faith per se, prayerful discussion continues regarding this subject in many Lutheran bodies. Therefore, while these are finally individual decisions, a discussion regarding these medical options is best pursued with the inclusion of an appropriate Lutheran pastor.

- **Vaccinations**: Lutherans teach that the use of vaccines is a proactive measure to protect life and lives.

- **Withholding/Withdrawing Life Support**: While withholding or withdrawing life support in medically futile cases may not violate teachings of the Lutheran faith per se, prayerful discussion continues regarding this subject in many Lutheran bodies. Therefore, while these are finally individual decisions, a discussion regarding these medical options is best pursued with the inclusion of an appropriate Lutheran pastor.

Gender and Personal Issues

- Other than generally accepted standards which respect personal modesty and dignity, there are no specific concerns to be considered in providing pastoral care or health care to an individual.

Principles for Spiritual Care through the Cycles of Life

Concepts of Living and Dying for Spiritual Support

- Life is created and sustained by God and so is sacred.
- Death is a result of humanity's sinfulness. The faithful may approach death with the hope of eternal life through faith in Jesus Christ by the grace of God.
- There will be a resurrection of the body. This resurrection will take place regardless of the disposition of the person's remains at the time of death.

During Birth

- Lutherans teach that a person is born in original sin. Therefore, the person is in need of God's grace which is most immediately available through baptism.
- Baptism would ordinarily be delayed in order that it may occur in the presence of the worshipping community. However, emergency baptism may and should be considered whenever the child's life is in jeopardy. If death should occur before baptism can be provided, there is consolation in God's love and mercy for it is generally accepted that it is the abuse not the lack of the sacrament that is of concern.
- As stated earlier, circumcision for male infants is a personal decision rather than a religious one.

During Illness

- During illness, an individual may struggle with the questions both of illness as direct retribution for a personal act taken or avoided and as a general sign of the state of her or his faith.
- Pastoral care may occur within the tension of the Christian being at once saint and sinner with the assurance that a person's sin cannot be more powerful than the forgiveness which is available by grace through faith in Jesus Christ.
- Holy Communion should be offered to the individual on a regular basis when they are in circumstances that keep them from participating in communal worship. Given the opportunity, an individual may choose to receive communion from a non-Lutheran pastor, priest, or other communion minister.
- Patients may receive comfort from the reading of scriptures or other devotional material, listening to religious music, or watching televised worship services of their own or a similar tradition.
- Patients may receive comfort and other benefits from prayer. Prayers from clergy are valued, but so also are prayers from any other person.
- Patients may request baptism. In an emergency, anyone may administer baptism, though in ordinary circumstances baptism would be provided by a Lutheran pastor. Lutheran practice allows for application of water by various means (sprinkling, pouring, or immersion). The Rite of Baptism may include a variety of words and actions, but should always include "You are baptized in the name of the Father, the Son and the Holy Spirit."

During End of Life

- End of life is a release from the burdens, infirmities, and other effects of sinfulness and yet a time of grief and loss. This ambiguity is compatible with Lutheran teaching regarding being at once saint and sinner as well as for instance a world that is a blessing as a creation of God yet a burden as it is affected by sinfulness. In other words, this ambiguity need not be a source of doubt regarding the individual's faith.

- All of the practices noted earlier in the "During Illness" section are also applicable at the time of death.
- Family may wish to view the body of the deceased in the hospital room or the chapel. Nurse and chaplain should be consulted for assistance.

Care of the Body

- At the time of death, the body should be handled with respect.
- Disposition and embalming are individual decisions. The chaplain and the funeral home director should be consulted for assistance.
- Autopsy is an individual decision unless required by law. The chaplain and/or nurse should be consulted for assistance.
- Donation for medical research is an individual decision. The chaplain and/or nurse should be consulted for assistance. Advance planning for such donations is required by most receiving organizations. Last-minute donations are usually not possible.
- There are no specific time considerations regarding the funeral.

Organ and Tissue Donation

- Organ and tissue donation is permitted and is an individual decision. It may be preferable for a chaplain and/or nurse who are trained designated requesters to be consulted for assistance.

Scriptures, Inspirational Readings, and Prayers

- For the Lutheran, scripture would be the commonly accepted 66 books of the Bible commonly referred to as the Old Testament and the New Testament. Very

few Lutherans would use the Bible in its original languages for devotional purposes. Rather, they would use the Bible in whatever is their primary language. For English-speaking Lutherans, the specific translation is something of a personal choice. The New Revised Standard Version would be familiar to many.

- Conversation with the patient or family may often identify reading from the Bible that will be particularly meaningful or comforting. Other suggestions for readings from the Bible may be found in the pastoral manuals or handbooks published by the various Lutheran bodies.
- Prayers may be offered from various texts such as the published pastoral manuals or handbooks provided by the various Lutheran bodies. An offer of prayer would be expected by the individual from anyone who is making a pastoral visit. On a more formal level, some of the Lutheran bodies may have some restrictions, especially regarding settings of communal prayer. Inviting the individual to join with the pastoral care provider and others present in saying together the *Lord's Prayer* would be appropriate. Use of the *Apostle's Creed* is appropriate especially when Holy Communion is being shared. A Trinitarian benediction or another blessing would ordinarily be familiar and meaningful.

The Apostles' Creed

I believe in God, the Father almighty,
    creator of heaven and earth,
I believe in Jesus Christ, His only
    Son, our Lord.
He was conceived by the power of the
    Holy Spirit;
and born of the virgin Mary.
He suffered under Pontius Pilate,

was crucified, died, and was buried.
He descended into hell (-or- He
 descended to the dead).
On the third day he rose again.
He ascended into heaven and is
 seated at the right hand of the
 Father.
He will come again to judge the living
 and the dead.
I believe in the Holy Spirit,
the holy catholic Church,
the communion of saints,
the forgiveness of sins,
the resurrection of the body and the
 life everlasting. Amen.

The Lord's Prayer

Our Father, who art in heaven,
hallowed be thy name.
thy kingdom come,
thy will be done, on earth as it is in
 heaven.
Give us this day our daily bread;
and forgive us our trespasses,
as we forgive those who trespass
 against us.
and lead us not into temptation,
but deliver us from evil.
For thine is the kingdom, and the
 power, and the glory,
Forever and ever. Amen.

or

Our Father in heaven,
hallowed be your name,
your kingdom come,
your will be done, on earth as in
 heaven.
Give us today our daily bread.
Forgive us our sins
as we forgive those who sin against
 us.
Save us from the time of trial
and deliver us from evil.
For the kingdom, the power,
and the glory are yours,
now and forever. Amen.

A Trinitarian Blessing

The Lord bless you and keep you.
The Lord make his face shine on you
 and be gracious to you.
The Lord look upon you with favor
 and give you peace. Amen.

Church of the Nazarene

Holiness unto the Lord[275]

Prepared by:
Darius Salter, PhD
Professor of Christian Preaching and Pastoral Theology;
Judith A. Schwanz, PhD
Professor of Pastoral Care and Counseling
Nazarene Theological Seminary
Kansas City, MO

History and Facts

On October 20, 1895, the Church of the Nazarene began with 82 charter members in Los Angeles, California. In 1907, the Church of the Nazarene merged with the Association of Pentecostal Churches of America to become the Pentecostal Church of the Nazarene. The present-day Church of the Nazarene considers its birthday as October 13, 1908, when the Pentecostal Church of the Nazarene united with the Holiness Church of Christ at Pilot Point, Texas. At that time, the denomination became a truly national church uniting eastern, western, northern, and southern factions which adhered to "holiness" theology and experience.

In 1919, the General Assembly dropped the word Pentecostal from the denomination's name. In 2009, the Church of the Nazarene was an international organization with 17 277 churches and 1.9 million members worldwide.

Several historical strains led to the beginning of the Church of the Nazarene: the nineteenth-century holiness movement especially as expressed in its hundreds of camp meetings; a reaction against the wealth of the Gilded Age Church which disregarded the poor; the increasing "worldliness" of Methodism of which the founder of the church of the Nazarene, Phineas Bresee, was a member; and the "entire sanctification" teaching of John Wesley, a theological stance that many Methodists perceived was being increasingly discredited in the church. Thus, the Church of the Nazarene is the spiritual child of the holiness revival of the nineteenth-century and the theological child of John Wesley, the eighteenth-century Anglican revivalist and reformer. The modern-day Church of the Nazarene is part of the worldwide Wesleyan holiness movement with its sister denominations: the Wesleyan Church, the Free Methodist Church, the Salvation Army, and other holiness denominations. It also considers itself a participant in the broader evangelical movement, hence its

---

275 Quote obtained from the Church of the Nazarene official logo, provided by Dr. Judith Schwanz, coauthor of this chapter.

membership in the National Association of Evangelicals.

Basic Teachings

Many Nazarenes affirm the content of the ancient *Apostles' Creed*, which is a brief statement of faith attributed to the early church.

The Apostles' Creed

I believe in God, the Father almighty,
  creator of heaven and earth,
I believe in Jesus Christ, His only
  Son, our Lord.
Who was conceived by the power of
  the Holy Spirit;
Born of the virgin Mary;
Suffered under Pontius Pilate;
Was crucified, died, and buried.
He descended into hell (or the realm
  of the dead).
On the third day he rose again.
He ascended into heaven and is
  seated at the right hand of the
  Father.
He will come again to judge the living
  and the dead.
I believe in the Holy Spirit,
The holy catholic (universal) church,
The communion of saints,
The forgiveness of sins,
The resurrection of the body and the
  life everlasting. Amen.

- All humans are fallen from an original state of innocence and are bent toward actions (i.e., sins) that disconnect them from God and others.
- All humans deserve just punishment for misdeeds.
- Humans can be rescued (i.e., saved) from just punishment through faith in the death, burial, and resurrection of Jesus.

- The final destination for those who have been saved from the consequences of their misdeeds is heaven, which is communion with God and all the redeemed in a state of peace, justice, and perfect love.
- The final destination of those who are not saved is hell, a state of punishment and disconnected-ness from God and the saved.
- Nazarenes affirm the Bible, or Holy Scriptures, which is a compilation of 66 different books written over a thousand-year period. These writings contain wisdom sayings, history, poetry, social commentary, and devotional literature from ancient Semitic Jewish, Hellenistic Jewish, and early Christian authors. Some Christians also include additional books from Hellenistic Jewish culture called the Apocrypha. The number of these books varies according to the different traditions.
- The full authority of the Bible as to the instruction of life in matters of ethics, piety, and theology is central to Nazarene belief and practice.
- The critical tenets of the Reformation, such as the priesthood of all believers and salvation by faith alone, are focal points of Nazarene theology.
- An ordained ministry is accountable to both local church and to a denominational system.
- Clergy and laity who hold church membership affirm the "articles of faith" as presented in the Manual of the Church of the Nazarene.
- God extends "prevenient" grace, which is God's love reaching out to all persons making it possible for them to recognize their need and accept God's gracious offer of salvation.
- Entire sanctification, which enables a person through the blood of Christ

and the power of the Holy Spirit to be wholly devoted to God and free from the dominion of sin, is the ultimate goal of the earthly existence of Christians.

- The faithful will be eternally rewarded at the triumphant return of Christ when evil will be destroyed and righteousness will forever triumph.
- All members of the church (also called the body of Christ) are ministers gifted by the Holy Spirit; God has called some to special roles as pastors, evangelists, and teachers for the equipping of the saints and leadership of the church.
- The practice of ministry and leadership by both clergy and laity is fully inclusive for gender, race, and socioeconomic status.

Basic Practices

- Nazarenes value communal worship, and will gather on Sundays and at other times to hear preaching, study scripture, sing hymns, and pray.
- The sharing of one's faith (evangelism) is of great importance to Nazarenes. This may be communicated through loving actions, talking about personal spiritual experiences, reading scriptures, distributing informational tracts and discussions of doctrinal positions.
- Prayer, meditation, and scripture are fundamental spiritual practices for many Christians. The many forms of these practices include reading and/or silent contemplation upon scripture or doctrinal beliefs and prayers of various kinds – petition, healing, repentance for unethical thoughts and actions, praise, worship, and thanksgiving to God.
- Mission work is important to Nazarenes. These acts of service take the forms of working for social justice with

marginalized peoples, charitable giving to provide food, building, and educational programs for the poor, volunteerism, and so forth. Mission work is also an intentional witness to one's faith through proclamation and teaching.

- While all of life is sacramental, God has designated particular rites, mainly Baptism and the Lord's Supper (i.e., Communion), to be integral events for Christian worship.
- Baptism signifies a declaration of faith in Jesus Christ as Savior and an intent to pursue holiness and righteousness. Baptism may be administered by sprinkling, pouring, or immersion. Children, at the request of their parents (or guardians), may be baptized or presented for dedication to God.
- Communion is a declaration of Jesus' sacrificial death. The sacrament of the Lord's Supper is reserved for those who have expressed faith in Christ, and is open to all who desire to repent of their sins and initiate faith in Christ. Nazarene communion is open to Christians of all denominations.
- The Church of the Nazarene had its beginnings with ministry to the poor and continues to encourage its membership to practice stewardship of distributive justice and economic responsibility.
- The Church of the Nazarene practices a worldwide compassionate ministry and missionary outreach, with an established presence in 154 countries as of the year 2009.
- The Nazarene "Covenant of Christian Character" prohibits the use of tobacco and alcohol. Nazarenes are to take seriously the biblical declaration that the body is the "temple of the Holy Spirit." Thus, the body, as God's gift, is to be taken care of with proper rest, diet, and exercise.

Principles for Clinical Care
Dietary Issues
- The Church of the Nazarene has no dietary restrictions with respect to religious beliefs.

General Medical Beliefs
- Nazarenes are appreciative of modern medical technology and are encouraged to take full advantage of it whenever the quality of life can be preserved and enhanced.
- Nazarenes believe in divine healing which emphasizes both the immediate touch of God and the use of medical science.
- Nazarenes refer to God as the Great Physician.
- Normal practices of birth control and fertility measures are encouraged.

Specific Medical Issues
- **Abortion**: Abortion and euthanasia are prohibited.
- **Advance Directives**: Nazarenes are encouraged to express their desires for end-of-life decisions in the form of "advance directives."
- **Birth Control**: The church has issued no statement on the use of birth control; it is an individual decision.
- **Blood Transfusions**: The church has issued no statement on the use of blood products; it is an individual decision.
- **Circumcision**: Circumcision for male infants may be chosen for cultural and health, not religious, reasons.
- **In Vitro Fertilization**: The church has issued no statement on in vitro fertilization; the matter is left to the discretion of individuals and/or families.
- **Stem Cell Research**: All medical practices, especially those such as cloning and stem cell research, must be examined in the light of biblical ethics and the realization that medical science is not the ultimate answer to human problems. The Church of the Nazarene strongly encourages the scientific community to aggressively pursue advances in stem cell technology obtained from sources such as adult human tissues, placenta, umbilical cord blood, animal sources, and other nonhuman embryonic sources. This has the righteous end of attempting to bring healing to many, without violating the sanctity of human life. The stand on human embryonic stem cell research flows from the affirmation that the human embryo is a person made in the image of God. Therefore, the church opposes the use of stem cells produced from human embryos for research, therapeutic interventions, or any other purpose. As future scientific advances make new technologies available, the church strongly supports this research when it does not violate the sanctity of human life or other moral, biblical laws. However, the church opposes the destruction of human embryos for any purpose and any type of research that takes the life of a human after conception. Consistent with this view, the church opposes the use, for any purpose, of tissue derived from aborted human fetuses.
- **Vaccinations**: The *Manual of the Church of the Nazarene* states that we believe God heals through the means of medical science. This would include accepting the use of vaccinations to prevent illness, although the statement does not specify a policy on vaccinations.
- **Withholding/Withdrawing Life Support**: Nazarenes are to exercise freedom of conscience concerning life-support systems.

Gender and Personal Issues

- The Church of the Nazarene encourages modesty as an expression of holiness. Personal standards of modesty may result in preferences for same-gender health care providers or in areas of personal hygiene.

Principles for Spiritual Care through the Cycles of Life

Concepts of Living and Dying for Spiritual Support

- Life is sacred.
- Death is something all must experience and should not be feared.
- Humans live in a "fallen world" victimized by disease. Even though sickness is the result of Adam's sin, God can use it for drawing people closer to Him. Holiness theology has historically emphasized sanctification through suffering. However, Christians are cautioned against making assumptions in relating sickness to the will of God. At no point should spiritual direction state that "God sent this on you because you have sinned" or "God is punishing you."
- The rites of passage – birth, baptism, marriage, and death – are to be celebrated within the context of the church. As individuals make covenantal commitments, for instance marriage and baptism, the church enters into covenantal commitment with the individuals or couple to pray for them, love them, and support them.
- Nazarenes have a linear concept of time which is moving toward a grand consummation, the ultimate triumph of Christ. The final entrance into that triumph is through physical death, if not preceded by the second advent of Jesus Christ.
- Knowing that life is limited motivates Christians to "redeem the time," to make every moment count for the glory of God, even in sickness, dying, and death.
- Nazarenes fully concur with the teachings of the *Apostles' Creed*, which affirms the "resurrection of the body" and "the life everlasting."
- The Wesleyan holiness movement has a rich tradition regarding the victory and spiritual confidence that can be celebrated at death. John Wesley's dying words were reportedly "best of all God is with us." Nazarenes believe that all suffering and death find their ultimate comprehension in the death and resurrection of Jesus Christ. As the Apostle Paul stated, "death has been swallowed up in victory" (1 Cor. 15:34).

During Birth

- Nazarenes practice both infant baptism and dedication, whichever the parents prefer. Neither of these acts are magical (i.e., guaranteeing salvation). They must be performed within the context of Christian families, dedicated parents, and covenantal communities.
- As stated earlier, circumcision for male infants may be chosen for cultural and health, not religious, reasons.

During Illness

- "Laying on of hands" and anointing with oil is practiced by Nazarenes for the purpose of healing according to James 5. Whether physical healing occurs in this life or ultimate healing occurs in the life to come is within the provision of sovereign grace according to the wisdom of God.
- Patients may find comfort in having their own personal Bible or other significant personal symbols in their room.
- Spiritual counsel may be provided by

family, friends, or clergy. Illness often raises issues of mortality, the meaning of life, and generativity.

- The playing of songs or devotional music, reading of scripture, prayer, and visits by family, friends, or clergy may provide comfort.

During End of Life

- Nazarenes are encouraged to express their desires for end-of-life decisions in the form of "advance directives."
- Christians must make all efforts to help the dying end life with dignity, part of which is accepting one's mortality.
- Many dying people find comfort in planning their own funeral with their own pastor and/or family members. Their wishes should be honored as much as is feasible.
- Family and loved ones present are meaningful sources of support for the dying person.
- Singing of hymns, reading of scripture, and praying are sources of spiritual support for the dying person.
- Fulfillment of any requests that the dying may have – hearing of confession, baptism, reconciliation with others, and receiving Communion, and so forth – is strongly advised. The chaplain or clergy should be consulted for assistance with communion or baptism.
- Those present, including the pastor, are to do whatever possible to help assure the patient of an eternity with God. However, people must respect the faith community to which that person belongs or would wish to belong if he or she was able to make a conscious decision and, therefore avoid any pressure to "convert."
- Physical touch is important to many of the dying.

Care of the Body

- Family members should be allowed to spend time with the body after the spirit of the deceased has departed. Saying goodbye, even though the person is dead, is important in facilitating closure on a relationship that has been radically altered.
- The body should be treated with respect at all times.
- Decisions regarding disposition of the body should be made according to the preferences of the family, in consideration of the wishes of the deceased.
- Decisions regarding donation of the body for medical research should be made according to the preferences of the family, in consideration of the wishes of the deceased.
- Decisions regarding autopsy should be made according to the preferences of the family, in consideration of medical and/or legal concerns.

Organ and Tissue Donation

- The Church of the Nazarene encourages its members who do not object personally to support anatomical organ donation. Within the basic concern for others, organ donation may help family members of the deceased find closure and meaning in their loved one's death. It may be preferable for a chaplain and/or nurse who are trained designated requesters to be consulted for assistance.

Scriptures, Inspirational Readings, and Prayers

READINGS DURING ILLNESS

These can be read by family, friends, clergy, and health care professionals. (All scripture quotations are from the New Revised Standard Version.)

The Lord is my shepherd I shall not want.
He makes me lie down in green pastures; he restores my soul.
He leads me in right paths for his name's sake.
Even though I walk through the darkest valley, I fear no evil;
for you are with me; your rod and your staff – they comfort me.
You prepare a table before me in the presence of my enemies;
you anoint my head with oil; my cup overflows.
Surely goodness and mercy shall follow me all the days of my life,
and I shall dwell in the house of the Lord my whole life long.

—Psalm 23

We know that all things work together for good …
For I am convinced that neither death, nor life, nor angels, nor rulers, nor things present, nor things to come, nor powers, nor height, nor depth, nor anything else in all creation, will be able to separate us from the love of God in Christ Jesus our Lord.

—Rom. 8:28a, 38–39

READINGS DURING END-OF-LIFE PROCESS

These can be read by family, friends, clergy, and health care professionals. (All scripture quotations are from the New Revised Standard Version.)

I am the resurrection and the life. Those who believe in me, even though they die, will live, and everyone who lives and believes in me will never die.

—John 11:25–26

Do not let your hearts be troubled. Believe in God, believe also in me. In my Father's house there are many dwelling places. If it were not so, would I have told you that I go to prepare a place for you? And if I go and prepare a place for you, I will come again and will take you to myself, so that where I am, there you may be also.

—John 14:1–3

PRAYER DURING END-OF-LIFE PROCESS

This prayer can be offered by family, friends, clergy, and health care professionals.

Holy and Merciful Father,
We thank you for the gift of your Son, Jesus, whom you sent to die that we might live. We thank you also that you raised Him from the dead, and that He is seated with you in heaven. We acknowledge that you are the Lord of Life and the Lord of Death. We ask that you send your holy angels to escort our brother/sister_____ through death into your presence. Give our brother/sister_____ peace and comfort the family who will be saddened by the loss.
In Jesus' precious name, we pray. Amen.

SONG FOR END OF LIFE OR AFTER DEATH

Christ the Lord is Risen Today[276]
Lives again our glorious King.
  Alleluia!
Where, O death, is now thy sting?
  Alleluia!
Dying once, He all doth save.
  Alleluia!

Where thy victory, O grave? Alleluia!
Soar we now where Christ has led.
  Alleluia!
Foll'wing our exalted Head. Alleluia!
Made like Him, like Him we rise.
  Alleluia!
Ours the cross, the grave, the skies.
  Alleluia!

—Charles Wesley

---

276 Bible, K. ed. (1993). *Sing to the Lord* [hymnal].
  Kansas City, MO: Lillenas Publishing, 260.

Presbyterian Church

What does the Lord require of you but to do justice, and to love kindness, and to walk humbly with your God.[277]

Prepared by:
Robert H. Meneilly, DD
Founding Pastor, Village Presbyterian Church
Prairie Village, KS

Reviewed and approved by:
Heartland Presbytery Executive Staff in the Synod of
   Mid-America
Kansas City, MO

History and Facts

The Presbyterian Church, one of the oldest denominations in the United States because her roots date back to the very first settlers in the colonies, is about life, not religion. The Presbyterian Church grew out of the "Reformed" movement when John Calvin became a convert to Protestantism. Hiding from the French Catholic authorities, Calvin wrote a book, *The Institutes of the Christian Religion*, which set forth the understanding of Protestant belief. John Knox, a Scottish Protestant established Presbyterianism in Scotland in 1559. The earliest settlers in the American colonies were primarily Reformed Protestant exiles from Scotland, Ireland, England, and the European Continent. Presbyterians were so much a part of the Revolutionary War that the English called it "the Presbyterian Rebellion." The Presbyterian Church is considered by many to be the rebirth of the early New Testament Church.

Basic Teachings

Presbyterians will affirm the content of the ancient *Apostles' Creed*, which is a brief statement of faith attributed to the early church.

The Apostles' Creed

I believe in God, the Father almighty,
   creator of heaven and earth,
I believe in Jesus Christ, His only
   Son, our Lord.
Who was conceived by the power of
   the Holy Spirit;
Born of the virgin Mary;
Suffered under Pontius Pilate;
Was crucified, died, and buried.
He descended into hell (or the realm
   of the dead).
On the third day he rose again.
He ascended into heaven and is
   seated at the right hand of the
   Father.
He will come again to judge the living
   and the dead.
I believe in the Holy Spirit,
The holy catholic (universal) church,
The communion of saints,
The forgiveness of sins,

---

277 Mic. 6:8 (New Revised Standard Version).

364

The resurrection of the body and the life everlasting. Amen.

- All humans are fallen from an original state of innocence and are bent toward actions (i.e., sins) that disconnect them from God and others.
- All humans deserve just punishment for misdeeds.
- Humans can be rescued (i.e., saved) from just punishment through faith in the death, burial, and resurrection of Jesus.
- The final destination for those who have been saved from the consequences of their misdeeds is heaven, which is communion with God and all the redeemed in a state of peace, justice, and perfect love.
- The final destination of those who are not saved is hell, a state of punishment and disconnected-ness from God and the saved. Opinions differ as to whether or not hell is eternal.
- Christians affirm the Bible, or Holy Scriptures, which is a compilation of 66 different books written over a thousand-year period. These writings contain wisdom sayings, history, poetry, social commentary, and devotional literature from ancient Semitic Jewish, Hellenistic Jewish, and early Christian authors. Some Christians also include additional books from Hellenistic Jewish culture called the Apocrypha. The number of these books varies according to the different traditions.
- The Presbyterian Church is a "confessional" church which means that the basic beliefs of the church are embodied in a series of creeds, doctrinal statements and confessions produced by the great councils of the church. The *Apostles' Creed* and the *Nicene Creed* unite the Presbyterian Church with most of Christendom.

- Presbyterian beliefs about God, grace, Jesus Christ, justification by faith, the Holy Spirit, the priesthood of all believers are similar to those held by other Protestants.
- Presbyterians have traditionally emphasized the sovereignty of God.
- Presbyterians believe the scriptures are inspired by God and are to be studied critically and in the context of their historical settings. God inspired persons, not words!
- God is experienced as the Father, the Son, and the Holy Spirit (the Trinity).
- Presbyterians believe in the doctrine of the incarnation – Jesus is God in the flesh … both fully human and fully divine.
- Two sacraments are recognized: baptism and the Lord's Supper.
- Baptism is offered to both infants of believing parents and to adults who will confess their faith publicly. Baptism is usually administered by the sprinkling of water.
- The Lord's Supper is open to all baptized members including "informed" children.
- The ministry of the church is carried out by properly educated and licensed men and women ministers of Word and Sacrament.
- The official board of the local congregation is called the Session, and is made up of duly elected and ordained laypersons with the pastor as the Moderator.

Basic Practices
- Presbyterians value communal worship, and will gather on Sundays and at other times to hear preaching, study scripture, sing hymns, and pray.
- The sharing of one's faith (evangelism) is of great importance to Presbyterians.

Some of the ways it is communicated is through loving actions, talking about personal spiritual experiences, reading scriptures, distributing informational tracts, and discussions of doctrinal positions.

- Prayer, meditation, and scripture are the fundamental spiritual practices for many Christians. The many forms of these practices include reading and/or silent contemplation upon scripture or doctrinal beliefs and prayers of various kinds – petition, healing, repentance for unethical thoughts and actions, praise, worship, and thanksgiving to God.
- Mission work is important to Presbyterians. These acts of service take the forms of working for social justice with marginalized peoples, charitable giving to provide food, building, and educational programs for the poor, volunteerism, and so forth. Mission work is also an intentional witness to one's faith through proclamation and teaching.
- Infant baptism, practiced by some Presbyterians, especially emphasizes the action of God in the life of the child. This tradition places a great responsibility upon the church community to raise the child to make responsible ethical and spiritual decisions and to influence the child to choose to follow God through the process of Confirmation, (summation of specific religious training – usually in early teens).
- Christening is the ceremonial act which includes naming of the child. It can be an official part of the ceremony of baptism or combined with infant dedication.
- The Presbyterian Church (USA) is very socially conscious and is deeply involved in peacemaking, seeking equal rights for all; the elimination of poverty, hunger, and discrimination; and securing the wall of separation of church and state as set forth in the First Amendment of the Constitution. Almost every congregation has a "Social Justice" Committee.
- The sacrament of the Lord's Supper is normally served quarterly, but more and more churches are now observing it monthly. It is also served to the homebound when requested. Common bread and fresh grape juice serve as the elements.
- The sacrament of baptism is offered throughout the year.
- Services of Healing and Comfort are also offered throughout the year.
- Pastoral care and counseling is offered throughout the year.
- Every Presbyterian congregation recognizes and honors the "connectional" church at all levels of church life and organization.
- Every congregation attempts to offer the best of Christian education for young and old alike.
- Worship is always the primary offering of every congregation.
- The church believes in mission, the practicing of its faith, walking the Christian talk at home and worldwide.
- The church emphasizes Christian stewardship of one's time, talents, and resources. It also emphasizes the stewardship of the planet.

Principles for Clinical Care
Dietary Issues
- The Presbyterian Church offers no dietary rules. If one finds that times of fasting serve to nurture one's spiritual life, so be it.

General Medical Beliefs

- Like most Christians, Presbyterians often refer to God or Christ as "The Great Physician."
- Presbyterians generally believe that God uses a variety of ways of healing including the best of today's medical practices. Good health is always God's will.
- Seek the best medical attention and care available.
- The church is pro-life – that is, pro-"quality" life.

Specific Medical Issues

- **Abortion**: The church believes that the matter of abortion is to be left to the counsel of the woman, her physician and spiritual counselor.
- **Advance Directives**: The church encourages its people to have final health care directives (living wills), durable power of attorney for health care decisions and an estate plan.
- **Birth Control**: The Presbyterian Church promotes equal access to birth control options.
- **Blood Transfusions**: The church has no stated position on the use of blood products. It believes this matter is for individuals and families to decide in determining the best means for health of the patient.
- **Circumcision**: Christians in Western societies have requested circumcision of male infants for cultural, not religious, reasons.
- **In Vitro Fertilization**: The church has no stated opinions on in vitro fertilization. It believes this is a matter for individuals and families as part of responsible and intelligent family planning, including the use of contraceptives.
- **Stem Cell Research**: The church urges legislative bodies to encourage stem cell research and all reasonable programs to result in the best of health and wholeness.
- **Vaccinations**: The Presbyterian Church USA endorses all vacinations recommended by the American Medical Association.
- **Withholding/Withdrawing Life Support**: The church has no stated positions on withholding/withdrawing life support in medically futile cases. It believes this matter is for individuals and families to decide in the context of one's right to have adequate pain management and the honor of dignity in dying.

Gender and Personal Issues

- The Presbyterian Church as a faith tradition has no prescriptions or proscriptions with respect to gender and personal issues.

Principles for Spiritual Care through the Cycles of Life

Concepts of Living and Dying for Spiritual Support

- Human life is sacred.
- Death is a part of life and is to be revered and not feared.
- The soul, the spirit dimension of life, is transposed to what is called "heaven" upon the death of the body. Heaven is understood to be a "state of being" and not a "place." It is understood to be "at-one-ment with God."
- Resurrection of the body and everlasting life are faith values.

During Birth

- Christening or baptism may be requested by family for a baby, living or deceased. The chaplain or clergy should be consulted for assistance.

- As stated earlier, Christians in Western societies have requested circumcision of male infants for cultural, not religious, reasons.
- Upon fetal demise, the remains should be respectfully handled and the grieving parents comforted with ongoing pastoral care.

During Illness

- Patients may receive comfort from the reading of scriptures or other devotional material, listening to religious music, watching televised worship services of their own or a similar tradition. Patients may request Holy Communion. The chaplain or clergy should be consulted for assistance.
- Patients may receive comfort from healing prayers. These can be offered by health care professionals. Patients from some traditions, however, may ask for healing prayer to be connected with "anointing with oil" or the "the laying on of hands." The chaplain or clergy should be consulted for assistance for these requests.
- Patients may request baptism. In the clinical setting, sprinkling is an acceptable mode of baptism, even for traditions that practice immersion. The chaplain or clergy should be consulted for assistance.
- Patients should exercise their religious faith to the fullest.
- Presbyterians have special trained laypersons, called Stephen Ministers, to attend the ill, offering support, prayer, and practical helps in the home.

During End of Life

- Patient or the family may request baptism. (Note: baptism signifies the beginning of life in Christ, not its completion.) The chaplain or clergy should be consulted for assistance.
- Patient or the family may request the Lord's Supper. The chaplain or clergy should be consulted for assistance.
- Hospice may be called in to give care to the critically ill.
- Family may wish to view the body of the deceased in the hospital room or the chapel. Nurse and chaplain should be consulted for assistance.
- Family may request prayers for the deceased. These can be offered by the chaplain, clergy, family, friends, and health care professionals.
- When a family member expires, the family should contact the pastor immediately to consult about final arrangements.

Care of the Body

- Disposition and embalming are individual decisions. Cremation is now the choice of many Christians. The chaplain and the funeral home director should be consulted for assistance.
- Autopsy is an individual decision unless required by law. The chaplain and/or nurse should be consulted for assistance.
- Donation for medical research is an individual decision. The chaplain and/or nurse should be consulted for assistance. Advance planning for such donations is required by most receiving organizations. Last-minute donations are usually not possible.
- Presbyterians have no instructions or traditions when it comes to handling the body of the deceased except that the body should be handled with dignity and respect because the body is the earthly housing for the human soul.
- Cremation and burial are both acceptable for Presbyterians.

Organ and Tissue Donation

- Organ and tissue donation is permitted and is an individual decision. It may be preferable for a chaplain and/or nurse who are trained designated requesters to be consulted for assistance.
- Presbyterians encourage organ and tissue donation as an act of final stewardship. The availability of such potential donations should be noted on one's driver's license and in advance directives so that donations may be available in a timely fashion without delay.

Scriptures, Inspirational Readings, and Prayers

- Ask the patient and/or family if there are favorite texts of scripture or devotional readings.

READINGS DURING ILLNESS

These can be read by family, friends, clergy, and health care professionals. (Scripture quotations are from the New Revised Standard Version.)

The Lord is my constant companion,
  There is no need that God cannot fulfill.
Whether God's course for me points
  to the mountaintops of glorious ecstasy
or to the valleys of human suffering,
  God is by my side. God is ever present with me
when I tread the dark streets of
  danger, and even when I flirt with death itself.
God will never leave me. When
  the pain is severe, God is near to comfort.
When the burden is heavy, God is
  near to lean upon.

When depression darkens my soul,
  God touches me with eternal joy.
When I feel empty and alone, God
  feels the aching vacuum with His power.
My security is in God's promise to be
  near to me always,
and in the knowledge God will never
  let me go.

—Paraphrase of Psalm 23

Be strong and courageous; do not
be frightened or dismayed, for the
Lord your God is with you wherever
you go.

—Josh. 1:9b

The Lord is my light and salvation;
  whom shall I fear?
The Lord is the stronghold of my life;
  of whom shall I be afraid?

—Ps. 46:10

Our help is in the name of the Lord,
who made heaven and earth.

—Ps. 124:8

Do not fear, for I am with you; do not
  be afraid, for I am your God;
I will strengthen you, I will help you,
  I will uphold you with my victorious
right hand.

—Isa. 41:10

Come to me, all you who are weary and are carrying heaven burdens, and I will give you rest.

—Matt. 11:28

Do not let your hearts be troubled. Believe in God, believe also in me.

—John 14:1

My grace is sufficient for you, for my power is made perfect in weakness.

—2 Cor. 12:9a

READINGS DURING END-OF-LIFE PROCESS

These can be read by family, friends, clergy, and health care professionals. (Scripture quotations are from the New Revised Standard Version.)

The eternal God is our dwelling place, and underneath are the everlasting arms.

—Deut. 33:27

Blessed are those who mourn, for they will be comforted.

—Matt. 5:4

Peace I leave with you and my peace I give you. I do not give to you as the world gives. Don't let your hearts be troubled, and do not let them be afraid.

—John 14:27

We believe that Jesus died and rose again; and so it will be with those who have died. God will raise them to be with the Lord forever.

—1 Thess. 4:14

Blessed are the dead who die in the Lord, says the Spirit.
They will rest from their labors, and their deeds will follow them.

—Rev. 14:13

I am convinced that neither death, nor life, nor angels, nor rulers, nor things present, nor things to come, nor powers, nor height, nor depth, nor anything else in all creation, will be able to separate us from the love of God in Christ Jesus our Lord.

—Rom. 8:38–39

PRAYER DURING END-OF-LIFE PROCESS

This prayer may be offered by family, friends, clergy, or health care workers.

Almighty God, Father of the whole family in heaven and earth: stand by those who sorrow, that, as they lean on your strength, they may be upheld, and believe the good news of life beyond life; through Jesus Christ our Lord.
In to your loving care we entrust one another, life without end. Amen.

Seventh-Day Adventist Church

A ministry of hope and healing[278]

Prepared by:
William G. Johnsson, PhD
Assistant to the World Church President for Interfaith Relations
World Church headquarters
Silver Spring, MD

History and Facts

With a presence in more than 200 nations, the Seventh-Day Adventist Church is the most widespread Protestant church in the world. The church now numbers some 15 million adherents and membership doubles about every 10 years. North America, where the church arose, accounts for about 1 million Adventists.

As an organized denomination, the Seventh-Day Adventist Church is young. She arose out of the eschatological expectation (i.e., the belief in the imminent return of Jesus to earth) of the nineteenth century, and was formally organized only in 1863. The early part of that century witnessed an upsurge in expectation that the Second Coming of Jesus Christ was near. In North America, this "revival movement" was spearheaded by William Miller, who, basing his calculations on prophecies in the biblical book of Daniel, predicted that Jesus would return to earth around the year 1840. When that year passed and Miller's prophecy was not fulfilled, other dates were proposed. The

last date set by the Millerites (followers of William Miller) for Jesus' second coming was October 22, 1844. After the October 22 date failed, the Millerite movement fell into disarray. One small group out of that movement, numbering only about 100 people, adopted the seventh-day Sabbath. From such unpromising soil arose the present global, vigorous Seventh-Day Adventist Church.

Seventh-Day Adventists are known worldwide for their involvement in health and education, as well as their efforts in relief and development. In North America, Seventh-Day Adventists own and operate some 62 health care facilities; worldwide, about 720 health-related facilities. Some of those institutions are very large, such as Loma Linda University Medical Center in southern California, which specializes in medical sciences. This center pioneered infant heart transplants ("Baby Fae") and constructed the world's first proton-beam treatment for cancer in a medical setting.

The church, which strongly promotes public health, owns and operates a network of health food factories around the world. Adventists themselves tend to be more

---

278 Quote provided by William G. Johnsson, author of this chapter.

conscious about health matters than many Christians. They counsel against drinking alcohol or smoking tobacco products, and many adhere to a vegetarian diet. Because of their higher life expectancies (due in large part to lifestyle considerations), Adventists have been the subject of large demographic studies.

Adventists operate one of the largest school systems in the world, with more than 100 universities and colleges and about 6000 schools altogether. The relief and development arm of the church works in more than 100 countries, providing disaster response and long-term help such as clean water supplies, nutrition, and economic independence.

The Seventh-Day Adventist Church has a centralized organization, with headquarters based in Silver Spring, Maryland, and 13 divisional administrative offices for the world body.

Basic Teachings

- Seventh-Day Adventists are a strongly biblical people. In the Christian scriptures (the Old and New Testaments), they find their rule of faith and practice.
- Adventists are orthodox Christians, believing in the Trinity, the virgin birth and deity of Jesus of Nazareth, His atoning death, His resurrection, and His heavenly ministry as high priest. The name, Seventh-Day Adventists, highlights the major features of their identity: observance of the Sabbath, Saturday, as the day of rest and worship; and belief in the literal return of Jesus to this earth.
- Adventists hold that God continues to lead His people to clearer understanding of truth. Thus, although their teachings have been codified into 28 Fundamental

Beliefs, these statements may be, and have been, revised from time to time.
- Adventists believe that the New Testament teaching concerning spiritual gifts was not restricted to the apostolic age; they further hold that the gift of prophecy was specifically manifested in the ministry and writings of one of their pioneers, Ellen G. White. During a long and fruitful ministry, Ellen White (1827–1915) counseled, preached, taught, traveled, and wrote extensively. She at no time assumed a formal leadership role, nor was she ordained as a minister; her counsels, however, helped shape the growing church. Continually pointing to the Bible as the judge of all her revelations, she refused to take any position that would raise her writings to the level of scripture.
- Adventists recognize all agencies that lift up Christ as part of the divine plan for the evangelization of the world. They rejoice in the advancement of God's kingdom through every means that He provides. They enter into fellowship with other Christians; they practice open communion; they rejoice in opportunities for dialogue with other Christian bodies.
- Adventists have a sense of destiny. They believe that God has given them a message to the world – to call men and women everywhere to worship Him, to put Him first, to accept the eternal gospel, to make the scriptures the foundation of their life.
- Adventists have a strong emphasis on missions and a global identity. While Adventists interact with other Christians on the local level, they have not formally joined the ecumenical movement.

Basic Practices

- The Sabbath, from sunset Friday to sunset Saturday, is the day set apart for rest and worship.
- Baptism is by immersion of an individual who has reached the age of understanding and responsibility. Infants are not baptized or "sprinkled."
- The Lord's Supper is open to all who believe in Jesus Christ. It is not observed on a strictly regulated basis, usually once every three months. Unfermented wine (grape juice) is used.

Principles for Clinical Care

Dietary Issues

- The Seventh-Day Adventist Church recommends a vegetarian diet, and many Adventists adhere to this practice. For nonvegetarians, Adventists restrict their diet to the "clean" (kosher) meats specified in the scriptures.

General Medical Beliefs

- Seventh-Day Adventists believe that God is the ultimate source of all life, health, and healing.
- Seventh-Day Adventists refer to God as the Great Physician.
- Seventh-Day Adventists affirm the validity of traditional Western medical procedures in the treatment of illness and disease.

Specific Medical Issues

- **Abortion**: Abortion is primarily a decision between woman and physician. While it is always regrettable, it is acceptable to protect the physical and mental health of the mother. It is not acceptable for birth control, sex selection, or convenience.

- **Advance Directives**: Use of advance directives does not violate teachings of the Seventh-Day Adventist Church. It is an individual decision.
- **Birth Control**: The Seventh-Day Adventist Church leaves the decision of birth control up to the individual.
- **Blood Transfusions**: The Seventh-Day Adventist Church has no reservations about blood transfusions.
- **Circumcision**: Adventists may request circumcision for cultural, not religious, reasons.
- **In Vitro Fertilization**: The Seventh-Day Adventist Church has no reservations about in vitro fertilization and birth control.
- **Stem Cell Research**: Stem cell research for therapeutic purposes does not violate teachings of the Seventh-Day Adventist Church. It is an individual decision.
- **Vaccinations**: The Seventh-Day Adventist church strongly supports and recommends vaccinations for its members, children included.
- **Withholding/Withdrawing Life Support**: Withholding/withdrawing life support in medically futile cases does not violate teachings of the Seventh-Day Adventist Church. It is an individual decision.

Gender and Personal Issues

- The Seventh-Day Adventist Church as a faith tradition has no prescriptions or proscriptions with respect to gender and personal issues.

Principles for Spiritual Care through the Cycles of Life

Concepts of Living and Dying for Spiritual Support

- Life is sacred.
- Death is something all must experience and should be not feared.
- Death is perceived as sleep, a time of peaceful comfort until the Second Coming of Jesus.
- Resurrection of the physical body will happen at the Second Coming of Jesus. Humanity, all living creatures, and the entire cosmos will be healed and restored to a state of perfection.

During Birth

- Christening or baptism will not be requested.
- As stated earlier, Adventists may request circumcision for cultural, not religious, reasons.

During Illness

- Patients may receive comfort from the reading of scriptures or other devotional material, listening to religious music, watching televised worship services of their own or a similar tradition.
- Patients may receive comfort from healing prayers. These can be offered by health care professionals. Patients may ask for healing prayer to be connected with "anointing with oil." The chaplain or clergy should be consulted for assistance for these requests.

During End of Life

- Patient may request baptism. The chaplain or clergy should be consulted for assistance.
- Patient or the family may request the Lord's Supper. The chaplain or clergy should be consulted for assistance.
- Patient or family may request Anointing of the Sick, and prayers for the dying. The chaplain or clergy should be consulted for assistance.
- Family may wish to view the body of the deceased in the hospital room or the chapel. Nurse and chaplain should be consulted for assistance.
- Family may request prayers of comfort. These can be offered by the chaplain, clergy, family, friends, and health care professionals.

Care of the Body

- Disposition and embalming are individual decisions. The chaplain and the funeral home director should be consulted for assistance.
- Donation for medical research is an individual decision. The chaplain and/or nurse should be consulted for assistance. Advance planning for such donations is required by most receiving organizations. Last-minute donations are usually not possible.

Organ and Tissue Donation

- Organ and tissue donation is permitted and is an individual decision. It may be preferable for a chaplain and/or nurse who are trained designated requesters to be consulted for assistance.

Scriptures, Inspirational Readings, and Prayers

READINGS DURING ILLNESS

These can be read by family, friends, clergy, and health care professionals. (All scripture quotations are from the New Revised Standard Version.)

The Lord is my shepherd I shall not
want.
He makes me lie down in green
pastures; he restores my soul.
He leads me in right paths for his
name's sake.
Even though I walk through the
darkest valley, I fear no evil;
for you are with me; your rod and
your staff – they comfort me.
You prepare a table before me in the
presence of my enemies;
you anoint my head with oil; my cup
overflows.
Surely goodness and mercy shall
follow me all the days of my life,
and I shall dwell in the house of the
Lord my whole life long.

—Psalm 23

We know that all things work
together for good …
For I am convinced that neither
death, nor life, nor angels, nor
rulers, nor things present, nor things
to come, nor powers, nor height,
nor depth, nor anything else in all
creation, will be able to separate
us from the love of God in Christ
Jesus our Lord.

—Rom. 8:28a, 38–39

READINGS DURING END-OF-LIFE PROCESS

These can be read by family, friends, clergy, and health care professionals. (All scripture quotations are from the New Revised Standard Version.)

I am the resurrection and the life.
Those who believe in me, even though
they die, will live, and everyone who
lives and believes in me will never die.

—John 11:25–26

Do not let your hearts be troubled.
Believe in God, believe also in me.
In my Father's house there are many
dwelling places. If it were not so,
would I have told you that I go to
prepare a place for you? And if I
go and prepare a place for you, I
will come again and will take you
to myself, so that where I am, there
you may be also.

—John 14:1–3

PRAYER DURING END-OF-LIFE PROCESS

This prayer can be offered by family, friends, clergy, and health care professionals.

Holy and Merciful Father,
We thank you for the gift of your
Son, Jesus, whom you sent to die
that we might live.
We thank you also that you raised
Him from the dead, and that He
is seated with you in heaven. We
acknowledge that you are the Lord
of Life and the Lord of Death.
We ask that you will keep our
brother/sister _____ safe
in your loving care and
give peace and comfort to the family
who will be saddened by this loss.
In Jesus' precious name we pray,
Amen.

United Church of Christ

That All May Be One[279]

Prepared by:
The Reverend Greg Heinsman, MDiv, BCC
Chaplain
Cape Girardeau, MO

History and Facts

The United Church of Christ, a united and uniting church, was born on June 25, 1957; it came from four groups.[280] Two of the groups were the Congregational Churches of the English Reformation with Puritan New England roots in America and the Christian Church with American frontier beginnings. These two denominations were concerned with freedom of religious expression and local autonomy. They united on June 17, 1931, and became the Congregational Christian Churches.

The other two denominations were the Evangelical Synod of North America, a nineteenth-century German-American church of the frontier Mississippi Valley, and the Reformed Church in the United States which unified in 1793 to become a synod. The parent churches of the two groups were of German and Swiss heritage and conscientious carriers of the Reformed and Lutheran traditions of the Reformation.

They united to form the Evangelical and Reformed Church on June 26, 1934.

The Evangelical and Reformed Church and the Congregational Christian Churches shared a strong commitment under Christ to the freedom of religious expression. Their union as the United Church of Christ forced accommodation between congregational and presbyterial forms of church government. This new denomination found its authority in the Bible and was more concerned about what unites Christians than what divides them. The denomination was broadened by a deep sense of covenant with Christ that embraced diversity and freedom.

Basic Teachings

The United Church of Christ affirms its faith through the Statement of Faith. This is not to be understood as a creed, but rather a statement of faith, which suggests a less rigid, less authoritarian document. It is a modest attempt to say what Christians believe and is to be understood as a testimony and not a test of faith.

---

279 Quote provided by Rev. Greg Heinsman, author of this chapter.

280 An abbreviated history of the United Church of Christ can be found online at: www.ucc.org/about-us/short-course/ (accessed 8 Sept 12).

United Church of Christ Statement of Faith-Adapted by Robert V. Moss

We believe in God, the Eternal Spirit, who is made known to us in Jesus our brother, and to whose deeds we testify:

God calls the worlds into being, creates humankind in the divine image, and sets before us the ways of life and death.

God seeks in holy love to save all people from aimlessness and sin.

God judges all humanity and all nations by that will of righteousness declared through prophets and apostles.

In Jesus Christ, the man of Nazareth, our crucified and risen Lord, God has come to us and shared our common lot, conquering sin and death and reconciling the whole creation to its Creator.

God bestows upon us the Holy Spirit, creating and renewing the church of Jesus Christ, binding in covenant faithful people of all ages, tongues, and races.

God calls us into the church to accept the cost and joy of discipleship, to be servants in the service of the whole human family, to proclaim the gospel to all the world and resist the powers of evil, to share in Christ's baptism and eat at his table, to join him in his passion and victory.

God promises to all who trust in the gospel forgiveness of sins and fullness of grace, courage in the struggle for justice and peace, the presence of the Holy Spirit in trial and rejoicing, and eternal life in that kingdom which has no end.

Blessing and honor, glory and power be unto God.[281]

Amen.

- The United Church of Christ believes in the triune God: Creator; resurrected Christ, the sole Head of the Church; and the Holy Spirit, who guides and brings about the creative and redemptive work of God in the world.[282]
- Each person is unique and valuable. It is the will of God that all people belong to a family of faith where they have a strong sense of being valued and loved.
- Each person is on a spiritual journey and at a different stage in that journey.
- Each person's search for God produces: an authentic relationship with God; engendering love; strengthening faith; dissolving guilt; and life-giving purpose and direction.
- Every baptized person belongs to the Lord and Savior, Jesus Christ. No matter where people are on life's journey, regardless of gender, race, sexual orientation, class, or creed, they are welcome in the United Church of Christ. All baptized persons – past, present, and future – are connected to each other and to God through the sacrament of baptism. The Church baptizes during worship when the community is present because baptism includes the promise of love, support, and care for the baptized.
- The United Church of Christ invites all to Christ's table for the sacrament of Holy Communion. The breaking of bread and the pouring of the wine reminds

---

281 Shinn, R. (1990). *Confessing Our Faith: An Interpretation of the Statement of Faith of the United Church of Christ*. Cleveland, OH: Pilgrim Press, xiii.

282 United Church of Christ beliefs can be found online at: http://ucc.org/about-us/what-we-believe.html.

individuals of the costliness of Christ's sacrifice and the discipleship to which they are called. In the breaking of the bread, people celebrate Christ's presence among them. It is a great mystery that is proclaimed by faith.

- The United Church of Christ is called to be a united and a uniting church: "That all may be one" (John 17:21); "In essentials – unity, in nonessentials – diversity, in all things – charity." Theses mottos touch core values deep within every person. The Church has no rigid formula or attachment to creeds or structures. The key is love and unity in the midst of diversity.
- God continues to speak and breaks forth light and truth from the scriptures. The Bible, though written in specific historical times and places, still speaks to people in their present conditions. The study of scriptures is not limited by past interpretations, but it is pursued with the expectations of new insights and God's help for living today.
- The Church is called to be prophetic. In the tradition of the apostles and prophets, God calls the church to speak truth to power, to liberate the oppressed, care for the poor, and comfort the afflicted.
- The United Church of Christ is a Just Peace Church. It is important to work for nonviolent solutions to local, national, and international problems. Just Peace is the relationship of friendship, justice, and common security from violence. It is grounded in covenant relationship with God and one another. When God's abiding presence is embraced, human well-being results and individuals experience Just Peace or *shalom*.
- The United Church of Christ is an "Open and Affirming Church." It welcomes all people, including persons who are lesbian, gay, transgender and bisexual. The Church believes in a gospel of inclusion which values all people. Church members are called to be agents of reconciliation and wholeness in the world and in the Church.

Basic Practices

- The United Church of Christ values communal worship, and will gather on Sundays and at other times to hear preaching, study scripture, sing hymns, and pray.
- Evangelism is communicated through loving actions, talking about personal experiences, and missions projects. The United Church of Christ in the Evangelical tradition has "Sausage Suppers," which is an opportunity for outreach to the community.
- Prayer, meditation, and scripture are spiritual practices for many Christians. The many forms include: reading and/or silent contemplation upon scripture and prayers of many kinds – petition, healing, repentance for unethical thoughts and actions, praise, worship, and thanksgiving to God.
- The Lord's Supper, also called Holy Communion or Eucharist (meaning "thanksgiving") is a powerful sacrament. It is a liturgical reenactment of the death, burial, and resurrection of Jesus, in which Christians eat bread (to commemorate the broken body of Jesus) and drink wine or grape juice (to symbolize Jesus' shed blood). This can be done during communal worship or in other settings and is administered by licensed or ordained clergy within the United Church of Christ. All who have been baptized are invited to receive communion.

Principles for Clinical Care
Dietary Issues
- The United Church of Christ has no dietary restrictions with respect to religious beliefs.

General Medical Beliefs
- The United Church of Christ believes that God is the ultimate source of all life, health and healing. The Church is appreciative of modern technology and takes advantage of it whenever the quality of life can be preserved and enhanced.
- The United Church of Christ views health care as a basic human right and supports equal assess to medical care.

Specific Medical Issues
- **Abortion**: The United Church of Christ has affirmed that access to safe and legal abortion is consistent with a woman's right to follow her own faith and beliefs. The Church's position is not pro-abortion, but a pro-faith, pro-family, and pro-woman position.
- **Advance Directives**: The United Church of Christ supports the use of advance directives for health care preplanning.
- **Birth Control**: The United Church of Christ believes it should be an individual choice.
- **Blood Transfusions**: The United Church of Christ believes it should be an individual choice. Most would support blood transfusions for life saving measures.
- **Circumcision**: Circumcision may be requested for cultural and not religious reasons.
- **In Vitro Fertilization**: The United Church of Christ has no reservations about in vitro fertilization or birth control.
- **Stem Cell Research**: The United Church of Christ supports the use of adult and embryonic stem cells. Embryonic stem cells may be used when there is informed consent by the couple. The United Church of Christ supports federally funded embryonic stem cell research within ethically sound guidelines (including concern for justice, privacy, and access to the benefits of the research for all).
- **Vaccinations**: The United Church of Christ believes it should be an individual choice and one that promotes health and healing.
- **Withholding/Withdrawing Life Support**: Dying persons and their families should avail themselves of all medical technology but are under no religious or moral obligation to continue life-sustaining treatments when they cease to be beneficial or are being used to prolong the dying process.

Gender and Personal Issues
- The United Church of Christ affirms the equal value and worth of women and men and rejects any practice that supports superiority of one over another. It believes in the ordination of women and men and that all should be treated with equity and justice. One's relationship with God is not based on race, gender, or sexual orientation; are all children of God.
- The United Church of Christ celebrates a diversity of thought as well as the understanding of covenant. Despite any differences, individuals are to work together for the glory of God and the common good of all. People can agree to disagree and recognize the importance of engaging in dialogue despite their differences.
- The United Church of Christ supports health care professionals regardless of one's sexual orientation.

Principles for Spiritual Care through the Cycles of Life

Concepts of Living and Dying for Spiritual Support

- Human life is God's wonderful creation, and it is sacred.
- Death is a sign of one's mortal life and human finitude. It is not to be feared, but rather is a time to celebrate the life that has been lived by recalling the memories and journey of faith.
- People are called to live life that is pleasing to God and are granted eternal life by their Savior, Jesus Christ.
- The rites of passage – birth, baptism, marriage, and death – are to be celebrated within the context of the church. As individuals make covenantal commitments, the church enters into a covenant with individuals or couples to pray, love, and support them.

During Birth

- United Church of Christ believes in infant baptism. This sacrament is performed by a minister of the United Church of Christ. Any Christian baptism is recognized by the United Church of Christ.
- Baptism may be requested by family for a baby. The chaplain or clergy should be consulted. Baptism would ordinarily be delayed so that it may occur before the worshipping community. However, emergency baptism should be done when a baby's life is in jeopardy. If death should occur before baptism can be provided, there is consolation in God's love and mercy.
- As stated earlier, circumcision may be requested for cultural and not religious reasons.

During Illness

- Patients may receive comfort from the reading of scriptures or other devotional material, listening to religious music, watching televised worship services.
- Patients may request Holy Communion. The chaplain or clergy should be consulted.
- Patients may receive comfort from healing prayers. These can be offered by health care professionals.
- Spiritual counsel may be provided by chaplain or pastor. Illness often raises questions about why people suffer, and the meaning and purpose of life.
- Patients may request baptism. In an emergency, anyone can administer baptism, although in ordinary circumstances baptism would be provided by a Church pastor. The Rite of Baptism may include a variety of words, but should always include "You are baptized in the name of the Father, Son, and Holy Spirit." (The Church will sometimes use gender inclusive language.)

End of Life

- Dying persons and their families should avail themselves of the best medical technology, but are under no moral obligation to continue life sustaining treatments when they cease to be beneficial or prolong the dying process.
- United Church of Christ supports palliative care and hospice when appropriate.
- Families may wish to view the body of the deceased in the hospital room. The nurse and chaplain should be consulted for assistance.
- Family may request prayers for the deceased. These can be offered by the chaplain or pastor.

Care of the Body

- Family members should be allowed to spend time with their deceased loved one. Saying goodbye, even though the person is dead, is important in bringing closure. It helps facilitate the grief process.
- The body should be treated with respect at all times.
- Disposition and embalming are individual decisions. Cremation is now the choice of many Christians. The chaplain and the funeral home director should be consulted for assistance.
- Autopsy is an individual decision unless required by law. The chaplain and/or nurse should be consulted.
- Donation for medical research is an individual decision. The chaplain and/or nurse should be consulted for assistance. Advance planning for such donations is required by most receiving organizations. Last-minute donations are usually not possible.

Organ and Tissue Donation

- The United Church of Christ encourages and supports its members to become organ and tissue donors as an expression of Christian ministry, generosity, stewardship, and love. The Church calls upon those providing pastoral care to provide information in helping individuals make informed decisions regarding organ and tissue donation; it also encourages individuals to sign organ and tissue donor cards and to include in their advance medical directives instructions for organ and tissue donation.

Scriptures, Inspirational Readings, and Prayers

READINGS DURING ILLNESS

These can be read by family, friends, clergy, and health care professionals. (Scripture quotations are from the New Revised Standard Version, unless specified differently).

The Lord is my shepherd I shall not want.
He makes me to lie down in green pastures; he restores my soul.
He leads me in right paths for his name's sake.
Even though I walk through the darkest valley, I will fear no evil;
For you are with me; your rod and your staff – they comfort me.
You prepare a table before me in the presence of my enemies
You anoint my head with oil; my cup overflows.
Surely goodness and mercy shall follow me all the days of my life,
And I shall dwell in the house of the Lord my whole life.

—Psalm 23

Our Father who art in heaven, hallowed be thy name.
Thy kingdom come; Thy will be done on earth as it is in heaven.
Give us this day our daily bread.
And forgive us our debts as we forgive our debtors.
And lead us not into temptation, but deliver us from evil.

For thine is the kingdom, and the
power, and the glory, forever.
Amen.

—The Lord's Prayer, Matt. 6: 9–13
(Authorized [King James] Version)

READINGS DURING END-OF-LIFE PROCESS

These can be read by family, friends, clergy, and health care professionals. (All scripture quotations are from the New Revised Standard Version.)

I am the resurrection and the life.
Those who believe in me, even
though they die, will live, and
everyone who lives and believes in me
will never die.

—John 11:25–26.

Do not let your hearts be troubled.
Believe in God, believe also in me.
In my Father's house there are many
dwelling places. If it were not so,
would I have told you that I go and
prepare a place for you? And if I
go and prepare a place for you, I

will come again and will take you to
myself, so that where I am, there you
may be also.

—John 14:1–3

PRAYER DURING END-OF-LIFE PROCESS

This prayer can be offered by chaplain or pastor. (The prayer is taken from the *Book of Worship* by the United Church of Christ Office for Church Life and Leadership.)

Almighty God,
By your gentle power you raised
Jesus Christ from death.
Watch over this child of yours, our
brother/sister _____.
Fill his/her eyes with light that he/
she may see beyond human sight,
a home where pain is gone and
physical frailty becomes glory.
Banish fear. Brush away tears.
Let death be gentle as nightfall,
promising a new day when sighs
of grief turn to songs of joy, and
we are joined again in the presence
of Jesus Christ in our Heavenly
reunion.
Amen.[283]

---

283 *Book of Worship United Church of Christ.* (1986).
New York, NY: United Church of Christ Office for
Church Life and Leadership.

United Methodist Church

284

"Love is the fulfilling of the law, the end of the commandment." Very
excellent things are spoken of love; it is the essence, the spirit, the life
of all virtue. It is not only the first and great command, but it is all the
commandments in one. "Whatsoever things are just, whatsoever things are
pure, whatsoever things are amiable," or honorable; "if there be any virtue,
if there be any praise, they are all comprised in this one word, – love."[285]

Prepared by:
Jeanne Hoeft, PhD
Associate Professor of Pastoral Theology and Pastoral Care
with assistance from Amanda Caruso
Saint Paul School of Theology
Kansas City, MO

History and Facts

Methodism in the United States began as an extension of a movement initiated by an Anglican priest, John Wesley (1703–1791), and his followers in Great Britain. One of the unique features of the Wesleyan movement was the formation of small groups or "societies," as they were first called, which served as a means of spiritual accountability and growth for the members (non-ordained).

Especially as the movement expanded to the United States, the lay (non-ordained) people have been central to the mission and organization of United Methodism. In the mid-eighteenth century, followers of Wesley in the United States designated "circuit riders" who traveled from place to place to preach and spread the gospel, often in the camp meeting revival style of the time. The lack of ordained priests from the Church of England, and therefore the lack of persons authorized to administer the sacraments, compelled the preachers in 1784 to organize a new church, The Methodist Episcopal Church in America. At about the same time, some primarily

---

284 Circuit rider, often associated with Methodism in America, was provided by the author of this chapter.

285 Wesley, J. (1733). Circumcision of the heart. In E. Sugden. ed. (1983). *John Wesley's Fifty-Three Sermons.* Nashville, TN: Abingdon Press, 192.

German-speaking people from the German Reformed, Mennonite, and Lutheran traditions organized to form the Church of the United Brethren in Christ and Evangelical Association. These two churches united in 1946 to form the Evangelical United Brethren Church. After divisions in the Methodist Episcopal Church over racial discrimination and slavery, and the leadership role of laypersons, several churches came together to in 1939 to form the Methodist Church. Many denominations have historical ties to Methodism, such as the African Methodist Episcopal Church and the Free Methodist Church, but they have no structural relationship. In 1956, the Methodist Church granted full clergy rights to women.

The United Methodist Church was created in 1968 with the merger of the 1939 Methodist Church and the 1946 Evangelical United Brethren Church. African American churches had been assigned to separate Central Conferences; those were abolished in the 1968 merger. United Methodism is the second largest Protestant Christian denomination in the United States. As of 2006, there are about 11 million United Methodists worldwide and approximately 8.5 million in the United States.

Basic Teachings

- All the teachings of "Christianity" apply with the following exceptions, clarifications and additions.
- In addition to the *Apostles' Creed*, the *Nicene Creed* is also significant to Methodist doctrinal heritage.

Nicene Creed

We believe in one God,
the Father, the Almighty,
maker of heaven and earth,
of all that is, seen and unseen.

We believe in one Lord, Jesus Christ,
the only Son of God,
eternally begotten of the Father,
God from God, Light from Light,
true God from true God,
begotten, not made,
of one Being with the Father;
through him all things were made.
For us and for our salvation
he came down from heaven,
was incarnate of the Holy Spirit and
the Virgin Mary
and became truly human.
For our sake he was crucified under
Pontius Pilate;
he suffered death and was buried.
On the third day he rose again
in accordance with the Scriptures;
he ascended into heaven
and is seated at the right hand of the
Father.
He will come again in glory
to judge the living and the dead,
and his kingdom will have no end.

We believe in the Holy Spirit, the
Lord, the giver of life,
who proceeds from the Father and
the Son,
who with the Father and the Son
is worshipped and glorified,
who has spoken through the prophets.
We believe in the one holy catholic
and apostolic church.
We acknowledge one baptism
for the forgiveness of sins.
We look for the resurrection of the
dead,
and the life of the world to come.
Amen.

- The basic tenets of the Reformation are central, especially salvation by God's grace through faith, and the priesthood of all believers.
- The Reign of God is both a present and future reality, rather than a "final destination" alone.
- Wesleyan theology emphasizes God's grace, the loving activity of God in human existence through the Holy Spirit revealed in Jesus Christ, rather than God's punishment of human depravity.
- Salvation is a process of growing in perfect love through the grace of God, lived out in acts of personal and social holiness. This is reflected in Methodism's strong emphasis on the inextricable tie between personal transformation and social concern, love of God and love of neighbor.
- Teachings are grounded in scripture, Christian tradition, experience, and reason, with scripture being primary. Methodists encourage the use of contemporary scholarship for the interpretation of scripture.

Basic Practices

- All the practices of "Christianity" apply with the following exceptions, clarifications and additions.
- United Methodist pastors are ordained in Annual Conferences, not individual congregations, or they are licensed to serve as a pastor in one particular United Methodist congregation.
- Pastors are appointed to ministry settings by a bishop. Historically, United Methodist pastors have participated in an "itinerate" ministry, which means that they often move from one congregation to another.
- There are two Sacraments: the Lord's Supper (or Holy Communion) and baptism. The sacraments are means of God's grace and available to anyone who expresses a desire for them.
- Infants or persons of any age may be baptized, not only as a mark of initiation into Christian faith, but as an act of new birth. United Methodists recognize any Christian baptism and will not rebaptize, although reaffirmation of baptism is encouraged.
- Participation in the Holy Communion is participation in the life, death and resurrection of Jesus Christ. In the giving and receiving of bread, symbolizing the body of Christ, and wine (or grape juice), symbolizing the blood of the new covenant in Christ, the church remembers and is once again prepared to be the body of Christ in ministry to the world.
- The sacraments may be presided over only by clergy who are ordained elders or other clergy who have been granted license for certain situations.
- Membership in the United Methodist Church is open to any baptized Christian who reaffirms her or his baptismal vows, promises loyalty to the United Methodist Church and faithful participation by prayer, presence, gifts, and service. No confessional statement is required as a prerequisite to membership. Methodists emphasize mission and holy living over doctrinal conformity.
- Children, usually at about 12 years of age, may be confirmed into full membership in the United Methodist Church.
- Members are bound by the policies set forth in the "Book of Discipline of the United Methodist Church" (UMBD), which is reviewed and revised every 4 years at General Conference, a conference of equal parts clergy and laity

from all over the world (UMBD 103.3, 120–141).[286]

Principles for Clinical Care
Dietary Issues
- The United Methodist Church does not have any specific teachings regarding eating habits and religious beliefs.

General Medical Beliefs
- United Methodists see health care as a basic human right and therefore support equal access to medical care (UMBD 162.T).
- The well being of persons' mental and physical health has been enhanced by medical science. However, United Methodists insist on caution in the use of new technologies, drugs, and human subjects to advance science (UMBD 162.L).
- Genetic technology is welcomed when it contributes to the well-being of persons and their environment. Human cloning and the genetic manipulation of an unborn child are opposed (UMBD 162.M).
- United Methodists oppose assisted suicide and euthanasia (UMBD 161.N).

Specific Medical Issues
- **Abortion**: United Methodists believe in the sanctity of unborn human life, but recognize that there may be certain situations in which an abortion may be justified, provided it is a legal option, performed under proper medical care and with pastoral counsel (UMBD 161.J).

- **Advance Directives**: Advance directives are encouraged (UMBD 161.M).
- **Birth Control**: The United Methodist Church affirms the importance of family planning and supports medically safe birth control methods. United Methodists are committed to the principle that every child coming into the world should be wanted, supported, and provided for.
- **Blood Transfusions**: United Methodists have no restrictions on the use of blood transfusions.
- **Circumcision**: Circumcision may be chosen for cultural, not religious, reasons.
- **In Vitro Fertilization**: United Methodists have no objection to in vitro fertilization that is consensual by the couple involved.
- **Stem Cell Research**: United Methodists have no objection to the use of adult or umbilical cord stem cells in research toward this end. Taking seriously the moral implications of certain genetic science, United Methodists cautiously support embryonic stem cell research that uses excess in vitro fertilization embryos when there is informed consent by the couple involved. Embryos should not be created for the sole purpose of research, nor with the intent of destroying them (UMBR, 102).[287]
- **Vaccinations**: United Methodists have issued no statement on vaccinations but have no objections to them. It is an individual decision.
- **Withholding/Withdrawing Life Support**: Dying persons and their families should avail themselves of all medical technology but are under no religious or moral obligation to continue

---

286 *The Book of Discipline of the United Methodist Church 2004.* (2004). Nashville, TN: The United Methodist Publishing House. Citations in the text will make reference to this document as "UMBD."

287 *The Book of Resolutions of the United Methodist Church 2004.* (2004). Nashville, TN: United Methodist Publishing House. Citations in the text make reference to this document as "UMBR."

life-sustaining treatments when they cease to be beneficial or are being used to prolong the process of dying (UMBD 161.M).

Gender and Personal Issues

- United Methodists affirm the equal worth of women and men and reject any notion or practice that supports superiority of one over the other or sets different standards for them (UMBD 161.F).
- Sexuality is a gift from God that is to be affirmed and celebrated. United Methodists are called to practice responsible stewardship of this gift (UMBD 161.F).
- Homosexual persons, like all persons, are persons of "sacred worth" and should be treated with care and respect. While United Methodists consider the practice of homosexuality to be incompatible with Christian teaching, full human and civil rights for homosexuals should be ensured, including full access to medical care. Violence against gay and lesbian persons is not tolerated (UMBD 161.F, 162.H).
- United Methodists denounce any rejection, discrimination, or condemnation of persons living with HIV or AIDS (UMBD 162.S).
- United Methodists celebrate a diversity of thought and practice in spite of a strong connectional structure. Local customs and culturally diverse expressions of faith and practice are encouraged. There are many local United Methodist churches in the United States that are strongly rooted in the unique cultural gifts of African Americans, Korean Americans, Spanish-speaking Americans, and Native Americans. Health care providers should inquire about customary rituals and

practices that are particular to the region or cultural tradition of the person.

Principles for Spiritual Care through the Cycles of Life

Concepts of Living and Dying for Spiritual Support

- Human life is God's good creation. All human beings are created in the image of God. The body, no less then the soul, is a gift of God.
- Therefore, all are called to faithful living in this earthly life, including care of the body as part of God's creation.
- Illness is not God's will for people or a sign that God has deserted them.
- Death is a sign of one's mortal life and human finitude. However, through the death and resurrection of Jesus Christ, people are assured of eternal life in perfect love, in body and spirit.
- Eternal life is assured through faith, evidenced in good works, but not dependent upon a sinless life. No sin or past mistake lies outside the possibility of God's redemption.
- While individuals may seek to prolong meaningful life, death, in and of itself, should not be feared.

During Birth

- United Methodists believe in infant baptism.
- This sacramental ritual is performed only by an ordained elder or licensed pastor preferably in the context of a local congregation, but may be done in a hospital setting.
- Any Christian baptism is recognized by the United Methodist Church.
- As stated earlier, circumcision may be chosen for cultural, not religious, reasons.

During Illness

- Patients may receive comfort from the reading of scriptures or other devotional material, listening to religious music, watching televised worship services of their own or a similar tradition. Patients may request Holy Communion. The chaplain or clergy should be consulted for assistance.
- Patients may receive comfort from healing prayers. These can be offered by health care professionals. Patients from some traditions, however, may ask for healing prayer to be connected with "anointing with oil" or the "the laying on of hands." The chaplain or clergy should be consulted for assistance for these requests.
- Patients may request baptism. In the clinical setting, sprinkling is an acceptable mode of baptism, even for traditions that practice immersion. The chaplain or clergy should be consulted for assistance.
- Because of the "itinerate" system, sometimes a patient in a health care setting may request a visit from a former pastor who is still in the area. The manner in which this is handled varies by region. Health care providers should be aware that in many areas a former pastor will not visit, even at the request of the patient, as a way to support the ministry of the person's congregation and current pastor.
- United Methodists have a multilayered system of spiritual leaders that includes ordained elders, ordained deacons, commissioned ministers, local pastors, and lay leaders. Any of these persons may be called upon to provide spiritual support to the sick. Only ordained elders or a licensed pastor may serve Holy Communion or perform a baptism.

During End of Life

- United Methodists seek to ensure the comfort and dignity of the dying and pastoral care for their families.
- Advance directives are encouraged.
- Dying persons and their families should avail themselves of all medical technology but are under no religious or moral obligation to continue life-sustaining treatments when they cease to be beneficial or are being used to prolong the process of dying.
- United Methodists support palliative care and the use of hospice when appropriate.
- Customs vary regionally. There are no required or sacramental rites for the dying, though persons and families may request Holy Communion. This should be performed by an ordained chaplain or local United Methodist pastor.
- Families may wish to gather for prayer with the body of the deceased. Their pastor or chaplain should be consulted.

Care of the Body

- Disposition and embalming are individual decisions. Cremation is now the choice of many Christians. The chaplain and the funeral home director should be consulted for assistance.
- Autopsy is an individual decision unless required by law. The chaplain and/or nurse should be consulted for assistance.
- Donation for medical research is an individual decision. The chaplain and/or nurse should be consulted for assistance. Advance planning for such donations is required by most receiving organizations. Last-minute donations are usually not possible.
- United Methodists have no specific rituals or beliefs regarding care of the deceased body.

Organ and Tissue Donation

- United Methodists urge organ and tissue donation as an act of self-sacrificing love, in an environment of respect for the dead and care for living, following standards to prevent the abuse or exploitation of donors. It may be preferable for a chaplain and/or nurse who are trained designated requesters to be consulted for assistance.

Scriptures, Inspirational Readings, and Prayers

- Most United Methodists will be used to hearing non-gendered language for humanity and God.
- United Methodists will be familiar with the Lord's Prayer from the Authorized (King James) Version of the Bible and often wish to recite it from memory.

Our Father, who art in heaven,
hallowed be thy name.
Thy kingdom come,
thy will be done on earth as it is in
    heaven.
Give us this day our daily bread.
And forgive us our trespasses,
as we forgive those who trespass
    against us.
And lead us not into temptation,
but deliver us from evil.
For thine is the kingdom, and the
    power, and the glory,
forever. Amen.

United Methodists will often have favorite hymns. Singing, or hearing these sung, can provide great comfort. Some of the more familiar, and more distinctively United Methodist are "O For a Thousand Tongues to Sing," "Love Divine, All Loves Excelling," "Christ the Lord is Risen Today" by Charles Wesley and "Hymn of Promise" by Natalie Sleeth.[288]

O For a Thousand Tongues to Sing

O for a thousand tongues to sing,
my great Redeemer's praise,
the glories of my God and King,
the triumphs of his grace!

—Words by Charles Wesley, 1739
(*United Methodist Hymnal*, 1989, #57)

Love Divine, All Loves Excelling

Love divine, all loves excelling,
joy of heaven, to earth come down;
fix in us thy humble dwelling;
all thy faithful mercies crown!
Jesus thou art all compassion,
pure, unbounded love thou art;
visit us with thy salvation;
enter every trembling heart.

—Words by Charles Wesley, 1747
(*United Methodist Hymnal*, 1989, #384)

Christ the Lord is Risen Today

Christ the Lord is risen today,
    Alleluia!
Earth and heaven in chorus say,
    Alleluia!
Raise your joys and triumphs high,
    Alleluia!
Sing, ye heavens, and earth reply,
    Alleluia!

—Words by Charles Wesley, 1739
(*United Methodist Hymnal*, 1989,
#302)

---

288 All songs were obtained from *The United Methodist Hymnal*. (1989). Nashville, TN: United Methodist Publishing House. Page numbers are cited with each song in the text.

Hymn of Promise

In the bulb there is a flower; in the
  seed, and apple tree;
in cocoons, a hidden promise:
  butterflies will soon be free!
In the cold and snow of winter there's
  a spring that waits to be,
unrevealed until its season, something
  God alone can see.

—Words and music by Natalie Sleeth
  (*United Methodist Hymnal*, 1989,
  #707)

In addition to readings named in "Christianity," these scripture readings may be familiar to United Methodists and especially appropriate for the dying:

READINGS DURING END-OF-LIFE PROCESS

These can be read by family, friends, clergy, and health care professionals. (All scripture quotations are from the New Revised Standard Version.)

Comfort, comfort my people,
says your God. Speak tenderly to
Jerusalem, and cry to her that she has
served her term, that her penalty is
paid, that she has received from the
LORD's hand double for all her sins.
A voice cries out: "In the wilderness
prepare the way of the LORD; make
straight in the wilderness a highway
for our God. Every valley shall be
lifted up, every mountain and hill
made low; the uneven ground shall
become level, the rugged places a
plain. And the glory of the LORD
will be revealed, and all the people
will see it together. For the mouth
of the LORD has spoken." A voice

says, "Cry out!" And I said, "What
shall I cry?" "All people are grass,
their constancy is like the flowers of
the field. The grass withers, and the
flower fades, when the breath of the
LORD blows upon it. Surely the
people are grass. The grass withers,
the flower fades; but the word of our
God will stand forever."

—Isa. 40:1–8

Then I saw a new heaven and a new
earth; for the first heaven and the first
earth had passed away, and the sea
was no more. And I saw the holy city,
the new Jerusalem, coming down
out of heaven from God, prepared
as a bride adorned for her husband.
And I heard a loud voice from the
throne saying, "See, the home of God
is among mortals. He will dwell with
them as their God; they will be his
peoples, and God himself will be with
them; he will wipe every tear from
their eyes. Death will be no more;
mourning and crying and pain will
be no more, for the first things have
passed away."

And the one who was seated on the
throne said, "See, I am making all
things new." Also he said, "Write this,
for these words are trustworthy and
true." Then he said to me, "It is done!
I am the Alpha and the Omega, the
beginning and the end. To the thirsty
I will give water as a gift from the
spring of the water of life.

—Rev. 21:1–6

PRAYER FOR THE DYING[289]

This prayer can be offered by family, friends, clergy, or health care professionals.

Gracious God, you are nearer than
hands or feet, closer than breathing.
Sustain with your presence our
brother/sister Name.
Help him/her now to trust in your
goodness and claim your promise of
life everlasting.
Cleanse him/her of all sin and remove
all burdens.
Grant him/her the sure joy of your
salvation,
through Jesus Christ our Lord.
Amen.

—*United Methodist Book of Worship*,
1992, p. 166

PRAYER WITH PERSONS WITH LIFE-THREATENING ILLNESS

This prayer can be offered by family, friends, clergy, or health care professionals.

Lord Jesus Christ,
we come to you sharing the suffering
that you endured.
Grant us patience during this time,
that as we and Name live with pain,
disappointment, and frustration,
we may realize that suffering is a part
of life,
a part of life that you know intimately.
Touch Name in his/her time of trial,
hold him/her tenderly in your loving
arms,
and let him/her know you care.
Renew us in our spirits,
even when our bodies are not being
renewed,
that we might be ever prepared to
dwell in your eternal home,
through our faith in you, Lord Jesus,
who died and are alive for evermore.
Amen.

—*United Methodist Book of Worship*,
1992, p. 628

---

289 All prayers were obtained from *The United Methodist Book of Worship*. (1992). Nashville, TN: United Methodist Publishing House. Page numbers for the individual prayers are cited in the text.

Unity

Culturally Christian, Spiritually Unlimited

Prepared by:
The Reverend Thomas W. Shepherd, DMin
Historical and Theological Studies Chair, Unity Institute
 and Seminary
Lee's Summit, MO

Reviewed and approved by:
The Reverend Phillip M. Pierson
Former Vice President for Education, Unity School of
 Christianity
Charlotte D. Shelton, EdD
President and CEO, Unity School of Christianity
Lee's Summit, MO

History and Facts

Unity cofounders Charles Fillmore (1854–1948) and Myrtle Fillmore (1845–1931) never intended to start a new church, and especially to add another denomination to the rolls of American Protestantism. Unity actually started as the result of a medical condition of one of its founders. In the 1880s, Myrtle Fillmore was diagnosed with advanced tuberculosis, which was considered terminal by nineteenth-century science. After trying the usual, impotent medicines of the day, Myrtle and her husband, Charles, attended a public lecture by Dr. E. B. Weeks in the spring of 1886. Sometime during the talk, Weeks said, "I am a child of God, and therefore I do not inherit sickness." Charles was apparently unaffected by the lecture, but that sentence stood out so vividly for Myrtle that she later said it felt like, "He said that especially for me."[290] Myrtle then began an intensive program of meditation on positive imagery and affirmative prayer. Here is her account, written in the gender-specific language of her era.

I have made what seems to me a discovery. I was fearfully sick; I had all the ills of mind and body I could bear. Medicine and doctors ceased to give me relief, and I was in despair when I found practical Christianity. I took it up and I was healed. I did most of the healing myself, because I wanted the understanding for future use. This is how I made what I call my discovery:

I was thinking about life. Life is everywhere – in worm and in man. "Then why does not the life in the worm make a body like man's?" I asked. Then I thought, "The worm has not as much sense as man." Ah! Intelligence, as well as life, is needed to make a body. Here is the key to my discovery. Life has to be guided by intelligence in making all forms. The same law works in my own body. Life is simply a form of energy and has to be guided and directed in man's body by his intelligence. How do we communicate intelligence? By thinking and talking, of course. Then it flashed upon me that I might talk to the life in every part of my body and have it do just

---

290 Freeman, J. (1987). *The Story of Unity.* Unity Village, MO: Unity Books, 44–45.

what I wanted. I began to teach my body and got marvelous results.

I told the life in my liver that it was not torpid or inert, but full of vigor and energy. I told the life in my stomach that it was not weak or inefficient, but energetic, strong and intelligent. I told the life in my abdomen that it was not longer infested with ignorant thoughts or disease, put there by myself and by doctors, but that it was all a thrill with the sweet, pure, wholesome energy of God. I told my limbs that they were active and strong. I told my eyes that they did not see of themselves but that they expressed the sight of Spirit, and that they were drawing upon an unlimited source. I told them that they were young eyes, clear, bright eyes, because the light of God shone right through them. I told my heart that the pure love of Jesus Christ flowed in and out through its beatings and that all the world felt its joyous pulsation.

I went to all the life centers in my body and spoke words of Truth to them – words of strength and power. I asked their forgiveness for the foolish, ignorant course that I had pursued in the past, when I had condemned them and called them weak, inefficient and diseased. I did not become discouraged at their being slow to wake up, but kept right on, both silently and aloud, declaring the words of Truth, until the organs responded. And neither did I forget to tell them that they were free, unlimited Spirit. I told them that they were no longer in bondage to the carnal mind; that they were not corruptible flesh, but centers of life and energy omnipresent.

Then I asked the Father to forgive me for taking His life into my organism and there using it so meanly. I promised Him that I would never, never again retard the free flow of that life through my mind and my body by any false word or thought; that I would always bless it and encourage it with true thoughts

and words in its wise work of building up my body temple; that I would use all diligence and wisdom in telling it just what I wanted it to do.

I also saw that I was using the life of the Father in thinking thoughts and speaking words, and I became very watchful as to what I thought and said. I did not let any worried or anxious thoughts into my mind, and I stopped speaking gossipy, frivolous, petulant, angry words. I would let a little prayer go up every hour that Jesus Christ would be with me and help me to think and speak only kind, loving, true words; and I am sure He is with me, because I am so peaceful and happy now …

I want everyone to know about this beautiful, true law, and to use it. It is not a new discovery, but, when you use it and get the fruits of health and harmony it will seem new to you, and you will feel that it is your own discovery.[291]

After 2 years of steady prayer work, Myrtle Fillmore was so completely healed that she would live another 45 years. Friends and neighbors learned of her recovery and asked her to teach them what she had done. Unity literally began over Myrtle's kitchen table as she talked with people and shared her "discovery" with an ever-expanding number of inquirers. Charles became interested, too, and soon they were publishing booklets and holding after-church meetings which eventually grew into the Unity movement. It is fair to say that Unity began as a healing ministry and continues to emphasize spiritual healing in its teachings today

Unity could be further described – although not without controversy – as a progressive Protestant denomination, an

---

291 Freeman. *The Story of Unity*, 47–49. Lengthy quote by Myrtle Fillmore.

expression of "metaphysical Christianity" with roots in American transcendentalism and the New Thought movement of the late nineteenth century. The Unity movement is more than a religious affiliation; it is a powerful, fulfilling, richly satisfying way of life. However, because Unity evolved from lay-led groups studying nineteenth-century transcendentalism and spiritual healing, the movement became a church almost by accident. The Fillmores initially encouraged people to continue attending their various churches and then come together afterward as a nondenominational group for prayer and spiritual studies. When these after-church experiences grew more important to the participants than their Sunday morning worship events, the study group insisted on organizing itself into a church. The process duplicated elsewhere, and Unity found itself a de facto branch of Protestantism, a kind of "nondenominational denomination." Even today, the word "church" remains controversial in some congregations, where the term "Unity Center" is preferred. These churches and centers have organized themselves into, what is today, a worldwide network called the Association of Unity Churches International.

Although Unity has its roots in Protestant thought, especially transcendentalism, many Unity people actually see themselves as trans-denominational, culturally Christian but spiritually unlimited. The Judeo-Christian scripture provides the main textbook for the Unity movement, although it is quite common for Unity worship services to include references from the sacred texts of non-Western traditions as well. The Bible is usually read in modern translations and interpreted with special attention to historical context and biblical symbolism.

As mentioned, Unity cofounders Charles and Myrtle Fillmore never intended their informal fellowship to grow into a formal denomination. At first, people from a hodgepodge of Christian traditions gathered for prayer and study on Sundays after attending their home churches. Bolstered by the prayers and encouragement of a growing number of people, Charles and Myrtle began publishing their understandings of the Jesus Christ teachings and founded *Modern Thought* magazine in 1889. This would later be renamed *Unity Magazine*, which is still published today. As the publication ministry grew, Charles invited readers around the world to join them in a *Society of Silent Help*, as it was first called. Members were asked to hold specific prayer thoughts each month during a period of silent prayer in the evening. This was later renamed the *Society of Silent Unity*, and the ministry quickly expanded to a spiritual helpline and hub of ongoing prayer, 24-7-365. Today, this worldwide ministry is called, simply, *Silent Unity*. Its distinctive nonsectarian prayer line was the first such ministry and has set the standard for all the live call dial-a-prayer systems to come after. By 2007, Silent Unity was answering 200 000 emails, 500 000 phone calls, and 1.3 million letters each year. One of the symbols of Silent Unity's eternal prayer vigil for the whole world is called "the light that shines for you," a lighted cupola tower that can be seen at a distance and never goes out, indicating that someone is currently at prayer in the Silent Unity prayer chapel.

Since it is an interdenominational, nonsectarian form of spiritual support, people from virtually every religious tradition on the face of the earth have contacted Silent Unity for prayer. It is a good resource which can help both Unity and non-Unity patients, staff and families in times when they need an affirmative, spiritual word. You may try this prayer ministry for yourself by calling 1-800-NOW-PRAY (1-800-669-7729).

In 1924 Silent Unity began publishing *Daily Word*, a hand-sized daily devotional guide featuring nonsectarian, affirmative prayer, and which again established the pattern for an array of daily devotional publications now available.

Unity Village, Missouri, located in the suburbs of Kansas City, is the headquarters and world center of the Unity movement, a place dedicated to prayer, education, and illumination. People from all over the world come to stroll the lovely rose garden and linger awhile beside one of the finest fountain systems in the United States. There are smaller prayer groves, an open-air "labyrinth" to walk, and even a golf course for spiritual recreation. Retreats and special events are held throughout the year, and visitors to the grounds are always welcome.

The Unity website describes its organizational goals with this inclusive, nonjudgmental affirmation:

Unity helps people of all faiths apply positive spiritual principles in their daily lives.[292]

As stated earlier, the majority of the work at Unity Village involves prayer, publishing, and education services to people of all faiths. These include the prayer ministry, Silent Unity, *Daily Word* (Unity's nonsectarian, inspirational monthly magazine), retreats, and continuing education classes that are open to everyone and teach Unity principles in trans-denominational settings.[293] Some of

these principles are reflected in a few self-descriptive summary statements published by Unity School of Christianity:

- Unity is a worldwide movement of prayer, education and publishing that helps people of all faiths apply positive spiritual principles in their daily lives.[294]
- Unity is positive, practical Christianity. We teach the effective, daily application of the principles of Truth taught and exemplified by Jesus Christ. We promote a way of life that leads to health, prosperity, happiness, and peace of mind.
- Unity has established centers of study and worship throughout the world where people discover and practice the Unity way of life. We address physical, mental, and emotional needs through affirmative prayer and spiritual education. We serve those who seek inspiration and prayer support as well as those who use Unity teachings as their primary path of spiritual growth.
- We believe that all people are created with sacred worth, and we strive to reach out to all who seek support and spiritual growth. Therefore, we recognize the importance of serving all people in spiritually and emotionally caring ways. Our ministries and outreaches are free of discrimination on the basis of race, gender, age, creed, religion, national origin, ethnicity, physical disability, and sexual orientation.[295]

Basic Teachings
The Unity belief system is deep and vast, but perhaps the best summary has been expressed in the following five basic ideas:

292 www.unity.org
293 http://content.unity.org/aboutunity/faq/index.html (accessed 16 Sept 2012).
294 www.unity.org (accessed 16 Sept 2012).
295 http://content.unity.org/aboutunity/faq/index.html (accessed 16 Sept 2012).

1. God is the source and creator of all. There is no other enduring power. God is good and present everywhere.

2. We are spiritual beings, created in God's image. The spirit of God lives within each person; therefore, all people are inherently good.

3. We create our life experiences through our way of thinking.

4. There is power in affirmative prayer, which we believe increases our connection to God.

5. Knowledge of these spiritual principles is not enough. We must live them.[296]

Principle 1: One Presence/One Power, God the Good

Unity's doctrine of God flows from a central pivotal belief, summarized by the affirmation: "There is only one Presence and one Power in the universe, God, the good omnipotent."[297] This statement, quoted here from the writings of Myrtle Fillmore, is frequently repeated in Unity publications. Theologically, Unity's form of Christianity is both *panentheistic* and *universalist*. Everything in the Cosmos is "in" God as a fish is in the water (*panentheism*), and everyone is destined to eventual union with the divine (*universalism*), an eternal state of creativity and love which Unity calls *Christ consciousness*. As mentioned, Unity holds an historical-allegorical approach to the scripture and a symbolic understanding of most traditional Christian doctrines, such as the Trinity, which is interpreted not as three divine persons but as three phases of consciousness – mind, idea, expression.

Principle 2: *Imago Dei*

Unity accepts the idea of humanity described in the opening chapter of Genesis: "So God created humankind in his image, in the image of God he created them; male and female he created them."[298] Unity wholeheartedly embraces the biblical theme of humanity as created *Imago Dei*, in the image and likeness of God. This belief comes without any hint of anthropomorphism, recognizing the fundamental "likeness" between God and *Homo sapiens* must be spiritual rather than physical. Unity's theology therefore flows from Creation-centered spirituality.

For a Unity person, it is not enough to say everyone has within them the *Imago Dei*, because this inner divine image is each person's true identity. Human consciousness is actually an outpicturing of the Divine, limited only by our degree of openness to its expression. Consequently, Unity sees theological anthropology – that which was formerly called the "doctrine of man" – as the study of unfolding awareness in human consciousness of the divine nature within every sentient being. Unity professes no belief in the metaphysical reality of sin or evil while acknowledging that human free will can certainly take people away from the good which God is trying to work through them. As the opening chapter of Genesis proclaims with its rapturous litany, "And God saw that it was good ... God saw everything that he had made, and indeed, it was very good."[299]

Not surprisingly, Unity interprets the Atonement much differently from the classical sense. The "work" of Jesus Christ was to serve as the Way-shower for humanity's

---

296 www.unityonline.org/discover_faq.htm (accessed February 8, 2007).

297 Fillmore, M. (1954). *Myrtle Fillmore's Healing Letters.* Unity Village, MO: Unity Books, 132.

298 Gen. 1:27 (New Revised Standard Version).

299 Gen. 1:25, 31.

path to God; there is no need to postulate an estrangement between the divine and the Cosmos. God has always been in harmonious relationship with Creation, because God is the very operating system by which the Universe functions. Certainly, as a child might wander in the wilds, poor choices can lead one off the path, away from the best way to happiness and growth. However, *sin* for Unity is error-belief, the attempt to negate a divine idea, missing the mark, or simply making a mistake – even a horrific mistake is a mistake no less. Unity theologians also tend to see sin as societal and institutional – racism, world poverty, sexism, homophobia, endless violence, genocide, and hatred in all its many self-defeating categories.

Humans themselves are not viewed as totally depraved, just totally free. Rather than fallen, flawed, and fouled, Unity tends to see human nature as evolutionary and unfolding: neither dysfunctional needing repair nor lost needing redemption, but simply embryonic, needing time to grow. Unity does not see humanity as broken, any more than a 7-year-old is "broken" because she can't do calculus or decline a German noun. She is not even truly *incomplete*, because she is doing what a 7-year-old is supposed to do at this stage of her development (i.e., learning the basic building blocks which will lead to higher things). An acorn is not an incomplete oak; it is seed en route to the treetops. Since it appears programmed into the nature of reality itself, one could argue that *growth* is the fundamental principle of life in the cosmos.

If humans are guilty of anything, it is a state of militant ignorance; yet humanity is nonetheless brimming with divine potential, like a child prodigy learning by trial-and-error. For Unity, sin is error-belief in action, which can only be overcome by denying

its power in the first place and affirming the universal divine nature of all sentient beings as expressed through the indwelling Christ. Although it cannot be denied that humans are capable of monstrous "evil" by exercising their divine powers to make ungodly choices, most people are neither Adolph Hitler nor Mother Teresa. Unity people find no virtue in aggrandizement of the trivial mistakes made along the road of life. Things take time, and human growth will be accomplished as the evolution of consciousness continues.

Principle 3: The Law of Mind Action

An oft-repeated New Thought Christian maxim goes, "Thoughts held in mind, produce after their own kind." Unity people believe they can attract positive or negative experiences to themselves by what they think about. So profound is this cause-effect relationship that many Unity people believe humanity literally creates in mind the world in which it lives. As one Unity website writes:

> Every effect we see and experience in our outer world is the result of a thought held in mind. As human beings, we create our experience by the activity of our thinking. Everything in the manifest realm has its beginning in thought.[300]

To apply this idea to medical conditions, the Unity person will often believe it is possible for healing to occur in any and all circumstances. Medical personnel will likely find this faith in the healing power of mind to be an asset in the patient's recovery process.

---

300 www.unitychurchofmemphis.com/UnityBasics.html (accessed 16 Sept 12).

Principle 4: Affirmative Prayer

Affirmative prayer is a useful tool for focusing our thoughts on the truth that we are spiritual beings, filled with vibrant energy and renewing life. We, too, can use this tool in our daily lives. When we pray affirmatively about a health challenge, we are recognizing the life of God within ... As we pray affirmatively, we assert our confidence in God's healing power within our minds and bodies. We affirm daily, even momently, that we are one with God and that the life of God is flowing freely within us.[301]

Unity people generally work with the prayer forms known as *denials* and *affirmations*. Metaphysical Christians use the word "denial" differently from the popularized psychological term, which often means refusing to look at or take responsibility for an unpleasant situation. What Unity means by *denials* is for the person to refuse to accept that there is any eternal truth in sickness, poverty, or any seemingly negative condition. Unity teaches people to deny the *power* of the dis-ease over them, not to deny that it hurts to hurt. Denials are another way of saying there is no Presence or Power but God, in Whom we trust completely.

Here are a few examples of denials:

- I deny the belief that I have inherited disease, sickness, ignorance, or any mental limitations whatsoever.[302]
- I deny that I inherit any belief that in any

way limits me in health, virtue, intelligence, or power to do good.[303]
- No person or thing in the universe, no chain of circumstances, can by any possibility interpose itself between you and all joy – all good.[304]

After *denials* have cleared the mind of fears and error-beliefs, Unity people turn to *affirmations* to remind themselves of that which is eternally true. Rather than telling God what is true about God, Unity people realize the faith-work is theirs to do. Since God obviously already knows everything, metaphysical Christianity teaches people to *affirm spiritual truth to themselves* in positive statements. Here are a few samples:

- With my heart open to God's renewing love, I accept my healing now.
- I am healthy and strong because I am one with God's healing, revitalizing presence.
- I am created in the image of God, blessed with strength and wholeness.
- The power of God sustains and blesses me with perfect health.
- I have instant access to God's healing power within. I am whole and well in mind, body, and spirit.[305]

Principle 5: Spiritual Principles Must be Lived

All that has already been mentioned should indicate how important it is to Unity people for their faith to be more than just a Sunday visit to church. Unity teaches spiritual principles as a life-long practice. In fact, the journey to Christ-consciousness continues

---

301 Cameron, D. (n.d.). Affirm Life! Online article on Unity School of Christianity website. Available at: http://content.unity.org/prayer/inspirational Articles/affirmLife.html (accessed 16 Sept 2012).

302 Fillmore, C. and C. D. Fillmore. (1941). *Teach Us to Pray.* Unity Village, MO: Unity Books, 184.

303 Ibid., 187.

304 Cady, H. (2005). *Lessons in Truth: Centennial 1903–2003 Edition.* Unity Village, MO: Unity Books, 53.

305 "Healing Affirmations," online at: http://content. unity.org/prayer/prayersAffirmations/healing PrayerAffirm.html (accessed 16 Sept 2012).

beyond life. Unity people generally believe that everyone has an individualized learning plan and will spend as much time as needed to learn whatever is necessary for spiritual growth. They call their faith a "movement" or a "way of life" and are sometimes uncomfortable with the notion of organized religion as a separate category from everyday experiences. For this reason, the practice of daily prayer and meditation is especially important, as is the ongoing study of spiritual principles and their application in everyday life.

Most Unity people practice some form of regular prayer and meditation. Often this will involve reading the *Daily Word* reading for that date, followed by a time of prayer, reflection, and sitting in the Silence.

Unity Minister

In Unity churches, the ministers are usually called *Reverend*, although many just prefer using their first name. Sometimes a shorthand version appears, such as "Reverend Tom" or "Reverend Susan" (written as RevTom, RevSusan). Ministers are typically ordained and licensed like other Protestants following a congregational polity, although all Unity ordinations must be centrally approved by the Association of Unity Churches International. Unity Institute, located at Unity Village near Kansas City, Missouri, is the main theological seminary for the movement. Ministers can also come into Unity through a field licensing program, which usually involves working as a Spiritual Leader of a congregation. The Unity movement also offers three opportunities for ministry which are somewhat unique: *Spiritual Leader*, *Licensed Unity teacher*, and *Unity Chaplain*.

1. **Spiritual Leader**: Usually a Licensed Unity Teacher who has been appointed to act as the local pastor when another minister is unavailable. The spiritual leader should be considered equivalent to a fully ordained minister, although this person is probably in the process of completing steps to achieve that official status.

2. **Licensed Unity Teacher (LUT)**: A layperson who has gone through a rigorous, somewhat lengthy course of study and can function as an assistant to the senior minister or in some cases as spiritual leader of a congregation. Not simply a teacher, the LUT can do virtually everything a minister can do – marry, bury, lead worship services, teach classes for Unity credit. The only difference is that LUTs normally work under the direction and support of a senior minister or spiritual leader rather than independently.

3. **Prayer Chaplain**: The term *chaplain* is somewhat misleading, because it suggests an ordained minister serving at an institution, which is not the case. The Unity Chaplain is a layperson who has some training in prayer ministry and spiritual counseling techniques, but with no professional functions (cannot marry, bury, serve as Spiritual Leader, etc.) Chaplains usually serve as prayer partners after worship for those who desire extra support in their spiritual lives, however they may also make hospital and nursing home calls to visit and pray with Unity people who are in those institutions. The important distinction for medical and professional staff is that Unity Chaplains are generally not ordained ministers, but trained laypeople with a heart full of love to share. Unity ministers sometimes serve as professional hospital chaplains, but

they will usually be identified by name tags and by the use of the title *Reverend*.

Basic Practices

- Unity people are quite like liberal Protestants in their basic practices. They ordinarily meet Sunday mornings for worship, which usually includes some combination of the following: affirmative prayer, guided meditation, sacred readings, music, some form of the Lord's Prayer, sermons/lessons, taking the offering, and closing with the "Prayer for Protection"[306] and the Peace Song ("Let There Be Peace on Earth").
- Lord's Supper/Communion is celebrated by some churches, but not by all. Sometimes it is done as a meditation exercise without elements; other churches do a modified version of the Lord's Supper indistinguishable from that which might be offered at a liberal Protestant church.
- Christening, baptizing, and name-giving are possible, almost any method and almost any age. These are generally viewed as rites of passage or declarations of allegiance to the church community, not as supernatural sacraments.
- Sacraments are generally understood as places where the normally invisible presence of God becomes discernible. When a person realizes he/she is expressing the God-within, or becomes aware that everything is in God, that is a sacramental encounter. It may happen in church, but more likely in a mountain cathedral, pillared by tall pines under a domed vault of blue-and-white sky.

- Unity people work at seeing the totality of life as a spiritual experience.

Principles for Clinical Care
Dietary Issues

- Like the cofounders, Charles and Myrtle Fillmore, many Unity people are vegetarians, although it is not required. Others eat fish, eggs, chicken, or other combinations of foods, while a great many people in Unity observe no food restrictions whatsoever. There are also quite a few people in various "recovery" programs who may have special needs.
- The best policy would be to ask for each Unity person's dietary preferences.

General Medical Beliefs

- Medical staff, clergy, and other helping professionals who work with Unity people will generally find them upbeat and positive, easy to approach, and filled with faith in God and trust in the healing process. They can generally be treated as progressive Protestants with no special restrictions.
- Individual consciousness, guided by prayer, informs the decisions of Unity people on spiritual and ethical issues, so the best course will be to ask each person individually about any questions on medical procedures or other matters.
- With a positive attitude and prayerful confidence in God as the Source of all healing, Unity people will usually present the helping professional with a congenial experience in patient-staff interactions.
- Unity has constantly held that all healing comes from the same Source, which includes both medical and spiritual healing. An old saying among metaphysical Christians – indicated by its outdated use

---

306 By James Dillet Freeman; *see* "Scriptures, Inspirational Readings, and Prayers" section.

of gender – is the following: "Go first to God, then to man, as God directs."[307]

- Unity people are taught to hold positive thoughts in mind, to see themselves as whole and well, surrounded by God's light and love and protection. Their prayer and meditation work will also envision the medical staff as extensions of God's hands, doing God's good work, allowing divine healing to work through their efforts. The following daily devotional provides a classic example of the metaphysical Christian approach to healing. It is drawn from Unity's best-read publication, *Daily Word*. (Note the prayer is in the form of *affirmation* rather than petition.)

Healing

Created in the image of God, I express pure life and energy. If I may have been holding thoughts of myself as sick or injured, I change that image and see myself healthy and whole. God loves me. Nothing can prevent me from feeling this love within me and knowing that love's healing energy is continually moving throughout my being. I am a divine creation, given shape and form according to God's perfect design. I am created for life, created to know love and joy and wholeness. There is no injury, no sickness that is beyond God's power to heal. I feel God's presence enfolding me. God and I are one, and a mighty healing work is taking place.[308]

---

307 Attributed to the Reverend Ernest C. Wilson (1896–1982), Unity minister.
308 *Daily Word* for Wednesday, February 7, 2007 (Unity Village, MO: *Daily Word* magazine, February 2007), 24.

- The Unity person will often believe it is possible for healing to occur in any and all circumstances. Medical personnel will likely find this faith in the healing power of mind to be an asset in the patient's recovery process.

Specific Medical Issues

- **Abortion**: Although some religious traditions limit their followers from receiving certain medical procedures there are no specific restrictions on abortion in Unity. Each person should be asked individually.
- **Advance Directives**: Unity has no stated position on use of advance directives in health care planning; individuals are free to make their own decisions.
- **Birth Control**: Again, Unity takes no "official" position on this issue. However, the practice of responsible sexual behavior – to include oral contraceptives for prevention of unplanned pregnancies and condoms to halt the spread of sexually transmitted diseases – is widely considered to be harmonious with spiritual principles.
- **Blood Transfusions**: Although some religious traditions limit their followers from receiving certain medical procedures there are no specific restrictions on blood transfusions in Unity. Each person should be asked individually.
- **Circumcision**: Circumcision of male infants is for cultural, not religious, reasons. It is an individual family decision.
- **In Vitro Fertilization**: Unity has no stated position on in vitro fertilization; individuals are free to make their own decisions.
- **Stem Cell Research**: Unity has no stated position on stem cell research for therapeutic purposes; individuals are free to make their own decisions.

- **Vaccinations**: Unity has no restrictions or requirements about vaccinations.
- **Wihholding/Withdrawing Life Support**: Unity has no stated position on withholding/withdrawing life support in medically futile cases; individuals are free to make their own decisions.

Gender and Personal Issues

- Unity has no prescriptions or proscriptions with respect to gender and personal issues.
- Individual preferences should be the guideline for gender and personal issues (i.e., hygiene issues, modesty and privacy concerns, and so forth).

Principles for Spiritual Care through the Cycles of Life

Concepts of Living and Dying for Spiritual Support

- Unity people see themselves as radiant spiritual beings, regardless of what their current bodily conditions portray.
- To the Unity way of thinking, sickness and death are not evil, nor are they divine punishment in any sense of the word.
- Unity teaches that life is eternal and speaks of its earthly end as *transition*, which is the preferred term for death.
- As theological universalists, Unity people believe all sentient beings will eventually realize their oneness with God and achieve a state of higher existence called *Christ consciousness*. The term *Christ* is not limited to Jesus of Nazareth, but represents the divine spirit in everyone.
- In trying to live according to the Jesus Christ teachings, Unity people are content to make their transition while affirming their status as beloved children of a loving Father-Mother God. While spiritual perfection will probably be realized sometime after this life, Unity people are nevertheless comfortable with affirming, in life and in death: "The love of God manifests through me, and I am filled with light wisdom, and peace."[309]

- Many Unity people believe in reincarnation, holding that this life is a schoolhouse where people come to learn specific lessons. If the schooling is not done by the time life ends, some form of remedial work seems logical, and reincarnation provides the mechanism. Unity generally does *not* teach transmigration of the soul, which is the belief that humans can return as simpler forms of life. Actually, there is no requirement to believe in reincarnation in Unity, but the idea of multiple lives for ongoing soul-work is probably held by a majority of New Thought Christians. The idea of *bad karma* (i.e., evil deeds that must be expiated by repeated lives, often involving suffering) is also not a widely held Unity belief, since this appears to give spiritual power to "evil" actions. More chances at missed opportunities? – perhaps. Remedial work for sin? – definitely not, according to the Unity worldview.
- Death can also be seen as a form of healing, since the consciousness of the person is released from its temporary condition of frailty and suffering to continue the eternal process of soul growth.

During Birth

- What is true about transition is also true about the beginning of life in this world. Life is good, God is good, and everything is in Divine Order – all is well – regardless of appearances to the contrary.

---

309 Bach, M. (1982). *The Unity Way*. Unity Village, MO: Unity Books, 163.

- No special birth rituals or baptism are required, although many Unity people bring their children to church for a christening or spiritual baptism. This may include anointing with water or simply be a name-giving ceremony with prayers and blessings.
- As stated earlier, circumcision of male infants is for cultural, not religious, reasons. It is an individual family decision.

During Illness

- Anyone can pray for a Unity person, although the most meaningful experience will follow the form of affirmative prayer.
- Readings from any positive scripture – especially anything that stresses God's gracious goodness and the peace which can come even in the presence of sadness and loss.

During End of Life

- The guidelines for Unity people who are facing end of life are basically the same as in any potentially frightening circumstance, such as disease or loss of a loved one. Affirmative prayer, positive imagery, and ultimate trust that God is wherever they are.
- Unity people will appreciate a positive approach to spirituality; however, they will be uncomfortable with any attempt at prompting a deathbed conversion to some other belief formula.

Care of the Body

- There are no specific Unity requirements for the care of the body after transition.
- There are no prohibitions against autopsy.
- Disposition of the body is an individual decision; ask families of the deceased for their preferences.
- Donation of the body for medical research is an individual decision; ask families of the deceased for their preferences.

Organ and Tissue Donation

- There are no prohibitions against organ donation.
- It is an individual decision; ask families of the deceased for their preferences. It may be preferable for a chaplain and/or nurse who are trained designated requesters to be consulted for assistance.

Scriptures, Inspirational Readings, and Prayers

READINGS DURING ILLNESS

These can be read by family, friends, clergy, and health care professionals. Health care professionals may find readings helpful and comforting for Unity people who are facing a health challenge. Here are some examples of affirmative prayers for healing:

In the stillness of Your presence, God, I feel Your healing life flowing through me now, bringing peace to my mind and energy to my body.

Enfolded in Your powerful healing love, God, I experience health and wholeness in mind, body, and emotions.

Thank You, God, for Your healing life that surges throughout every cell of my entire being, strengthening me and restoring me to wholeness.

To You, dear God, I release any concern about my health. I trust Your healing love and Your life-giving presence to renew me.

Dear God, I am open and receptive to Your healing power. Your light and

life energize every cell of my being,
and I am grateful.

PRAYERS FOR DURING ILLNESS OR END-OF-LIFE PROCESS

These prayers can be offered by family, friends, clergy, and health care professionals. Perhaps the best-known and most-repeated Unity prayer is by Unity author James Dillet Freeman, the "Prayer for Protection," which was taken aboard Apollo 11 for the first moon landing in July 1969 by pilot Edwin E. Aldrin Jr. Apparently, James Dillet Freeman's work was popular within the astronaut community, since 2 years later astronaut James Irwin left a copy of another Freeman work, "I Am There," on the moon for future space travelers. The complete texts of both the "Prayer for Protection" and "I Am There" are provided here.

Prayer for Protection
The light of God surrounds us;
The love of God enfolds us;
The power of God protects us;
The presence of God watches over us;
Wherever we are, God is!

—James Dillet Freeman

I Am There
Do you need Me?
I am there.

You cannot see Me, yet I am the light
you see by.
You cannot hear Me, yet I speak
through your voice.
You cannot feel Me, yet I am the
power at work in your hands.

I am at work, though you do not
understand My ways.
I am at work, though you do not
recognize My works.
I am not strange visions. I am not
mysteries.

Only in absolute stillness, beyond
self, can you know Me as I am, and
then but as a feeling and a faith.

Yet I am there. Yet I hear. Yet I
answer.
When you need Me, I am there.
Even if you deny Me, I am there.
Even when you feel most alone, I am
there.
Even in your fears, I am there.
Even in your pain, I am there.

I am there when you pray and when
you do not pray.
I am in you, and you are in Me.
Only in your mind can you feel
separate from Me,
for only in your mind are the mists of
"yours" and "mine."
Yet only with your mind can you
know Me and experience Me.

Empty your heart of empty fears.
When you get yourself out of the way,
I am there.
You can of yourself do nothing, but I
can do all.
And I am in all.

Though you may not see the good,
good is there, for I am there.
I am there because I have to be,
because I am.

Only in Me does the world have
meaning; only out of Me does the

world take form; only because of
Me does the world go forward.
I am the law on which the movement
of the stars and the growth of living
cells are founded.

I am the love that is the law's
fulfilling. I am assurance.
I am peace. I am oneness. I am the
law that you can live by.
I am the love that you can cling to.
I am your assurance.
I am your peace. I am one with you.
I am.

Though you fail to find Me, I do not
fail you.
Though your faith in Me is unsure,
My faith in you never wavers,
because I know you, because I love
you. Beloved, I am there.[310]

—James Dillet Freeman

PRAYER FOR END-OF-LIFE PROCESS

This prayer can be offered by family, friends,
clergy, and health care professionals. An
additional prayer by James Dillet Freeman,
"The Traveler," may be especially helpful to
Unity families at the time of loss of a loved
one. Since it refers to the transition of a
specific, gendered person, this prayer is
available in male and female versions. The
female adaptation follows:

The Traveler

She has put on invisibility.
Dear Lord, I cannot see –
But this I know, although the road
ascends
And passes from my sight,
That there will be no night;
That You will take her gently by the
hand
And lead her on
Along the road of life that never ends,
And she will find it is not death but
dawn.
I do not doubt that You are there as
here,
And You will hold her dear.

Our life did not begin with birth,
It is not of the earth;
And this that we call death, it is no
more
Than the opening and closing of a
door –
And in Your house how many rooms
must be
Beyond this one where we rest
momently.

Dear Lord, I thank You for the faith
that frees,
The love that knows it cannot lose its
own;
The love that, looking through the
shadows, sees
That You and he and I are ever
one![311]

—James Dillet Freeman

---

310 James Dillet Freeman, http://content.unity.org/
prayer/prayersAffirmations/iAmTherePoem.html
(accessed 16 Sept 2012).

311 Ibid.

Quakerism: General Introduction

Prepared by:
Chel Avery
Director, Quaker Information Center
Philadelphia, PA

The Religious Society of Friends emerged in mid-seventeenth-century England as part of the religious upheaval and turmoil that comprised the Protestant Reformation. Yet, Friends (or Quakers, as they have generally been called, at first derisively, and then as a neutral, informal name) have been reluctant to consider themselves Protestants. Early generations of Friends were persecuted by Anglicans, Catholics, and Puritans in Britain and in the American colonies, and were the subject of frequent rebuke by Baptists and other emerging denominations. Although today most branches of Friends lack a formal creed, early Friends disputed with other Christians over such matters as human perfectibility, the Trinity and the nature of biblical authority. Some Friends describe themselves as a "third tradition," departing both from the ultimate authority of the church hierarchy in Catholicism and from the ultimate authority of Christian scripture maintained by Protestants, but instead emphasizing the primacy of "unmediated revelation" or direct encounter with Christ.

Friends began to establish themselves in various American colonies in the mid-1650s. In 1682, they began to settle in large numbers in Pennsylvania, a commonwealth founded by Quaker William Penn as the first political entity in the Western world to offer equal rights to all religions. In 1827, Pennsylvania Quakers separated into two divisions, followed the next year by further separations in other parts of the country. As Friends migrated westward and came under the influence of other religious and cultural trends, particularly the Methodist revival, there were further separations. Today, despite the fact that Friends in the mid-Atlantic and New England regions have reconciled and healed their divisions, there are at least four branches of Friends across the United States.

The characteristics that distinguish these modern branches of Friends most recognizably from each other are the degree of emphasis on Christian scripture versus the degree of emphasis on the "Inward Light" (which may or may not be interpreted as Christian in nature by those Friends who emphasize it); the manner of worship, ranging from "unprogrammed" worship based on silence and led by the Holy Spirit rather than any individual person, to "pastoral" worship which includes the leadership of a pastor and many traditional liturgical elements, though not sacramental rituals such as baptism; the degree of emphasis on Christian evangelism versus inward mystical experience; and the religious response to various social issues such as same-sex marriage.

The two chapters on Quakers in this book represent the two major variations in American Quakerism: "Liberal" Friends (which tend to be theologically universalistic and politically liberal, and which practice unprogrammed worship) and "Pastoral" Friends (which place stronger emphasis on Christian scripture and have pastor-led church services). The much smaller "Conservative" branch practices unprogrammed worship but acknowledges scriptural authority, and the "Evangelical" branch is in many ways similar to other Evangelical Christian churches today. Sometimes a fifth "Beanite" (or Western Independent) branch is identified, which is similar to Liberal Friends, but which evolved in the western states independently of the Liberal Friends in the eastern and middle United States.

Today there are approximately 87 000 Quakers in the United States and 359 000 worldwide. Outside of the United States, Friends in Europe and former British colonies are most similar to Liberal Friends, while those in Africa and Latin America continue the traditions of mission work by Pastoral and Evangelical Friends. There are many exceptions, however, to this generalized overview.

Liberal Quakers (Friends)

Walk cheerfully over the world, answering that of God in every one.[312]

Prepared by:
Chel Avery
Director, Quaker Information Center
Philadelphia, PA

History and Facts

In the United States, Quakers or Friends (the words are interchangeable) have separated into four major "branches," which in some ways are quite different from each other. The material in this chapter (beginning with the section entitled "Basic Teachings") refers to "liberal" Quakers, which predominate in the northeastern United States, but can be found throughout the country. Liberal Friends may also identify themselves with various other terms, such as "nonpastoral" or "unprogrammed" Friends, as "FGC-affiliated" (Friends General Conference is a networking body for many liberal Friends in North America), or occasionally as "Hicksite" (a historic term, now obsolete).

The Religious Society of Friends originated in mid-seventeenth century England as an attempt to revive the experience of early Christians and as an alternative to corruption and stagnancy that disillusioned

seekers encountered in the state church. George Fox, a traveling preacher, is the best known of the early leaders of this movement. "Quakers," originally a term of derision, were much persecuted and many were imprisoned, but there was nonetheless a period of rapid, enthusiastic growth. Immigration to the Americas and West Indies began in the 1650s. In North America, beginning in 1827, Friends began to separate into significant divisions, leading to the diverse branches we have today.

Although originally a "plain" people, Quakers no longer resemble the stereotype represented by the "Quaker Oats man." They are known for their pacifism and peace work, as well as for leadership in the movements to abolish slavery, for women's suffrage, and for prison reform and social justice.

Today, according to Friends' own membership counts, there are approximately 338 000 Friends worldwide, with 87 000 in the United States, of which 32 000 are liberal Friends. The American Religious Identification Survey, which relies on self-report data, gives the figure of 217 000 Quakers in the United States.

---

312 Nickalls, J. ed. (1975). *The Journal of George Fox.* Philadelphia, PA: Philadelphia Meeting of the Religious Society of Friends, p. 263, with permission of the London Yearly Meeting of the Religious Society of Friends (copyright holder). London Yearly Meeting is now known as the Britain Yearly Meeting. This quote was attributed to George Fox, who founded the Quakers in 1656.

Basic Teachings

- There is "that of God in everyone" – all people are sacred; all people are potential recipients of Divine visitation and intervention; all people are potential ministers of God through the leading of the "Inward Light" or "Christ Within."
- All people have the capacity for direct revelation from God, unmediated by ritual, clergy, or text, which they call "continuing revelation."
- Guidance from such revelation is valued above all other teachings, although a person's interpretation of it is not infallible and must be tested, both individually and with the faith community.
- Friends eschew the practices of paid clergy, the use of symbols or ritual (including outward sacraments, such as water baptism), and have no formal creed.
- Individuals are expected to seek God's direct guidance individually and as a community in the conduct of their lives. "Queries" (prepared questions considered during silent worship) are used for examining whether one's conduct is faithful to the teachings of the Light.
- Certain principles, called "**testimonies**," are recognized as having consistently emerged in Friends efforts to live faithfully. Commonly identified testimonies include: **peace** (including pacifism with respect to war and capital punishment), **simplicity**, social **equality**, **integrity**, **community**, and, increasingly, environmental **stewardship**. Individual interpretations of how to apply these testimonies in one's own life vary from person to person.
- Though Christian by tradition, some liberal Quakers today do not consider themselves Christian but, rather, universalists.

Basic Practices

- Outwardly, most Friends are no longer readily distinguishable from the mainstream by dress, speech, or behavior. Many Friends, however, are attentive to the aforementioned testimonies above in the daily choices they make.
- Friends worship by gathering in silence and "waiting expectantly" for Divine visitation. Any inspired individual may rise and speak a message during meeting for worship, after which silence resumes.
- Since Friends do not divide the world into the sacred and profane, preferring to seek the sacred in all times, places, and people, no day of the week is set aside as a "Sabbath." Worship is usually held on Sundays for convenience. Traditionally, Friends did not celebrate religious holidays, although Christmas and sometimes Easter have entered the cultural practice of most modern Quaker families.
- Friends traditionally avoid the use of "honorifics" in speech. They often use first and last names to address people, rather than "Mr." "Mrs." or "Dr." They are unlikely to refer to an ordained chaplain as "Reverend." This is a religious testimony (equality), as well as part of Quaker culture.
- Traditionally, Quakers do not take oaths. They will affirm rather than swear. This is a religious testimony (integrity – not having a dual standard of truth) as well as conformation to Jesus' instructions in the Sermon on the Mount.
- Congregations are called "meetings" or "monthly meetings" (because business is conducted once a month). Larger regional groupings are called "quarterly meetings" and "yearly meetings." Each of the 17 liberal yearly meetings in the United States is its own highest

authority, with no governing body above them. Decisions are reached without voting through "sense of the meeting," or a search for spiritual unity.

- Unprogrammed friends have no pastors. All members are considered to be ministers, and the work of the meeting is handled by committees. The person who coordinates the administrative business of the meeting, and who serves as the communication touchstone, is called the "clerk." Large meetings may have a full or part time secretary who handles communication for the community, but in the majority of meetings, it is the clerk who is contacted at home when someone needs to reach the meeting.

- Many meetings have committees that coordinate pastoral care, such as visiting the sick. These committees are often called "overseers," but go by many other names, such as "care of members," "ministry and counsel," or "nurture."

- Any leadership function is likely to be filled by a man or a woman; nor is it unusual for gay Friends to serve in leadership roles.

- Quakers practice no outward rituals or sacraments, such as baptism. Ritual and the use of symbols are generally held in suspicion among Friends, although sometimes individuals may create private ceremonies.

Principles for Clinical Care
Dietary Issues

- There are no religious dietary issues for Friends, although many are vegetarians.

General Medical Beliefs

- Quakers generally respect science and are receptive to the use of most medical technologies.

- Many Friends also explore alternative sources for healing, and may want to hold "meetings for healing," in silent worship with other Friends.

- Interpretation of the testimonies listed earlier (*see* "testimonies," penultimate bulleted item in "Basic Teachings" section) may vary from one person to the next in health care decisions, as Friends are expected to seek personal guidance from God. For example, a cancer patient may choose a treatment that will not produce toxic waste (environmental stewardship), while another individual might choose a generic medication, even when their health insurance covers a more expensive drug (simplicity; economic justice).

Specific Medical Issues

- **Abortion**: Friends differ on the subject of abortion, and there are strong feelings at both ends of the spectrum.

- **Advance Directives**: There is no particular Quaker teaching on the use of advance directives for health care preplanning. This is an issue for individual discernment, although community support may be sought in making that discernment.

- **Birth Control**: There is no particular Quaker teaching about birth control, although Friends are generally approving of any individual choice. Note that Quakers are sometimes confused with Shakers, a now-extinct sect that practiced complete celibacy. This has never been a Quaker tradition.

- **Blood Transfusions**: There is no particular Quaker teaching on the use of blood products. This is an issue for individual discernment, although community support may be sought in making that discernment.

- **Circumcision**: A decision about whether to have a son circumcised is one that Quaker parents would make based on reasons other than religion; Quakers have no tenets on that matter. It is an individual or family decision. However, the majority of Quakers would object to female circumcision.
- **In Vitro Fertilization**: There is no particular Quaker teaching on in vitro fertilization. This is an issue for individual discernment, although community support may be sought in making that discernment.
- **Stem Cell Research**: There is no particular Quaker teaching on stem cell research for therapeutic purposes. This is an issue for individual discernment, although community support may be sought in making that discernment.
- **Vaccinations**: Quakers have no religious teachings about vaccinations. It is an individual decision.
- **Withholding/Withdrawing Life Support**: There is no particular Quaker teaching on withholding/withdrawing life support in medically futile cases. This is an issue for individual discernment, although community support may be sought in making that discernment.

Gender and Personal Issues

- Friends pride themselves on a long tradition of gender equality. Similarly, most Friends strive for equality with respect to race, age, sexual identity, language, and immigration status.

Principles for Spiritual Care through the Cycles of Life
Concepts of Living and Dying for Spiritual Support

- Life is considered sacred.
- Dying is a natural part of the cycle of life, not to be feared.

During Birth

- There are no specific restrictions or requirements regarding birth, stillbirth, or miscarriage. Individuals may have different ways of spiritually addressing these experiences.
- Friends differ on the subject of abortion, and there are strong feelings at both ends of the spectrum.

During Illness

- Friends are usually open to spiritual care and support from those of other faiths. Offers of spiritual companionship from another faith tradition (e.g., prayers or songs), may be accepted or not, but they will usually be appreciated.
- Quakers often use the phrase "to hold someone in the Light" as the equivalent to praying for someone.
- When making difficult decisions, the following may be important to Friends:
  ○ Extended periods of silence for worship.
  ○ A worship group or "clearness committee" (a group that provides spiritual and practical help in decision making) from their meeting. Please recognize that such "informal" groups may be as important to Friends as pastors are to other denominations.
  ○ Time. Quakers make decisions slowly, and when in a group, they wait for unity rather than voting or deferring to a human authority. Even if a person has intellectually identified the most

sensible course of action, he or she will often seek spiritual confirmation through worship and waiting.

During End of Life
- There are no special traditions surrounding the end of life.
- Friends have no particular teachings about the afterlife. A typical attitude is that one should live one's life as faithfully as possible, and leave the rest in God's hands.
- In hospice situations or during "final days," many members of the community may visit to participate with the dying person and their family in the experience of life's completion.

Care of the Body
- There are no specific restrictions or requirements. Many choose cremation.
- Donation of the body for medical research is not uncommon.

Organ and Tissue Donation
- Organ and tissue donations are not uncommon.
- It is an individual/family decision. It may be preferable for a chaplain and/or nurse who are trained designated requesters to be consulted for assistance.

Memorials
- Memorial meetings for worship in memory of a deceased person are sometimes scheduled weeks or even months after the death. Health care personnel are welcome to attend, but may not learn of the event through standard channels, such as newspaper obituaries. Feel free to express an interest in being notified to a member of the family or the Friends meeting.

Scriptures, Inspirational Readings, and Prayers
GENERAL PRINCIPLES ABOUT SCRIPTURE
- The most fundamental "scripture" for liberal Friends is what emerges inwardly from the experience of shared silence.
- Although Quaker tradition excludes the use of planned words, a scriptural or other passage, poem, or song may be welcomed when offered out of an unpremeditated inspiration that occurs in the moment.
- Friends are often eclectic in their choice of sources for inspiration or comfort, drawing on the Bible, the journals of early Friends, scriptures of non-Christian traditions, poetry, music, or secular writings.
- No particular readings are suggested, for the reasons mentioned in the previous point. It is usually acceptable, however, for a visitor to bring a text that he or she finds personally meaningful, and to offer to share it, if wanted.

Pastoral (Programmed) Quakers

Jesus said, "You are my friends if you do what I command you."[313]

Prepared by:
Brenda McKinney,
Friends North Carolina Yearly Meeting
Ararat, NC

Reviewed and approved by:
Max Carter, Director
The Friends Center at Guilford College
Greensboro, NC

History and Facts

The Religious Society of Friends (Quakers) grew out of the yearnings of George Fox and other radical English Christians in the mid-1600s to find more meaning and purpose to life. After a period of intense seeking for a profession of Christian faith that had integrity, he personally experienced the living Christ and in his journal wrote of hearing a voice saying "there is one, even Christ Jesus, that can speak to thy condition." His experience convinced him that what he had been seeking was present inwardly. He then found communion with God through the Holy Spirit, the inward light of Christ.

Preceding his experience of the inward Christ, he was dismayed by what he saw occurring in the Church of England as friends and acquaintances practiced pious rituals on Sunday mornings and involved themselves in brawls in the taverns during the week. After his conversion, he began leading worship services based on silent, expectant waiting in homes, open fields, taverns, and other noninstitutional locations (as he believed God was not confined to a building) where the gathered worshipped by centering their thoughts on God and listening to His voice. In these gatherings (unlike services in the Church of England) if people felt led by the Holy Spirit to share aloud what God had laid on their hearts, they did so. These early followers of George Fox's new movement were known as "children of the light" and later became "Friends" in reference to the teaching of John 15:14: "you are my friends if you do what I command you."

During the early years of the movement, there were many young, enthusiastic converts and the "valiant 60," a group of young men and women convinced by Fox, scattered throughout England to preach the gospel and attend to the sick and needy and those in prisons. However, there was not wide acceptance within traditional religious or civic circles. For example, one early story reports the name "Quaker" was originally a form of derision given to a group of Friends who found themselves in court, and the judge remarked how they "quaked with the spirit of the Lord." Subsequently, many Quakers found themselves in prison when they did not conform to the social and religious norms of the day. Their belief that God created everyone and that there

---

313 John 15:14 (New Century Version).

should be equality among all people with no distinctions of gender, class, or power was not widely accepted in England.

In the early 1670s, George Fox brought his message of the power of the gospel and the personal experience of the living Christ to America. Ann Austin and Mary Fisher had already made the first missionary venture to Virginia in 1656, and countless others had come to the colonies, including those hanged by the Puritans in Boston in 1659/1660. William Penn, an early Quaker, was instrumental in writing the "frame of government" for the colony which became Pennsylvania, and this document developed into a model for the United States Constitution. By the dawn of the American Revolution, Quakers were numerous in the American colonies. The Quaker belief in peace (that war is inconsistent with the spirit and teaching of Christ) led to disagreements when many Friends refused to take up arms in the War for Independence. This also led to a diminishment in their influence, and they never regained their place among the top American denominations following the Revolution. The Quaker belief in equality led to the Underground Railroad as Quakers helped slaves escape to freedom prior to and during the Civil War.

Distinctive emphases and practices of Friends have been articulated as "testimonies." Primary among the ones they are most noted for socially are integrity, simplicity, peace, community, and equality. Quakers are known and respected for their honesty (integrity). They believed one should do as the Bible says when Jesus said "let your nay mean nay and your yea mean yea"; a handshake was the contract. Even today, Quakers "affirm" in court rather than swearing on the Bible. There is no need to swear because one should always tell the truth.

Quakers have also had a great love for education: George Fox encouraged the establishment of schools for boys and girls at the very beginning of the Quaker movement; Quaker schools were established in Philadelphia by 1689; the first public school in North Carolina was established by Friends at Symon's Creek in 1703; numerous colleges and universities were established by Friends as well as schools for black children after the Civil War and overseas in places like Ramallah, Palestine, where a girls' school was established in 1869 and the Friends' Theological College in Kenya in 1946 to train the Kenyans to become pastors. When a Friends meeting was established, a school was soon to be in place.

Today, Friends United Meeting, the largest organization of programmed, pastoral Friends, with offices in Richmond, Indiana, and Kaimosi, Kenya, numbers 45 000 Quakers in the United States and 300 000 around the world, including Canada, Cuba, Jamaica, Mexico, Belize, Uganda, and Kenya.

Basic Teachings

- Programmed Quakers believe the scriptures are inspired by God and each person can draw new insight and meaning as the Holy Spirit continues to help them understand and interpret the written Word.
- Programmed Quakers believe Jesus is the son of God who was sent to save people from their sins and if they believe in him and confess their sins, they will have eternal life. Salvation is a personal experience between a person and God and a life led by the Spirit is guided and directed to obey Him.
- All believers are baptized in the Spirit (1 Cor. 12:13) and should feel a part of

Christ at all times, not just on special occasions. Friends do not observe the outward sacraments.

- George Fox stated there is "that of God in everyone." He also spoke of "the Light within," the belief there is a light in the soul of divine origin that enables an individual to move beyond self to respond to the Holy Spirit. Quakers speak now of "holding people in the Light," praying with them and for them.

- The meeting for worship is the ideal place for the power of the Holy Spirit to be experienced as Jesus promised; where two or three are gathered His presence can be made known.

- Quakers are rare among Christians in their emphasis on the Holy Spirit and the inward presence of Jesus Christ guiding us to become more like Him. George Fox was concerned that people were more focused on ritual than their meanings. Quakers are to be led beyond ceremony to a transformed life.

- The Quaker principles are *simplicity*, *peace*, *equality*, *integrity*, and *community*.
  - Simplicity in speech, dress, and manner of living were early ideals of living to show stewardship of the resources God has blessed all with and no concern for worldly prestige or power.
  - The peace testimony stems from the belief that all human life is sacred and Quakers cannot bring themselves to inflict violence on anyone as there is "that of God in everyone."
  - Each individual has worth, dignity, freedom, and responsibility before God.
  - Living in the light causes inner examination and truth becomes a way of life. Early Friends became well known for their honesty; their word and a handshake were as good as a contract.

  - Christlike love and concern for others finds expression in humanitarian service – to preach and to heal, to pray and to go forth and change the world.

Basic Practices

- "Un-programmed" meetings occur in silence and the worshippers "center down," focusing on God. His presence is made known and believers are led by the Holy Spirit to speak as directed.

- "Programmed" meetings are similar to other Protestant churches with a pastor delivering a sermon and songs of praise and worship, including a choir. There is also a time of open worship when the congregation is invited to silently wait upon the presence and power of the Holy Spirit and share vocally if so led.

- In programmed meetings, there is no hierarchy of leadership. However, the pastor is the spiritual leader. Pastors spend much of their time visiting the sick and shut-ins and praying for them.

- Elders are chosen for their gifts of discernment and leadership and view caring for the sick as an integral part of their duties and responsibilities.

- The clerk determines the sense of the meeting in business sessions. The nature of Quaker decision making involves a gathering of the "sense of the meeting" by the clerk; no votes are taken; an emphasis is placed on unity and group discernment of truth.

- The local group (called a "monthly meeting") meets monthly for worship and business concerns, in addition to Sunday morning services and, for many, Wednesday evening services as well. The monthly meeting groups in a particular region come together for a quarterly meeting, which meets four times a year, and all gather annually as a yearly meeting and at other times of the year as well.

- Individual meetings have lengthy prayer lists for members and the community of individual needs, both physical and emotional.

- Quakers believe in their actions demonstrating their faith. They believe Jesus has called them to minister to a hurting world and are instructed to leave their comfort zones and, with the guidance and help of the Holy Spirit, called to love far beyond human capabilities. George Fox encouraged Friends to "let your lives preach."

- Friends believe their relationship with God is more important than any outward symbol. Friends do not baptize with water or celebrate the Lord's Supper. John the Baptist says in John 1:33 that while he came to baptize with water, Christ has come to baptize with the Holy Spirit. The accurate translation from the original language of Matt. 28:19 refers to a change of heart, not water baptism. All of life can be sacramental if truly lived in God's light.

- Daily scripture reading is encouraged, to learn more about God as the Holy Spirit reveals himself to us through the written word. George Fox is reputed to have so memorized the Bible that he could recreate it from memory should all copies be lost.

Principles for Clinical Care
Dietary Issues

- Quakers have no specific practices or diet restrictions. Many Friends practice a vegetarian or even vegan diet in response to the testimonies on peace, integrity, and simplicity.

- In accordance with simplicity, many Quakers in rural areas continue to grow their own fruits and vegetables with many practicing organic or "permaculture" techniques.

General Medical Beliefs

- Quakers believe in the power of individual and corporate prayer. There are many documented cases of cancer and other serious illnesses being completely eradicated, without medical explanation, through prayer. Modern scientific studies have concluded that prayer is beneficial for those facing surgery and extended hospitalizations.

- Quakers accept technological advances in medicine.

- Some Quakers practice holistic therapies.

Specific Medical Issues

- **Abortion**: Quakers believe in the sanctity of life and do not believe in abortion, but typically it is left up to the individual conscience rather than dictated by organizational decree.

- **Advance Directives**: Advance directives are an individual choice.

- **Birth Control**: Quakers believe children are a gift from God and parents are encouraged to rear them in a Christlike manner. There is no doctrine or statement regarding birth control which is considered an individual's choice.

- **Blood Transfusions**: Quakers are not averse to blood transfusions.

- **Circumcision**: Quakers have no official position on this issue. People may choose to circumcise their infant sons for cultural, not religious, reasons; it is an individual decision.

- **In Vitro Fertilization**: Quakers believe in the sanctity of life and have no official position or doctrine on in vitro fertilization. This issue is an individual decision. People are to seek direction in this matter through the leading of the Holy Spirit.

- **Stem Cell Research**: Quakers believe in the sanctity of life and have no official position or doctrine on stem cell research for therapeutic purposes. This issue is an individual decision. People are to seek direction in this matter through the leading of the Holy Spirit.
- **Vaccinations**: Quakers do not have a formal statement or policy on health care and vaccinations per se, leaving it up to individual members to make the best judgment with the advice of their physicians on such matters.
- **Withholding/Withdrawing Life Support**: Quakers believe in the sanctity of life and have no official position or doctrine on withholding/withdrawing life support in medically futile cases. This issue is an individual decision. People are to seek direction in this matter through the leading of the Holy Spirit.

Gender and Personal Issues

- Quakers believe in equality and, therefore, are very accepting of nontraditional roles for men and women. Women have been ministers from the beginnings of Quakerism.
- Quakers have been forerunners in their belief that women should have the same rights as men.
- Many people prefer same sex health care providers as their primary care provider, but are willing to be referred to specialists of either gender.

Principles for Spiritual Care through the Cycles of Life
Concepts of Living and Dying for Spiritual Support

- Programmed Quakers believe in heaven where they will live eternally praising God with no sorrow or concerns. Friends don't obsess about the afterlife; John Greenleaf Whittier says it best (in his poem "The Eternal Goodness"):

I know not what the future hath of marvel or surprise, assured alone that life and death God's mercy underlies; I know not where God's islands lift their fronded palms in air; I only know we cannot drift beyond God's love and care.

- Quakers believe in the sacredness of human life.
- Dying is a time to be surrounded by family and friends
- Death is something all must experience; there is a time appointed for everyone.
- While a time of great sorrow for those left behind, death is considered a time of celebration for the departed one, and often a relief if there has been much suffering.
- Friends live in the hope of an eternity with God, but believe the priority must be put on the here and now, living in His presence daily. The end of life is seen as a transition from work here on earth to the natural reward in heaven for that obedience to God's will.

During Birth

- Quakers believe in the sanctity of life and do not believe in abortion, but typically it is left up to the individual conscience rather than dictated by organizational decree.

- The Christian nurture of children is a sacred duty of the home and church. Many meetings have baby dedications in which the congregation is encouraged as are the parents/family to instruct the child in the Bible and its teachings.
- The birth of a child is a joyous occasion with many prayers of thankfulness for this gift from God. The death of an infant is heartbreaking for anyone. A caring word or prayer would be welcome.

During Illness

- Laying on of hands by the elders is welcomed.
- Prayer is always welcome by anyone who feels led.
- Scripture reading is also comforting.
- Many in the church family provide meals for the sick and offer to help with chores.
- Pastors and elders visit the hospitals and homes frequently offering encouragement and support.
- Health care providers should listen for the patient's questions and fears and understanding of the problem and respect the patient's decisions. Encourage patients to draw on their spiritual resources, allowing God to be their source of strength, comfort, and hope. Physicians treat; God heals.

During End of Life

- Family is essential at this time and the church family often shows their support by spending time with the family.
- Pastors are usually present for prayer with and for the family.
- Health care providers can encourage the family to talk about their feelings, their memories, and gratitude for the life of their loved one.
- The traditional Quaker memorial service includes a time of silence and open worship and can be an occasion of much joy and telling of stories as friends are led by the Holy Spirit to share.

Care of the Body

- Disposition of the body, burial, or cremation, is an individual choice.
- There is no prohibition concerning autopsy.
- Hospital personnel are welcome to care for and prepare the body of the deceased.
- Clergy need not be involved, although they may be present.
- Donation of the body for research is a personal or family decision.

Organ and Tissue Donation

- Organ and tissue donation is a personal or family choice. It may be preferable for a chaplain and/or nurse who are trained designated requesters to be consulted for assistance.

Scriptures, Inspirational Readings, and Prayers

- There are no standard prayers.
- Much of scripture is comforting and individuals usually have favorite passages.
- Psalms 6, 39, 41, and 67 and Isaiah 26 are encouraging when one is sick or in pain. Quakers use a variety of texts, including the Authorized (King James) Version, the New International Version, and Holman Christian Standard Bible. The following passages are from the New Century Version.

READINGS DURING ILLNESS

These can be read by family, friends, clergy, and health care professionals.

Lord, have mercy on me because I
am weak. Heal me, Lord, because my
bones ache. The Lord has heard my
cry for help; the Lord will answer my
prayer.

—Ps. 6:2, 9

The Lord is my shepherd; I have
everything I need.
He lets me rest in green pastures.
He leads me to calm water.
He gives me new strength.
He leads me on paths that are right
for the good of his name.

Even though I walk through a very
dark valley,
I will not be afraid,
because you are with me.
Your rod and your walking stick
comfort me.

You prepare a meal for me in front of
my enemies.
You pour oil on my head; you fill my
cup to overflowing.
Surely your goodness and love will be
with me all my life,
and I will live in the house of the
Lord forever.

—Psalm 23

Lord, tell me when the end will
come and how long I will live.
You have given me only a short
life; my lifetime is like nothing to
you.
Everyone's life is only a breath.
So, Lord, what hope do I have?

You are my hope.
Lord, hear my prayer, and listen to
my cry.
Do not ignore my tears.

—Ps. 39: 4–12

Happy is the person who thinks about
the poor. When trouble comes, the
Lord will save him.
The Lord will protect him and spare
his life and will bless him in the
land. He will not let his enemies
take him.
The Lord will give him strength when
he is sick, and he will make him well
again.

—Ps. 41:1–3

God have mercy on us and bless us
and show us your kindness so the
world will learn your ways, and all
nations will learn that you can save.
God, the people should praise you;
all people should praise you. The
nations should be glad and sing
because you judge people fairly.
You guide all the nations on earth.
God, the people should praise you;
all people should praise you. The
land has given its crops. God, our
God, blesses us. God blesses us so
people all over the earth will fear
him.

—Psalm 67

You, Lord, give true peace to those
who depend on you, because they

419

trust you. So, trust the Lord always, because He is our Rock forever.

—Isa. 26:3–4

The true Light that gives light to all was coming into the world!

—John 1:9

You say, "What can I bring with me when I come before the Lord, when I bow before God on high? Should I come before him with burnt offerings, with year-old calves?

Will the Lord be pleased with a thousand male sheep? Will he be pleased with ten thousand rivers of oil? Should I give my first child for the evil I have done? Should I give my very own child for my sin?"

The Lord has told you, human, what is good; he has told you what he wants from you: to do what is right to other people, love being kind to others, and live humbly, obeying your God.

—Mic. 6:6–8

Then wolves will live in peace with lambs, and leopards will lie down to rest with goats. Calves, lions, and young bulls will eat together, and a little child will lead them. Cows and bears will eat together in peace. Their young will lie down to rest together. Lions will eat hay as oxen do. A baby will be able to play near a cobra's hole, and a child will be able to put

his hand into the nest of a poisonous snake. They will not hurt or destroy each other on my holy mountain, because the earth will be full of the knowledge of the Lord, as the sea is full of water.

—Isa. 11:6–9

READINGS DURING END-OF-LIFE PROCESS

John 11, 17, 20; 2 Corinthians 5, and 1 Cor. 15:54–56 are helpful to those who may be apprehensive about death. The following passages are from the New Century Version. These can be read by family, friends, clergy, and health care professionals.

Jesus said to her, "I am the resurrection and the life. Those who believe in me will have life even if they die. And everyone who lives and believes in me will never die."

—John 11:25

After Jesus said these things, he looked toward heaven and prayed, "Father, the time has come. Give glory to your Son so that the Son can give glory to you. You gave the Son power over all people so that the Son could give eternal life to all those you gave him. And this is eternal life: that people know you, the only true God, and that they know Jesus Christ, the One you sent … I have given these people the glory that you gave me so that they can be one, just as you and I are one. I will be in them and you will be in me so that they will be completely one. Then the world will know that you sent me and that you loved them just as much as you loved me."

—John 17:1–3, 22–23

"I am going back to my Father and your Father, to my God and your God."

—John 20:17

We know that our body – the tent we live in here on earth – will be destroyed. But when that happens, God will have a house for us. It will not be a house made with human hands; instead, it will be a home in heaven that will last forever. But now we groan in this tent. We want God to give us our heavenly home, because it will clothe us so we will not be naked. While we live in this body, we have burdens, and we groan. We do not want to be naked, but we want to be clothed with our heavenly home. Then this body that dies will be fully

covered with life. This is what God made us for, and he has given us the Spirit to be a guarantee for this new life. So we always have courage. We know that while we live in this body, we are away from the Lord. We live by what we believe, not by what we can see. So I say that we have courage. We really want to be away from this body and be at home with the Lord. Our only goal is to please God whether we live here or there.

—2 Cor. 5:1–9

Possibly the best scripture for end of life is found in Paul's prayer.

"Death is destroyed forever in victory. Death, where is your victory? Death, where is your pain?"

Death's power to hurt is sin, and the power of sin is the law. But we thank God! He gives us the victory through our Lord Jesus Christ.

—1 Cor. 15:55–57

Confucianism

A complete person thinks of righteousness over personal gain, accepts responsibility
even when endangered, and remembers promises made throughout life.[314]

Prepared by:
Edward R. Canda, PhD, Professor
Director of the Office for Research on Spiritual Diversity in Social Work
The University of Kansas School of Social Welfare
Courtesy Professor, Department of Religious Studies
Lawrence, KS[315]

History and Facts

Confucianism is a philosophical and religious tradition that originated in China about 2500 years ago. It has had major impact on the worldviews of people throughout East Asia and other people of East Asian descent, especially Chinese, Japanese, Koreans, and Vietnamese. It is named for the founder, Kongzi or Kong Fuzi (孔子), anglicized as Confucius, who lived about 551–479 BCE. Over many centuries and through various countries, Confucianism has taken various forms. Therefore, this summary only presents basic ideas that are rooted in the significant traditional Confucian writings along with related common contemporary customs.

Few contemporary East Asians or Asian Americans identify as Confucians and few have formally studied the philosophical texts. However, it directly or indirectly influences the worldviews, social ethics, and health practices of many millions of people.

Confucius did not claim to found a new religion. He described himself as the transmitter of wisdom from ancient sages. He hoped to apply long-rooted wisdom to rectify various social and political problems of his time. His main role was as a teacher who tried to show students and social administrators how to apply the *Dao* (or Way 道) of humane benevolence to relations with self, family, the wider society, and world. The second-most eminent teacher in this tradition was Mengzi (孟子 anglicized as Mencius), who lived in China from about 371–289 BCE. Mencius was especially concerned about political corruption. He elaborated Confucius' teachings about human nature and social justice. Over the centuries, Confucianism was alternately embraced, suppressed, or neglected by governments in East Asia. In contradiction to

---

314 Li, D. trans. (1999). *The Analects of Confucius: A New Millenium Translation.* Bethesda, MD: Premier Publishing, 166.

315 Thanks to my wife, Hwi-Ja Canda, LSCSW, Social Work Coordinator at Lawrence Memorial Hospital (Kansas, United States), for helpful information and suggestions. Thanks also to Professor Woochan Shim, PhD, of Daejeon University Department of Social Welfare (South Korea) for provision of Chinese characters.

Confucius' and Mencius' concerns about justice, traditional royalty and bureaucrats sometimes selectively emphasized authoritarian versions of Confucianism, leading to many people's association of Confucianism with patriarchal and authoritarian social controls. Other Confucian scholars protested social policies that injured public and personal health and well-being. Yet, because of long periods of governmental promotion of Confucianism through social policies and education, the influence of Confucianism became very widespread.

Since it would be rare for a health care provider in the West to encounter a patient who identifies as a Confucian, the ideas in this summary should be used only as hints for beliefs and behaviors that might be relevant to some more traditionally minded people of East Asian descent. Conversation with the patient and family is the only way to know the actual significance of Confucianism for them. In general, if concepts of benevolence, filial piety, ancestor honoring, and holistic healing based on *yin* (陰) and *yang* (陽) energies are important to the patient, then Confucianism is probably an important influence. These concepts will be explained in the following sections. The term "Confucian" is used broadly here to refer to people who are significantly influenced by Confucian worldview, directly or indirectly, even if they formally affiliate with some other religion or with no religion.

Basic Teachings

- **Benevolence and Virtue**: The main purpose of Confucianism is to help people become aware of their inherent nature of *ren* (仁) (all special terms are in Chinese, using the *pinyin*, 拼音, system) which means benevolence, humanity, or humane-heartedness. Benevolence should express in relations with family, society, the wider world, and all in heaven and earth. For example, Mencius said that anyone who notices that a child is in danger of falling into a well would naturally rush to save the child, regardless of ulterior motives. Further, Confucianism teaches that when people look into their own hearts with sincerity, they recognize their own genuine needs and understand that these needs are shared by everyone. The benevolent person wishes to attend to the needs of everyone and seeks harmony in relationships. Confucian teachers recognize that it is not easy for most people to do this, however. So individuals need to exert effort to keep the benevolent nature clear in mind and action. One can begin by sincerely cultivating wisdom in oneself and by extending that outward in larger spirals of relationship through family, community, society, and world. Benevolence is the basis of all other cardinal virtues, such as *li* (禮), which means proper conduct of rituals as well as propriety in daily life. Health in a holistic sense is fostered through the cultivation of virtue (*de*, 德), which can be considered both a quality of character and a positive force of influence on the well-being of oneself and others. Mencius explained that the best way to keep one's vital energy (*qi*, 氣) flowing in a healthy way is to develop virtue through diligent yet gentle effort.

- **Reciprocity**: The recognition of the essential relatedness and interdependency of all people and things leads to the principle of reciprocity (*shu*, 恕). Human social relations are traditionally organized in partnerships of related persons, for example, royalty and common people, teacher and student, leader and subordinate, husband and wife, parents and children, elder and younger siblings, friend and friend. In traditional societies, many of these relationships were hierarchical, with greater authority given to those in the superior position. Ideally, the principle of reciprocity means that those with more authority should use it for the care and benefit of their juniors, while the juniors should relate to their superiors with respect. Thus, benevolent reciprocity should create a mutually beneficial relationship. If this pattern is violated, then those in lesser positions of power may be exploited or oppressed. Health at both personal and social levels depends on harmony and benevolent reciprocity in all these relationships.

- **Filial Piety**: The relationship between parents and children is the most basic building block of traditional East Asian societies. Therefore, great attention is given to this relationship and the virtue of filial piety (*xiao*, 孝). It is the model for other types of hierarchical relationships. For example, the king and queen are like the parents of their subjects. A special teacher or mentor is like a parent to her or his students.

On the most concrete level, parents have given life to their children. This is a gift that can never be equaled. Therefore, children are expected to have a natural and abiding respect and appreciation for their parents. In fact, when parents are elders, the adult children (especially the oldest son and his wife) are expected to return care and support for their parents. This presumes that parents should have raised their children with guidance and loving attentiveness. Confucian inspired parents often use great effort, resources, and personal sacrifice to raise their children in a healthy way and to educate them. Traditional people live in extended families, often including grandparents, parents, and adult eldest son with his spouse and children. Other family members remain closely connected.

By extending the parent child analogy, filial piety has implications for relations with everyone. Younger people should respect their elders, while receiving their encouragement and support. Further, heaven and earth are like our spiritual parents. Therefore, all people and all creatures are our brothers and sisters. People owe greatest respect and care to heaven and earth. We should care for people in need and for all creatures. Confucian philosophers did not promote anthropomorphic ideas about heaven. Heaven (*tian*, 天) refers both to the sky and to a metaphysical force. Heaven is regarded as the source of human nature, the creative power behind all things, and the determiner of personal destiny. Earth is respected for its nurturing bounty and beauty. Traditionally, it is thought that human disharmony with heaven and earth leads to natural disasters like drought, famine, and endemic illnesses. The workings of heaven and earth reflect the dynamics of yin and yang energies.

- ***Yin, Yang, Qi,* and *Taiji*:** Ideas about *yin* and *yang* originated before Confucianism. They influenced the philosophies of Confucianism and Taoism. They also have a significant impact on health care beliefs and practices. *Yin* and *yang* are qualities or types of vital energy (*qi*). They are complementary opposites that work together to produce everything. *Yin* is the receptive, yielding, birthing quality. *Yang* is the creative, proactive, generating quality. The concepts are related to the play of shadow and light. On a bright day, one side of a tree is shaded and the other is brightened. As the sun moves, the shade and light shift. Shade is not possible without light. *Yin* is not possible without *yang*. In the process of all changes, *yin* and *yang* qualities interact. Sometimes *yin* is more prominent and sometimes *yang*. For example, each human body has organ and energy systems (addressed in acupuncture and herbal medicine, for example) that are affected by *yin* and *yang*. If either energy quality is too extreme or too faint, or if they are not in harmony, illness results. *Qi* and its aspects of *yin* and *yang* are said to emerge from the Great Primal Beginning or Supreme Ultimate (*Taiji*, 太極) which is boundless and beyond any division, name or form. Health in the deepest sense involves both a practical harmonization of *yin* and *yang* in the body and in relationships, plus a profound realization of the oneness of everything in the Supreme Ultimate.

Basic Practices

Most contemporary people influenced by Confucianism do not frequently or regularly engage in formal Confucian religious institution-based practices such as rituals or prayers that existed in ancient times. However, many people influenced by Confucianism are members of other religions, such as Buddhism or Christianity, through which they may engage in formal religious practices. Many others do not consider themselves to be formally religious. In these two cases, such people consider Confucianism to be more an ethical or philosophical system than a religion.

Yet, the Confucian tradition emphasizes that personal health and public health are rooted in the cultivation of virtue within oneself and extension of it throughout the wider society and world. Various Confucian inspired practices may be used to this end. Some of these are listed here.

- **Constant Learning**: The Confucian Way emphasizes that people should approach each moment as an opportunity for learning, including times of illness and distress. Many practices promote constant learning, such as daily reflecting on the quality and results of one's intentions and actions; maintaining a consistently sincere attitude; seeking to understand both the practical details of how things work and the deeper principles beneath them; intensive study of the Five Classics and Four Books; and pursuit of formal education that should round the whole person and develop skills for human service. People who are teachers or doctors are highly respected because of their commitments to learning and to teaching and serving others.

- **Quiet Sitting or Meditation**: Many Confucians practice a form of quiet sitting. This involves resting in simple quiet that allows the mind to still and one's true nature to emerge clearly. It does not involve use of strong mental force, extreme postures, or overly intense techniques of concentration. Intentions and disturbing thoughts and feelings are released, so that the true nature becomes clear of its own accord. Quiet sitting can aid the process of learning and cultivating virtue. It also promotes physical health and overall well-being.

- **Vital Energy Movement (*Qigong*, 氣功)**: Some Confucians employ meditative movements and breathing exercises, such as *qigong*, to stimulate vital energy (*qi*) and promote health. But as Mencius advised, such practices should be done in the context of cultivating and expressing virtue, not merely for selfish health gains. Confucius explained that the benevolent person protects and cares for one's own health in order to be able to serve others well.

- **Celebration of Significant Days**: In some countries, Confucians hold a major national celebration and local celebrations to honor the teachings of Confucius, Mencius, and the other sages and highly honored scholars. These occur at the spring and autumn equinoxes, the exact date of which varies by year according to the lunar calendar. Confucians may also visit the graves of previous famous scholars on special commemorative days or whenever convenient in order to honor their contributions and to reflect on their teachings.

The principle of filial piety requires that descendants honor their ancestors. This means that people influenced by Confucianism perform rites to memorialize their deceased parents, grandparents, and other close deceased relatives (generally for three or four generations). These involve offerings of food and bows of respect before the grave or an offering table set at home. These rites may be performed on anniversaries of the death and on special holidays, such as Autumn Harvest Thanksgiving Day.

Principles for Clinical Care
Dietary Issues

- Diet should be balanced in terms of nutritional content and vital energy qualities. Each type of food has a predominant quality of *yin*, *yang*, or neutral energy. Good

health can be supported by harmonizing these energies in relation to one's specific body type at each meal. Some people's bodies are more *yang* energy (sometimes described metaphorically as hot), so they may need more *yin*-type foods. Others are more *yin* (sometimes described as cold), so they may need more *yang*-type foods. Examples of *yin* predominant foods are duck, fish, and tofu. Examples of *yang* predominant foods are beef, chili, garlic, and onions. Examples of neutral foods are bread and white rice. But this system is complicated and not everyone agrees on the food type designations. It is best to consult the patient or patient's parent or caregiver for food preferences. If the family wishes, a traditional Eastern medicine practitioner can be consulted.

- Diet may be supplemented by a wide variety of herbal medicines, such as ginseng, and other kinds of traditional medicines. East Asian traditional medicines are very numerous. Physicians should be aware of the ways patients may combine traditional and conventional Western medications, for possible helpful or harmful interactions.

- Confucians are not typically vegetarian. However, all plants and animals should be treated humanely and the environment should not be destroyed in food production.

- In general, a healthy, balanced diet should be part of an overall lifestyle of moderation. Specifics of dietary style (such as focus on rice, meats, seafood, types of spice) are determined by cultural norms and personal preferences. Hospital food providers and dieticians should discuss with the patient about food preferences based on culture and concerns about balanced *yin* and *yang*.

General Medical Beliefs

- There is no centralized religious hierarchy in Confucianism. Therefore, there is no single authority to dictate medical ethics. Cultural and family values and particular circumstances will have significant influence on medical care preferences.
- In general, Confucians highly respect medicine as a profession of human service. Medical care providers should place first priority on benevolent, respectful, and skilled service to patients. Issues of profit and prestige should not drive medical care. Due to this respect, many traditional people from Confucian influenced cultures expect medical care providers to demonstrate expert authority and may tend to have a deferent, rather than proactive, approach to the patient/doctor relationship.
- Most people influenced by Confucianism recognize that physical illness can be caused by many factors, such as injury, infection, genetic predisposition, poor sanitation and environmental pollutants. Most are likely to be comfortable with blending conventional Western style medicine and other medical interventions with traditional medical practices, such as acupuncture, herbs, breathing exercises, and *qigong*.
- Traditionally, it is believed that health is threatened by disharmony (such as extreme emotions, thoughts, and behaviors) and distress within oneself and in relationships with other people, heaven, and earth. Most fundamentally, failure to properly cultivate virtue results in poorly operating vital energy, mental and physical problems, and disrupted relationships. This relates to a popular belief that illness can result from fate as determined by heaven or as a result of cosmic retribution for misconduct of oneself or one's family members.
- Any disruption or imbalance of *yin* and *yang* qualities of vital energy can cause illness. Traditional medical practices seek to maintain and restore proper balance and flow of vital energy. (These practices and their related medical theory are also influenced by Taoism.)
- Cultivation of virtue, balanced and moderate lifestyle, clear mind, and service to others all contribute to health and well-being for oneself, society, and the world.
- Many people influenced by Confucianism will accept conventional medical determinations of death. Medical personnel should explain standards for determining death and solicit family responses. Confucius did not make strict pronouncements about what happens at or after death. He said that most people do not even understand what it is to live, so it is better to focus on learning that than to speculate about what happens after death. Accordingly, many Confucian scholars do not hold a firm idea about what occurs at or after death. However, there are common cultural beliefs that a person's soul continues to exist after death and must be properly respected through ancestor honoring rites. For many Confucians, the ancestor honoring rites are more significant for the intrinsic value of sincere remembrance and family solidarity than for literal contact with a deceased spirit.

Specific Medical Issues

- **Abortion**: Abortion may be acceptable when considered necessary based on careful considerations. Traditionally, full human life (personhood) was considered to begin at birth and welcoming into family and society. Yet each individual and family will have their own opinions about this.

- **Advance Directives**: End-of-life care and advance directives should be discussed clearly with elders, those with serious health challenges, and their loved ones, if they are willing. Such discussion should be sensitive to family-based decision making, including the roles of patient and family members and their comfort levels in discussing death. People who are serious practitioners of Confucian self-cultivation may have no hesitance about this. But some people might feel that discussing death or advanced directives might imply lack of willingness to do everything possible to help their loved ones. For example, some adult children might feel that failure to take extreme life saving measures for sick parents could violate filial piety.

- **Birth Control**: Confucianism encourages parents to have children in order to continue the generations, to honor their own parents, and to help maintain society at large. Since many people who are influenced by Confucianism come from patrilineal cultures, they often have a special interest in continuing to have children until at least one is male, in order to continue the family name and line. Confucianism also encourages moderation and harmony, so large numbers of children is not a standard ideal. There are no specific restrictions on birth control if it contributes to well-being of the family and society. But individual opinions vary. For example, someone might be influenced by Confucianism and also be a Catholic, in which case Catholic principles would apply.

- **Blood Transfusions**: Beliefs about euthanasia, abortion, blood transfusion, surgical interventions, and transplantation will vary by person, family, and culture. In general, Confucianism teaches respect for the body, which is considered a great gift from heaven and one's parents. Any abuse of the body is unwelcome. For very traditional Confucians, even cutting the hair can be an offense. However, given clear medical reasoning, any medical intervention that has a likelihood of prolonging a healthy life for oneself and loved ones may be welcome.

- **Circumcision**: Some Confucians view circumcision as a violation of the body. However, it is a common medical practice for Korean male infants and youth.

- **In Vitro Fertilization**: Fertility treatments and artificial means of conception (such as in vitro fertilization) may be acceptable and even desirable to Confucian influenced parents. This is because bearing children (especially sons in patrilineal cultures) to continue the family line is extremely important. However, this must be balanced with the principle of harmonizing with natural processes. Adoption is beginning to increase as an option for infertile couples in some East Asian countries.

- **Stem Cell Research**: Stem cell research is too recent for any consensus to be clear. However, it is noteworthy that South Korean scientists have been promoting stem cell research, given that Korean culture is strongly influenced by Confucianism. Traditionally, human life was considered to begin at birth, so stem cells may not be considered human. If there is likelihood that stem cell research can lead to widespread human benefits, it might be desirable.

- **Vaccinations**: Attitudes about vaccinations vary among individuals and cultural groups influenced by Confucianism. To the extent that vaccinations may contribute to personal health, they would be consistent with the Confucian emphasis on protecting the body in order to fulfill filial duty, since one's body is a precious gift from one's parents and as a means of keeping in good physical condition so as to be able to serve others. Vaccinations are common in industrialized East Asian countries.

- **Withholding/Withdrawing Life Support**: It might be difficult for some to consider termination of life-sustaining treatments for parents or other family members, if this appears to be a violation of virtues of filial piety, caring for children and siblings, or spousal affection. However, it might be considered benevolent to allow someone to die in a natural and dignified way with least amount of pain.

Gender and Personal Issues

- Ideally, women and men should be held in equal dignity. However, many people influenced by Confucianism come from patriarchal cultures and may give preferential treatment to males.
- Traditionally, adult men were expected to have primary authority and activity outside the home, while adult women were to have primary authority and activity within the home. The roles were to be complementary. This may still manifest in men (particularly family elders) being most outspoken in public discussions about medical issues for their families. However, the role of women as family nurturers and behind-the-scenes decision makers is significant.
- Traditionally, boys and girls were separated into different activities around the age of 6 years. Following this pattern, many Confucian-influenced people gather socially with members of their own gender. It may be uncomfortable for some men when a female physician or nurse intrudes on their bodies and private medical matters.

Principles for Spiritual Care through the Cycles of Life
Concepts of Living and Dying for Spiritual Support

- Death is a natural part of the cycle of change in human life and the cosmos. Although the loss of loved ones is cause for mourning, death itself is not necessarily to be feared. If one lives one's life moment to moment in a sincere and benevolent manner, then one's own death can be accepted more easily. Confucius said that if a benevolent person hears about the *Dao* (the Way of Benevolence) in the morning, then one can accept death in the evening. People who are out of harmony with themselves and do not understand the cycle of change are more likely to experience fear of death.
- There are common cultural beliefs that a person's soul continues to exist after death and must be properly respected through proper treatment of the body at death, proper location of an auspicious burial site, and ancestor honoring rites. Some elder immigrants might prefer to be buried in their country of origin near to their ancestors. For some Confucians, the ancestor honoring rites are more significant for the intrinsic value of sincere remembrance and family solidarity than for literal contact with a deceased spirit.

During Birth

- Specific customs surrounding birth are rooted in the person's culture. Confucianism celebrates birth as a great event supporting the continuity of generations and as the beginning of a person's journey on the *Dao*.
- In some cultures influenced by Confucianism, there is a special party to celebrate at birth or 100 days after birth and on the first birthday.
- Artificial contraception is generally acceptable, but this cannot be assumed.
- Ideally, birthing should occur in a harmonious environment, attended by loved ones, especially mothers or grandmothers.
- Fertility treatments and artificial means of conception (such as in vitro fertilization) may be acceptable and even desirable to Confucian influenced parents. This is because bearing children to continue the family line is extremely important. However, this must be balanced with the principle of harmonizing with natural processes. Adoption is beginning to increase as an option for infertile couples in some East Asian countries.
- Traditionally, parents preferred to give birth at home. Midwives (who might be kinship related women) often assisted. With the increase of hospital-based births, the presence of nurturing family is still important. The parents should be consulted about culture-specific rituals and beliefs concerning birth.
- If a baby dies in the hospital, parents or family members should be consulted for how they wish to respond.
- As stated earlier, some Confucians view circumcision as a violation of the body. However, it is a common medical practice for Korean male infants and youth.

During Illness

- There are no Confucian clergy per se. Patients may wish to seek advice and support from respected family elders, mentors or scholars. Medical or pastoral care providers can inquire with the patient or family about this.
- Situations of illness, dying, and personal crises can be powerful opportunities to learn about the nature of human existence and the cycles of change in nature. They can stimulate progress on the Way of benevolence if viewed in this way. Some Confucians study the Chinese Book of Changes to gain such insights.
- Recovery can be promoted through a harmonious environment, loving attention of family members, resumption of balanced diet, and use of complementary healing practices such as acupuncture, massage, herbal medicines, *qigong*, and quiet sitting.
- Many Confucian-influenced people are interested in wise and inspiring readings from a variety of traditions.
- Prayers and religious texts that do not fit the patient's interest and comfort should not be imposed.
- If a person will stay in the hospital for more than a brief period, she or he could be invited to decorate the room to make it feel meaningful, beautiful, and full of healing energy. This might include pictures (such as family photos), meaningful calligraphy, flowers, or other items.
- Many Confucian-influenced people participate in some other formal religion, such as Christianity. If this is true for a patient, then explore whether any religious images or a shrine might be appropriate.

During End of Life

- The best way to prepare for death is to live a life of virtue.
- Death is a natural part of the cycle of change in human life and the cosmos. Although the loss of loved ones is cause for mourning, death itself is not necessarily to be feared. If one lives one's life moment to moment in a sincere and benevolent manner, then one's own death can be accepted more easily. Confucius said that if a benevolent person hears about the *Dao* (the Way of benevolence) in the morning, then one can accept death in the evening. People who are out of harmony with themselves and do not understand the cycle of change are more likely to experience fear of death.
- Parents are especially concerned to leave a legacy of material support, love, and family tradition to their children. Helping dying parents to engage in such life review and to share their thoughts with their children can support the entire family in the letting go process.
- Many Confucian-influenced people are interested in wise and inspiring readings from a variety of traditions.
- Prayers and religious texts that do not fit the patient's interest and comfort should not be imposed.
- Standards about pain control vary by person and family. In general, reduction of unnecessary pain is benevolent. It is also desirable for pain management to allow the patient to maintain mental clarity if possible.
- Traditionally, most people preferred to die at home with care from family members. Hospice care might facilitate this. If this is not possible, then a home-like environment with a feeling of harmony and family support should be created in a hospital setting with palliative or hospice care.
- When a person dies far away from home or under traumatic and disfiguring conditions, the shock to the surviving family may be greater. Special family counseling may be necessary.
- It may be difficult for some adult children (especially the eldest son) influenced by the Confucian virtue of filial piety to consider withdrawing or withholding of life-sustaining treatments for parents, even when there appears no hope of recovery of consciousness. Active euthanasia that causes an early death even when a person is conscious would be most controversial. However, Confucianism places high priority on moral quality of life and harmony with the natural course of change. If a person's suffering is needlessly prolonged by unnatural medical interventions, this may not be desirable. When there are clear signs of the body's natural tendency to die, artificial life sustenance may be inappropriate. Good palliative care, allowing natural death process with maximum pain relief and opportunities for patient self-reflection and connection with family would likely be consistent with Confucian principles. End of life care and advance directives should be discussed clearly with elders, those with serious health challenges, and their loved ones, if they are willing.
- The place where a person is dying, including a hospital room, should be maintained with a sense of respect, dignity, and beauty. If a person is committed to Confucian style self-cultivation, the room should not be excessively noisy or distracting. A dying patient or family members could decorate the room as discussed previously.
- Medical care providers should respect

the culture-specific ways of showing grief at the time of death. In some Confucian influenced cultures, expressions of grief may be loud and intense, varying in style according to the relationship of person to the deceased.

- The family should be supported in making plans for the funeral and memorial. For example, in South Korea, some hospitals include both patient care areas and rooms for funeral/memorial service according to a specific religion. A Confucian style memorial room may be used immediately after the death so that relatives, friends, and others may come to pay respect in bows for the surviving immediate family members and the deceased person. A memorial table may be arranged that includes a photograph of the deceased and other items. Such details depend on family and culture.

Care of the Body

- The family's particular customs should be consulted ahead of time regarding care of the body immediately after death and preparation for burial.
- Immediately at death, in the hospital or elsewhere, family members may express grief and lamentation in a culturally specific style. However, at least among Confucian Koreans, visitation of the body for quiet viewing in a procession is not traditional.
- In some cultures (such as Korean), there is a designated family member or members who wash the body.
- It is common for a deceased person to be memorialized in a photograph and/ or calligraphy, displayed at a funeral or memorial service. Western style embalming and displaying of the body is not traditional.

- The body should not be unnecessarily damaged or treated disrespectfully during autopsy.
- Most Confucians prefer burial to cremation and some may wish to be buried in family plots, even if this means an immigrant's body must be returned to the country of origin.
- Donation of the body for medical research might be acceptable if the benefit to society outweighs the injury to the individual's body. Such a decision would require careful family discussion. The family should be informed that burial could be delayed.

Organ and Tissue Donation

- Damage to the body is undesirable, since the body is a gift from heaven and one's parents. However, organ and tissue donation might be acceptable if benefit to others is significant. Such a decision would require careful family discussion. It may be preferable for a chaplain, social worker or nurse who is trained to be culturally and spiritually appropriate to assist with this discussion.
- Planning for advance directives with a person prior to death can make this decision more clear.

Scriptures, Inspirational Readings, and Prayers
GENERAL PRINCIPLES ABOUT PRAYER
- In Confucianism, formal prayers and prayers to spiritual beings for personal benefit are not typical. Confucius said that his life was his prayer. It is most important to discern the will of heaven and to live a virtuous life on a daily basis.
- In ancient times, Confucian governments maintained rituals and prayers for spirits associated with the sky and earth. These are no longer common. They are

not inherent or necessary to Confucian philosophy. In fact, Confucius advised keeping a respectful distance from spirits.

- During rites of honor for sages and ancestors, participants may express their intentions of respect as well as wishes for family well-being.
- Many Confucian-influenced families keep a home altar to commemorate their deceased family members, especially parents or grandparents.
- Quiet sitting and *qigong* are practices to help with spiritual attunement, but they do not rely on formal prayers.
- Some Confucians keep a painting in their home of Confucius and/or other sages. These show respect for the teachings of the sages and inspire people to emulate them.
- Serious practitioners of Confucianism fervently study the writings of past sages and scholars. These may even be memorized and chanted.

GENERAL INFORMATION ABOUT SCRIPTURAL TEXTS

- There are numerous books, essays, and poems in Chinese and other East Asian languages that are significant for Confucians. Patients or family members can be asked to recommend to health care providers readings that might help them to understand the patient. Some patients may wish to read inspiring books during hospital stays or convalescence at home. If a patient is interested, a health care provider, pastoral counselor, or family member may read to the patient.
- Many Confucian-influenced people are interested in wise and inspiring readings from a variety of traditions.
- Prayers and religious texts that do not fit the patient's interest and comfort should not be imposed.

- There are no Confucian clergy per se. However, a patient may wish to seek guidance and spiritual counsel from a trusted elder, friend, or scholar.
- All Confucians recognize the importance of the foundational Chinese classics. These were composed in China from around the time of Confucius through the Han dynasty (until around 200 CE). These include the Five Classics: The Book of Changes (*Yi Jing*, 易經), the Book of History (*Shu Jing*, 書經), the Book of Poetry or Songs (*Shi Jing*, 詩經), The Record of Rites (*Li Ji*, 禮記), and the Spring and Autumn Annals (*Chun Qiu*, 春秋) plus the Four Books: The Great Learning (*Da Xue*, 大學), The Doctrine of the Mean (*Zhong Yong*, 中庸), the Analects of Confucius (*Lun Yu*, 論語), and the Book of Mencius (*Mengzi*, 孟子).
- Patients, family members, or health care professionals may be able to read these in the original classical Chinese, or in translations of contemporary Chinese, Korean, Japanese, Vietnamese, English, and other languages. It is easy to find English translations of the Four Books and the classic, The Book of Changes. Some of these are available online and can be found using a search engine with the title of the book or the term "Confucianism."

INSIGHTS FROM THE CHINESE CLASSICS

The following are paraphrases based on comparing various translations. Various translations may have different chapter divisions. It is best to read the original texts.

From: *The Analects of Confucius*[316]
A noble minded person eats without

---

316 Li. *The Analects of Confucius*. Page numbers cited in the text.

excess, lives without craving luxury, works diligently, and is careful with words. These are the steps to learn and move toward the Dao. (p. 17)

When your parents are alive, serve them properly. When they are deceased, bury them and memorialize them properly. (p. 22)

If you serve food to parents without reverence, this is not different from feeding dogs and horses. (p. 23)

If you learn of the Dao in the morning, you can be content to die at evening. (p. 46)

When parents are misguided, plead respectfully a few times.

If the pleas are rejected, respect their decision without complaint. (p. 50)

Heaven endowed me with virtue. (p. 88)

If you do not even understand life, then how can you know about death? (p. 128)

That which you do not like, do not do to others. (p. 139)

When you assess yourself and find no regrets, why would you need to be anxious? (p. 139)

A complete person thinks of righteousness over personal gain, accepts responsibility even when endangered, and remembers promises made throughout life. (p. 166)

A noble person learns the Dao in order to love people. (p. 147)

From: *The Great Learning*[317]
Great learning means to manifest virtue, to renovate society, and to rest in excellence. When the point to rest is known, the goal is clear. Then calmness and repose develop. In this repose, you may carefully deliberate and attain your desired goal … If you wish to manifest virtue throughout the world, first harmonize your own region. If you wish to regulate your region, first harmonize your family. Wishing to harmonize your family, you must first cultivate yourself by rectifying your heart and making your thoughts sincere.

Wishing to make your thoughts sincere, you must extend your knowledge to the utmost by investigating things. (pp. 356–358)

From: *The Doctrine of the Mean*[318]
Equilibrium results when the mind is not disrupted by pleasure, anger, sadness, or joy. When such feelings arise, but are expressed in proper degree, there is harmony. Equilibrium is the great root of all human action. Harmony is the universal path that all should pursue. Perfect the conditions of equilibrium and harmony; then a happy order will pervade heaven and earth, and all things will flourish. (pp. 384–385)

---

317 Legge, J. Trans. (1960). *The Chinese Classics in Five Volumes*. Hong Kong: Hong Kong University Press. Page numbers cited in text.

318 Legge. *The Chinese Classics in Five Volumes*. Page numbers cited in text.

From: *The Book of Mencius*[319]

Keep your will firm and whole; then
   you can guide your vital energy.
But never oppress it. Nurture your
   vital energy and protect it from
   harm.
Then it will fill heaven and earth.
   (pp. 47–48)

Don't fret about dying young or living
long. Just cultivate yourself well and
let come what may. Then you will be
secure in your destiny. (p. 235)

All things are within me. The greatest
   joy is to look within and find them.
Devote yourself to treating others as
   you wish to be treated.

That is the direct way to benevolence.
   (p. 235)

Cultivate virtue and benevolence
   when you are poor and lonely.
Succeeding in that, share virtue with
   all. (p. 238)

Special Days: Confucianism

There are no fixed days for celebration that all Confucians in all countries would follow consistently. Furthermore, there are days for ceremonies at the national Confucian shrine and shrine for kings in South Korea, but most people are not involved. Also, some of these holidays are spread over more than 1 day.

February 7 *New Year's Day* – For countries that follow the traditional lunar calendar, such as China and Korea, the lunar new year (e.g., beginning February 10 in 2013) is a significant time for celebration, enjoying family, and respecting ancestors. The exact day changes because of the fluctuations in the lunar calendar.

September 15–16 *Chuseok* – This event, also known as Autumn Harvest Day, is a major holiday in Korea for visiting the graves of ancestors, celebrating harvest, and enjoying family. It is held variably, on the fifteenth day of the eighth lunar month. Otherwise, each family keeps records of the days to commemorate individual ancestors.

September 27/28 *Confucius' Birthday* – This day, also regarded as Teacher's Day, to honor Confucius is celebrated in Taiwan on September 27 or 28. It has been proposed for September 28 in the United States.

---

319 Hinton, D. trans. (1999). *Mencius*. Washington,
   DC: Counterpoint. Page numbers cited in the text.

Glossary of Confucianist Terms (*Pinyin*)

Dao: (Also commonly spelled *Tao*) The way or order of the cosmos, especially as expressed in benevolence and virtuous human relationships.

de: Virtue, meaning the power inherent in a person or thing existing in harmony with the *Dao*, considered both a quality of character and a positive force of influence on the well-being of oneself and others.

li: The virtue of proper conduct of rituals as well as propriety in daily life.

pinyin: A system to represent Standard Mandarin pronunciations in the Latin alphabet rather than Chinese characters.

qi: Literally, "breath" or "energy," this refers to the vital energy of the universe. According to Mencius, the quality of a person's vital energy is closely related to how well they cultivate and express a virtuous life. In traditional Chinese medicine, *qi* is understood to flow in lines through earth and the body, and it can be affected by meditation, exercises, acupuncture, herbal and other traditional medicines, and the features of local geography or placement of objects in a room.

ren: The cardinal virtue of benevolence, humanity, and humane-heartedness.

shu: Principle of reciprocity or mutual benefit in relationships.

Taiji: Great Primal Beginning or Supreme Ultimate which is boundless and beyond any division, name or form, yet gives rise to *yin* and *yang* energies and the creation of all things.

tian: Concept of heaven that refers both to the sky and to a metaphysical force that imparts virtue into human nature and affects fate.

xiao: The virtue of filial piety that can be summarized as respect of parents by children, since parents have given the ultimate gift of life. This principle can be extended to respect of elders generally, and to respect of heaven and earth as being like the parents of humans and all creatures.

yang: The assertive, creative, and bright quality of vital energy; most prominent quality of heaven/sky and the masculine; *yin* and *yang* are complementary aspects of *qi*.

yin: The receptive, nurturing, and shaded quality of vital energy; most prominent quality of the earth and the feminine; *yin* and *yang* are complementary aspects of *qi*.

Additional information can be found online by entering the search term "Confucianism" plus other relevant terms such as "*yin*," "*yang*," "medical ethics," "euthanasia," and "diet."

Hare Krishna

Religion without philosophy is sentimentalism, Philosophy
without religion is dry speculation.[320]

Prepared by:
Kathleen Buckley
Los Angeles, California

History and Facts

In 1965, A.C. Bhaktivedanta Swami
Prabhupada, a holy man came from
India, journeyed to the United States, and
in 1966, in New York City, he founded
the International Society for Krishna
Consciousness (ISKCON), popularly
known as the Hare Krishna movement.
The Society bases its teachings and practices on ancient Vedic texts of India, such
as the Bhagavad Gita and the Srimad
Bhagavatam, as taught by the Lord Himself,
who appeared in East India about 500 years
ago as Caitanya Mahaprabhu. Prabhupada
translated dozens of volumes of Sanskrit and
Bengali works which have been published
in dozens of languages and distributed by
the tens of millions.

Prabhupada's goal was to teach the world
the timeless practice of bhakti yoga (devotion to Krishna, God). Followers dedicate
their thoughts and actions to Krishna and
thus awaken their dormant love for Him.

ISKCON has grown into a worldwide
society with over 400 temples and centers
around the globe, including farm communities, educational institutions, vegetarian
restaurants, and hospitals. Prabhupada
established a Governing Body Commission,
composed of a few dozen leaders from
around the world, who constitute ISKCON's
highest administrative body.

Basic Teachings

Isvara paramah krsnah sac-cid-
ananda-vigrahah, anadir adir govindah
sarva-karana-karanam. "Govinda, Krishna
is the cause of all causes. He is the primal
cause and He is the very form of eternity,
knowledge and bliss"[321]

Krishna, God, is the source of all. He exists
eternally, in His eternal, blissful, omniscient form. He expands Himself into many
other plenary forms. Yogis, mystics and
devotees realize God in three stages: first,
one may realize Him as an impersonal,

---

320 Srila Prabhupada. Available at www.prabhupada
nugas.eu/?p=8843 (accessed 16 Sept 2012).

321 Brahma-samhita. Available at http://harekrishna.
com/col/books/RP/BS/bs-fir.html (accessed
16 Sept 2012).

all-pervading spiritual light. Above this, He exists as the all-pervading witness within all creatures and all things. Ultimately, God is the Supreme Person, existing forever in His own abode. In this supreme form of Krishna, God manifests fully His six divine opulences: (1) infinite beauty, (1) strength, (3) knowledge, (4) detachment, (5) wealth, and (6) fame.

God is not only masculine. The complete Godhead includes the feminine aspect, known as Radha, Laksmi, Sri, or simply *the goddess*. Thus the Absolute Truth the supreme male and female principle.

Every living being is an eternal fragmental part of God. Although various species and genders of bodies cover the innumerable souls, they are spiritually one as siblings of the supreme parents, Radha-Krishna.

Souls possess the same quality of existence as God, though the quantity of their consciousness and power is infinitesimal compared to the infinite consciousness and power of God. Analogously, a drop of ocean water has the same chemical composition as the ocean, but in a far lesser quantity. We are eternally both one with, and subordinate to God.

Living, conscious souls are the superior energy (*shakti*) of God, whereas matter constitutes His inferior energy. Material forms are temporary, and ever changing, but the soul, though sometimes covered by illusion, is eternally the same. A sleeping person forgets his or her real identity, but the identity does not change.

The temporary pleasures of the body do not satisfy the spiritual soul, who needs to be in touch with God to be happy. Beyond our human needs of physical and mental health, justice, economic sufficiency, and so forth, we can only find final satisfaction in our spiritual love for God.

Originally, each soul has a direct relationship with God. Life's highest purpose is to revive this forgotten relationship through bhakti yoga. Human life uniquely affords a full opportunity to achieve this goal.

In the Bhagavad Gita after describing various kinds of yoga Lord Krishna declares, "Of all yogis, one who abides in Me with great faith, worshiping Me in transcendental service (*bhakti*) is most intimately united with Me in yoga and is highest of all."[322]

Similarly, after explaining various religious and spiritual practices, He states "One can understand the Supreme Personality as He is only by devotional service. And one in full consciousness of the Supreme Lord by such devotion, can enter into the kingdom of God."[323]

Basic Practices

- Those who worship God in the forms of Vishnu, Krishna, and so forth, are called Vaishnava. Although there are various Vaishnava traditions, all basically agree on the importance of chanting God's holy names, most famously exemplified by the chanting of the Hare Krishna mantra: Hare Krishna, Hare Krishna, Krishna Krishna, Hare Hare/Hare Rama, Hare Rama, Rama Rama, Hare Hare. This 16-word mantra, known as the "mahamantra" or "great mantra" features three Sanskrit names of God: Krishna means "all-attractive," Rama means "the source of pleasure," and Hare calls upon the feminine aspect of the Godhead.
- This mantra is either sung out loud in a

---

322 Bhagavad Gita. At http://bhagavad-gitaasitis.com/?g=157420 (accessed 25 Aug 2012).

323 Bhagavad Gita. At www.harekrsna.com/sun/editorials/07-12/editorials8822.htm (accessed 25 Aug 2012).

group (*kirtan/bhajan*) or chanted softly on beads (*japa*). God and His powers are held to be fully present in His names, which are thereby identical to Him. In fact we find that religious traditions throughout the world recognize the presence of God in His names.

- Devotees choose to serve the Lord within four possible *ashramas*, or social orders: a *brahmacari*, or female *brahmacarini*, is a celibate student who often lives and serves directly under the guidance of a spiritual teacher. The *grihastha*, or married person, practices bhakti yoga within the family circle. Having raised their children, married people then enter the third order, *vanaprastha*, in which, having fulfilled their domestic duties, the couple dedicates themselves fully to spiritual practice and service. The complete renunciant, the *sannyasi*, engages exclusively in teaching spiritual knowledge.

- Vaishnavas anoint their bodies with sacred clay in 12 places, most notably the forehead, thus acknowledging the body as God's temple and one's self as His devotee. Followers wear strands of small neck beads made from the sacred *tulasi* plant. They carry a cloth bag that holds their chanting beads. Congregational members and householders often dress in Western attire, but may dress in traditional Indian clothing when attending temple services.

- Krishna's devotees strive to purify their consciousness of material attachments, by hearing and chanting the names, glories and activities of Krishna. Temple ceremonies center on worship of a Krishna Deity, to whom the devotees offer sumptuous food, lovely garments, incense, water, and so forth. Vaishnava tradition claims, with sophisticated ontological arguments, that Krishna is present in the Deity form.

- The daily worship begins around 4:15 a.m. with an offering of food especially prepared with devotion by a priest. The devotees gather for *Arati*, a ceremony to greet the Lord with offerings of incense, lamps, waters, and so forth, while everyone chants the Hare Krishna Mantra in a spirit of joyous, prayerful devotion. There are about six such daily offerings in larger temples, though most of the devotees only attend one or two per day. After the early morning arati, devotees perform their individual, meditative chanting called *japa* on a strand of 108 beads. In ISKCON, formally initiated devotees chant 16 rounds a day on their beads, which takes approximately 2 hours. Next the temple offers a class on Srimad Bhagavatam, followed by breakfast. Devotees then disperse to carry out their respective duties. Some go to outside jobs, others engage in public outreach, others attend to the internal temple management and worship.

- In the evenings many devotees gather again for Arati and Bhagavad Gita class.

- *Prasadam* indicates any item, such as food, flowers, and so forth, that has been offered to Krishna, and thus spiritualized. Contact with such sanctified articles purifies the devotee. Krishna states in the Bhagavad Gita: "What ever you do, whatever you eat, whatever you offer or give away and whatever austerities you perform – do that, as an offering to Me" (Bg 9:27). Devotees only eat vegetarian food first offered with devotion to Krishna. A devotee does not taste, smell or enjoy anything before offering it to the Lord for His pleasure, since all that exists emanates from Him.

- The Vaishnava calendar includes many special days, most of which celebrate the appearances of incarnations of God, and the appearances and disappearances of great personalities. Twice a month, devotees observe *ekadasi*, a day when devotees fast from grains and beans.

- One of the most important activities of a devotee is the distribution of books and devotional literature. Book distribution is considered to be the greatest service to humanity because it shares with people bhakti yoga and the science of God, thus giving humanity the knowledge and the tools to put an end to the soul's continued cycle of birth, death, old age, and disease, and reconstitute its eternal position with Krishna. In addition, devotees chant in the streets and have *kirtan* for the general population, who benefit spiritually by hearing the Holy Name.

- Devotees believe in reincarnation, the passage of the soul through different species of life. Reaching the human life is critical to making spiritual advancement and stopping the reincarnation cycle. Leading a degraded life can cause the soul to take birth in lower forms of life like animals, insects, or plants. The laws of karma explain this: sinful and degraded activities yield bad results and lower births; pious activities yield good results and higher births. Leading a life of pure love of Godhead and devotional service, on the other hand, breaks the reincarnation cycle and our bondage to the laws of karma, and takes us back to Krishna. This is the ultimate goal of life.

Principles for Clinical Care
Dietary Issues

- Devotees follow a strict lacto-vegetarian diet, with no meat, fish, or eggs allowed. There is also no consumption of onion or garlic. Devotees prefer organic fresh vegetables and fruits. They prefer to eat food cooked by other devotees and will only eat food that is first offered to Krishna. Devotees generally prefer natural processes of healing – ayurvedic, herbs, acupuncture, and homeopathy. Srila Prabhupada's instructions were to be practical. Allopathy is not discouraged. Twice a month, on *ekadasi*, devotees fast from grains and beans. There are other fasts throughout the year, but exceptions are made for health reasons. Some very austere followers eat very little or very simply.

Specific Medical Issues

- **Abortion**: Abortion is strongly prohibited. It is believed that the soul enters the womb at the time of conception.
- **Advanced Directives/Living Wills**: These are encouraged, especially if other family members are not of the same belief.
- **Birth Control**: Abstinence is the recommended method.
- **Blood Transfusions**: Blood transfusion is an acceptable practice.
- **Circumcision**: Circumcision is not regulated by scripture but according to the parents' desire.
- **In Vitro Fertilization**: This is a personal decision.
- **Stem Cell Research**: This is acceptable as long as an abortion is not involved.
- **Vaccinations**: Vaccinations are not regulated but are a personal decision.
- **Withholding/Withdrawing Life Support**: This is preferred to prolonging death.

Gender and Personal Issues

- Treatment is preferred from a health professional of the same sex; however, the qualification of the professional is more important to a devotee. Devotees are chaste and keep their private parts covered at all times.

- Cleanliness is important. Devotees wash their hands and mouth after eating and shower after passing stool. Devotees take two showers a day, one when they rise and one in the afternoon.

Principles for Spiritual Care through the Cycles of Life

During Birth

- The birth of a child is a celebrated moment from the time of conception. Devotees use abstinence for birth control. The time of conception is a very special time, as the parents' consciousness attracts the soul to the mother's womb. Prayers, fasting, and mantra chanting is preformed for all phases of the birth cycle.
- Prenatal care is advised.
- During pregnancy women are advised to follow a wholesome diet with moderate regular exercise and a healthy and positive state of mind.
- There is no dancing after the fourth month of pregnancy and no traveling after the seventh month.
- The child becomes conscious in the seventh month, so it is important to read aloud or have devotional music for the child.
- Prabhupada recommended that the first child be born in a hospital. If there are no complications, parents may choose a midwife thereafter.
- Who is present during the birth is a personal choice.
- Many devotees prefer a natural birth with no drugs.
- If possible the mother will want to keep the child near her.

- The mother should rest in bed for at least 3 weeks.
- Nursing is preferred to bottle-feeding.

During Illness

- Depending on their nature, some devotees may have many visitors; others only a few.
- Patients should be offered *prasadam* (food cooked by Vaishnavas and offered to Krishna)
- Patients should be allowed to chant the maha mantra on *japa* beads.
- Patients should be encouraged through visits by other devotees.
- Patients should have access to scriptures written by His Divine Grace A.C. Bhaktivedanta Swami Prabhupada
- Patients may wish to engage in devotional service, as they are able to, in order to aid in diminishing any spiritual anxieties.
- Tradition declares that spiritual association, taking *prasadam*, chanting *japa*, worship of deities, and reading scriptures are all beneficial methods that lead to enlightenment as well as mental and physical well-being.
- Health care providers should keep the devotee's room free of outside noise (TVs, radios, loud talking)
- The patient's room should be kept free of cooking odors, especially meat and garlic.
- Visits from clergy members can be encouraged to participate in the chanting and reading. They may bring flowers and *prasadam*.
- According to the individual, a terminal illness can be a time for intense emotional closure with loved ones and friends. However, it is considered a blessing to have this time to prepare for one's death. Hospice and palliative care is encouraged as well as emotional and spiritual support from the congregation.

- It is appropriate for clinicians to offer emotional and spiritual support to the patient, family, and friends during an acute or terminal illness.
- It is appropriate to ask visitors to step out of the patient's room when a procedure must be performed.
- It is extremely important for devotees of Lord Krishna to hear the chanting of the Holy Names of God (maha mantra) in life as in death. Family and friends may offer to sing this mantra for the patient or to read to them from the Bhagavad Gita or other Vedic scriptures, as it gives solace to the patient and relatives. They may wish to have an audio recording continuously playing.
- Incense is allowed if it does not irritate their illness or other people.
- Devotees see the body as a source of suffering. Karma may manifest through disease. Distress is an opportunity to increase devotion to God.
- Krishna says in the Bhagavad Gita: "Always think of Me, become My devotee, worship Me and offer homage unto Me. Thus you will come to Me without fail. I promise you this because you are My very dear friend" (Bg 18:65).
- **Never remove the beads around the neck or the sacred string around a male devotee's body.**

During End of Life

- Death is seen as a transition to one's next birth or an opportunity to end the cycle of birth and death (reincarnation) by going back to Godhead. A strong emphasis is placed on one's thoughts (consciousness) at the time of death.
- Devotees prefer to be at home or in a Hare Krishna hospice facility.

- Friends and family members will want to know when the time is near.
- There will be a *kirtan* (singing of the maha mantra).
- Devotees will want their bodies anointed with holy water from the Ganges or the Yamuna.
- Flower garlands from the Deities should be placed on the devotee.
- Allow for and encourage expressions of feelings and emotions concerning impending death so that the patient can become at peace and focus on Lord Krishna.
- It is best for dying patients to have a private room to ensure quiet and undisturbed rest.
- Dying patients can be comforted by being reminded that the Lord will never leave them.
- Health care providers who are good nonjudgmental listeners can aid patients in releasing their anxieties.

The following are some things health care professionals can do or facilitate in the care of the patients.

- Provide the opportunity to hear lectures, chant *japa*, or listen to other spiritual media.
- Offer visitors to have kirtan (chanting mantras and prayers with musical accompaniment).
- Talk about spiritual matters.
- Read aloud from the revealed scriptures or songs by Srila Narottama dasa Thakura, Srila Bhaktivinoda Thakura, and other Vaishnava *acaryas* (spiritual masters who taught by example), who have provided poems for meditation.
- Reassure patients that their life has made a difference in the world.

- Patients should leave their body remembering Lord Krishna. To this end, patients should hear the name of Krishna without cessation until death and be surrounded with images, scents, sights, and sounds that will help their minds remain fixed on Krishna before, during, and after the time of departure. This includes the use of chanting, singing, burning incense, reading scriptures aloud, and so forth.
- Being able to die in the holy *dhama* (abode) in Vrindavan, India (place where Lord Krishna descended from heaven and spent time on Earth) provides great spiritual benefits. This may not be possible because of the expense and difficulty for the ill to travel.
- Help patients experience a "good death" by doing everything possible to manage physical, emotional, and mental pain, so the patient can focus more completely on spiritual matters.
- A *tulasi* leaf should be placed in the devotees' mouth just before they leave their bodies.

Care of the Body
- Preparation of the body for cremation includes bathing it with pure water (in India, the body is bathed in a holy river – Ganges or Yamuna), dressing it in new clothes, using *tilaka* (holy clay used to mark body and forehead. A *tulasi* leaf dedicated to the Lord is placed in the deceased's mouth as well as *caranamrita* (water from bathing the Deity of the Lord). A garland from the Deities can be placed around the deceased's neck, and a small piece of the Deities' clothing is pinned to the deceased's clothes. Water from holy rivers, if available, is sprinkled over the body.

- Cremation is the preferred means of disposition of the body.
- Autopsies are not desirable unless required by law.
- Devotees do not donate their bodies for medical research.
- Family members may view the body, but cremating the body as soon as possible is preferred, as the soul may linger with the dead body.
- The chanting of the maha mantra is very important during this process.

Organ and Tissue Donation
- This is a personal choice. There is no scriptural recommendation.

Scriptures, Inspirational Readings, and Prayers
READING DURING ILLNESS

Hearing and chanting about the transcendental holy name, form, qualities, paraphernalia, and pastimes of Lord Vishnu, remembering them, serving the lotus feet of the Lord, offering the Lord respectful worship with sixteen types of paraphernalia, offering prayers to the Lord, becoming His servant, considering the Lord one's best friend, and surrendering everything unto Him – these nine processes are accepted as pure devotional service. One who has dedicated his life to the service of Krishna through these nine methods should be understood to be the most learned person, for he has acquired complete knowledge.

—Srimad Bhagavatam, 7:5:24

READINGS DURING END-OF-LIFE PROCESS

The wise, engaged in devotional service, take refuge in the Lord, and free themselves from the cycle of birth and death by renouncing the fruits of action in the material world. In this way, they can attain that state beyond all miseries.

—Bhagavad Gita, 2:51

Whoever at the time of death quits his body remembering Me alone at once attains My nature. Of this there is no doubt.

—Bhagavad Gita, 8:5

Hearing and chanting about the transcendental holy name, form, qualities, paraphernalia, and pastimes of Lord Vishnu, remembering them, serving the lotus feet of the Lord, offering the Lord respectful worship with sixteen types of paraphernalia, offering prayers to the Lord, becoming His servant, considering the Lord one's best friend, and surrendering everything unto Him — these nine processes are accepted as pure devotional service. One who has dedicated his life to the service of Krishna through these nine methods should be understood to be the most learned person, for he has acquired complete knowledge.

—Srimad Bhagavatam, 7:5:24

Further Reading and Resources

- All books by A.C. Bhaktivedanta Swami
- *Songs of the Vaisnava Acaryas.* Available at (accessed 25 Aug 2012)
- Pattison, S. *The Final Journey.* Torchligh Publishing; 2011
- www.krishna.com

Hinduism

Religion is not in doctrines, in dogmas, nor in intellectual argumentation. It is being and becoming. It is realization.[324]

Prepared by:
Anand Bhattacharyya
with contributions from Arvind Khetia, Kris Krishna,
and Roy Hegde
Overland Park, KS

Reviewed and approved by:
Swami Chetanananda
Minister-in-Charge, Vedanta Society of St. Louis
St. Louis, MO

History and Facts

Hinduism, originally called the "Eternal Religion," is one of the oldest of all living religions. Unlike other major religions, Hinduism has no prophet as its founder.

Scriptures

Vedas are the principal and the most authoritative scriptures, and are often referred to by the term *Shruti* (As Revealed). The composers of Vedas were the sages of ancient India. These sages, in their meditation, attained transcendental consciousness and realized the eternal and the universal truths. These were later compiled in books, called Vedas. There are four Vedas – *Rig, Sama, Yajur,* and *Atharva.* Later sections of Vedas are called Upanishads. The Upanishads, also known as Vedanta, are the "Knowledge Parts" of the Vedas. These philosophical treatises explain that in this ever-changing world of cause and effect, *Brahman* (Impersonal,

Transcendental God) is the ultimate and absolute reality.

The scriptures variously describe *Brahman* as Infinite Existence, Infinite Consciousness, Infinite Bliss and Supreme Self. They also explain the identity of *Brahman* with *atman*, the in-dwelling self (soul) of all beings. In addition to these revealed scriptures, there are many auxiliary scriptures, called *Smriti* (As Remembered). These scriptures were composed subsequent to Vedas to analyze, explain, and illustrate the spiritual truths contained in Vedas. The most popular of these scriptures is the Bhagavad Gita (The Song of the Lord) which explains the practical applications of the teachings of Upanishads in day-to-day life.

The following paragraphs relate the significant accomplishments of and movements within Hinduism throughout different periods of history.

The *Vedic* Period (5000–600 BCE)

During this period, Vedas and the principal Upanishads were composed. Most

---

324 Vivekananda, S. (1987). *Vedanta: Voice of Freedom.* Mayavati, India: Advaita Ashrama, 87.

scholars believe that the earliest hymns in the *Rigveda*, which is the earliest of four Vedas, were composed between 5000 and 4000 BCE. The literature of this period shows three successive stages in which were recorded the *Samhitas* (the hymns), the *Brahmanas* (the codes of conduct), the *Aranyakas* (forest treatises), and the Upanishads (the philosophical texts). A distinct philosophical system, known as Jainism, emphasizing nonviolence, attainment of supreme purity, and self-liberation as its goal, was also developed during this period. Twenty-four Jain *Tirthankaras* (Messengers of God) appeared from time to time, *Rsabha* being the first, and *Mahavira* the last.

The *Sutra* Period (600–300 BCE)

During this period, the manuals of ritualism (the *Kalpa Sutras*) were developed. These manuals contain the description of various religious rites and oblations performed in the sacrificial fire. The manuals also include detailed descriptions of the duties of the king and the duties of the people belonging to all four castes. Also, Buddha was born in India as a Hindu prince during this period (563 BCE). He retained the moral and ethical ideas of Hinduism, but repudiated the authority of Vedas and emphasized the monastic life. However, the agnosticism of Buddhism never took a firm root in the land of its birth.

The Epic Period (400 BCE–750 CE)

This period is marked by the creation of two great epics, *Ramayana* and *Mahabharata*. *Ramayana*, composed by Sage *Valmiki*, is the inspiring story of the life of God-incarnate *Rama*, who was an ideal son, an ideal husband and an ideal king. He had a fierce fight with *Ravana*, the demon-king who abducted his wife, *Sita*. *Rama* finally slayed him, rescued *Sita* and reestablished the religious and moral laws. *Mahabharata*, composed by Sage *Vyasa*, is the story of an epic struggle between the two branches of the *Kuru* clan – *Kauravas* and *Pandavas*. *Kauravas* were the evil and the unrighteous. *Pandavas* were the good and the righteous. The struggle culminated in the great battlefield of *Kurukshetra*. God-incarnate *Krishna* took the side of *Pandavas*. Ultimately, *Pandavas* won the war. Justice and righteousness (*dharma*) finally prevailed. The Bhagavad Gita, which contains the "cream" of Hindu philosophy, was composed as a part of *Mahabharata* in the form of a dialogue between *Krishna* and *Arjuna*, one of the *Pandava* brothers. The historical facts narrated in the stories of *Ramayana* and *Mahabharata* are believed to be 5000–7000 years old. But the existing version of the epics can be traced to 400–100 BCE. In addition, the Laws of *Manu*, the minor Upanishads, and the philosophical sutras (aphorisms) were composed. Because of these auxiliary scriptures, the teachings of Upanishads were brought home to the people in a form they could understand. This period also marked the composition of *Puranas*, full of stories and legends. These scriptures became the instruments of education bringing Hindu ideals and Hindu codes of ethics to the masses.

The *Darsana* Period (750–1000 CE)

The establishment of the Monistic (*Advaita*) system of philosophy by *Sankara* is a great landmark in this period. Sankara's commentaries on the Upanishads, Gita, and *Brahma Sutras* formed the basis of the Monistic theory. The Bhagavata Purana, an ecstatic love of exceptional beauty between Krishna and shepherdesses (*gopis*) embodying the quality of divine love, was also created during this period. This work which postulated a great spiritual unfoldment through love made a profound impression on the people's minds.

The Medieval Period (1000–1800 CE)

The medieval period in Hinduism is characterized by the spread of the Devotional (*Bhakti*) movement, known as *Vaisnavism*. This movement laid stress on the ideals of all-consuming love for God. A whole-hearted lover of God can realize mystic union with God. The movement first started in the southern part of India and then spread to the northern part. This period also witnessed the two important philosophical systems. These are the Dualistic (*Dvaita*) system of *Madhva* and the Qualified Monistic (*Vishishtha Advaita*) system of *Ramanuja*. In the latter stages of this period, stagnation began to creep into Hinduism. This led to the need for reform.

The Modern Period (1800 CE–Present)

Raja Rammohan Roy was at the forefront of the modern Hindu reform movement. He fought against the conservative elements in Hindu society and all the social evils practiced in the name of religion. He formed *Brahmo Samaj*, a socioreligious movement, and tried to revitalize the real quintessence of Hinduism. *Arya Samaj*, established by *Swami Dayananda*, tried to unify all sections of Hindu society. *Ramakrishna* was able to infuse into his followers a true spirit of Hinduism, the harmony of religions and a sense of service to humanity. His followers, led by *Swami Vivekananda* founded the *Ramakrishna* Order and spread the messages of Vedanta throughout the world. He represented Hinduism at the Parliament of Religions in Chicago in 1893. During the nineteenth and twentieth centuries, enormous contributions were made by several spiritual luminaries to popularize the spiritual values of Hinduism in India and abroad – *Shirdi* and *Satya Sai Baba, Bhagwan Shree Swaminarayan (BAPS), Prabhupada Bhaktiacharya* (International Society of Krishna Consciousness), *Pandurang Shastri Athavale (Swadhaya), Paramhansa Yogananda* (Self-Realization Fellowship) – just to name a few.

Worldwide, there are approximately 800 million Hindus, a great majority of them live in India. Hindus comprise less than 1% of the US population.

Basic Teachings

Thousands of years ago, the sages (seers of truth), some of whom were women, realized eternal truths in their meditation. The primary emphasis of Hindu teachings is to experience these truths in one's daily life. Thus, for the Hindus, religion is a way of life. The main tenets of Hinduism are from the philosophical texts of the Vedas and are briefly summarized as follows:

- **The Divinity of the Soul**: Hinduism believes in God's omnipresence and recognizes every human soul as divine. The goal of human life is to manifest this inner divinity by the practice of spiritual disciplines. The divinity of the soul is the "real nature" of humans. Therefore, it is called "Self" (*Atman*).

- **The Unity of Existence**: One of the Upanishads says, "All this, whatsoever moves in this moving universe, is permeated by God." Thus, the Upanishads explain that behind all names and forms, there is only one Reality (*Brahman*).

- **The Oneness of the Godhead**: Hindus believe that God is one, but He has many names and manifestations. In the *Rig Veda*, it is stated, "Truth is one; sages call it by various names."

The whole world is pervaded by Me (GOD), yet my form is not seen. All living things have their being in Me, yet I am not limited by them, and they don't consciously abide in Me.

—Bhagavad Gita, 9:4

- **The Harmony of Religions**: Hindus believe that all religions are pathways to the
- same goal; as different streams having their sources in different places, all mingle their water in the sea.

The following is some of the additional information pertinent to overall Hindu religious thoughts.

- **Creation**: The universe goes through endless cycles of creation, preservation and dissolution. Therefore, Vedanta contends that creation cannot be out of nothing.
- **Doctrine of Karma**: The universal law of karma is the law of cause and effect by which one creates one's own destiny. Thus, the doctrine of karma provides the impetus for accountability for one's thoughts, words, and deeds and gives moral incentive to act justly.
- **Reincarnation**: The individual soul goes through many cycles of birth and death until all karmic results are exhausted. One has to continue to strive for liberation from the cycle of birth and death in this life by pursuing the spiritual disciplines.
- **Four Stages in Life**: The Hindus generally view one's life span composed of four distinct stages (*ashramas*). These are (1) a student's life pursuing studies to prepare

for the future, (2) a life of a householder, (3) a life of retirement for spiritual pursuits, and (4) a life of renunciation. All these stages are guided by specific duties, known as *dharma*, to provide a moral organization to one's life.

- **Four Goals of Life**: These are *Dharma, Artha, Kama,* and *Moksha*. For an average person, life's pursuits include *Artha* – one's need for material goods and *Kama* – one's legitimate desire for fulfillment of the pleasure of the senses. But these pursuits need to be guided by *Dharma* – one's intrinsic duty to oneself and to the society, guided by truth and unselfishness. Even while living a normal life, one has to remember to pursue the ultimate goal of human life, which is to attain *Moksha* (Liberation). The "four stages in life" and the "four goals of life," governed by *dharma*, provide the necessary organization and stability to the Hindu way of life.
- **Rituals and Prayers**: Divine presence is invoked through rituals and prayers. Although God is worshipped by many names and in many forms, Hindus believe they all are the manifestations of one Reality (*Brahman*).
- **Quotes from the Scriptures**: The essence of Vedanta philosophy is stated in four great declarations (*Maha Vakya*) of the Vedas. All of these statements direct one's mind to the fact that there is one Reality (*Brahman*) behind the individual soul and the personal God.
  - *"Consciousness is **Brahman**"* – The individual consciousness is the same as the cosmic consciousness (*Brahman*). It is in all beings and pervades everything. Once this truth is understood, a spiritual teacher explains to a disciple the next statement.
  - *"That Thou Art"* – This explains the

ultimate identity of Thou (individual soul) and That (*Brahman*). Thus, one knows the true meaning of religion, which is to realize the eternal oneness of the eternal God and the eternal Soul. The disciple then realizes that the ind-welling Self is *Brahman*.

- o *"This Self is **Brahman**"* – A disciple meditates on the aforementioned truth and concludes that the Self (*Atman*) within is *Brahman*, and declares the ultimate truth.
- o *"I am **Brahman**"* – Thus, a disciple experiences the ultimate truth that he or she is not limited by mind and body, but in essence, is *Brahman*.
- The moral and ethical life of the Hindus is also guided by the teachings expressed in some of the very simple yet enlightening statements found in different scriptures. A few of these statements are:
  - o The whole world is a family.
  - o Truth always triumphs.
  - o Non-Violence is the supreme ideal.
  - o Always speak the truth.
  - o Always do your duty.
  - o Treat mother as God.
  - o Treat father as God.
  - o Treat teacher as God.
  - o Treat guest as God.
  - o Let noble thoughts come to us from all directions.
- Hindus' strong belief in the universal law of karma, gives them necessary motivation for being good and doing good in the present life. An honest and unbiased examination of history, of prevailing personal and social problems due to crumbling moral values, and problems of decaying environment, clearly reveals the law of karma to be true.
- All Hindu teachings are tuned to one supreme goal, and that is to realize one's

inner divinity by raising one's consciousness to the highest level.

- The ultimate goal of human life is to realize the divine nature and for *Atman* (Self) to find unity with *Brahman* (Ultimate Reality, that is God). This is called *Mukti* (Liberation) – freedom from birth-death-rebirth cycles.

Basic Practices

Hinduism, based on the philosophy of Vedanta, provides a unified and integrated vision of life, because it is based on eternal and universal truths. The primary emphasis of Hindu teachings is not confined to any doctrine or dogma. On the contrary, it provides freedom of interpretation and insists on verifying these truths through one's own life experience. The insistence on experience makes it imperative that these religious values are integrated into daily living.

The Hindu epic, *Mahabharat*, states that every human being has three types of energy. The first is the physical energy, the second is the intellectual energy, and the third, and the most important one, is the spiritual energy emanating from the *Atman*. The practice of yoga and meditation as spiritual disciplines, as discussed shortly, are pertinent in the manifestation of this third type of energy. Interestingly, these practices are gaining wide acceptance outside the Hindu community.

- **The Four *Yogas*** – As stated earlier, the ultimate goal of human life is the unity of *Atman* with *Brahman*. This Divine Nature is realized through the four paths of *yoga*, which means "Union with God." Although one may choose a specific *yoga* depending on one's mental trait, one is encouraged to explore and glean wisdom from the different *yogas*.

- *Jnana Yoga* – *Jnana yoga* is the "way to God through knowledge or intuitive discernment." This discernment is the growing awareness that one's essential being is the Ultimate. *Jnana yoga* is said to be the shortest path to divine awareness, but also the steepest, for it requires total control of and stilling of the mind and is for very reflective individuals.
- *Bhakti Yoga* – *Bhakti yoga* is the "way to God through love and devotion." It is the most common of the four pathways and centers upon loving God wholeheartedly, instead of worldly attachments, through one or more of the many concepts of the Ultimate provided by Hinduism's magnificent myths.
- *Karma Yoga* – *Karma Yoga* is the "way to God through selfless work or through sacred duty." Actions are taken with thoughtfulness and without attachment. Loving, unselfish service diminishes the disconnected-ness with the divine until the barriers between the Ultimate and one's personal ego disappear altogether.
- *Raja Yoga* – *Raja Yoga* is the "way to God through spiritual discipline of meditation." Through physical and psychic exercises, the adherent becomes skilled at shutting out the phenomenal universe and becoming alone with a stilled mind. When this is attained, it is called *samadhi*, utter oneness with the Ultimate and dissolution of the personal self.
- **Prayers**: Hindu prayers always seek peace and prosperity for all. A typical daily prayer for Hindus is: "May there be welfare to all beings; may there be fullness and wholeness to all people; may there be constant good and auspicious life to

everyone; may there be peace everywhere ... *Om*. Peace! Peace! Peace!"

- **Worship Practices**: The main worship practices of Hinduism vary from one community to another. There are, however, a few major religious festivals, such as, birth anniversaries of Lord *Rama* and Lord *Krishna*, *Diwali* (Festival of Lights) that are common to most Hindus. On those days, collective worship is usually performed in a temple where the priests perform the rituals and chant verses from scriptures in Sanskrit. In some communities, *Satsang* is popular. *Satsang* is collective singing of devotional songs (*bhajan*) by all in attendance, accompanied by musical instruments. These are similar to spirituals (hymns) sung in churches. Hindus also do individual worship at their homes. Many Hindu homes have a small prayer room with the family's chosen deities and pictures of spiritual icons for worship. Meditation is usually conducted here.
- **Hindu Greetings**: The traditional Hindu greeting (*namaste*) is to fold the hands, join the two palms and bow the head to the person who is being greeted. This is the same way a Hindu prays to God. The reason for this custom is that when a Hindu greets another person, he or she greets not just the body of the person, but the person's inner soul, which is divine.
- **Interfaith Dialogue**: Hindus actively participate in interfaith dialogues and refrain from spreading misinformation about other faiths.
- **Rites of Passage (The *Samsakaras*)**: The following are the important stages in a person's development from birth to death.
  - *Conception* (**Garbadhana**): During the time of conception, parents perform fervent prayers for the child to

be conceived in order to fulfill their obligation to continue the human species. Scriptures and hymns are recited by both parents during this sacrament as well as prayers for mutual love, kindness, compassion, cooperation, and enjoyment of their married life.

○ *Fetal Protection* (**Punsavana**): This is a sacrament performed to promote protection and safety for the unborn child during the third or fourth month of pregnancy. Priests recite Vedic hymns to invoke divine qualities in the child.

○ *Birth* (**Jatakarma**): This is the ritual welcoming of the child into the family. Mantras are recited for a long and happy life. Circumcision is not a part of the tradition, although may be requested by parents.

○ *Naming Ceremony* (**Namakarma**): The name of the infant is selected according to spiritual principles to inspire the child to follow the path of righteousness.

○ *Introduction to the Outdoors* (**Nishkramana**): Performed during the fourth month after birth, the child is taken outside and introduced to the outdoors.

○ *Introduction to Solid Food* (**Annaprasanna**): During the sixth or seventh month, after teeth begin to appear, the child is introduced to solid food for the first time.

○ *Shaving of Head* (**Mundan**): This is done during either the first or the third year. The tradition maintains that this will help to ensure a healthy growth of new hair. It is a time of familial festivity and celebration.

○ *Ear Piercing* (**Karnaveda**): This is done between 3 and 5 years of age. Girls may also get nose piercing.

○ *Sacred Thread Ceremony* (**Upanayana**):

This ceremony takes place when the male child enters the adolescent stage.

○ *Marriage* (**Vivaha**): This ceremony is performed to start the second stage of life, which is the life of a householder.

○ *Retirement Life* (**Vanaprastha**): At age 50 (the age differs in various cultures), a person enters the third stage of life, a life of retirement which is dedicated in the pursuit of spiritual progress.

○ *Detachment from Material Life* (**Sannyasa**): At age 75, a person enters the final stage of life, a life of complete renunciation of the material world to perform spiritual practices.

○ *Funeral Services* (**Antyesthi**): At death, the soul leaves the body, and the body is cremated by the family members. The family members collect the ashes and at a later time scatter the ashes into a holy river, such as the Ganges. Thus, the ashes are returned to nature.

○ *Post Funeral Service* (**Shraddha**): The relatives of the deceased observe "*sutak*," for 10 days. During this time, the bereaved family sings devotional songs, reads scriptures, does not receive or give any gifts, does not perform any rituals and eats simple food. Male members do not shave, or cut their hair. After the 10 days, a ceremony, called *shraddha* is performed by the family with the aid of a priest to help the departed soul rest in peace.

Principles for Clinical Care
Dietary Issues

• Fasting is common for people who offer *pujas* (worship services) to Hindu deities, as well as for the priests who conduct these services. After the services, the devotees break their fasting by eating *prasad* which is the food offered to the deities during the services. The family of a sick person in a hospital ward may wish to bring *prasad* from home or from the Hindu temple and share with the patient. Some Hindus fast on certain days during lunar cycles. However, fasting is not obligatory for a sick person. For some fasting persons, eating fruits, raw vegetables, like salad, tea, milk is permitted for health reasons.

- Most Hindus do not eat beef. Many are strictly vegetarian. Dietary preferences for vegetarians are rice, wheat products such as pita bread, falafal, vegetables, curries, fruits, yogurt, and so forth. Some vegetarian Hindus may eat eggs. Those who are nonvegetarians may prefer chicken, turkey or fish, but no beef.
- At different stages in one's life and in different emphases in one's life, one can follow dietary practices that are suitable. For example, a nonvegetarian may turn vegetarian after initiation by a guru (spiritual teacher). At older age for health reasons, a nonvegetarian may eat fish and white meat, but no red meat. Dietary preferences of a patient should always be checked with the patient or family members before serving any meal.

General Medical Beliefs

- *Ayurveda*: *Ayurveda*, which means "Life Science," is the Vedic system of health care developed many thousands of years ago. It is still practiced in India and is gradually expanding into other countries, including the United States. This ancient life science takes into consideration the patient's entire nature – physical, mental, and spiritual.
- *Ashtanga Yoga*: *Ashtanga Yoga* literally means "eight-limbed Yoga." This system of

Yoga was outlined by Sage *Patanjali* in the *Yoga Sutras*. In *Ashtanga Yoga*, the eight practices are specified for the purification of body, mind, and soul. These are *Yama* (Moral codes), *Niyama* (Self-purification and study), *Asana* (Posture), *Pranayama* (Breath control), *Pratyahara* (Sense control), *Dharana* (Concentration), *Dhyana* (Meditation) and *Samadhi* (Absorption). A practitioner of *Ashtanga Yoga* obtains a healthy, strong and flexible body, improved blood circulation, relief of joint pain, control of the mind, and ability to concentrate on thoughts of the holy.

- Assisted suicide and euthanasia: Hindu ethics generally are against assisted suicide or involuntary euthanasia. Suicide for selfish reason is a great sin. However, a distinction is made between suicide and voluntarily ending one's life by fasting. For example, it is not considered a suicide if a terminally ill patient wants to end his or her life by fasting.

Specific Medical Issues

- **Abortion**: Abortion except for medical reasons, such as when the mother's life is at risk, is discouraged. Hindus believe that life is sacred.
- **Advance Directives**: An advance directive should be prepared for each member of the family and kept in family's secured possession. This document will be very helpful for the caregivers as well as for the family to make decisions for the patient in a critical situation.
- **Birth Control**: Hindus have no religious objection to the practice of birth control.
- **Blood Transfusions**: There is no religious objection to such procedures.
- **Circumcision**: Circumcision is not practiced as a part of the faith. It can be done only at the parents' request.

- **In Vitro Fertilization**: When the normal method of conception has failed, in vitro fertilization or artificial insemination is generally acceptable to a couple if the egg and sperm belong to the wife and the husband.
- **Stem Cell Research**: Hindus generally have no problem in applying genetic engineering to cure a disease. Stem cell research for therapeutic purposes is acceptable, provided a growing fetus is not killed to harvest stem cells. Killing a fetus is a great sin.
- **Vaccinations**: Hindus generally have no problem with vaccinations when taken on doctor's advice to prevent a disease.
- **Withholding/Withdrawing Life Support**: Generally speaking, keeping a patient on artificial life support for a prolonged period in a vegetative state is not encouraged. Always check with the nearest family member before removing any life support system.

Gender and Personal Issues

- Hindu women patients may prefer to be medically examined by a female doctor. If that is not possible, the presence of a female nurse is required. It is appropriate to provide a long hospital gown to a female patient, especially during examinations.
- Hindus (male or female) would prefer to wear garments under the hospital gowns.
- Special under clothing during the procedures like cardiac catheterization would be appreciated by Hindus. Such under clothing would cover the genitals and still allow access to the groin while preserving the modesty.
- Hindu patients may wish to wash their body with water after using the toilet facilities. Though the use of toilet paper for cleaning is becoming a common practice, making water easily accessible near the toilet will be appreciated.

Principles for Spiritual Care through the Cycles of Life
Concept of Spiritual Support for the Living and the Dying

- The physical body is a material product, subject to birth, growth, and decay. The embodied soul, the source of consciousness, the luminous self, the divinity within the person is eternal. It activates the physical body through the medium of the subtle body. At death, the embodied soul leaves only the physical body, but departs with the subtle body with all its components and the impressions of the person's karma.
- The dying person's accumulated karma determines what will happen after death. The impressions of the person's karma, comprising his or her merits and demerits, his or her good and evil deeds, his or her tendencies and capacities go with the individual soul. These impressions are contained in the subtle body.
- Just as a person's inner attitude and thoughts determine his or her life's course before his or her death, so do they after his or her death. The person's immediate course depends on what thought prevails in his or her mind at the time of death.
- The Hindu scripture, Bhagavad Gita, says, "Thinking of whatever object at the time of death a person leaves the body, that very object the person attains." So, the goal of the spiritual caregivers, who may be family, friends, temple priest, hospital chaplain or nursing staff, is to raise the spiritual consciousness of the dying

patient through various means that are described in the "During End of Life" section.

- The cycle of birth, death, and rebirth continues until the individual soul is liberated and unites with God in eternal bliss. So, death is not the end of everything and should not be feared. Each subsequent birth provides an opportunity to advance spiritually until the final liberation takes place.

- A good death is when a person dies at old age, peacefully and voluntarily, after doing all his or her life's duties, without any desire or attachment to material possession, and with the name of God on his or her lips.

During Birth

- Women generally prefer female physicians and nurses to deliver babies.

- As stated earlier, circumcision is not practiced as a part of the faith. It can be done only at the parents' request.

- Traditionally, the mother is required to take rest for 40 days after childbirth. During this time, mother and child are not separated, except for medical reasons. If hospital procedures require moving the baby into a nursery, that should not be a problem to modern Hindu families.

- In the home birth, traditionally the delivery of the baby is done by a midwife. The husband is not allowed to stay in the delivery room. But in a hospital delivery room, that prohibition is lifted.

- Hindu tradition for naming a child varies greatly. In some traditions, the naming ceremony is performed on the twelfth day after the child is born. A mixture of honey and clarified butter is put on the baby's tongue. Then, the naming ceremony follows. In other traditions, the naming

ceremony is performed 3 months after the child is born. In still other traditions, it can be done any time before the first birthday anniversary. In a hospital, the naming of the child can be done in the hospital as soon as possible for the purpose of medical records and birth certificates.

During Illness

- It is a common practice that the friends and relatives of the sick person visit in groups.

- Visitors often bring flowers as a token of their "get well" wishes.

- The family or friends may wish to provide *prasad* (food blessed from religious service) for the patient to eat. The family or friends may call the local Hindu temple, and arrange to bring *prasad* from Hindu temple or from home. Check with nurse for dietary restrictions.

- The family or friends may wish to play devotional music, spiritual discourses or lectures on the spiritual life for spiritual comfort of the patient. If there is another patient in the room, the nurse's permission is required.

- As a general rule, the nearest family member is the primary spokesperson. All questions or other dialogue should be directed to him or her.

- It is important to create a spiritual atmosphere in the patient's room by placing holy pictures and flowers. It creates joy to the patient's mind and that helps facilitate a quicker recovery.

During End of Life

- The practices described under "During Illness" are also applicable here. The following are the additional practices for a dying patient.

- It is important to fulfill small wishes the

dying patient may have for a particular food.

- The family may wish to put holy water (water from the sacred river, Ganges, or any other sacred river) into the mouth of the patient. Consult chaplain for assistance to contact the local Hindu temple or other sources.

- The family may wish to place a picture of a Personal Deity or Spiritual Guru in the hospital room near the patient's bed.

- When death is imminent, the family may wish to have the Hindu temple priest come to the hospital to provide spiritual support to the dying patient. If the temple priest is not available, the family may call any person who has some knowledge of spiritual care giving to a Hindu patient. The priest or the spiritual caregiver can perform any or all of the following practices:
  - chant mantras from scriptures
  - sing devotional songs
  - touch head or arms as a gesture of affection and pray silently
  - encourage patient to think of his or her favorite image of God.

- Some typical spiritual support practices are listed here (these may vary from one tradition to another):
  - tying a thread blessed in a religious service around neck/wrist of the dying patient
  - sprinkling of holy water
  - placing a basil leaf on the tongue (basil leaf, called *tulsi*, is considered sacred)
  - having the dying patient touch money that will be given to a charity
  - lighting incense to create holy atmosphere, if the nurse permits
  - repeating mantram in the ears of the patient

  - reminding the dying person that *Atman*, the real Self, is immortal.

- Some patients may prefer to die at home. The hospital should give reasonable consideration if such a request comes from the family.

- At the time of death, always expect the nearest family members, especially women, to weep loudly as an expression of grief.

Care of the Body

- The deceased's body may be washed and dressed by the family (especially in the case of a female) or by the hospital at the request of the family. The family should use disposable gloves provided by the hospital to remove jewelry and so forth worn by the patient. (Note: Do not remove sacred thread or other religious objects from the body.)

- The body should be covered with a white sheet. Head may be kept uncovered, eyes closed and limbs straightened at the request of the family.

- Autopsies are allowed, if required by law.

- Cremation is the preferred method of the disposition of the body. Infants, up to 27 months, and stillborn and miscarriage babies are not cremated but, rather, should be buried. No services are required in such cases. In all other cases the body should be cremated within 24 hours. However, this is always not possible for various reasons (scheduling a funeral service may take time; the priest may not be available on a short notice; some waiting time may be required for close relatives to arrive before funeral service). If organ donation is permitted, allow additional time. The body may be kept in cold storage for preservation. Embalming the body is discouraged unless required by law.

- Appropriate ways to support the bereaved:
  - Visit the grief-stricken family and offer any kind of help to the family, such as, bringing cooked food, buying products to meet current needs, and so forth.
  - Hug the bereaved family members. (Note: Hindu tradition generally does not allow hugging between opposite genders.)
- The family should call or visit the local Hindu temple for the advice of funeral home selection as well as to schedule funeral services (*Antyesthi*) by the Hindu temple priest. The scripture, *Garuda Purana*, describes in detail various observances and procedures to be followed before cremation. The family should seek advice from the Hindu temple priest who advises the family of all requirements for the service. (Note: Requirements may be found on a temple website.)
- Where possible, clay pots with sesame seeds, milk, *ghee* (clarified butter), and so forth, are to be ceremonially given away. Such proper observance of the procedures, before and after cremation, means the soul of the deceased reaches satisfaction and peace.
- Normally, the Hindu temple priest goes to the designated funeral home and performs funeral services. Alternatively, with a hospital's permission, funeral services can be performed in the hospital chapel, and the body may be sent directly for cremation after the service. See chaplain for assistance to coordinate things with the temple priest.
- Families wishing to collect ashes in urns to preserve and/or to place or immerse in a holy river at a later date should give this requirement to the funeral home before cremation.

- Donation of the body for medical research is an individual decision. Planning in advance for such donation is required.

Organ and Tissue Donation

- Organ and tissue donation is an individual decision. Some Hindus consider it good karma to donate body parts to others as gifts of life. It may be preferable for a chaplain and/or nurse who are trained designated requesters to be consulted for assistance.
- The intending donor should make his or her wishes known beforehand through a health care directive or driver's license.
- Organ transplantation: Hindu views vary on this subject. Some think that it is an artificial way to keep a person alive. To some, organ transplantation is acceptable if the prospect for a quality life after transplant is good. To many, heart transplantation is not favored because the heart is understood as the "seat of the soul." It is important to discuss organ transplantation with the patient's family before performing the procedure. Hindus dislike unethical trade in human organs.

Scriptures, Inspirational Readings, and Prayers
CHANTING, READING, AND SINGING FOR THE DYING PATIENT

Maha Mrityunjaya Mantra
om trayambakam yajaamahe
   sugandhim pustivardhanam urvaaru
   kamiva bandhanaat mrutyor
   muksheeya maamritaat
"We worship the three eyed One (Lord Shiva), who is fragrant, and who nourishes well all beings. As the cucumber is severed from its bondage (to the creeper), may He

liberate us from death for the sake of immortality."

—Yajur Veda 3:60

Bhagavad Gita

In the Bhagavad Gita, Lord Krishna mentioned the immortality of the Soul from verses 11 to 30, chapter 2.[325]

"Even as the embodied Self (soul) passes, in this body, through the stages of childhood, youth and old age, so does It passes into another body.
Calm souls are not bewildered by this."

—2:13

"It is never born, nor does It ever die. Nor having once been, does It again cease to be. Unborn, eternal, permanent, and primordial, It is not slain when the body is slain"

—2:20

"Just as a person casts off worn-out clothes and puts on others that are new, so the embodied Self casts off worn-out bodies and enters into others that are new."

—2:22

"This Self is said to be unmanifest, incomprehensible, and unchangeable. Therefore, knowing it to be so, you should not grieve."

—2:25

Katha Upanishad

For the consolation of the dying, it is good to read the Katha Upanishad where *Yama*, the God of Death, unveiled the mystery of death to *Naciketa*.[326]

"When all desires that dwell in the heart fall away, then the mortal becomes immortal and here attains Brahman (God). When all the knots of the heart (to the material desire) are destroyed, even while a man is alive, then a mortal becomes immortal. This much alone is the teaching (of all Upanishads)."

—II:iii:14–15

"The Purusha, the indwelling Self, not larger than a thumb always dwells in the hearts of men. Let a man unerringly separate Him from his body like a stalk from a blade of grass. Let him know that Self is pure and immortal; yes, let him know that Self is pure and immortal. Naciketa, having gained this knowledge imparted by the God of Death, as also the process of yoga in its totality, became free and attained Brahman.

325 Nikhilananda, S. (1992). *The Bhagavad Gita*. New York, NY: Ramkrishna-Vivekananda Center. Chapters and verses are cited with each selection in the text.

326 Easwaran, E. (1987). *The Upanishads*. Tomales, CA: Nilgiri Press. Chapters and verses are cited with each selection in the text. This includes the *Katha*, *Brihadaranyaka* and *Chhandogya Upanishads*.

Any one, who becomes a knower (like Naciketa) of the indwelling Self, attains Brahman."

—II:iii:16–17

Brihadaranyaka Upanishad

"Lead me from the unreal to the real. Lead me from darkness to light. Lead me from death to immortality."

—I:iii:28

"You can not see the Seer of seeing; you can not hear the Hearer of hearing; you can not think the Thinker of thinking; you can not know the Knower of knowing. This is your Self that is within all; everything else but This is perishable."

—III:v:1

Chhandogya Upanishad

"This (the physical body) is being left by the living Self. But the living Self dies not."

—VI:xi:3

"A knower of Self goes beyond grief."

—VII:i:3

DEVOTIONAL SONGS[327]
This hymn repeats the name of Lord Hari, Lord Rama, and Lord Krishna in great devotion:

Maha Mantra
Hare Ram, Hare Ram, Ram Ram Hare Hare
Hare Krishna, Hare Krishna, Krishna Krishna Hare Hare.

This song is to be chanted repeatedly:

I Bow to Lord Shiva
Om, namah Shivaya, Om, namah Shivaya,
Om, namah Shivaya, Om, namah Shivaya.

This song is to be chanted repeatedly:

Victory to Rama
Shri Ram, jay Ram, jay jay Ram Shri Ram, jay Ram, jay jay Ram.

This is Mahatma Gandhi's favorite prayer song:

Ram Dhun
Raghupati Raghav Raja Ram,
Patita Pavana Sita Ram.

(Chant the name of Rama – "Lord of Raghu clan,
Raghav, King Rama,
Savior of the fallen and the depraved")

---

327 These songs have been handed down through the centuries by oral tradition; as such, there is no actual bibliographic information.

Special Days: Hinduism

January 14 *Makara Sankranti* – *Makara* literally means "Capricorn" and *Sankranti* is the day when the sun passes from one sign of the zodiac to the next. The *Sankranti* of any month is considered auspicious as it signifies a fresh start. However, *Makara Sankranti* is celebrated in the month of Magha when the sun passes through the winter solstice, from the Tropic of Cancer to the Tropic of Capricorn; the day on which the sun begins to move northward is called *Makara Shankranti*. (In the south of India, this same event is the *Pongal* festival. It is closely connected with agriculture, and the first harvest is symbolically offered to God.)

(Note: Makara Sankranti always occurs on January 14; it is the only Hindu event based on a solar calendar. All other festival dates vary from year to year based on the lunar calendar. The months in which the day of the other festivals fall are in parentheses.)

Vasanta Panchami *(January–February)* This is the festival that marks the first day of spring which all Hindus observe; the day is also known as *Magh Sukla Panchami* as it falls on the fifth day after the new moon in the month of *Magh* (January–February). Saraswathi, the Goddess of education, music, art, and speech, is worshipped on this day commemorating Brahma's creation of Saraswati to dislodge the plainness of the creation. She is the symbol of purity and wisdom.

Maha Shivaratri *(February–March)* This is a festival of worshipping Lord Shiva, one the great gods of the Hindu Trinity. This event is celebrated with great devotion by Hindus all over the world. The festival continues through the night when devotees make offerings of food, flowers, and incense to the Lord.

Holi *(February–March)* *Holi* is the time when people from all castes and social strata come together forgetting all past differences and grievances. The festival is a favorite with most Indians for being the most colorful and joyous of all. *Holi* bears close resemblance to the important ancient festival called *Vasantotsava*. *Holi* is not celebrated in the south of India, but a similar festival in the honor of the god of love, Kama, takes place there at the same time. While there does not seem to be a direct link between the two rituals, both occasions are examples of an age-old tradition of celebrating the arrival of spring. Young men throw colored powder and colored water on women, using hand pumps. The origin of this custom can be found in the pranks of Krishna, who used to drench milkmaids in the village with water and play various other tricks on them. The singing of lewd songs, shouting, and dancing also marks *Holi* celebrations. The main ritual on this day centers around a bonfire ceremoniously kindled at the time of the rising moon. According to mythology, the *Holi* fire is regarded as a funeral pyre, for it is understood to have destroyed Holika, a demoness.

Rama Navami *(March–April)* This event celebrates the birthday of Lord Rama, the incarnation of Lord Vishnu, which falls on the ninth day after the new moon of the month *Chaitra* (March–April). Rama was the son of King Dasaratha of Ayodhya, but He is also the divine omnipresent, omnipotent and omniscient God.

Hanuman Jayanti *(March–April)* Hanuman Jayanthi is celebrated to commemorate the birth of Hanuman, the son of Vayu (God of winds) and Anjana. Hanuman was an ardent devotee of Rama and is worshipped for his unflinching devotion to the god. On this holy day, people worship Sri Hanuman and read the *Hanuman Chalisa*. He is worshipped in folk tradition as a deity with magical powers and the ability to conquer evil spirits.

Gurupurnima *(July–August)* The day of the full moon in the month of *Ashad* (July–August) is an extremely auspicious and holy day of Guru Purnima. On this day, sacred to the memory of the great sage, Bhagavan Sri Vyasa, gurus or teachers are worshipped. The best form of worship of the Guru is to follow his teachings, to shine as the very embodiment of his teachings and to propagate his glory and his message.

Raksha Bandhan *(August)* Raksha Bandhan, called *Avani Avittam* in the south of India, falls on the day of the full moon of the month of *Sravan* (August-September). It is an important festival during which Hindus wear a new holy thread and offer libations of water to the ancient Rishis on this day. This festival is also known as *Upakarmam*, and is especially sacred to the *Brahmins*, who have been invested with the sacred thread. It is also a celebration of emotional bonding with brothers and sisters. This part of the celebration takes place by tying a holy thread around the wrist, which signifies a bond of protection.

Krishna Janmashtami *(August–September)* This day, one of the greatest of all Hindu festivals, is the birthday of Lord Krishna, the Divine incarnation of Lord Vishnu. A fast observed on this day (eighth day after the full moon) and broken at midnight is indicative of the time of Lord Krishna's birth - midnight.

Ganesh Chaturthi *(August–September)* Ganesh Chaturthi, the birthday of Lord Ganesha, is one of the most popular of Hindu festivals. Lord Ganesha, the elephant-headed God, is the Lord of power and wisdom. His names are repeated first before any auspicious work is begun, before any kind of worship is begun. The celebration of his birth is observed throughout India, as well as by devoted Hindus in all parts of the world. Clay figures of the Deity are made and after being worshipped for 2 days, or in some cases 10 days, they are immersed in water.

Navaratri, Dussehra (September–October) *Durga Puja* or *Navaratri* is held in commemoration of the victory of Durga over Mahishasura, the buffalo-headed demon. Hinduism is one of the few religions that emphasize the motherhood of the deity. One's relationship with one's mother is the dearest and the sweetest of all human relations. Hence, it is proper to look upon God as mother. Durga represents the Divine Mother. She is the energy aspect of the Lord. Without Durga, Shiva has no expression and without Shiva, Durga has no existence. The Durga Puja is celebrated in various parts of India in different styles. One basic aim of this celebration is to propitiate Shakti, the Goddess in Her aspect as Power, to bestow upon man all wealth, auspiciousness, prosperity, knowledge (both sacred and secular), and all other potent powers. The festivities culminate on the tenth day, called variously Vijayadashmi or Dussehra. In the eastern part of India, this period is celebrated as Durga Puja. In the western part of the country, this is the time for the joyous Garba and Dandia dances and people pour out at night to participate in this community festival. In the southern part of India, the first 3 days of the festival are dedicated to Lakshmi, the next 3 days to Durga, and the last 3 days to Sarasvati.

Diwali (October–November) *Deepavali* or *Diwali*, which means a row of lights, is the most important festival in India. Originally celebrated by Hindus, it has now crossed the boundaries of religion and is celebrated by all in India with fervor and gaiety. This day is a public holiday all over India. The celebrations include the lighting of lamps and candles, and the bursting of firecrackers. Friends and neighbors exchange special sweets. People buy new clothes. For some it is a 3-day festival. There are various alleged origins attributed to this festival. Some hold that it celebrates the marriage of Lakshmi with Lord Vishnu. In some traditions, the festival is dedicated to the worship of Kali. It also commemorates the day on which Lord Rama returned to Ayodhya after defeating Ravana. On this day also Sri Krishna killed the demon Narakasura. Diwali in India is equivalent to Christmas among

Christians. The dazzle of the occasion ushers in an all pervading and overpowering spirit of happiness and laughter and an inescapable feeling of joy.

The Gita Jayanti   *(December–January)* The birthday of the Bhagavad Gita (popularly referred to as Gita), is celebrated throughout India by all the admirers and lovers of this most sacred scripture. On this day nearly 6000 years ago, Sanjaya narrated to King Dhritarashtra the dialogue between Sri Krishna and Arjuna on the battlefield of Kurukshetra, and thus made the glorious teachings of the Lord available to us, and to people of the world. The teachings of the Gita are broad, sublime, and universal. They do not belong to any particular cult, sect, creed, age, place, or country. The Gita has a message for the solace, peace, freedom, salvation, and perfection of all human beings.

Glossary of Hindu Terms

Advaita: Monistic system of philosophy composed by Sankara in the *Darsana* Period (750–1000 CE). His commentaries on the Upanishads, Gita, and *Brahma Sutras* formed the basis of the Monistic theory. This concept of "*Advaita*" (oneness) conveys the idea that *Atman* and *Brahman* comprise a single entity of absolute reality. The apparent world is in the shadow of illusion (*Maya*) because it disappears in the light of knowledge of Brahman.

Antyesthi: The last rite (i.e., funeral service) for sanctifying the body in this material world before cremation.

Aranyakas: Term literally meaning "forest treatises" and contained in the "Work Part" of the *Vedas*. During Vedic time these treatises, because of their philosophical contents, were studied in quiet wooded areas, away from the hustles and bustles of populated areas. Because of their content, they have been associated with mystical, ascetic groups as to their origin and composition.

Arya Samaj: Reform sect of modern Hinduism (1800 CE–Present), established by *Swami Dayananda*, who tried to unify all sections of Hindu society; movement rejects use of images and traditional rituals in worship and instead focuses on social justice.

ashrama: View of one's life span composed of four distinct stages which are: (1) a student's life pursuing studies to prepare for the future; (2) a life of a householder; (3) a life of retirement for spiritual pursuits; and (4) a life of renunciation. All these stages are guided by specific duties, known as *dharma*, to provide a moral organization to one's life.

Atman: Term used as way to describe one's true self; often translated into English as "self" or "soul."

Ayurveda: Vedic system of health care, which means "Life Science," developed many thousands of years ago; still practiced in India and gradually expanding into other countries, including the United States. This ancient life science takes into consideration the patient's entire nature – physical, mental and spiritual.

Bhagavad Gita: One of secondary, and most popular, scriptures that were composed subsequent to *Vedas* to analyze, explain and illustrate the spiritual truths contained in Vedas. The Bhagavad Gita (The Song of the Lord) explains the practical applications of the teachings of Upanishads in day-to-day life. In this text, Lord Krishna instructs Arjuna about progression on the spiritual path.

bhajan: Devotional song of praise or chant as an expression of worshipping God.

Bhakti Yoga: "Way to God through love and devotion." It is the most common of the four pathways and centers upon loving God wholeheartedly.

Brahman: Impersonal, Transcendental God who is the ultimate and absolute reality. The scriptures variously describe *Brahman* as Infinite Existence, Infinite Consciousness, Infinite Bliss and Supreme Self.

Brahmanas: codes of conduct, sacrificial rites and specific duties in daily life included in the "Work Parts" of the Vedas.

dharma: Right way of living, proper conduct, duty or righteousness.

Diwali: Event, called "Festival of Lights," celebrated by Hindus, Jains, and Sikhs.

Dvaita: Dualist school of Hindu philosophy of Madhva (twelfth-century philosopher); concept of "twoness" teaches that all things are different from another, which includes the distinction between God and individual soul. Individual souls are distinct from one another. Matter is distinct from God and from the individual soul. God is the ruler of the universe. The universe is real, because it is perceived as real.

Garuda Purana: Scripture, which, in part, describes various observances and procedures to be followed before cremation.

ghee: Clarified butter, offered in many Hindu rituals.

guru: Term used in Hinduism to refer to religious or spiritual teacher. In Sikhism, the term is used to refer to the early inspired leaders of the faith; it also is contained in the title of the Sikh Holy Scriptures.

Jnana Yoga: "Way to God through knowledge or intuitive discernment." This discernment is the growing awareness that one's essential being is the Ultimate. *Jnana Yoga* is said to be the shortest path to divine awareness, but also the steepest, for it requires total control of and stilling of the mind and is for very reflective individuals.

Kalpa Sutras: Manuals of ritualism containing the description of various religious rites and oblations performed in the sacrificial fire; they also include detailed descriptions of the duties of the king and the duties of the people belonging to all four castes.

Karma Yoga: "Way to God through selfless work or through sacred duty." Actions are taken with thoughtfulness and without attachment. Loving, unselfish service diminishes the disconnected-ness with the divine until the barriers between the Ultimate and one's personal ego disappear altogether.

Moksha/Mukti: liberation from the cycle of birth, death, and rebirth and all of the suffering and limitation of worldly existence.

namaste: Traditional Hindu greeting folding the hands, joining the two palms and bowing the head to the person who is being greeted. This is the same method a Hindu employs when offering prayers to God. The reason for this custom is that when a Hindu greets another person, he or she greets not just the body of the person, but the person's inner soul, which is divine.

prasad: Food or other objects that have been offered to deities during worship services and blessed by the services.

Puja: An offering of worship in a show of respect for or paying homage to a deity or some revered personage.

Puranas: Composition of literature full of stories and legends during the Epic Period

(400 BCE–750 CE); these scriptures became the instruments of education bringing Hindu ideals and Hindu codes of ethics to the masses.

Raja Yoga: "Way to God through spiritual discipline of meditation." Through physical and psychic exercises, the adherent becomes skilled at shutting out the phenomenal universe and becoming alone with a stilled mind. When this is attained, it is called *samadhi*, utter oneness with the Ultimate and dissolution of the personal self.

Ramakrishna Order: *Ramakrishna* was able to infuse into his followers a true spirit of Hinduism, the harmony of religions and a sense of service to humanity. His followers, led by *Swami Vivekananda* founded the *Ramakrishna* Order and spread the messages of Vedanta throughout the world. He represented Hinduism at the Parliament of Religions in Chicago in 1893.

Samhitas: Collection of hymns composed, praising one or the other personal deity and included in the "Work Parts" of the Vedas.

Tirthankara: Term for "Messenger of God" in Jainism; 24 *Tirthankaras* have appeared throughout history, *Rsabha* being the first, *Mahavira* the most recent. These inspired teachers, who were capable of breaking out of the cycle of birth, death, and rebirth, made their appearances to instruct humanity how to do the same.

tulsi: Basil leaf, considered sacred.

Upanishads: The "Knowledge Parts" of Vedas. These philosophical treatises explain that in this ever-changing world of cause and effect, *Brahman* (Impersonal, Transcendental God) is the ultimate and absolute reality. They also discuss the concepts of karma, *samsara* and reincarnation. They also explain the identity of *Brahman* with *atman*, the in-dwelling self (soul) of all beings.

Vaisnavism: Also known as Devotional (*Bhakti*) movement, is a movement of the Medieval Period (1000–1800 CE) in Hinduism; this movement, which first started in the southern part of India and later spread to the northern part, laid stress on the ideals of all-consuming love for God: a wholehearted lover of God can realize mystic union with Him.

Vedanta: Term that literally means "end of the Vedas"; system of philosophy based on the Upanishads, systematized in *Brahma Sutras* and explained in practical terms in the Bhagavad Gita. Vedanta is the "culmination of the Vedas" (knowledge).

Vedas: The principal and the most authoritative scriptures of Hinduism; often referred to by the term *Shruti* (As Revealed). The composers of the Vedas were the sages of ancient India. These sages, in their meditation, attained transcendental consciousness and realized the eternal and the universal truths. These were later compiled in books, called Vedas. There are four Vedas – *Rig, Sama, Yajur*, and *Atharva*. Later sections of Vedas are called Upanishads.

Vedic: Period dating from approximately 5000 to 600 BCE during which the Vedas and principal Upanishads were written; term used to designate the seers, sages, or scriptures of that period.

Vishishtha Advaita: Qualified monistic system of Ramanuja (eleventh-century philosopher) viewed as a philosophy of love and devotion which taught *Bhakti Yoga* as the correct way to attain Truth. In this philosophy, the relationship between Brahman, individual soul, and the universe is considered like this: the universe is the body of God, Brahman is the Supreme Soul of that body, and the individual souls are the innumerable cells of that body.

yoga: Common meanings include "joining" or "uniting," and related ideas such as "union" and "conjunction"; in the religious sense, yoga is associated with various practices for the purpose of "uniting with God."

Islam

In the Name of God, Most Gracious, Most Merciful[328]

Prepared by:
A. Rauf Mir, MD[329]
Past President, Islamic Medical Association of North America
Leawood, KS;
Mahnaz Shabbir
President, Shabbir Advisors
Overland Park, KS

Reviewed and approved by:
Imam Hassan Qazwini
Religious Leader, Islamic Center of America
Chicago, IL

History and Facts

The Arabic word "Islam" simply means submission to the will of God. It also conveys the means to achieve peace – peace with God, peace with oneself, and peace with the creations of God – through wholly giving oneself to God and accepting His guidance. People who practice the religion of Islam are called Muslims. The Arabic word "Muslim" is a person who submits to the will of God.

Islam is a qualitative term – the quality of accepting God's supreme authority above one's own. As such, being a Muslim does not mean having to give up one's culture or traditions; rather it means adopting the simple and logical principles of Islam to better one's life and attain peace.

Islam is not a new faith. The name of the religion was revealed to Prophet Muhammad (Peace be upon Him)[330] via the Archangel Gabriel from God in 610 CE. "He (God) has sent down to you the Book (the Qur'an) with truth, confirming what was revealed before; And He sent down the Torah (of Moses) and the Gospel (of Jesus) before this as a guide to humankind; and He sent down the Criterion (the Qur'an)" (Qur'an 3:3–4).

During his lifetime, the Prophet Muhammad worked very hard in bringing the people together in what is called the **ummah** (the Muslim community). During the Prophet's lifetime, there were no variations from what he taught. Following his death, a difference in opinion on who should lead the Islamic faith resulted in

---

328 Quote provided by A. Rauf Mir, MD, and Mahnaz Shabbir, authors of this chapter.

329 The authors of this chapter represent the Sunni (Mir) and Shia (Shabbir) sects of Islam.

330 Muslims will include a salutation "may peace be upon him" every time any Prophet's name is mentioned. Shia Muslims will also mention this phrase after any member of the Prophet's family. To avoid interrupting the flow of ideas, this phrase has not been included after each reference. It is requested that Muslim readers include the salutation after each Prophet's name.

two major sects, Sunni and Shia. These were later divided into five different schools of thought based on interpretation of religious laws. However, these five schools can be generally categorized by Sunni and Shia (sometimes referred to as Shiite) Muslims. Sunni Muslims have the largest number of Muslims who believe that they follow the example of Prophet Muhammad and his companions. Shia Muslims believe that, prior to his death, Prophet Muhammad had declared his son-in-law Ali as his successor and the descendants of Ali and Fatima, Prophet Muhammad's daughter, the rightful leaders of Islam. The four Sunni schools of thought are Hanafi (approximately 31%), Maliki (25%), Shaf'i (16%), and Hanbali (4%). The Hanafi came to predominate in the Arab world and South Asia; the Maliki in North, Central, and West Africa; the Shaf'i in East Africa and Southeast Asia; and the Hanbali in Saudi Arabia.

Most Shias (approximately 24% of the 1.2 billion) are from the Ja'fari School, also known as "Twelvers" (i.e., they recognize the 12 Imams who are the descendants of Prophet Muhammad. The first Imam was Ali, Prophet Muhammad's son-in-law. The last, twelfth, Imam is Mehdi who is in Occultation or hidden and will reappear before the end of the World). There are also Ismaili Shias (also known as "Seveners" that recognize seven Imams) and Zaidi Shias (also known as "Fivers" that recognize five Imams).

Although these schools of thought are different in some ways, they recognize each other as Muslims and agree on the fundamental Islamic beliefs. One becomes a Muslim by believing and proclaiming the testimony of the faith (Shahadah, see definition in Basic Teachings section). By this declaration, the believer announces his or her faith in all of God's messengers, and in the scriptures revealed to them.

Muslims believe that their faith is the same truth that God revealed through all His prophets to every people. Biblical prophets mentioned in the Qur'an include: Adam, Enoch, Noah, Abraham, Lot, Ishmael, Isaac, Job, Ezekiel, Jacob, Joseph, Jonah (Yunus), Jethro (Shoaib), Moses, Aaron, Elijah (Ilyas), Elisha (Alyasa), David, Solomon, Zechariah, John the Baptist, and Jesus; peace be upon them all. In addition, the Qur'an devotes an entire chapter to Mary, the mother of Jesus. Many books· were revealed to the Prophets over time. Four books that are important to Muslims are: (1) Tawrah (Torah) was revealed to Prophet Musa (Moses); (2) Zabur (Psalms of David) was revealed to Prophet Dawood (David); (3) Injeel (Gospel) was revealed to Prophet Isa (Jesus); and (4) the final book (Qur'an) revealed to Muhammad through the Archangel Gabriel, confirmed and finalized all previous revelations that were sent to humankind through God's previous messengers.

The Qur'an was revealed over a period of 23 years and was memorized by Prophet Muhammad and his followers and written down by scribes, during the Prophet's lifetime. Not one word of its 114 *surahs* (chapters) has been changed over the centuries. The Qur'an is in every detail the same unique and miraculous text that was revealed to Muhammad (peace be upon him) over 14 centuries ago. The Qur'an is the principle source of every Muslim's faith and practice. It deals with all subjects that concern human beings, including wisdom, doctrine, worship, and law; but its basic theme is the relationship between God and His creatures. At the same time, the Qur'an provides guidelines for a just society, proper human conduct and equitable economic principles.

Muslims believe in the One, Unique, Incomparable, Merciful God – the Sole Creator, Sustainer and Cherisher of the Universe – and in the Angels created by Him. Muslims also believe in: the prophets through whom His revelations were brought to humankind; the Day of Judgment and in individual accountability for actions; and in God's complete authority over destiny (be it good or bad) and in life after death.

Today, there are approximately 1.2 billion Muslims living all over the world. The largest concentration of Muslims lives in Indonesia, followed by Pakistan and India. The Arab population is approximately 20% of the 1.2 billion. Significant Muslim minorities are found in China, India, Russia, Europe, North America, and South America. There are over 7 million Muslims in the United States. Of that number, approximately 38% are African American. American Muslims, who live in the United States, represent every race, ethnicity, and culture. They come from all social demographics. The first Muslims in America were West Africans who were captured and brought to the United States as slaves.

For a faith tradition that encompasses a fifth of the world's population, Islam is not just a personal religion, but also a complete way of life. Muslims come from all races, nationalities, and cultures across the globe. They have varied languages, foods, dress, and customs; even the way they practice some aspects of Islam may differ. Yet, they all consider themselves Muslims.

Basic Teachings

The Qur'an is the prime source of every Muslim's faith and practice. It provides guidelines for a just society, proper human conduct and an equitable economic system. In addition, Muslims use the *sunnah* (Prophet Muhammad's example as recorded in the *hadith*), the practice and example of the Prophet, as another authority for Muslims. A *hadith* is a reliable transmitted report of what the Prophet said, did or approved. The source of various *hadiths* will vary among the Islamic schools of thought.

From a Sunni perspective, the "five pillars" of Islam are:

1. **Shahadah** (declaration of faith): The basic testimony of faith is the first and foremost of Islam.

   "There is no deity except God; Muhammad (peace be upon him) is the messenger of God."

   This simple declaration of faith is required of all those who accept Islam as their chosen way of life. The words have to be uttered with sincere conviction and under no coercion. The significance of this testimony is the belief that the only purpose of life is to serve and obey God; and this is achieved through following the example of Prophet Muhammad. Muslims believe that, throughout history, God sent His chosen messengers to guide humankind. The testimony that these prophets taught was similar. The first commandment found in the Hebrew Bible is "I am the Lord, thy God; thou shalt not have other gods before Me" (Exod. 20: 2–3). This belief in the Oneness of God is central to Islam and permeates all of Muslim life.

2. **Salat** (prayers): The five obligatory prayers contain verses from the Qur'an and recited in Arabic. A key element

of Muslim life is the obligatory, ritual prayer. These prayers are a direct link between the worshipper and God. This very personal relationship with the Creator allows one to fully depend, trust, and love God, and to truly achieve inner peace and harmony, regardless of the trials one faces. Prophet Muhammad said: "Indeed, when one of you prays, he speaks privately with his Lord" (Book of Hadith). Prayers are performed before dawn, and sunrise, early afternoon, late afternoon, after sunset, and nightfall to remind one of God throughout the day. The morning prayer is the shortest, while the two afternoon and nightfall prayers are the longest. Regular prayer helps prevent destructive deeds and gives one the opportunity to seek God's pardon for any misgivings. Prayers are performed facing the Kabbah in Mecca (Makkah) no matter where a Muslim lives. So, in the United States, the prayer direction is approximately northeast. Prayers involve standing, kneeling, and prostration. Friday is the day of congregation for Muslims. The mid-day prayer on Friday is different from all other prayers in that it includes a sermon. Prayers at other times are relatively simple; they include verses from the Qur'an and take only a few minutes to complete. Muslims are greatly encouraged to perform their five daily prayers in congregation and in a mosque. A mosque, in its most basic form, is simply a clean area designated for prayers. A translation of the call to prayer comes from the teachings of Prophet Muhammad from Allah.

God is Great, God is Great;
God is Great, God is Great.
I testify that there is no deity except God;
I testify that there is no deity except God.
I testify that Muhammad is the messenger of God;
I testify that Muhammad is the messenger of God.
Come to prayer! Come to prayer!
Come to success! Come to success!
God is Great! God is Great!
There is no deity except God.[331]

A translation of the obligatory prayer:

In the Name of God, the Merciful, the Compassionate
Praise belongs to God, Lord of the World, the Merciful, the Compassionate, Master of the Day of Judgment;
We worship only You, and from You alone do we seek help.
Lead us on the straight path, the path of those whom You have blessed, not of those on whom is [Your] Wrath, nor of those who have gone astray.[332]

In the Name of God, the Merciful, the Compassionate
Say: "He is God, the One,
God the Eternal and Besought of all,
Neither begetting nor begot, Nor is there anything
comparable or equal to Him.[333]

---

331 Book of Hadith.
332 Qur'an 1:1–7.
333 Qur'an 112:1–4.

God is Great

Glory be to my Lord, the Great, and
praise belongs to Him

God hears the one who praises Him

God is Great

Glory be to my Exalted Lord, and
praise belongs to Him

I ask forgiveness of God, my Lord,
and turn towards him

God is Great

With God's help and through His
power I stand and sit

O our Lord! Bestow upon us good
in this world and good in the
Hereafter, and protect us from the
torment of the fire

God is Great."[334]

To Allah! You alone deserve all
veneration, worship and glory.
O Prophet! Peace be on you and the
mercy of Allah and His blessings.
Peace be upon us and on virtuous
servants of Allah. I bear witness that
none is worthy of worship save Allah
and I bear witness that Muhammad
(peace be upon him) is His chosen
servant and His Messenger.

3. **Zakat** (charity): An important principle of Islam is that everything belongs
to God; wealth is, therefore, held by
human beings in trust. Obligatory
charity or *zakat* means both "purifica-
tions" and "growth." One's possessions
are purified by setting aside a proportion for those in need and for society in
general. Like the pruning of plants, this
cutting back balances and encourages
new growth. Each Muslim calculates his

or own *zakat* individually. This involves
the annual payments to those in need of
2.5% of the net assets, excluding such
items as primary residence, car and
professional tools. *Zakat* is a unique
concept, compared to other forms of
giving, in that it redistributes the wealth
of society; when applied correctly, it
could effectively eliminate poverty.
God places great emphasis on taking
care of the needy in society; He says in
the Qur'an: "Those who spend of their
wealth (in charity) by night and by day,
and in secret and in public have their
reward with their Lord, on them there
shall be no fear, nor shall they grieve"
(2:274). Giving beyond the obligatory
charity expected of every Muslim is
called *saddaqah* and may take many
forms. The Prophet said, "Even meeting
your brother with a smile is an act of
charity" (Book of Hadith). The Prophet
further said that when one has nothing
to give, he can stay away from evil; that
too is charity.

4. **Saum** (fast): The annual fast takes place
during the holy month of Ramadan
(ninth month in the Islamic lunar calendar; the dates change each year because
the Islamic calendar is based on cycles of
the moon, not the sun), which is a time
of sacrifice, self-examination, and self-
improvement. Ramadan is a month of
spiritual consciousness and an elevated
sense of social responsibility. Muslims
believe that fasting is an opportunity for
them to focus on improving their short-
comings, building on their strengths,
becoming more self-aware and spiritually conscious, achieving greater
self-control, becoming more thankful, gaining greater sympathy for those
who are less fortunate and becoming

---

334 Muslims bend and prostrate during the recitation
of this part of the prayer.

more proactive in honoring and assisting the needy. During the month of Ramadan, Muslims fast from dawn until sundown, abstaining from food, drink, and marital relations. Those who are sick, elderly, or on a journey, and women who are pregnant or nursing are excused, but are required to make up those days at another time. If they are physically unable to do this, they must feed a needy person for every day missed. Children begin fasting from puberty, but some start earlier. A fasting person gains true sympathy with those who go hungry as well as growth in one's spiritual life. Muslims believe that Ramadan is the month in which the Qur'an was revealed to the Prophet Muhammad. Thus, Muslims make special efforts to recite and reflect on the entire Qur'an during this holy month and congregate to stand together in ritual prayer during part of each night. At the end of Ramadan, Muslims celebrate *Eid al-Fitr* (the feast of the breaking of the fast), a festive holiday which begins with a congregational prayer and address by a learned person. Muslims make it a point to wear their finest new clothes and apply their best scents when attending the congregation. Afterward, people greet each other and proceed to share meals with family and friends. Children typically are recipients of gifts on this festive occasion. Remembering that Muslims follow a lunar calendar, Ramadan begins 11 days earlier than previous years and completes a full year cycle in 30 years.

5. *Hajj* (pilgrimage): Every Muslim is expected to make a pilgrimage to Mecca once during one's lifetime, if financially and physically able. Approximately over 2 million Muslims complete this pilgrimage annually. The *Hajj* begins on the eighth day of *Dhul-Hijjah* (month for *Hajj*), the twelfth month of the Islamic year, and lasts for as long as 6 days. Pilgrims wear special clothes: simple garments that strip away distinctions of class and culture, so that all stand equal before God. The rites of the *Hajj*, which are of Prophet Abrahamic (*Ibrahim*) origin, include circling the *Ka'ba* (the cube-shaped shrine in Mecca built by Prophet Abraham and before that Prophet Adam) seven times, and going seven times between the mountains of Safa and Marwa as did Hagar during her search for water. Then, the pilgrims stand together on the wide plain of Arafa and join in prayers for God's forgiveness, in what is often thought of as preview of the Day of Judgment. The *Hajj* includes *Eid al-Adha*, which is celebrated with prayers and exchange of gifts in Muslim communities everywhere. This event observes the would-be sacrifice of Prophet Abraham's son, Ishmael. *Eid al-Adha* and *Eid al-Fitr*, a feast day commemorating the end of Ramadan, are the main festivals of the Muslim lunar calendar.

For the Shia perspective, one can use the metaphor of a tree to describe the teachings of Islam: the roots of Islam are called **Usul-e-deen** and the branches of Islam are called **Furoodeen**.

Usul-e-deen are as follows.

1. **Tawheed (Shahadah)** (could be viewed as declaration of faith): "*There is no deity except God; Muhammad (peace be upon him) is the messenger of God.*"

2. **Adl** (Justice of God): This means that

God is just and not a tyrant. Everybody's rewards will depend upon their own deeds. *Allah affirms that there is no God but He; and so do the angels, and these endued with knowledge, He is standing firm in justice. (Qur'an 3.18)*

3. **Nabuwwat** (Prophethood): This concept is derived from the premise that: it is the will of God that every human being should pursue a defined code of life and follow certain principles of conduct; that God sent Prophets to acquaint humanity with these principles and the code of life. According to Islam, Allah sent 1 240 000 prophets in all with Prophet Muhammad being the last Prophet.

4. **Imamat** (vicegerency of the Prophet): Shias believe that Prophet Muhammad announced that the guidance for Muslims after his death will be certain named persons as ordained by God. These persons are known as Imams, vicegerents of the Prophet. The first Imam was his son-in-law, Ali and the remaining Imams are from the descendants of his only surviving daughter Fatima.

5. **Quyamat** (Day of Judgment). There is life in the Hereafter. After death, an individual gets the reward or the punishment of the deeds he/she performed before death. For this purpose, on a certain day, called the Day of Judgment, all the dead would be resurrected from their graves and awarded Heaven or Hell depending on the merits of their actions in this world.

Furoodeen are as follows.

1. **Salat** (prayers). This is similar to the Sunni description given earlier except Shias can combine the afternoon

prayers together and the evening prayers together. The evening prayers are performed 17 minutes after sunset. A translation of the obligatory prayer:

In the Name of God, the Merciful, the Compassionate
Praise belongs to God, Lord of the World, the Merciful, the Compassionate, Master of the Day of Judgment;
We worship only You, and from You alone do we seek help.
Lead us on the straight path, the path of those whom You have blessed, not of those on whom is [Your] Wrath, nor of those who have gone astray.[335]

In the Name of God, the Merciful, the Compassionate
Say: 'He is God, the One,
God the Eternal and Besought of all,
Neither begetting nor begot, Nor is there anything
comparable or equal to Him.[336]

God is Great
Glory be to my Lord, the Great, and praise belongs to Him
God hears the one who praises Him
God is Great
Glory be to my Exalted Lord, and praise belongs to Him
I ask forgiveness of God, my Lord, and turn towards him
God is Great
With God's help and through His power I stand and sit
O our Lord! Bestow upon us good

335 Qur'an 1:1–7.
336 Qur'an 112:1–4.

in this world and good in the Hereafter, and protect us from the torment of the fire

God is Great.[337]

2. **Saum** (fast). This is similar to the Sunni description given earlier except Shias first perform their evening prayers 17 minutes after sunset and then break their fast.

3. **Hajj** (pilgrimage): This is similar to the Sunni description given earlier.

4. **Zakat** (charity): This is similar to the Sunni description given earlier.

5. **Khums** (additional charity): An additional one-fifth of the amount of a year's net savings is given to the poor, various charities, and religious leader (qualified) to support religious teachings.

6. **Jihad** (struggle: internal and external). The word *jihad* has its origin in the verb *jahada*, which means to struggle. The word has a few different connotations, since struggle can occur on several levels. For most Muslims, it is an intimate struggle to purify the soul of satanic influence, or inner struggle of the soul to obey what God has said is good and forbid what is evil, speaking of truth in the face of a tyrant, and to defend against oppression. This latter self-defense aspect of *jihad* has been grossly misunderstood in today's world. The Qur'an and teaching of Islam have placed severe restrictions on the latter form of *jihad*. When fighting, Muslims are required to follow strict rules of warfare and spare unarmed people. Killing innocent civilians, women, children, and the old is strictly prohibited. In addition, Muslims are not to destroy property, burn crops, pollute water supply, or cut down trees. The concept of "Holy War" is a western definition. In Islam, war is not considered holy.

7. **Amr Bil Maaroof**: This refers to enjoining the good and staying on the right path.

8. **Nahiy anil Munkar**: This refers to staying away from what is prohibited by Allah (i.e., any sin), forbidding evil.

9. **Tawalla**: This refers to expressions of affection toward the Prophet and his family by remembering their teachings.

10. **Tabarra**: This refers to staying away from those who are not supportive of the Prophet and his family by not associating with them.

Basic Practices

(Individual Practice May Vary)

- Muslims (Sunni and Shia) perform the "pillars" of the faith.
- Muslims gather on Fridays for congregational worship. It is held midday on Fridays. There is a formal sermon. The purpose is to bring the Muslim community together in prayer at a mosque.
- Ideally, it is best to have a religious leader known as an Imam to help with religious issues, but family members and close friends can also provide services as needed when an Imam is not available.
- Mosques (places of prayer and worship) throughout the world have taken on various architectural forms and reflect local cultures. They range from detached pavilions in China to elaborate courtyards in India; from massive domes in Turkey to glass and steel structures in the United

---

337 Muslims bend and prostrate during the recitation of this part of the prayer.

States. However, one unique and obvious feature of all mosques remains a place for the "call to prayer."

Principles for Clinical Care
Dietary Issues
- The few exceptions of which one needs to be aware in the Muslim dietary guidelines are: consumption of alcohol, pork, blood, and any intoxicants (any form of alcohol or any illicit drug) all are prohibited.
- Muslims eat *halal* food (permitted food). For patients, if *halal* meals are not available, allow patients to bring food from home if there are no medical dietary restrictions. Slaughtered meat becomes *halal* per Islamic law when Allah's name is said at the time of slaughter. In the Shia School of thought, four other conditions are required: (1) cutting four veins, (2) slaying toward Qibla (Mecca), (3) using a sharp knife, and (4) the slaughter must be done by a Muslim. Muslims should be served *halal* (lawful) food, which includes animals and poultry that has been ritually prepared and some seafood. In particular, pork, alcohol, and any foods containing these products are not allowed for Muslims. Alternatively, food prepared to vegetarian standards will be suitable for Muslims, provided that utensils used are clean of non-*halal* ingredients.
- Muslims fast once a year (from dawn to dusk) during the month of Ramadan. In general, fasting is exempt in illness and pregnancy.

General Medical Beliefs
- Muslims accept life as a trust from God and as trustees are required to take the very best care of their bodies in terms of both prevention and health care.

Eat and drink and be not prodigal.
—Qur'an 7:31

Do not let your own hands throw you into destruction.
—Qur'an 2:195

Your body has right over you. Seek treatment. Oh subjects of God … For God has created a remedy for every ailment, some known and some not.
—Book of Hadith

The most beloved by God, of the things he is asked to grant, is good health.
—Book of Hadith

If you hear that the plague is in place, do not enter it; and if it is in your place, do not run away from it.
—Book of Hadith

(Note: this is an example of a quarantine prescribed for the first time in history.)

Specific Medical Issues
Islam teaches that seeking the best medical treatment available is mandatory for all Muslims.
- **Abortion**: Abortion is not permitted except for saving the life of the prospective mother. Planning family and procreation within the institution of marriage is highly regarded.
- **Advance Directives**: Muslims live by the laws of their faith and the laws of the land. Given the concept of advance directives is a western concept and used in the health care field, Muslims are highly encouraged

to have an advance directive in order that their faith practices are honored.

- **Autopsy** is not encouraged. However, it is permitted if required by law for forensic or medical reasons.
- **Birth Control**: Preventive measures for birth control, if necessary, are acceptable; there is no role of abortion for birth control.
- **Blood Transfusions**: There is no prohibition against blood transfusions.
- **Conception**: Within the confines of marriage and use of spousal sperms, ova, or uterus, any necessary technological help is acceptable. Surrogate parenting is prohibited.
- **Circumcision**: Circumcision of male babies is required at time of birth. It may be delayed to the seventh day during the *aquiqah* (feast, naming ceremony, and prayer in honor of newborn). The concept of female circumcision is alien to the Islamic faith.
- **In Vitro Fertilization**: If during the in vitro fertilization process, fertilized eggs were destroyed, this would be considered an abortion and not allowed.
- **Organ Transplant**: Much like any professionally accepted medical procedure, transplantation of organs with all necessary precautions is permitted. This practice will vary among Muslims. Some Muslims may not allow organ donation. Shia religious scholars have determined that organ donation is allowed if two conditions are met: (1) donated organ should be internal, not external, and (2) life should not be dependent on it.
- **Stem Cell Research**: Muslims believe that life begins with conception. Terminating a fertilized ovum would be considered an abortion; thus, if stem cell research is conducted on a fertilized ovum, this would not be allowed. Whenever possible, though, research on stem cells taken from umbilical cord or from adults should be encouraged. Furthermore, no in vitro fertilization may be performed for the purpose of supplying stem cells for research. However, as fertility clinics are forced to fertilize more than one ovum so as to increase the chances of success, unused embryos may be used for research instead of destroying them, provided that this is done in the first few days after fertilization and provided further that the unused embryos are denoted without any financial return.
- **Vaccinations**: Preventive health care is core of Islamic health beliefs. As such, all vaccinations that are duly tested and recommended by reliable medical professionals are not only allowed but strongly encouraged to be used, especially in the care of infants and children.
- **Withholding/Withdrawing Life Support**: Comfort care measures and pain control are necessary in the care of a terminally ill person, but euthanasia and physician-assisted suicide are completely prohibited. According to Sunni scholars, withholding/withdrawing life-sustaining therapy is acceptable. Futile care and unnecessary measures of prolonging death are not permitted. Maintaining a terminal patient on artificial life support for a prolonged period in a vegetative state is not encouraged. According to Shia religious scholars, withholding care is acceptable, but withdrawing care is not acceptable. Also, maintaining terminal patient on artificial life support is encouraged.

Gender and Personal Issues

- Muslim women prefer female health care providers as their first choice.

- The generally expected greeting is "*As sala'amu alaikum*" (peace be upon you) and the generally expected reply is "*walaikum as sala'am*" (and unto you also, peace).
- In principle, shaking hands with women outside of one's family is prohibited. Men should not touch a woman's hand except if she is a close family member.

Principles for Spiritual Care through the Cycles of Life
Concepts of Living and Dying for Spiritual Support
For a Muslim, the concept of life and death has immense religious significance.

- Muslims believe that the soul passes from the present life into the next; death is not to be feared.
- Generally speaking, a Muslims' attitude toward death is captured by the words of condolence that Muslims are encouraged to speak: "We belong to God, and to Him is our return." As mentioned earlier, Judgment Day awaits every dying soul. Muslims perform daily prayers, supplication and Qur'an recitation anticipating their last day on earth. As death approaches, a Muslim will seek forgiveness and prepare to meet God.
- An important aspect of Muslim practice is the final enunciation of the Declaration of Faith "There is nothing worthy of worship except God," for its sincere pronouncement ultimately earns a believer an everlasting place in Heaven.

During Birth
- After childbirth, the call for prayer is recited softly in the both ears of the newborn. It is incumbent on the parents to give a meaningful name to the newborn.

- Breast-feeding for up to 2 years is recommended.
- As stated earlier, circumcision of male babies is required at time of birth. It may be delayed to the seventh day during the *aquiqah* (feast, naming ceremony, and prayer in honor of newborn). The concept of female circumcision is alien to the Islamic faith.
- Muslims require that no males are present in the delivery room except the husband of the patient.
- Funeral prayer is also recommended over a baby born dead after completing 4 months inside the mother's womb. However, no funeral prayer is required over a baby born dead before completing 4 months inside the mother's womb. Shias will perform prayer on a fetus 4 months and older. Shias will wash and wrap the body in a shroud for immediate burial
- In case of fetal demise or death of a baby, the baby's remains should be given to the parents. If the fetus is at least 4 months and has formed features of a child, the washing must be done. If it has not, it should be wrapped up in a cloth and buried in the Muslim tradition without the washing.

During Illness
- Illness is commonly accepted as a test and trial. Prayers, by the patient and on behalf of the patient by friends and family, for a full recovery and forgiveness are greatly appreciated.
- Reading scripture from the Qur'an is comforting to patients.
- Respect for modesty and privacy is of utmost importance; care should be given to covering "private parts" as much as possible.
- Muslims prefer that health care personnel

be the same sex as the patients for whom they are providing care.

- The primary spokesperson for the family will vary but traditionally it will be the spouse and/or the eldest child of the patient.

During End of Life

- Upon death and when someone first hears of the person's death, a Muslim will recite:

Inna Lillah wa inna Ilaihe Rajeoon

"Verily we belong to Allah, and truly to Him shall we return."

- Prayers, recitation of the Qur'an (especially Surah Yaseen 36) by family, friends, and clergy are offered during and immediately after dying.
- Remind dying patients of the importance of reciting the testimony of faith as a way of reaffirming their belief in God.
- Care of the dying at home is preferred by Muslims.
- Place patients in a position where Mecca is on their right side (facing toward Mecca by feet – that is, if the person was sitting down, he would face Mecca by face), if at all possible.
- Remind patient to think well of God and believe in the reality of the afterlife.
- Remind patient to not despair of God's mercy but to ask for His forgiveness.
- Help patient not to desire the hastening of death because of pain, but to ask God to prolong life if it would be good or to end life if that is the better course.
- Help patients to leave the world with no regrets by reminding them to pay their debts and complete an estate plan if they have not yet taken care of this important element of life.

- It is important that funeral and burial arrangements be made in advance in consultation with the family and according to the wishes of the dying or deceased patient if possible.

Care of the Body

- Upon death, the patient's eyes are to be closed, limbs straightened, and the entire body is covered with a sheet of cloth.
- Cremation and embalming are prohibited.
- Autopsy is allowed only if required by law or for forensic reasons.
- Donation of the body for medical research is prohibited. If a Shia puts this in his or her will, then it is allowed.
- Another important principle is prompt washing and burial of a Muslim, ideally achieved within a day of passing. Upon death, the proper care of a Muslim's body is a duty to which members of the Muslim community are entrusted (no need for health care staff to attend to this); formal washing of the body is followed by wrapping the body in two pieces of white cloth. (The washing can only be performed by Muslims.) Deference to their wishes would be appropriate and greatly appreciated.
- All Muslims in the area should make it a point to attend the funeral prayer. Formal prayers "Janaza Prayers" (see "Scriptures, Inspirational Readings, and Prayers" section) are conducted by a member of clergy and the body is taken to the cemetery for burial.
- No casket or vaults are used for burial. If state law prohibits burial without casket then wooden or bio-degradable casket can be used.

Organ and Tissue Donation

- Organ and tissue donation is considered an expression of goodness in that it saves or improves the quality of life of other human beings. However, it is an individual's decision.
- It may be preferable for a chaplain and/or nurse who are trained designated requesters to be consulted for assistance.

Scriptures, Inspirational Readings, and Prayers

READING DURING END-OF-LIFE PROCESS
This is a chapter in the Qur'an and can be read by anyone. It would be best for it to be read in Arabic, but the English translation is given here:

Surah Yaseen

In the Name of God, the Merciful, the Compassionate

Yasin.
By the wise Qur'an.
No doubt, you.
Have been sent on straight path.
Sent down by the Dignified, the Merciful.
So that you may warn a people whose fathers were not warned so they are unaware.
Undoubtedly, the word has been proved against most of them, so they shall not believe.
We have put on their necks chains reaching to their chins, so they remained raising up their faces.
And We have set a barrier before them and a barrier behind them and covered them from above, therefore they see nothing.
And it is equal for them whether you warn them or warn them not, they are not to believe.
You warn only him who follows admonition and fears the Most Affectionate without seeing, so give him glad tiding of forgiveness and a respectable reward.
Undoubtedly, We shall give life to the dead and We are noting down what they have sent forward and what signs they have left behind and We have already kept counted every thing in a clean Book.

SECTION: 2
And narrate them the signs of the people of a city; when there came to them sent ones.
When We sent to them two.
Then they belied them, so We strengthened them with a third, now they all said; verily we have been sent to you.'
They said, 'you are not, but a man like us and the Most Affectionate has sent down nothing, you are only lying.
They said, "our Lord Knows that undoubtedly, we have necessarily been sent to you."
And on us is not but clear deliverance.
They said, we augur ill of you, undoubtedly, if you desist not, we shall then surely stone you, and a painful chastisement from us will certainly fall you.
They said, "your ill star is with you. Do you start on it that you are made to understand? Nay, you are a people exceeding the limit."
And from the remote part of the city.

there came a man running He said, "O my people, follow the sent ones."

Follow those who do not ask any reward of you and they are on the right course.

And what is to me that I should not worship Him Who created me and you are to return only to Him.

Shall I take, besides Allah, other gods that if the Most Affectionate intends any harm, their intercession shall not be of any use to me and nor would they save me?

Undoubtedly then I am in a clear error.

Undoubtedly I believed in your Lord, so listen to me.

It was said to him, enter the garden. He said, "would that my people knew."

As my Lord has forgiven me and has made me of the honored ones.

And We sent not against his people after him any army from the heaven and nor We ever to send down there any army.

It was but only a shriek, hence they remained extinguished.

(And it was said) Ah! Woes on those bondmen, when any Messenger comes to them, they merely mock at them.

Have they not seen that how many generations before them We have destroyed? Now they are not to return to them.

And all of them shall be made to appear before Us.

SECTION: 3

And a sign for them is the dead earth We gave life to it and We brought forth grains from it. then they eat there from.

And We made therein gardens of dates and vines and We caused to gush forth springs therein.

In order that they may eat the fruits thereof and it is not made of their hands. Will then they not be grateful?

Sanctified is He who has made all pairs of what the earth grows, of themselves, and of those things of which they have no knowledge.

And a sign for them is the night, We draw off the day there from, hence they are in darkness.

And the sun runs to its appointed resting-place. This is the commandment of the Dominant, the Knowing.

And We have appointed stages for the moon till it becomes again like an old branch of palm tree.

It is not for the sun that it might catch the moon and nor the night may supersede the day. And each one is floating in an orbit.

And a sign for them is that We bore their offspring in a laden Ark.

And We have created for them similar (vessels) on which they ride.

And if We please, We may drown them, then there will be none to reach to their cry nor they shall be rescued.

But a mercy from Us and a convenience for a time.

And when it is said to them, "fear what is before you and what is to come behind you that perchance you may receive mercy, then they turn their faces."

And whenever there comes to them any sign out of the signs of their Lord, they turn their faces from it.

And when it is said to them, "spend something out of that with which Allah has provided you," then the infidels say to the Muslims, "shall we feed those whom Allah would have fed, if He had so willed? You are not but in a manifest error."

And they say, "when this promise will come, if you are truthful?"

They wait not but for a shriek that will seize them when they will be busy in worldly disputes.

Then neither they will be able to make a will nor will they return to their homes.

SECTION: 4

And the trumpet shall be blown, henceforth they will walk running towards their Lord from their graves.

They will say, "Ah, woe to us," who has awakened us from our sleeping. This is what the Most Affectionate had promised and the Messengers told the truth.

It will not be but a horrible shrieking, henceforth they all shall be presented before Us.

So today no soul shall be wronged, and you shall not be recompensed but what you have done.

Undoubtedly, the inmates of Heaven are enjoying their, entertainment comfortably.

They and their wives are in shades reclining on raised couches.

There is a fruit therein for them and there is for them whatever they ask for.

Peace will be on them, a word from the Merciful Lord.

And to day, be separate, O you culprits!

O children of Adam, Had I not made covenant with you that you should not worship the devil (Satan), verily he is your manifest enemy.

And that you should worship Me. This is the straight path.

And undoubtedly, he has led astray a great number of people from you. Had you then no wisdom?

This is the Hell, which you were promised.

Enter it today, the recompense of your infidelity.

Today, We shall set seal on their mouths and their hands will talk to us and their feet will bear witness of their doings.

If We willed, We would have obliterated their eyes, then they would have rushed towards the path but they would see nothing.

If We willed, We would have mutilated their faces sitting in their homes, they could not be able to go on or could return.

SECTION: 5

And to whosoever We give long life, We revert him in creation. Do they then not understand?

And We have not taught him to compose verses and nor it is befitting to his dignity. It is not but admonition and luminous Qur'an.

In order that it may warn him who is alive and the word may be proved against the infidels.

And have they not seen that We have

created from them Our hand made
cattle, so they are their owners?

And We have subjected the same for
them that some of them they ride
and some others they eat.

And there are in them various other
benefits and drinks for them. Will
they not be thankful?

And they have taken besides Allah
other gods that perhaps they may be
helped.

They cannot help them, but they
and their army all shall be brought
before arrested.

Therefore let not their speech grieve
you, Undoubtedly, We know what
they conceal and what they disclose.

And has the man not seen that We
have made him from a sperm,
henceforth he is an open disputant?

And he says for Us a similitude and
has forgotten his creation. He said,
"who will give life to the bones
when they are totally rotten."

Say you, He will give life to them,
Who made them the first time. And
He Knows every creation.

Who produced fire for you out of the
green tree, Henceforth, you kindle
there from.

And what! He who created the
heavens and the earth cannot make
the like of them. Why not, and He is
the Great Creator, all Knowing.

For Him is this only that whenever
He intends any thing, then He says
to it, "Be" and it becomes at once.

Therefore, Sanctified is He in Whose
hand is the control of every thing,
and towards Him, you will be
returned.

—Qur'an, Surah 36:1–83

PRAYERS FROM THE QUR'AN

Muslims communicate with Allah (God) in
prayers called *dua* (supplication, personal
requests to Allah can be said in silence or
aloud).

Suratul Fathiha

In the name of Allah, the Beneficent,
the Merciful. All praise is due to
Allah, the Lord of the Worlds. The
Beneficent, the Merciful. Master of
the Day of Judgment. Thee do we
serve and Thee do we beseech for
help. Keep us on the right path. The
path of those upon whom Thou hast
bestowed favors. Not (the path)
of those upon whom Thy wrath is
brought down, nor of those who go
astray.[338]

Suratul Qadr

In the Name of Allah, the Most
  Beneficent, the Most Merciful
Verily, We sent it down in the night of
  al-Qadr.
And what will make you know what
  the night of al-Qadr is?
The night of al-Qadr is better than a
  thousand months.
Therein descend the angels and the
  Spirit by their Lord's permission
  with all Decrees. Peace! Until the
  appearance of dawn.[339]

Ayatul Kursi

In the Name of Allah, the Most
Beneficent, the Most Merciful
  Allah is He besides Whom there
is no god, the Ever living, the Self-
subsisting by Whom all subsist;

---

338 Quran 1:1–7.
339 Quran 97:1–5.

slumber does not overtake Him nor sleep; whatever is in the heavens and whatever is in the earth is His; who is he that can intercede with Him but by His permission? He knows what is before them and what is behind them, and they cannot comprehend anything out of His knowledge except what He pleases, His knowledge extends over the heavens and the earth, and the preservation of them both tires Him not, and He is the Most High, the Great.[340]

Surah An-Nas (Mankind)

In the Name of Allah, the Most
  Beneficent, the Most Merciful
Say: I seek refuge with the Lord of
  An-Nas.
The King of An-Nas.
The God of An-Nas.
From the evil of the whisperer who
  withdraws.
Who whispers in the breasts of
  An-Nas.
Of Jinn and An-Nas.[341]

PRAYERS DURING ILLNESS

Al-Sahifat Al-Sajjadiyya, the oldest prayer manual for Shia Islamic sources, was composed by the Prophet's great grandson, 'Ali ibn al-Husayn, known as Zayn al-'Abidin.[342]

---

340 Quran 2:255.
341 Quran 114:1–6.
342 http://humanity.com/islamia/psalms_of_islam.htm (accessed 30 Aug 2012) *Al-Sahifat Al-Sajjadiyya* is the oldest prayer manual in Islamic sources and one of the most seminal works of Islamic spirituality of the early period. It was composed by the Prophet's great grandson, 'Ali ibn al-Husayn, known as Zayn al-'Abidin ("the adornment of the worshippers"), and has been cherished in Shia sources from earliest times. Zayn al-'Abidin was the fourth of the Shia Imams, after his father Husayn, his uncle Hasan, and his grandfather 'Ali, the Prophet's son-in-law.

These prayers can be used for Shias and Sunnis, but mostly Shias refer to these prayers. These prayers can be read by a non-Muslim, but are best read by a Muslim.

Supplication when Sick (Supplication 15)

O God, to Thee belongs praise for the
  good health of my body which lets
  me move about,
and to Thee belongs praise, for the
  ailments which Thou causest to
  arise in my flesh!
For I know not, my God, which of
  the two states deserves more my
  thanking Thee
and which of the two times is more
  worthy for my praise of Thee:
the time of health, within which Thou
  makest me delight in the agreeable
  things of Thy provision,
through which Thou givest me the
  joy to seek the means to Thy good
  pleasure and bounty,
and by which Thou strengthenest
  me for the acts of obedience which
  Thou hast given me success to
  accomplish;
or the time of illness through which
  Thou puttest me to the test
and bestowest upon me favors:
lightening of the offenses that weigh
  down my back,
purification of the evil deeds into
  which I have plunged,
incitement to reach for repentance,

Shia tradition considers the *Sahifa* a book worthy of the utmost veneration, ranking it behind only the Qur'an and 'Ali's *Nahj al-balagha*. These prayers can be used for Shias and Sunnis, but mostly Shias refer to these prayers. The prayers listed with the designation "supplication" are taken from this source.

reminder of the erasure of misdeeds through ancient favor;

and, through all that, what the two writers write for me:

blameless acts, which no heart had thought,

no tongue had uttered, and no limb had undertaken, rather, as Thy bestowal of bounty upon me

and the beneficence of Thy benefaction toward me

O God, bless Muhammad and his Household,

make me love what Thou hast approved for me,

make easy for me what Thou hast sent down upon me,

purify me of the defilement of what I have sent ahead,

erase the evil of what I have done beforehand,

let me find the sweetness of well-being, let me taste the coolness of safety,

and appoint for me a way out from my illness to Thy pardon,

transformation of my infirmity into Thy forbearance,

escape from my distress to Thy refreshment,

and safety from this hardship in Thy relief!

Thou art gratuitously bountiful in beneficence,

ever gracious in kindness, the Generous, the Giver,

Possessor of majesty and munificence!

Supplication for Well-Being (His Supplication when he Asked God for Well-Being and Thanked Him for it) (Supplication 23)

O God,

bless Muhammad and his Household, clothe me in Thy well-being,

wrap me in Thy well-being, fortify me through Thy well-being,

honor me with Thy well-being, free me from need through Thy well-being,

donate to me Thy well-being, bestow upon me Thy well-being,

spread out for me Thy well-being, set Thy well-being right for me,

and separate me not from Thy well-being in this world and the next!

O God,

bless Muhammad and his Household and make me well with

a well-being sufficient, healing, sublime, growing,

a well-being that will give birth to well-being in my body,

a well-being in this world and the next!

Oblige me through health, security, and safety in my religion and body,

insight in my heart, penetration in my affairs, dread of Thee,

fear of Thee, strength for the obedience which Thou hast commanded for me,

and avoidance of the disobedience which Thou hast prohibited for me!

O God,

oblige me through the hajj, the umra, and visiting the graves of Thy Messenger

(Thy blessings, mercy, and

benedictions upon him and upon his Household)

and the Household of Thy Messenger (upon them be peace)

for as long as Thou causest me to live, in this year of mine and in every year,

and make that accepted, thanked, and mentioned before Thee and stored away with Thee!

Make my tongue utter Thy praise, Thy thanksgiving, Thy remembrance, and Thy excellent laudation, and expand my heart toward the right goals of Thy religion!

Give me and my progeny refuge from the accursed Satan,

the evil of venomous vermin, threatening pests, swarming crowds, and evil eyes,

the evil of every rebel satan, the evil of every refractory sovereign,

the evil of everyone living in ease and served, the evil of everyone weak or strong,

the evil of everyone born high or low, the evil of everyone small or great,

the evil of everyone near or far, the evil of everyone, jinn or man,

who declares war on Thy Messenger and his Household, and the evil of every crawling creature that Thou hast taken by the forelock! Surely Thou art on a straight path.

O God,

bless Muhammad and his Household and if someone desires ill for me turn him away from me, drive away from me his deception,

avert from me his evil, send his trickery back to his own throat,

and place before him a barricade, so that Thou mayest

blind his eyes toward me, deafen his ears toward my mention,

lock his heart toward recalling me, silence his tongue against me,

restrain his head, abase his exaltation, break his arrogance,

abase his neck, disjoint his pride, and make me secure from all his injury,

his evil, his slander, his backbiting, his faultfinding,

his envy, his enmity, his snares, his traps,

his foot soldiers, and his cavalry! Surely Thou art Mighty, Powerful!

PRAYER DURING END-OF-LIFE PROCESS

Supplication when Death was Mentioned (Supplication when Someone's Death was Announced to him or when he Remembered Death) (Supplication 40)
O God,
Bless Muhammad and his Household, spare us drawn out expectations
and cut them short in us through sincerity of works, that we may not hope expectantly

For completing an hour after an hour, closing a day after a day,
joining a breath to a breath, or overtaking a step with a step!

Keep us safe from the delusions of expectations, make us secure from their evils,
set up death before us in display; and let not our remembering of it come and go!

Appoint for us from among the
righteous works a work through
which we will feel the homecoming to
Thee as slow
and crave a quick joining with Thee,
so that death may be
our intimate abode with which we are
intimate, our familiar place
toward which we yearn, and our next
of kin whose coming we love!

When Thou bringest it to us and
sendest it down upon us,
make us happy with it as a visitor,
comfort us with its arrival,
make us not wretched through
entertaining it, degrade us not
through its visit,
and appoint it one of the gates to Thy
forgiveness and the keys to Thy
mercy!

Make us die guided, not astray,
obedient, not averse,
repentant, not disobedient or
persisting, O He who guarantees
the repayment of the good-doers and
seeks to set right the work of the
corrupt!

PRAYERS FOR FUNERAL[343]

Janaza Prayer

The prayer over the deceased person takes
the following form (this reflects the Sunni
Janaza Prayer; the Shia *Janaza* Prayer is
slightly different.)

- The funeral prayer has no *Adhaan* (call
  to prayer).
- The deceased is laid down in a casket (for
  the purpose of the prayer only), with the
  face directed toward the *Ka'ba*.
- If the deceased is a man, the Imam would
  stand facing toward the head of the dead
  body; if the deceased is a woman, the
  Imam would stand facing the middle part
  of the dead body. Meanwhile, the congregation would be standing behind him
  in rows.
- The funeral prayer is performed with
  one standing only and has neither bows
  (*rukuus*) nor prostration (*sujuuds*).

343 Adam, N. (1996). *Kitab Al-Salaat* (*The Book of Prayer*). Riyadh: Cooperative Office for Call and Guidance; 2002.

Special Days: Islam

Al Hijra   The Islamic New Year also called *Muharram*, is the first day of the month of *Muharram*, the first month of the Islamic year. It marks the *Hijra* in 622 CE when Muhammad moved from Mecca to Medina. In fact, the Islamic calendar counts from the *Hijra*, which is why Muslim dates have the suffix AH (After *Hijra*). There is no specific religious ritual required on this day, but Muslims will often think about the general meaning of *Hijra* and regard this as a good time for "New Year's Resolutions." The Qur'an uses the word *Hijra* to mean moving from one place or state of affairs to a better one.

Aashura   Meaning "ten," this is an Islamic holiday observed on the tenth of *Muharram*. According to Sunnis, after the *Hijra*, Prophet Muhammad designated *Aashura* as a day of fasting to commemorate the day Moses was saved from the Egyptians by Allah. It also commemorates the death of Husayn (also spelled Hussein), son of Imam Ali and grandson of Prophet Muhammad, on the tenth of *Muharram* (October 10, 680) in Karbala, Iraq. This event, of central importance to Shias, is an important event to observe.

Mawlid al-Nabi   This holiday celebrates the birthday of Prophet Muhammad. *Mawlid* means birthday of a holy figure and *al-Nabi* means prophet. The day is commemorated with recollections of Muhammad's life and significance.

Lailat al Miraj   The festival is celebrated by telling the beautiful story of how the Prophet Muhammad fell asleep and traveled from Mecca to Jerusalem in a single night on a winged creature called *Buraq*. From Jerusalem he ascended into heaven where he met the earlier prophets. During his time in heaven Muhammad was told of the duty of Muslims to recite *Salat* (ritual prayer) five times a day.

Lailat al Bara'h   *Night of Forgiveness* – A night of prayer to Allah for forgiveness of the dead and preparation for Ramadan through intense prayer. The Night of Forgiveness takes place 2 weeks before Ramadan. Muslims spend the night in prayer seeking God's guidance and forgiveness for their sins. It is an opportunity to put the past behind them and forgive each other. Many Muslims believe that a person's destiny is fixed for the coming year by God on this night. For the Shias, it is also believed to be the twelfth Imam's birthday.

Ramadan   The annual event on Islamic calendar, devoted to the commemoration of Prophet Muhammad's reception of the divine revelation recorded in the Qur'an. It begins on the ninth month of the lunar calendar where fasting is observed by adults from dawn to sunset. The Qur'an was revealed to Prophet Muhammad during this month.

Lailat al Qadr   Night of Power – This date called Night of Destiny is observed during the last 10 days of Ramadan. Prayers are offered to Allah for a good destiny. Because of the importance of this night, Muslims strive harder to worship God and to do good deeds. They often pray extra prayers on this day, particularly the night prayer.

Jum' at al-Wada   "Farewell Friday" is the last Friday of the month of Ramadan and the Friday immediately preceding *Eid al-Fitr*.

Eid al-Fitr   It is the day after Ramadan. It is a festival of thanksgiving to Allah for enjoying the month of Ramadan which involves wearing finest clothing, saying congregational prayers, having feasts, and giving gifts to children.

Hajj   The *Hajj* is the annual pilgrimage to Mecca. Every able-bodied Muslim who can afford to do so is obliged to make the pilgrimage to Mecca at least once in his or her lifetime.

Eid al-Adha   Is a 3-day festival recalling Prophet Abraham's willingness to sacrifice his son Ishmael in obedience to Allah. Muslims sacrifice a domestic animals (usually sheep, but also camels, cows, and goats) as a symbol of Prophet Abraham's sacrifice. A large portion of the meat is given to the poor. Muslims wear their finest clothing, say congregational prayers, have feasts, and give gifts to children.

Eid al-Ghadeer   This is another *Eid* celebrated by Shias who believe that Prophet Muhammad appointed his son-in-law Ali to be his successor. Shias wear their finest clothing, say congregational prayers, have feasts, and give gifts to children.

Glossary of Islamic Terms

Al Fatihah: First chapter of the Qur'an. Its seven verses are a prayer for God's guidance and stress the lordship and mercy of God. This chapter has a special role in traditional daily prayers, being recited at the start of each unit of prayer.

Allahu Akbar: Translated "God is great" or "God is [the] greatest," it is a common Arabic expression, used as both an informal expression of faith and as a formal declaration. This phrase is recited by Muslims in numerous different situations. For example, when they are happy or wish to express approval, when an animal is slaughtered in a halal fashion, when they want to praise a speaker and even times of extreme stress or euphoria. The phrase is said during each stage of both obligatory prayers, which are supposed to be performed five times a day. The Muslim call to prayer, adhan, and to commence the prayer, iqama, also contains the phrase, which is heard in cities all over the Muslim world.

aquiqah: Religious ceremony in Islam including a feast, naming ceremony, and prayer in honor of newborn.

Eid al-Adha: Muslim festival that commemorates the willingness of Abraham to sacrifice his son Ishmael at the command of Allah. *Eid al-Adha* takes place on the tenth day of *Dhu al-Hijja* on the Islamic lunar calendar.

Eid al-Fitr: Muslim holiday that marks the end of Ramadan, the Islamic holy month of fasting. Eid is an Arabic word meaning "festivity," while *Fitr* means "to break the fast." *Eid al-Fitr* starts the day after Ramadan ends. *Eid al-Fitr* is a joyous occasion with important religious significance, celebrating the achievement of enhanced piety. It is a day of forgiveness, moral victory, fellowship, brotherhood, and unity. Muslims not only celebrate the end of fasting but also thank God for the self-control and strength that Muslims believe God gave them. It is a time of giving and sharing, and many Muslims dress in holiday attire.

Five Pillars of Islam: Five practices of Muslims (*Shahada, Salat, Saum, Hajj*, and *Zakat*). The definitions of each are as follows.

1. *Shahadah*: One of the Five Pillars of Islam; Muslim declaration of belief in the oneness of God and acceptance of Prophet Muhammad as his final prophet. Recitation of the **Shahadah** is the most important of the Five Pillars of Islam for Muslims and is performed daily

2. *Salat*: One of the Five Pillars of Islam; the obligatory prayers are a sign of submission and humility and adherence to the Islamic community.

3. *Saum*: One of the Five Pillars of Islam; ritual fasting is an obligatory act during the month of Ramadan. All Muslims must abstain from food, drink, and sexual intercourse from dawn to dusk during this month, and are to be especially mindful of other sins. The fast is meant to allow Muslims to seek nearness to Allah, to express their gratitude to and dependence on him, to atone for their past sins, and to remind them of the needy. Fasting during Ramadan is not obligatory for several groups for whom it would be excessively problematic. These include prepubescent children, those with a medical condition such as diabetes, elderly people, pregnant women, breast-feeding women, and travelers. Observing fasts is not permitted for menstruating women. Missing fasts usually must be made up soon afterward, although the exact requirements vary according to circumstance.

4. *Hajj*: One of the Five Pillars of Islam; pilgrimage that occurs during the Islamic month of Dhu al-Hijjah in the city of Mecca. Every able-bodied Muslim is obliged to make the pilgrimage to Mecca at least once in their lifetime. When the pilgrim is around 6 miles from Mecca, he must dress in Ihram clothing which consists of two white sheets. The main rituals of the *hajj* include walking seven times around the *Ka'ba*, touching the Black Stone, traveling seven times between Mount Safa and Mount Marwah and symbolically stoning the Devil in Mina. The *hajj* should be an expression of devotion to Allah, not a means to gain social standing. Believers should be self-aware and examine their intentions in performing the pilgrimage.

5. *Zakat*: One of the Five Pillars of Islam; the practice of charitable giving by Muslims

based on accumulated wealth and is obligatory for all who are able to do so. It is considered to be a personal responsibility for Muslims to ease economic hardship for others and eliminate inequality. *Zakat* consists of spending a fixed portion of one's wealth for the benefit of the poor or needy, including slaves, debtors, and travelers. A Muslim may also donate more as an act of voluntary charity (sadaqah) in order to achieve additional divine reward. There are two main types of *zakat*. First, there is the *zakat* which is a fixed amount based on the cost of food that is paid during the month of Ramadan by the head of a family for himself and his dependents. Second, there is the *zakat* on wealth, which covers money made in business, savings, income, and so forth.

Furoodeen: Ten practices that Shia Muslims must perform; called the "branches" of the religion.

1. **salat** (*See* Five Pillars of Islam).
2. **saum** (*See* Five Pillars of Islam).
3. **hajj** (*See* Five Pillars of Islam).
4. **zakat** (*See* Five Pillars of Islam).
5. **khums**: Arabic word for one-fifth. According to Shia Islamic legal terminology, it means one-fifth of certain items that a person acquires as wealth must be paid as an Islamic tax to be given to the poor and support religious teachings.
6. **jihad** (*See jihad* in main body of Glossary).
7. **ami-Bil Maaroof**: To persuade toward good deeds.
8. **nahiy anil munkar**: To restrain from bad deeds.
9. **tawalla**: Expressions of affection toward the Prophet and his family by remembering their teachings.
10. **taharra**: Staying away from those who are not supportive of the Prophet and his family by not associating with them.

hadith: Written record of the oral traditions passed down from the Muslim to Muslim of Prophet Muhammad's life, actions and deeds. It is second in authority only to the *Qur'an*.

halal: Arabic term meaning "permissible." In the English language it most frequently refers to food that is permissible according to Islamic law. The use of the term varies, though, between Arabic-speaking and non-Arabic-speaking communities. In Arabic-speaking countries, the term is used to describe anything permissible under Islamic law, in contrast to haraam, that which is forbidden. This includes human behavior, speech communication, clothing, conduct, manner and dietary laws. In non-Arabic-speaking countries, the term is most commonly used in the narrower context of just Muslim dietary laws, especially where meat and poultry are concerned, although it can be used for the more general meaning, as well.

jihad: The word *jihad* has its origin in the verb *jahada*, which means to struggle. The word has a few different connotations, since struggle can occur on several levels. For most Muslims, it is an intimate struggle to purify the soul of satanic influence, or inner struggle of the soul to obey what God has said is good and forbid what is evil, speaking of truth in the face of a tyrant, and to defend against oppression. This self-defense aspect of *jihad* has been grossly misunderstood in today's world. The Qur'an and teaching of Islam have placed severe restrictions on the later form of *jihad*. When fighting, Muslims are required to follow strict rules of warfare and spare unarmed people. Killing innocent civilians, women, children, and the old is strictly prohibited. In addition, Muslims are not to destroy property, burn crops, pollute the water supply, or cut down trees.

Ka'ba: Cubical structure located in Mecca. The *Baqara* verse, revealed to the Prophet

Muhammad, established the *Ka'ba* as the direction toward which Muslims must address their five daily prayers and as the destination of the annual *hajj*, required once in the lifetime of every Muslim. Each year, worshippers gather in the courtyard of *Masjid al-Haram* and encircle the *Ka'ba* seven times during which they kiss and touch the Black Stone, a Muslim object of veneration embedded in the eastern corner of the *Ka'ba*. As it stands today, the cubical structure is about 43 feet tall and measures approximately 36 by 42 feet on the exterior. It is oriented such that its four corners align roughly with north, south, east, and west.

Qur'an: Sacred scripture of Islam, regarded by Muslims as the infallible word of Allah (the Arabic word for God), revealed to the Prophet Muhammad. The Qu'ran, consists of 114 chapters (*surahs*) of varying length, written in Arabic. It includes stories of the Prophets. This message was given to Prophet Muhammad in pieces over a period spanning approximately 23 years (610–632 CE). Prophet Muhammad was 40 years old when the Qur'an began to be revealed to him, and he was 63 when the revelation was completed.

Ramadan: Muslim religious observance that takes place during the ninth month of the Islamic calendar, believed to be the month in which the Qur'an began to be revealed. The name "Ramadan" is taken from the name of this month; the word itself derived from an Arabic word for intense heat, scorched ground, and shortness of rations. It is considered the most venerated and blessed month of the Islamic year. Prayers, fasting, charity, and self-accountability are especially stressed at this time; religious observances associated with Ramadan are kept throughout the month.

Shia: Second-largest Muslim denomination, comprising about 20% of the Muslim population. Shias emerged out of a dispute over the succession to Prophet Muhammad. After the Prophet's death, supporters of Ali, claimed that it had been Ali's right to succeed Prophet Muhammad directly. They maintained that only the descendants of Ali and his wife, Fatima, Prophet Muhammad's daughter, were entitled to rule the Muslim community. Ali's followers are known as the Shia (partisans) or Shiites.

sunnah: Arabic word literally meaning "trodden path," and therefore the *sunnah* of the Prophet means "the way of the prophet." *Sunnah* in Sunni Islam means those religious actions that were instituted by the Islamic prophet Prophet Muhammad during the 23 years of his prophethood and which Muslims initially received through consensus of companions of Prophet Muhammad and further, through generation-to-generation transmission. In Shia Islam, *sunnah* means the deeds, sayings, and approvals of Prophet Muhammad and the 12 Imams who Shia Muslims believe were chosen by Prophet Muhammad to lead the world Muslim community.

Sunni: Largest denomination of Islam, comprising about 80% of the Muslim population. Sunnis, also known as *Ahl as-Sunnah wa'l-Jamā'h* (people of the example of Prophet Muhammad and the community). The word Sunni comes from the Arabic word *sunnah*, which means the words and actions or example of Prophet Muhammad. Sunnis have "the rightly guided caliphs" are Abu Bakr, Umar, Uthman, and Ali. The *Caliphs* were both political and religious leaders of the *theocracy*.

surah: Arabic term literally meaning "something enclosed or surrounded by a fence or wall." The term is commonly used to mean a "chapter" of the Qur'an, each of which is traditionally ordered roughly in order of decreasing length. Each *surah* is named for a word or name mentioned in a section of that *surah*.

ummah: Word used to mean the "community of the believers" and thus the whole Muslim world.

Usul-e-deen: Five articles of faith that forms the basis for Shia belief; called the "roots" of the religion, and it is from these articles that the "branches" of the religion are derived.

1. **Tawheed**: One of the *usool* of Shia Islam; Islamic conception of monotheism. *Tawheed* refers to the act of believing and affirming that God is one and unique. In Islam, recognition of this principle is achieved by the first of the Five Pillars of Islam, the Shahadah.

2. **Adl**: One of the *usool* of Shia Islam; Arabic term roughly meaning justice. In Islamic theology, it refers to God's divine justice.

3. **Nabuwwat**: One of the *usool* of Shia Islam; this concept of prophethood is derived from the premise that: it is the will of God that every human being should pursue a defined code of life and follow certain principles of conduct; that God sent Prophets to acquaint humanity with these principles and the code of life. According to Islam, Allah sent 1 240 000 prophets in all with Prophet Muhammad being the last Prophet.

4. **Imamat**: One of the *usool* of Shia Islam; concept of vicegerency of the Prophet: Shias believe that Prophet Muhammad announced that the guidance for Muslims after his death will be certain named persons as ordained by God. These persons are known as Imams, vicegerents of the Prophet. The first Imam was his son-in-law, Ali and the remaining Imams are from the descendants of his only surviving daughter, Fatima.

5. **Quyamat**: One of the *usool* of Shia Islam; concept of Day of Judgment. There is life in the Hereafter. After death, an individual gets the reward or the punishment of the deeds he or she performed before death. For this purpose, on a certain day, called the Day of Judgment, all the dead would be resurrected from their graves and awarded Heaven or Hell depending on the merits of their actions in this world.

Jainism

All things breathing, all things existing, all things living, all beings whatever should not be slain or treated with violence, nor insulted, nor tortured, nor driven away.[344]

Prepared by:
Christopher Key Chapple, PhD
Doshi Professor of Indic and Comparative Theology
Loyola Marymount University
Los Angeles, CA;
Gulab Kothari,
Overland Park, KS

Reviewed and approved by:
Dilip V. Shah[345]
President of the Jain Associations in North America
Philadelphia, PA

History and Facts

The word "Jain" comes from *Jina* which means "conqueror"; one who has overcome and defeated the weaknesses that prevent people from realizing their true spiritual potential. The Jain tradition revived in India more than 2500 years ago. According to the tradition, a foundational principle of Jainism is that karmic particles adhere to the soul, obscuring its true nature. By the progressive application of five great ethical vows (nonviolence [*ahimsa*], truthfulness [*satya*], not stealing [*asteya*], celibacy [*brahmacarya*], and nonpossession [*aparigraha*]), one is able to diminish and eventually expel the influence of karma, resulting in spiritual liberation. Twenty-four great spiritual teachers (*Tirthankaras*) are said to have attained this goal and set an example through their teachings for others. The first of these great teachers is known as Adinath, or Rishibha, who is said to have established agriculture, kingship, marriage, and the spiritual path. The most recent of these teachers is Mahavira Vardhamana (ca. 500 BCE); his immediate predecessor was Parshvanatha (ca. 800 BCE).

Mahavir, the last of the *Tirthankaras*, was a contemporary of the Buddha and both taught a doctrine grounded in renunciation of worldly concerns. Starting around 300 BCE, two strands of Jainism arose: the Digambara group, found mainly in south and central India and the Svetambara group, found mainly in western and northern India. The Digambara require total nudity for their most advanced monks

---

344 *Acharanga Sutra 1:4:1*, cited in *Pure Freedom* by Amar Salgia as the "Eternal Law" of Jainism.

345 Mr. Shah also had the document reviewed by two former presidents of the Jain Associations in North America (JAINA), a cardiologist from Phoenix, Arizona, who writes extensively on ethical issues in bioscience based on Jain principles, and several other notable Jain experts. They are as follows: Dr. Sulekh Jain, Texas, Former President of JAINA; Dr. Dilip Bobra, Arizona, a cardiologist; Naresh Jain, New Jersey, Chair, Interfaith Committee of JAINA; Anop Vora, New York, Former President of JAINA; Prakash Modi, Toronto, Member, Interfaith Committee of JAINA; and Dr. Pravin Shah, North Carolina, Chair, JAINA Education Committee.

and claim that women must be reborn as men to achieve liberation (*Moksha*). The Svetambara allow their monks and nuns to remain clothed in white and allow for the possibility of women's ascent to the highest spiritual realms.

The authentic scriptures agreed upon by both Jain sects are the *Purvas* (which have been lost), a collection of 14 texts that contained the teachings of Lord Mahavira. Other scriptures include the *Angas*, *Upangas*, *Mulasutras*, the *Satkhandagama*, and the *Anuyogas*. The earliest extant Jain text is the *Acaranga Sutra* (ca. 400 BCE), written in the Prakrit language and revered by the Svetambara community. It provides detailed instructions on how to practice the five great vows: Both traditions agree on the intricate Jain theory of karma and cosmology outlined by the scholar Umasvati in his *Tattvartha Sutra*, a Sanskrit text written in the fifth century BCE.

This text proclaims that countless individual life forces (*jiva*) have existed since beginningless time. They take many interchanging forms, and are found in (one sensed) the four forms of earth, water, fire, and air, as well as in microorganisms (*nigodha*), plants, and animals (from 2, 3, 4, and 5 sensed). At the point of death, the life force moves from one body to the next, depending on its karmic constitution. The life force attached to an earth body does not move, whereas the life force found in an insect or microorganism moves on very quickly. The goal of Jainism entails an elevation of consciousness about one's karma, leading to birth in a human body, and the adoption of a nonviolent lifestyle that will ultimately free a person from all karmic entanglements. At this final stage of blessedness, one ascends to the realm of perfection (*siddha-loka*) wherein one dwells eternally observing the machinations of the world but never again succumbing to its allurement. The 24 great teachers (*Tirthankaras*) of Jainism all are said to have attained this state, along with an undetermined number of saints.

Umasvati categorized life according to the number of senses it carries. Earth bodies hold only the sense of touch, as do plants. Worms add taste to the sense of touch. Bugs possess touch, taste, and the capacity to smell. Winged insects add the ability to see. More complex beings such as reptiles, mammals, and fish can also hear and think. As such, these life forms develop moral agency, and can make clear decisions about their behavior.

Jain cosmology proclaims that all aspects of the world that surrounds us have feelings and consciousness. The earth feels and responds in kind to human presence. The earth we tread upon, the water we drink, the air we inhale, the chair that supports us, the light that illumines our day; all these entities feel us through the sense of touch, though we might seldom acknowledge their presence. Humans, as living, sensate, sentient beings, have been given the special task and responsibility of growing in awareness and appreciation of these other life forms, and to act accordingly. Humans have the opportunity to cultivate ethical behavior that engenders respect toward the living, breathing, conscious beings that suffuse the universe. Consequently, the Jain community maintains thousands of animal shelters (*pinjrapole*), particularly in western India.

Jain cosmology further asserts that the world consists of myriad souls each seeking their own way. Through acts of malevolence, their karma becomes thick and entrenched. Through acts of benevolence, their karmic burden becomes lighter. By the adoption of a strict moral code grounded in nonviolence, Jains seek to shed their karmic cloak. This practice requires a clear understanding of what constitutes life and how one can cultivate care and concern in one's encounters with life. By carefully attending to what one consumes through dietary observances and restrictions of one's acquisitiveness, the soul gradually detaches itself from the clutches of karma.

In Jainism's later history during the period of the Islamic incursion into India, the Jain community was often in a place of retreat, with some of its temples taken over and converted into mosques. However, some Jain monks helped exert some nonviolent influence within the Islamic world. Jinacandrasuri II (1531–1613), a leader of the Khartar Gacch of the Svetambaras, traveled to Lahore in 1591 where he greatly influenced the Mughal Emperor, Akbar the Great. He gained protection for Jain pilgrimage places, as well as legal protection ensuring that Jain ceremonies would not be hindered. He even lent support to Jain advocacy for animals, and forbad the slaughter of animals for 1 week each year during *Paryushan* (Jain holy days).

Mahatma Gandhi, who liberated India from British colonialism through the enactment of nonviolent principles, was deeply influenced by the Jain tradition. He eschewed all forms of violence and even titled his lengthy autobiography after the second Jain vow: *Satyagraha or My Experiments with Truth*. He learned Jainism from his Jain mother during his childhood in Gujarat – an Indian state with a large Jain presence, and from Raichandra, a prominent Jain lay teacher.

A modern-day example of Jain activism can be found in the work of Acarya Tulsi (1914–1997), and his successor, Acarya

Mahaprajna, leaders of the Svetambara Therpanthi movement. Tulsi was appointed to the leadership of his order in 1936, when he was 22 years old. For 58 years, he served as its leader and preceptor and worked tirelessly at promulgating the Jain teachings of nonviolence. In June of 1945, deeply disturbed by World War II, he issued a nine-point declaration of the basic principles of nonviolence: (1) nonviolence should be widely propagated; (2) one must overcome anger, pride, deceitfulness, and discontent; (3) all persons should pursue education; (4) governments must become just; (5) science must not be used for purposes of war; (6) government information should promote "universal fraternity instead of national solidarity"; (7) people must not hoard; (8) the weak must not be oppressed; and (9) religious freedom should be granted to all.[346] In 1949, Acharya Tulsi issued an 11-point call for action, asking his followers, laypeople, and monastics to manifest the following characteristics: (1–2) not to kill or attack; (3) not to engage in destructive activities; (4–5) to subscribe to the ideals of human unity and religious toleration; (6) to follow good business ethics; (7) to limit acquisitions; (8) not to engage in falsification of elections; (9–10) to abstain from bad habits and addictions; and (11) to always be alert to the problem of keeping the environment pollution-free.[347]

The Jain community remained within India exclusively until the twentieth century, when many Jains migrated to east Africa, Britain, and North America. Most Jains follow a lay life and have excelled in business, particularly in publishing, pharmaceuticals,

---

346 Kumar, M. and M. Prakash. Anuvrat Anushasta Saint Tulsi: A glorious life with a purpose. *Anuvibha Reporter*. 2007; 3(1): 42.
347 Ibid, 71.

the diamond trade, marble, and textiles. Due to the strict adherence to the principle of nonviolence, several trades like farming were restricted. Although many Jains self-identify with the larger Hindu tradition, census figures place the Jain population at between 4 and 6 million. Approximately 100 000 of that number live in the United States. The first important Jain scholar to visit the United States was Veerchand R. Gandhi who addressed the first world Parliament of Religions in Chicago in 1893. Gurudev Shri Chitrabhanuji and Acharya Sri Sushil Munijis were the first Jain monks to arrive in the United States during the 1970s and both of the monks worked hard to unify the Jain communities in North America.

Basic Teachings

- Deeply committed laypersons manage liturgical and other temple activities. Monks and nuns travel frequently, offering Jain teachings in private homes and in temples.
- Jainism stresses the importance of adherence to the "five great vows": (1) nonviolence (*ahimsa*), (2) truthfulness (*satya*), (3) not stealing (*asteya*), (4) celibacy (*brahmacarya*), and (5) non-possession (*aparigraha*).
- Jainism places special emphasis on the teaching of nonviolence (*ahimsa*) as its "golden rule": live and let live.
- The universe in which the "soul" exists operates on fixed and impartial laws beyond the control of any outside influence. Jain teachings about the soul are:
  - the soul exists
  - the soul is eternal and independent
  - the soul is responsible for its own actions – mental, verbal, and physical

  - the soul experiences repercussions from its actions
  - the soul can attain liberation, the highest human attainment
  - there is a way to liberation – following the paths of right worldview, right knowledge, and right conduct.[348]
- The Jain concept of God is not one of creator, judge, savior, punisher, supreme being, power, or anything outside of a person. God (*Bhagavan*) is a word that describes one's own state of existence as soul. Jainism's perception of God is found in the following "pure soul" attributes:
  - infinite happiness and self-reliance
  - infinite power to know reality (i.e., omniscient)
  - infinite spiritual strength and willpower
  - infinite perception and vision
  - inherent immunity to any attraction (attachment) or repulsion (aversion)
  - incompatibility with the processes of birth, death, and rebirth
  - having no material properties
  - being neither superior nor inferior relative to any other soul.[349]
- Every soul is equal. There is a strong emphasis by Jainism on equality of souls. All souls differ only in the quantity of the "karmas" that they have accumulated as a result of their thoughts, speech, and action. Even the smallest living being on the planet should be treated with utmost respect because the underlying soul of all is the same.
- Destroy one's own "karma" and achieve

---

348 Salgia, A. (2002). *Pure Freedom: The Jain Way of Self Reliance*. Self-published (can be found at: www.faithresource.org/showcase/Jainism/jainismbooks.htm. (accessed 1 Sept 2012) author can be contacted at: asalgia@yahoo.com), 11–13.

349 Ibid, 14.

salvation (freedom from the cycle of life and death).

Basic Practices

- One is considered a Jain not on the basis of whether he or she is born into a Jain family but on the basis of what he or she practices.
- Customary Jain greeting is *Jal Jinendra,* meaning "Honor to Jina."
- With great detail, the Jain tradition emphasizes the perils of karma and urges people to avoid all forms of harm. A traditional tale warns against the wanton destruction of trees, while simultaneously explaining the mechanics of karma:

> A hungry person with the most negative black lesya karma uproots and kills an entire tree to obtain a few mangoes. The person of blue karma fells the tree by chopping the trunk, again merely to gain a handful of fruits. Fraught with gray karma, a third person spares the trunk but cuts off the major limbs of the tree. The one with orangish-red karma carelessly and needlessly lops of several branches to reach the mangoes. The fifth, exhibiting white or virtuous karma, "merely picks up ripe fruit that has dropped to the foot of the tree."[350]

- Again, trees were not to be regarded covetously for their fruits, but were to be given respect and treated without inflicting harm. This ethic of care may be extended to the entire biotic community, engendering an awareness and sensitivity in regard to the precious nature of life.
- Jains practice nonviolence by adhering

---

350 Jaini, J. (1916). *The Outlines of Jainism.* Cambridge: Cambridge University Press, 47.

to a vegetarian diet. Many of their religious holidays entail fasting, meditation, contemplation on self, and asking for forgiveness from those who have been harmed and granting forgiveness to others.
- Like Hindus, Jains cremate their dead.
- Many Jains practice various forms of yoga and meditation.
- Many Jains make regular temple visits to worship and to listen to lectures by learned monks.
  ○ Some Jains go every morning and evening to offer prayers to the spiritual masters, whose idols are in the temple.
  ○ Sermons, along with rituals are part of daily temple worship services.
- Jains are to:
  ○ practice truthfulness in behavior and speech
  ○ abstain from stealing anything
  ○ practice self-control over one's five senses (touch, taste, smell, sight, and hearing)
  ○ practice self-contentment.
- Many Jains wear face coverings to prevent the accidental inhalation and killing of insects. Some advance Jain monks go without clothing as an adoption of non-possesiveness; most wear simple white or saffron color garments.

Principles for Clinical Care
Dietary Issues

- All Jains are vegetarian. Vegetarian means would not eat meat, fish, chicken, or eggs. Most are lacto-vegetarian and very observant, avoiding eggs, even in cakes, and gelatin, which is often included in processed yogurts. Only rennet-free cheese is consumed. Wine and honey are other restricted items. Some Jains are now becoming vegan, in protest of the poor treatment of cattle in factory farming environments and because of the ill effects of a milk-heavy diet. Many Jains, particularly as they grow older, will avoid root vegetables and vegetables with an abundance of seeds, such as eggplant. Food cooked overnight is also avoided.

- Observant Jains refrain from eating and drinking between sunset and sunrise.

General Medical Beliefs

- For over 2800 years, there has been a tradition among some Jains to choose to voluntarily fast at the end of one's life, for which one needs to obtain permission from a religious authority.
- The practice known as *sallekhana* or *santhara*, "fast unto death" (i.e., abstention from food and drink), is permitted when the body becomes just a burden and no longer capable of functioning in celebration of a life well lived. It also helps in burning residues of karma that could impede the soul on its journey toward liberation.
- Jains will prefer to avoid animal-based medicines whenever possible.
- Heart valves, arteries, joints, or other devices derived from animals should be explained to Jains prior to using them, as most Jains will prefer alternatives if available.

Specific Medical Issues

- **Abortion**: Jain religious leaders, as individuals, have stated that if the mother's life is at risk, only then abortion can be permitted.
- **Advance Directives**: It would be in keeping with the principles of truth and nonviolence for Jains to fully disclose their intentions regarding extraordinary measures, hydration, and other issues.

- **Birth Control**: Because Jainism does not have one central authority, it must be surmised that conscience must be one's guide on the contemporary topic of artificial birth control. For monks and nuns, this would not be an issue, because strict celibacy is to be observed. For married persons, certain holy days require abstention from sexual activity. Because of the overarching ideal of nonviolence, care would be taken to ensure that sexual activity entails no harm, physical or emotional.
- **Blood Transfusions**: There are no specific pronouncements on blood transfusions. It is an individual decision.
- **Circumcision**: Circumcision is not required unless requested by parents or elders.
- **In Vitro Fertilization**: There are no stated objections to this procedure.
- **Stem Cell Research**: There is no unified objection to this form of research, though the Jain emphasis on nonviolence would urge prudence.
- **Vaccination**: There are no specific prohibitions on vaccinations.
- **Withholding/Withdrawing Life Support**: As noted earlier, there has been a long history of "inviting death," known in the Jain tradition as *sallekhana* or *santhara*. Many Jains have been known to refuse extraordinary medical treatment.

(Note: All of these specific medical points are guided by the principle and observance of nonviolence – that violence is absolutely necessary, minimum, and unavoidable.)

Gender and Personal Issues

- As with followers of the Hindu faith, most Jain women would prefer treatment from a female gynecologist/obstetrics specialist. Modesty will be of utmost importance particularly for Jain women. Particularly if the patient is from India, there might be an increased sensitivity to cold temperatures. Many Jains follow the "water method" for cleansing after toileting. Availability of a small pitcher in the bathroom would be helpful.

Principles for Spiritual Care through the Cycles of Life

Concepts of Living and Dying for Spiritual Support

- The physical body is just a materialistic support to the soul and subject to growth and decay.
- The soul never dies. It is immortal, imperishable, invincible, and indivisible.
- Death is just the end of the "current" life. It is viewed as the beginning of a new life of the soul. Depending on one's karma, the soul is reborn in a different place, in a different body until it frees itself from all karmas.
- Until salvation, the cycle of life and death is endless.

During Birth

- As stated earlier, circumcision is not required and not practiced unless requested by parents or elders.
- Naming ceremony is performed, typically after 12 days from birth.
- Friends and family will gather in the event of serious illness or death to offer support and prayers.

During Illness

- Some patients may receive moral and emotional support during illness by the playing of devotional music and songs.
- Some patients may benefit from the reading of selected portions of text from scriptures.
- Fasting for purposes of purification might be undertaken during illness by the patient.
- Health care professionals should remain respectful of fasting and dietary requests during times of illness.

During End of Life

- Place a picture or an idol of *Tirthankara* near the bed so that the dying person can easily see it and contemplate upon his virtues.
- It would be helpful to create a peaceful ambience for devotional songs and music.
- Some patients may benefit from the reading of selected portions of text from scriptures.
- It would be helpful to have a *Sadhu* (Jain monk) or a *Sadhvi* (Jain nun) or a Jain devotee present to chant religious mantras.
- Encourage patients to dissolute all and any grudges they might have had with anybody during their lifetimes.
- Encourage patients to strive to maintain their concentration steady on the *Arihants* and *Siddhas*.
- Elders in the family generally provide guidance on proceeding further to perform the last rites and suggestions on funeral homes.
- Some patients might refuse food and water when they anticipate that death is near. Health care professionals should be informed about this practice and, as with other situations, be mindful and respectful of Jain dietary practices.

Care of the Body

- Family may wish to wash the body and cover it with a plain white sheet.

- Cremation is the most common means of disposition. Dead body is to be cremated as early as possible but cremation is not permitted after sunset.
- An autopsy would generally not be conducted, unless required by law.
- Donation of the body for medical research is an individual decision.

Organ and Tissue Donation

- There are no prohibitions against organ and/or tissue donation; it is an individual or family decision.

Scriptures, Inspirational Readings, and Prayers

- The primary prayer would be the *Namokkhara* (also known as the *Namaskar Mantra* and the *Mahamantra* and the *Navkar Mantra*) in honor of the *arhats* (*tirthankaras*/teachers), the *siddhas* (liberated ones), the *acaryas* (ascetic leaders), the *upadhyayas* (ascetic preceptors), and the *sadhus* (ascetics).
- The *Namokkhara* is the most sacred mantra in Jainism and is applicable to every aspect of life – from birth to death. The text is provided here with the English translation of each verse in parentheses.

Namo Arihantanam
(I bow to the *Arihants*.)
Namo Siddhanam
(I bow to the *Siddhas*.)
Namo Ayariyanam
(I bow to the *Acharyas*.)
Namo Uvazzayanam
(I bow to the *Upadhyays*.)
Namo loye Sav Sahunam
(I bow to the *Sadhus*.)

- The primary teachings of Jainism are contained in the *Tattvarthasutra* of *Umasvat*, considered by many to be the Jain Bible. The *Tattvarthasutra* of *Umasvat* (ca. second century CE) is a systematization of Jain doctrine into concise aphorisms in the style of the Hindu Vedanta sutras. The *Tattvarthasutra* is recognized as authoritative, with only minor differences, by both Digambara and Svetambara sects.

Special Days: Jainism

March *Mahavira Jayanti* – Birth Anniversary of Lord Mahavira (also called *Janma Kalyanak*). Lord Mahavira was the twenty-fourth and the last *Tirthankara*; he was born in 599 BCE.

Late August, Early September *Paryushan* – An 8-day time of reflection and penance, including fasting; most revered festival among Jains.

October *Diwali* – Day marking the nirvana of Lord Mahavira, which occurred in 527 BCE.

September/October *Ksamavani* – Day of forgiveness during which one apologizes to friends and family for any suffering that one has caused during the past year.

October/November *Jnana Panchmi* – Celebration of knowledge; may involve a 36-hour fast.

October/November *Lokasha Jayanti* – Full moon celebration of great teachers and celebration of the New Year.

November/December *Maunajiyaras* – Day of fasting, silence, and meditation in honor of the five holy beings: monks, teachers, religious leaders, *Arihants* (*Jinas*, enlightened masters), and *Siddhas* (liberated souls); also regarded as the anniversary of the birth of many of the *Tirthankaras* or Pathfinders.

Glossary of Jain Terms

ahimsa: Nonviolence

aparigraha: Nonpossession

asteya: Not stealing

brahmacarya: Celibacy

Digambara: Sect of Jainas mainly in central and southern India

jiva: Soul

karma: Material substance that occludes the luminosity of the soul

lesya: Coloration of karma

Moksha: Spiritual liberation

Namokkhara: Most widely used prayer of the Jain faith. (Also known as the *Namaskar Mantra* and the *Mahamantra* and the *Navkar Mantra*.)

nigodha: Microorganisms

Paryushan: Week of repentance and fasting

pinjrapole: Animal shelters

satya: Truthfulness

siddha-loka: Realm of perfection

Svetambara: Sect of Jainas found mainly in western and northern India

Tattvarthasutra: Summary text of Jain philosophy (ca. 200–450 CE)

Tirthankaras: Twenty-four great spiritual teachers

Judaism

The world rests on three things – on Torah, on service of God, and on deeds of love.[351]

Prepared by:
Amy Wallk Katz, PhD
Senior Rabbi, Temple Beth El
Springfield, MA

Reviewed and approved by members of the
Rabbinical Association of Greater Kansas City
Kansas City, MO

History and Facts

The history of Judaism is more the story of a people than a religion. It is less focused on faith and belief than on *mitzvot* (commandments that include both ethical behavior and the observance of rituals).

Jewish history begins with the patriarchs Abraham, Isaac, and Jacob approximately 3500 years ago. Abraham embraced one **God**. He and his wife, Sarah, produced two sons, Esau and Isaac. Isaac's son Jacob had 12 sons, as well as a daughter, who formed the 12 tribes from which the entire Jewish people descend. Ten of Jacob's sons sold their brother Joseph into slavery in Egypt. Joseph rose to a leadership position under the pharaoh. Eventually, to escape famine, the other brothers led their families to Egypt, only to have their descendants become slaves for the next 400 years.

Moses led the people out of slavery in Egypt to Mount Sinai, where they received the **Torah** (Five Books of Moses [Hebrew Bible]). During the trek in the desert, the people were unfaithful to God. They had trouble believing in God, even though they witnessed the miracles of the Exodus. After 40 years of wandering in the desert, Joshua led the Israelites into the Promised Land or *Eretz Yisrael*, the Land of **Israel**. With the 12 tribes united under King David, the capital was established in Jerusalem. During David's son Solomon's reign, the First Temple was built. The 10 tribes who settled in the north of the country were conquered by the Assyrians and exiled, never to reappear in history. They are the Ten Lost Tribes. The First Temple was destroyed by the Babylonians in 586 BCE and the Judeans, the members of the two remaining tribes, were exiled. Upon return from exile, approximately 70 years later, the Judeans constructed the Second Temple and flourished as a people until resistance to Roman rule led to catastrophe. In 70 CE, Roman troops besieged Jerusalem, destroyed the Second Temple, and exiled the Jewish population. Upon conquering Judea, the Romans renamed the area Palestine, as an attempt to erase any Jewish connection with the land.

While the destruction of the Temple was

---

351 *Pirkei Avot* 1:2; a teaching of Shimon ha-Tzaddik. Available at www.myjewishlearning.com/texts/ Rabbinics/Talmud/Mishnah/Seder_Nezikin_ Damages_/Pirkei_Avot/Chapter_One.shtml (accessed 2 September 2012).

catastrophic, Judaism adapted itself to life outside of Judea. For the next nineteen centuries, most Jews lived in lands ranging from Europe to North Africa, Mesopotamia, and Persia. Rather than making offerings at the Temple, Jews expanded the already existing practice of synagogue prayer and worshipped God through prayers. In addition, the study of sacred texts became central to Judaism. Without a Temple, the priests became irrelevant and were replaced by a new kind of leader known as the sages or rabbis. These were not men who were born into their position; rather, these were men who studied and demonstrated leadership ability. Many of their teachings are recorded in rabbinic literature that is known as the Mishnah, the Gemara, and the responsa literature. This literature represents the academic activities of the sages.

Beginning in the eighth century CE, Jewish life flourished in Spain under Muslim rule. However, the "Golden Age of Spain" ended in 1492 with the expulsion of the Jews who refused to convert to Christianity (the number is in dispute). The Jews of England and France had already been expelled by the rulers of those countries. The Jewish population of Europe shifted to Central and Eastern Europe, and by the late 1500s, Jewish life thrived in Poland, Lithuania, and Eastern Europe. Most Jewish communities were founded by immigrants fleeing persecution in the West. Their culture produced a rich legacy of Jewish scholarship. Their devotion to study and Kaballah (Jewish mysticism) opened new paths to understanding God and the universe.

As a result of the Emancipation and the Enlightenment after the turn of the nineteenth century, European Jews gained access to secular as well as Jewish education. In Eastern Europe, a secular Jewish culture emerged, characterized by the growth of Hebrew literature as well as Yiddish newspapers, literature, music, and theater. Still, anti-Semitism (i.e., anti-Jewish sentiment) escalated. Vast numbers of Jews immigrated to the United States. Theodor Herzl proposed that the Jewish people build a future of their own making by returning to their homeland. Beginning in 1880, waves of Jewish immigration radically transformed the population of Palestine.

Between 1939 and 1945 in Europe under the Nazis, a third of the Jewish people (70 per cent of European Jewry) perished in the Holocaust. Of the survivors, few remained in Europe. Some went to the United States. The majority, despite British colonial opposition, went to Palestine.

In November, 1947, the United Nations adopted, and the Jews accepted, a resolution for the partition of Palestine into two independent states, one Arab and one Jewish. Six months later, on May 14, 1948, David Ben Gurion proclaimed the establishment of the State of Israel. The next day, five Arab armies invaded Israel. Their defeat turned hundreds of thousands of Palestinian Arabs into refugees. Israel became and remains the only Western-style democracy other than Turkey in the Middle East.

There are four main denominations within North American Judaism and to a lesser extent in other regions of the world. These are Orthodox, Reform, Conservative, and Reconstructionist. The differences are most pronounced in the way they relate to and practice ritual. A fifth group, although not a denomination, in American Jewish life is the Renewal movement.

1. **Orthodox**: Jews who adhere strictly to traditional beliefs and practices consider themselves Orthodox. Orthodox Jews hold that both the Written (Torah)

and Oral (Mishnah, Gemara, and rabbinical interpretations of Torah codified later in the Shulkhan Arukh) texts are immutably fixed and remain the basis for religious observance. Orthodox Judaism has held fast to such practices as daily worship, dietary laws, intensive study of the Torah, strict observance of the Sabbath, and separation of men and women in the synagogue.

2. **Reform**: The Reform Movement *reformed* or abandoned many traditional Jewish beliefs and practices in an effort to adapt Judaism to the modern world. It originated in Germany in the early 1800s and spread to the United States later that century. Reform Judaism permits men and women to sit together in the synagogue and does not require daily public worship, strict dietary laws, or the restriction of normal activities on the Sabbath. The premise of Reform Judaism is that Jewish ritual law is not binding, and the individual must make informed decisions about his or her religious observances. Observance of the ethical teachings is of course obligatory.

3. **Conservative**: The ideological roots of the Conservative Movement began in nineteenth-century Germany among German-Jewish theologians who advocated change, but found Reform positions too extreme. The goal of Conservative Judaism is to *conserve* Jewish tradition and rituals, while embracing modernity. Founders of Conservative Judaism accepted the Reform emphasis on critical scholarship, but wished to maintain a stricter observance of Jewish law. Conservative Judaism grapples with the tension between tradition and change. The premise of Conservative Judaism is that there is a need to change, but there is also a strong need to preserve Jewish law. In 1886, rabbis of this centrist persuasion founded the Jewish Theological Seminary of America, leading to the development of Conservative Judaism as a religious movement.

4. **Reconstructionist**: Reconstructism is a liberal form of Judaism developed in the United States in the 1920s. It is based on the belief that a person's individual autonomy should generally override tradition. At the same time, Reconstructionist Judaism believes that the changes must take into account communal consensus. A key aspect of Reconstructionist Judaism is that Judaism is an evolving religious civilization. Miracles and theism are generally not accepted. God is not personal and all anthropomorphic descriptions of God are viewed, at best, as imperfect metaphors.

5. **Renewal**: In the last several decades, the Renewal movement has begun to impact American Jewish life. Renewal is a nondenominational (sometimes referred to as trans- or post-denominational) Judaism. It honors the important and unique role of each denomination, and does not seek to become a denomination itself. Jewish renewal seeks to bring creativity, relevance, joy, and an all-embracing awareness to spiritual practice.

Basic Teachings

Three essential components comprise Jewish teachings: **God, Torah,** and **Israel**. While denominations may follow different principles and practices around these concepts, they would agree that authentic understanding of the Jewish people and religion is not possible without them.

1. **God**: A central theme of Judaism from its beginning is the belief that there is a Supreme Being, the Creator of all things, who loves humanity and with whom humanity can communicate in prayer and worship. While some Jews consider themselves completely secular, with no belief in God, traditional Judaism assumes there is a God. Opinions differ about the nature of God. Still, the classic literature – the Bible, prayer books, Passover *Haggadah* (which recounts the liberation from Egyptian slavery), poems, songs, and philosophical treatises of the Middle Ages – would be unintelligible without the strongest belief in God. There are many worthwhile resources for individuals who are struggling to believe in God. There has always been a place for those individuals who are uncertain about the nature of God. One of the most important Jewish teachings with respect to God is that each human being is created in the image of God, following the description of the creation of the first human being in the Book of Genesis. Historically, this teaching was revolutionary and, indeed, remains so today in many parts of the world. The Hebrew Bible insists that the intrinsic value of each individual life is the same. God's image does not grow or diminish with income or social status. Many questions arise regarding Jewish perspectives on Jesus. The belief in a messiah and messianic age is deeply rooted in Jewish tradition, which affirms that the messiah will be a descendant of King David, gain sovereignty over the Land of Israel, gather the Jews from the four corners of the earth, restore them to full observance of Torah and bring peace to the whole world. Jesus was an important teacher and leader during the first century. He was crucified by the Romans because his teachings were so controversial. According to Judaism, Jesus was a teacher, but he was not a prophet and nor was he the Messiah.

2. **Torah**: The *Tanakh*, or Hebrew Bible, is the foundational document of the Jewish people. It is comprised of three categories of books: (1) Torah (also known as *Chumash*, Five Books of Moses, or Pentateuch); (2) Prophets (24 books that trace Jewish history and monotheism from Moses' death until the exile in 586 BCE, as well as the books named for the prophets whose visions they contain); and (3) Writings (including historical books, as well as Psalms, Proverbs, Job, and Esther). Jews do not refer to the Hebrew Bible as the "Old Testament," which implies that it has been replaced by something "new." Once exiled from their homeland, the Jewish people survived as a people because of their deep commitment to Torah and its teachings about God and moral duty. From these texts, they spun endless commentaries, digests, laws, psychological insights, remedies, prophecies, and dramas.

3. **Israel**: The Romans conquered the Land of Israel and, seeking to erase its Jewish connection, renamed it Palestine. The Jews were thus faced with the challenge of surviving and thriving as a people in exile. Together with belief in God and commitment to study Torah, the Land of Israel is central to understanding Judaism. The name Israel itself is

significant. In Genesis 32, Jacob wrestled with a man until the break of dawn. As this man was about to depart he said: "Your name shall no longer be Jacob, but Israel, for you have striven with beings divine and human and have prevailed" (32:29). The name Israel in the Bible was popularly derived from *sarita* (you struggled), referring to Jacob's struggle and triumph. For the past 2000 years, wherever Jews are, they remember Israel. They yearn for it in their daily prayers; under the wedding canopy, they face Jerusalem and break a glass to recall the bitterness of exile; and at the end of every Passover Seder, they say, "Next year in Jerusalem!" A movement to reestablish a Jewish state gained momentum in the late 1800s under the leadership of Theodor Herzl. Vision became reality in 1948 when the modern state of Israel was born.

Basic Practices

- **Shabbat**: The Jewish Sabbath begins at sundown on Friday night. On Friday evening, families gather for Shabbat dinner, which includes the lighting of candles, blessing the children, blessings over two *challot* (loaves recalling the sacrifices in the First and Second Temples) and wine, washing of hands, the meal, songs, and grace after the meal. Saturday is a day of rest, worship at the synagogue, and visiting friends. Traditional Jews refrain from any form of work that involves production, creation, or transformation, as God refrained from creation on the seventh day. Less traditional Jews might do some of these activities, but set aside the day for family. Of course, there are many Jews who do not observe the Sabbath.

- **Holidays**: The Jewish calendar is filled with holidays, punctuated weekly by Shabbat. There are three pilgrim festivals mentioned in the Torah. These were agricultural in origin but evolved to mark important historical events of the Jewish people: (1) Passover (spring) commemorates the Exodus from Egypt; (2) *Sukkot* (autumn) recalls the sojourn in the desert; and (3) *Shavuot* (early summer) celebrates the giving of the Torah. *Rosh Hashanah*, which marks the New Year, and *Yom Kippur* (Day of Atonement), an opportunity for growth and reflection and to seek forgiveness, are also biblical holidays occurring in the autumn.

- There are three ancient, post-biblical holidays. *Tisha Ba'Av*, occurs in the mid-summer and commemorates the destruction of the Temple. *Purim*, which occurs in the early spring, recalls how Haman tried to kill all the Jews of Persia and Queen Esther and Mordecai saved the Jews from annhiliation. Finally, *Chanukah*, commemorates the post-biblical victory of the Jews over Greeks and rededication of the Temple in the second century BCE.

- There are also modern holidays, including *Yom HaShoah*, the day for remembering the Holocaust; *Yom HaZikaron*, Israel's Memorial Day; and *Yom HaAtzmaut*, Israel's Independence Day.

Principles for Clinical Care
Dietary Issues

- Dietary restrictions are associated with holiness in the Torah and are an integral part of traditional Jewish observance. The laws of keeping kosher (*kashrut*) regulate what foods are permitted and how they must be prepared. Only kosher animals are permitted and must be ritually slaughtered. As a rule, permitted animals are herbivorous. In three places, the Torah legislates: "You shall not seethe a kid in its mother's milk." The rabbis deduced from this that it is forbidden to prepare or eat meat and milk products together. This is why traditional Jews have two sets of dishes: one for meat (*fleishig*), the other for dairy (*milchic*). Foods that are neither meat nor dairy are considered *pareve* (food prepared without meat, milk, or their derivatives and therefore permissible to be eaten with both meat and dairy dishes according to dietary laws).

- Within the Jewish community, there is extraordinary variation in the way dietary laws are observed. During Passover, additional dietary laws pertaining to bread products come into play. Many Jews who do not keep kosher throughout the year will refrain from eating bread products during Passover.

General Medical Beliefs

Physician's Prayer
Inspire me with love for my art and
    for Thy creatures.
In the sufferer, let me see only the
    human being.

    —Attributed to Moses Maimonides
      (for full text, *see* "Scriptures,
      Inspirational Readings, and
      Prayers" section)

- The body belongs to God. Given the understanding that all people are created in the image of God, Jews believe that the body must be treated with great respect and sanctity.
- The body is neutral with respect to good and evil. It is neither inherently sinful nor pure. It is capable of acts of both good and evil.
- Sexuality is viewed as God-given and not to be shunned.
- Judaism stresses life and healing. Jews see life as a gift to be cherished and preserved – to live even when life begins to end. The traditional Jewish toast is "To life!" (*le chaim*). Jews believe God created humans with the imperative to use their God-given gifts to heal and repair the world (*tikkun olam*). This is one reason why, for generations, disproportionate numbers of Jews have become scientists and doctors.

Specific Medical Issues

- **Abortion**: There is a clear bias for life within the Jewish tradition. Indeed, it is considered sacred. Consequently, although abortion is permitted in some circumstances and actually required in others, it is not viewed as a morally neutral matter of individual desire or an acceptable form of post factor birth control. Contrary to what many contemporary Jews think, Jewish law restricts the legitimacy of abortion to a narrow range of cases; it does not give blanket permission to abort.
- **Advance Directives**: The advance directive is an important document for all Jews to complete. It lists a variety of medical decisions that commonly confront patients at the end of life and asks the person filling out the directive to indicate what she or he would like to have done under such circumstances. In the directives published by the four movements in Judaism, the options indicated are those that patients may elect according to the particular movement's interpretation of Jewish law and tradition.

- **Birth Control**: Despite the command to have two children and the ideal of having more, contraception is permitted and even required under certain circumstances. Because the command to propagate is legally the obligation of the male and not the female in Jewish law, and because of the traditional prohibition against "wasting the seed," whatever its basis, male forms of contraception are treated less favorably in the sources than female ones. Jewish sources from as early as the second century CE describe methods of contraception and prescribe when they may or should be used. Until the latter half of the twentieth century, though, Jews never contemplated using contraceptives for purposes of family planning. Judaism, after all, values large families. Moreover, if one wanted even two children to survive to adulthood, one had to try to have children continually, for many such attempts would be frustrated in miscarriages or in stillbirths, and many of the children who survived birth would die of childhood diseases or infections before being ready to propagate themselves. In judging the permissibility of contraceptives, then, we must recognize that we are asking an entirely new question. Not only have the techniques of contraception improved considerably, but the very purpose for which Jewish couples use them has changed. Thus although the use of contraceptives in our time may bear some formal resemblance to their use in times past, these changes in method and purpose must be kept clearly in mind as we examine traditional sources on contraception.
- **Blood Transfusions**: While Jews are prohibited from eating blood, they are permitted, indeed required, to have blood

transfusions if necessary. From Talmudic times on, Jews, in contrast to Jehovah's Witnesses, have not considered the insertion of blood through tubes to be a case of "eating" interdicted by the law.
- **Circumcision**: On the eighth day, the birth of a boy is celebrated with the rite of circumcision (*brit milah*), which is performed by a person trained in the procedure (*mohel*). This is the oldest ritual in Judaism, going back to Abraham, and should be viewed as more than a medical procedure. Most circumcision ceremonies take place in the home or at the synagogue on the eighth day. Some parents will, however, choose to have their child circumcised in the hospital by their obstetrician or pediatrician without the associated ritual.
- **In Vitro Fertilization**: Although Judaism regards having children as a great good, preserving the woman's life and health clearly takes precedence. We are permitted to take some risks in life, however, even for entertainment and certainly for the sacred goal of producing children. Since current medical research affirms that the risk involved in hyperovulation is not prohibitively high, infertile Jewish women may undergo that procedure, assuming, of course that no other factor in the woman's medical history would make that unwise. A serious objection to in vitro fertilization (IVF) is selective abortion. Because the rate of success with IVF is currently as low as 10% and only as high as 17%, the standard practice in North America among infertility specialists is to implant four or five sets of gametes (GIFT) or zygotes (IVF or ZIFT) each cycle in the hope of raising the odds of success to 25% or so. In most cases, the couple is lucky if even one of the implants

"takes." But, in some instances all four or five attach themselves to the uterus and begin to develop. Since women can generally safely carry up to three healthy children, it is a common practice to abort all but three fetuses if more than that successfully implant in the uterus. This practice is problematic for many reasons. To avoid the need for selective abortions as much as possible, Jews in the first place should have only two, or at most three, zygotes implanted for IVF or ZIFT and should use only two, or at most three, eggs for GIFT.

- **Stem Cell Research**: Life-saving procedures such as those resulting from stem cell research and organ transplantation are almost universally encouraged within all Jewish denominations.
- **Vaccinations**: The Jewish faith supports vaccinations for children and adults as a means to improve the general health of the community.
- **Withholding/Withdrawing Life Support**: Withholding and withdrawing treatment are dealt with on a case by case basis. Consult the patient's rabbi to determine treatment most consistent with the patient's and family's religious beliefs.

Gender and Personal Issues
- Ultra-Orthodox Jews will most likely prefer caregivers of the same gender.
- For Jews who do not identify themselves as ultra-Orthodox, this is a personal rather than religious issue.

Principles for Spiritual Care through the Cycles of Life
Concepts of Living and Dying for Spiritual Support

If I am not for me, who will be?
If I am only for myself alone, what
am I?
And if not now, when?[352]

- Traditional Judaism assumes that death is not the end. There is an afterworld, although no one knows anything about what that world is like.
- Judaism teaches that the soul is eternal.
- Death is viewed as part of life and not a punishment.

During Birth
- Jews rejoice in the birth of a child of either sex.
- As stated earlier, on the eighth day, the birth of a boy is celebrated with the rite of circumcision (*brit milah*), which is performed by a person trained in the procedure (*mohel*). This is the oldest ritual in Judaism, going back to Abraham, and should be viewed as more than a medical procedure. Most circumcision ceremonies take place in the home or at the synagogue on the eighth day. Some parents will, however, choose to have their child circumcised in the hospital by their obstetrician or pediatrician without the associated ritual.
- Many Jews have embraced the custom of celebrating the arrival of a new daughter with a ceremony anywhere from 8 days to a year after the birth.
- Jewish law does not require burial in the case of fetal demise. A baby, once

---

352 *Pirke Avot* 1:14; a teaching of Hillel.

born, that dies, however, would be buried according to the same rules and procedures as any other Jewish person.

During Illness

- The patient or family may request a visit from a rabbi.
- The religious needs and desires of a Jewish patient will vary greatly by individual. Ask how you might be helpful concerning spiritual matters.
- It is important to contact the patient's rabbi or, if they are not affiliated with a synagogue, the Jewish community chaplain (if there is one in the community).
- In Judaism, visiting and caring for the sick (*bikur cholim*) and providing support to their families is highly valued and considered a great *mitzvah*.
- Jewish law encourages whoever visits the sick, or hears about another's illness, to offer a prayer on behalf of the ailing person. A model for this is Moses' prayer for his sister Miriam: "O Lord, please heal her."
- Some patients will be very pleased to be visited by a non-Jewish volunteer or chaplain, while others may see it as intrusive.

During End of Life

- The patient or family may request a visit from a rabbi.
- Near death, some Jews may wish to say the confessional prayer (*vidui*).
- Some Jews may also recite the *Sh'ma*, which comes closest to a Jewish credo and is actually a verse from Deuteronomy: "Hear, O Israel, the Lord Is Our God, the Lord Is One" (6:4).
- The traditional words recited upon hearing the news that someone has died are "Blessed is the Judge of Truth" (*Baruch dayan ha-emet*).

Care of the Body

- When a Jewish person dies, out of respect, their eyes are to be closed immediately.
- The body is not left unattended until burial.
- The family of the deceased generally makes funeral and burial arrangements in consultation with their rabbi or the Jewish community chaplain.
- If the deceased is traditional, the body will be ritually prepared for burial by a group of volunteers called the *chevra kadisha* (holy society). Most funerals will be held at the funeral home or at the graveside. A few may be in the synagogue.
- Jewish tradition views open caskets as disrespectful to the deceased, who can no longer participate in this world.
- Traditional Judaism rejects cremation as a desecration of the body, although among some Jews the practice has gained wider acceptance in recent years.
- Autopsy is very rare, but may be accepted on an individual basis.
- Donation of the body for medical research is very rare among the Orthodox, but may be accepted on an individual basis.
- In Orthodox Judaism, *kohanim* (men who can trace their lineage to the priests who served in the Temple) are forbidden to come in contact with dead bodies, but they are commanded to do so for close relatives. Some but not all *kohanim* today continue to observe these laws.

Organ and Tissue Donation

- Because Jews place an enormous value on choosing life, organ donation among nearly all Jews is accepted and even encouraged. It may be preferable for a chaplain and/or nurse who are trained designated requesters to be consulted for assistance.

Scriptures, Inspirational Readings, and Prayers

Jewish law prefers that Jews pray communally rather than privately. In the synagogue, during the reading of the Torah, the *Mi-Shebeirakh* prayer is recited, petitioning God for the speedy recovery of an ill person. Those who are unable participate in communal worship should feel free to pray privately. God hears prayers whether people are in the synagogue or by themselves. It is just that when one prays alone, they do not receive the support of the community and that is a loss.

PRAYER FOR HEALING OF THE SICK

Mi-Shebeirakh

May God who blessed our ancestors, Abraham, Isaac and Jacob, Sarah, Rebecca, Rachel and Leah, bless those who are ill or recovering from illness.

May God who blessed our ancestors, Abraham, Isaac and Jacob, Sarah, Rebecca, Rachel and Leah, heal those who are ill (our brother/sister _____).

May the Holy One, blessed be He, show mercy unto them, restore their health, heal them, strengthen them and give them life.

And may God send them a speedy recovery.

Judaism does not seek to silence doubts about God's relevance or even existence, particularly in the face of illness. At the same time, the tradition encourages Jews to understand and reach out to God for strength and comfort. The following prayers are contemporary texts which may be useful for individuals who need help finding the words to petition God. It is appropriate and often useful for patients or family to simply pray spontaneously.

PRAYER BEFORE SURGERY

Compassionate God, as You have always sent angels to do your healing work, You send men and women as instruments of your healing. Bless all who will attend to me that their knowledge and skill might bring Your perfect healing.

All my days are in Your loving care. Amen.

PRAYER OF THANKSGIVING

God, Your mercies are new to me every day! I give You thanks for the renewing of my health; for the relief from my pain and worry. Continue Your healing within me that I may return to the work You have given me to do. Amen.

PRAYER FOR PAIN DURING ILLNESS OR END OF LIFE

God of compassion, You know my pain. Strengthen me and my faith in You. Even in this pain, help me experience Your presence; strengthen my faith when I despair. Give me the assurance of Your eternal love. Amen.

PRAYER FOR END OF LIFE

Adonai our God and God of our ancestors, we acknowledge that all life is in Your hands. May it be Your will to send healing to our brother/sister_____. Yet if the end is imminent, may it reflect Your love and atone for all those times our brother/sister_____ could have done better. Grant our brother/sister_____the reward of the righteous and give our brother/sister_____ eternal life in Your Presence. Amen.

READINGS FOR END OF LIFE

Shema

Hear O Israel, the Lord is our God, the Lord is One. May His name of Glory and majesty be blessed forever. You shall love the Lord your God with all your heart, with all your soul and in all your ways. These words that I am commanding you today shall be in your heart. You should teach them to your children, speak them while returning home, while traveling on your way and while dwelling in your place. You shall tie them as a sign upon your hand and as frontlets between your eyes. You should write them upon the doorposts of your houses and gates.

—Deut. 6:4–9

I lift my eyes to the mountains; what is the source of my help? My help comes from Adonai, maker of heaven and earth. God will not let your foot give way; your Protector will not slumber. See, the Protector of Israel neither slumbers nor sleeps! God is your Guardian; God is your protection at your right hand. The sun will not strike you by day, nor the moon by night. God will guard you from all harm; God will guard your soul, and your coming and going, now and forever.

—Psalm 121

God is my shepherd, I shall not want. God makes me to lie down in green pastures, leads me beside still waters and restores my soul. You lead me in right paths for the sake of Your Name.
Even when I walk in the valley of the shadow of death I shall fear no evil, for You are with me. Your rod and Your staff – they comfort me.
You have set a table before me in the presence of my enemies.
You have anointed my head my head with oil; my cup overflows.
Surely goodness and mercy shall follow me all the days of my life, and I shall dwell in the house of God forever.

—Psalm 23

Physician's Prayer (Full Text)
Almighty God, Thou has created the human body with infinite wisdom. Ten thousand times ten thousand organs hast Thou combined in it that act unceasingly and harmoniously to preserve the whole in all its beauty the body which is the envelope of the immortal soul. They are ever acting in perfect order, agreement and accord. Yet, when the frailty of matter or the unbridling of passions deranges this order or interrupts this accord, then forces clash and the body crumbles

into the primal dust from which it came. Thou sendest to man diseases as beneficent messengers to foretell approaching danger and to urge him to avert it.

Thou has blest Thine earth, Thy rivers and Thy mountains with healing substances; they enable Thy creatures to alleviate their sufferings and to heal their illnesses. Thou hast endowed man with the wisdom to relieve the suffering of his brother, to recognize his disorders, to extract the healing substances, to discover their powers and to prepare and to apply them to suit every ill. In Thine Eternal Providence Thou hast chosen me to watch over the life and health of Thy creatures. I am now about to apply myself to the duties of my profession. Support me, Almighty God, in these great labors that they may benefit mankind, for without Thy help not even the least thing will succeed.

Inspire me with love for my art and for Thy creatures. Do not allow thirst for profit, ambition for renown and admiration, to interfere with my profession, for these are the enemies of truth and of love for mankind and they can lead astray in the great task of attending to the welfare of Thy creatures.

Preserve the strength of my body and of my soul that they ever be ready to cheerfully help and support rich and poor, good and bad, enemy as well as friend. In the sufferer let me see only the human being. Illumine my mind that it recognize what presents itself and that it may comprehend what is absent or hidden.

Let it not fail to see what is visible, but do not permit it to arrogate to itself the power to see what cannot be seen, for delicate and indefinite are the bounds of the great art of caring for the lives and health of Thy creatures. Let me never be absent-minded. May no strange thoughts divert my attention at the bedside of the sick, or disturb my mind in its silent labors, for great and sacred are the thoughtful deliberations required to preserve the lives and health of Thy creatures.

Grant that my patients have confidence in me and my art and follow my directions and my counsel. Remove from their midst all charlatans and the whole host of officious relatives and know-all nurses, cruel people who arrogantly frustrate the wisest purposes of our art and often lead Thy creatures to their death.

Should those who are wiser than I wish to improve and instruct me, let my soul gratefully follow their guidance; for vast is the extent of our art. Should conceited fools, however, censure me, then let love for my profession steel me against them, so that I remain steadfast without regard for age, for reputation, or for honor, because surrender would bring to Thy creatures sickness and death.

Imbue my soul with gentleness and calmness when older colleagues, proud of their age, wish to displace me or to scorn me or disdainfully to teach me. May even this be of advantage to me, for they know many things of which I am ignorant, but let not their arrogance give me pain. For they are old and old age is not master of the passions. I also hope to attain old age upon this earth, before Thee, Almighty God!

Let me be contented in everything except in the great science of my profession. Never allow the thought to arise in me that I have attained to sufficient knowledge, but vouchsafe to me the strength, the leisure and the ambition ever to extend my knowledge. For art is great, but the mind of man is ever expanding.

Almighty God! Thou hast chosen me in Thy mercy to watch over the life and death of Thy creatures. I now apply myself to my profession. Support me in this great task so that it may benefit mankind, for without Thy help not even the least thing will succeed.

—Attributed to Moses Maimonides[353]

Special Days: Judaism

The Jewish calendar has a different number of days than the Gregorian calendar because the Jewish calendar is tied to the moon's cycles instead of the sun's. As a result, the Jewish calendar loses about 11 days relative to the solar calendar every year, but it makes up for it by adding a month every 2 or 3 years. Because of this, the holidays do not always fall on the same day, but they always fall within the same month or two. Jewish holidays actually occur on the same day every year: the same day on the Jewish calendar!

Hanukkah   The story of Hanukkah is preserved in the books of the First and Second Maccabees. The miracle of the 1-day supply of oil miraculously lasting 8 days is first described in the Talmud. Hanukkah marks the defeat of Seleucid Empire forces that had tried to prevent the people of Israel from practicing Judaism. Judah Maccabee and his brothers destroyed overwhelming forces, and rededicated the Temple in Jerusalem. The 8-day festival is marked by the kindling of lights – one on the first night, two on the second, and so on – using a special candle holder called a Chanukkiyah, or a Hanukkah menorah. There is a custom to give children money, also known as "gelt" on Hanukkah to commemorate the learning of Torah in guise of Jews gathering in what was perceived as gambling at that time since Torah was forbidden. Because of this, there is also the custom to play with the dreidel (called a sevivon in Hebrew). Hanukah is also called the Festival of

Lights and Feast of Dedication. The holiday is always observed in the winter months sometime between late November and late December.

Lag B'Omer   The 33rd day in the Omer count which began on the second night of Passover. The mourning restrictions on joyous activities during the Omer period are lifted on Lag B'Omer and there are often celebrations with picnics, bonfires, and bow and arrow play by children. In Israel, youth can be seen gathering materials for bonfires.

Passover   A 7- or 8-day observance of the Jews' "exodus" from slavery in Egypt from the time of the Patriarch Joseph to Moses (approximately 400 years). The name of the festival derives its name from the Hebrew term *pesach*, which means "to pass over." Passover is a celebration of freedom for a group of Jewish people from antiquity. That story is recounted during this season, but Passover is also about freedom for all people of the present day who are in bondage of various types. Passover is 1 month after Purim. The book of Deuteronomy demands that Passover is observed in the spring.

Purim   Festival (also called the Festival of Lots) celebrating the "miraculous" salvation from certain death of the Jewish people in Persia at the hands of Haman, a minister in the court of King Ahasuerus. The biblical book of Esther records the story of how Mordecai, cousin of Queen Esther, and the Queen herself "turned the tables" on Haman's plot, and he was the one who died. Purim is celebrated in late February to mid-March.

Rosh Hashanah   Jewish New Year beginning a 10-day period known as the "High Holy Days," which concludes with the Day of Atonement; this celebration of the start of a new year begins a time of introspection, self-examination, and repentance. It also calls to mind the creation of the world found in the biblical text of Genesis. Rosh Hashanah always comes in September or early October.

Rosh Hodesh   The first day of each month and the thirtieth day of the preceding month, if it has 30 days, is (in modern times) a minor holiday known as Rosh Chodesh (head of the month). The one exception is the month of Tishrei, the beginning of which is a major holiday, Rosh Hashanah. There are also special prayers said upon observing the new moon for the first time each month.

Shabbat   A day of rest celebrated on the seventh day of each week. Jewish law accords Shabbat the status of a holiday, and defines a day as ending at nightfall, which is when the next day then begins. Thus,

Shabbat begins at sundown Friday night, and ends at nightfall Saturday night. In many ways halakha (Jewish law) gives Shabbat the status of being the most important holy day in the Jewish calendar. It is the first holiday mentioned in the Tanakh (Hebrew Bible), and God was the first one to observe it. The liturgy treats Shabbat as a bride and queen. The Torah reading on Shabbat has more sections of parshiot (Torah readings) than on Yom Kippur, the most of any Jewish holiday. There is a tradition that the Messiah will come if every Jew observes Shabbat perfectly twice in a row.

Shavuot Festival that concludes the period of the "counting of the omer" is sometimes called the "Feast of Weeks"; commemorates the giving of the Torah at the foot of Mount Sinai, which included the Ten Commandments. Shavuot is celebrated 7 weeks after Passover. As a result, the holiday always falls in late May or early June.

Simhat Torah Day symbolizing the conclusion of Sukkot and the reading cycle of the Torah.

Shemini Atzeret Festival that falls on the day following Sukkot; holiday dedicated to the love of God. It also was a time when people prayed for rain and a hearty growing season for crops.

Sukkot A 7-day festival, also known as the Feast of Booths, the Feast of Tabernacles, or the Festival of Ingathering. It is one of the three pilgrimage festivals mentioned in the Bible. The word *sukkot* is the plural of the Hebrew word *sukkah*, meaning booth. Jews are commanded to "dwell" in booths during the holiday. This generally means taking meals, but some sleep in the sukkah as well. There are specific rules for constructing a sukkah. The seventh day of the holiday is called *Hoshanah Rabbah*. Sukkot begins in the evening of the fourth day following Yom Kippur.

Tisha B'Av A fast day that commemorates two of the saddest events in Jewish history: the destruction in 586 BCE of the First Temple, originally built by King Solomon, and destruction of the Second Temple in 70 CE. Other calamities throughout Jewish history are said to have taken place on Tisha B'Av, including King Edward I's edict compelling the Jews to leave England (1290) and the Jewish expulsion from Spain in 1492. Tisha B'Av falls in the summer months of July or August. Seven weeks following Tisha B'Av, the Jewish new year begins.

Tu B'shvat The new year for trees. According to the Mishnah, it marks the day from which fruit tithes are counted each year, and marks the time from which the biblical prohibition on eating the first 3 years of fruit and the requirement to bring the fourth-year fruit to the Temple in Jerusalem were counted. In modern times, it is celebrated by eating various fruits and nuts associated with the Land of Israel. During the 1600s, Rabbi Yitzchak Luria of Safed and his disciples created a short seder, called Hemdat ha-Yamim, reminiscent of the seder that Jews observe on Passover, that explores the holiday's Kabbalistic themes. Traditionally, trees are planted on this day. Many children collect funds leading up to this day to plant trees in Israel. Trees are usually planted locally as well.

Yom Ha'Atzmaut   Day celebrating independence of Israel and her recognition as a free nation among the nations of the world on May 14, 1948; known as Israel's Independence Day.

Yom HaSho'ah   Day for remembering the Holocaust when approximately 6 million Jews were executed by the Nazis until the end of World War II in 1945.

Yom Kippur   The most holy day in Judaism concludes the High Holy Days; it is a day of confession and repentance. Typically it is a day of fasting and praying for forgiveness of sins committed during the past year. The day ends with the blowing of the *shofar* (ram's horn). Yom Kippur is always 10 days after Rosh Hashanah.

Glossary of Jewish Terms

bikur cholim: Ministry of visiting and caring for the sick; considered a great mitzvah and highly valued in Judaism.

brit milah: Oldest religious ritual within Judaism, dating back to Abraham, in which Jewish infant boys are celebrated into life through circumcision on the eighth day following birth; its counterpart for newborn girls, without the surgical procedure, is baby naming.

challot: Loaves recalling the sacrifices in the First and Second Temples; today, it is the name given to the twisted loaves used on Sabbath and holidays which are commemorative of that ancient sacrifice.

chevra kadisha: Group of volunteers, called the "Holy Society," who ritually prepare the body of a Jew for burial. Acts relating to burial are considered *mitzvot* of the highest order; these would be acts of loving kindness without expectation of reward. The "Holy Society" fulfill these *mitzvot*.

Chumash: Another name for the Torah.

Eretz Yisrael: Hebrew phrase meaning the land of Israel.

Kaballah: Traditional term for mysticism in Judaism, which is very normative.

Kaddish: "Mourners' prayer" recited daily by those who have recently lost a loved one or who are marking the anniversary of a loved one's death. The prayer (which means "sanctification of") has no mention death in it, but rather its contents are doxology or praises to God.

kashrut: Refers to Jewish laws of keeping kosher; these laws (which pertain to animals, fowl and sea life) regulate what foods are permitted to be eaten and how they are to be prepared.

kohanim: Orthodox Jewish men who can trace their lineage to the priests who served in the Temple, dating from the Aaronic Priesthood. *Kohanim* are forbidden to come in contact with dead bodies, nor are they permitted to perform the customary mourning rites. They are commanded, however, to become "defiled" for their closest relatives: father, mother, brother, unmarried sister, child, or wife. Some *kohanim*, today, continue to observe these laws.

Mi-Shebeirakh: "Prayer of healing" recited during services or at a bedside of someone ill; the prayer calls upon God to hear the prayer of those asking for healing blessings for the ill.

mitzvot: Commandments (613 in the Torah) that include both ethical behavior and the observance of rituals; *Mitzvah* also connotes a good deed which may not be the specific fulfillment of a commandment.

mohel: Person trained in the procedure (medically and religiously) who performs the ritual circumcision, which is usually conducted in the home or synagogue.

pareve: Food prepared without meat, milk, or their derivatives and therefore permissible to be eaten with both meat and dairy dishes according to dietary laws.

Shema: Section of the Torah (Deut. 6:4–6) that come the closest to being a Jewish credo; it derives its name from the first word in the Hebrew text, *Shema*, which means "hear."

Tikkun olam: Hebrew phrase which means "repairing the world"; Judaism stresses life and healing and believes God created humans, endowed with gifts to bring about positive change in the world. The traditional Jewish toast "*le chaim*" (To life!) confirms this concept.

Torah: Five books of Moses in the Hebrew Bible; also referred to as the Pentateuch.

Yiddish: One of the major spoken and written languages of the Jewish people; even though Germanic in origin, Yiddish is written in Hebrew and from right to left.

Paganism

Prepared by:
Caroline Baughman
Priestess, Member of Gaia Community
Pagan Representative on the Greater Kansas City
** Interfaith Council**
Merriam, KS

Reviewed and approved by:
Mike Nichols
Priest, Founding Member of Coven of New Gwynedd
** and**
First Wiccan member on the Greater Kansas City
** Interfaith Council**
Kansas City, MO

History and Facts

Paganism is a term that dates from antiquity with a variety of meanings.[354] The operative meaning of Paganism for this paper is Neo-Paganism which can be described as a "twentieth-century revival of interest in the worship of nature, fertility, and so forth, as represented by various deities."[355] Therefore, paganism is understood as an umbrella term that encompasses many traditions and personal belief systems with no one founder or individual point of origin. The Paganism of today draws on the wisdom of both modern and ancient teaching traditions. The term "tradition" (or path) in Paganism refers to either a preestablished set of beliefs that provide spiritual meaning and structure (e.g., Druid, Wiccan, Dianic) or an individualized set of beliefs that provide spiritual meaning. However, a specific tradition may trace its lineage back to a particular place or person because many traditions of Paganism are "reconstructionist" faiths of their ancient historical counterparts (e.g., Druids associated with the British Isles; Kemetic Orthodox associated with Egypt; Hellenic associated with Greece; Asatru associated with the Germanic region; Gardnarian Wicca/Alexandrian Wicca associated with England; and Eclectic associated with beliefs inspired from many sources). The various paths will be discussed later in the chapter.

The understanding of deity in Paganism varies. Some traditions are polytheistic (belief in many gods); others are monotheistic (belief in one god). Still others are monistic (belief in a single guiding force) or animistic, which is understood in multiple ways: (1) belief in the existence of individual spirits that inhabit natural objects and phenomena – including rocks, trees, water, animals; (2) belief in the existence of spiritual beings that are separable or

---

354 *The American Heritage® Dictionary of the English Language*, Fourth Edition, defines paganism thusly:

Middle English, from Late Latin pāgānus, from Latin, *country-dweller*, from pāgus, *civilian*, *country*, rural district; "a member of a group professing a polytheistic religion or any religion other than Christianity, Judaism, or Islam."

Retrieved February 21, 2008, from Dictionary.com website: http://dictionary.reference.com/browse/paganism.

355 Dictionary.com Unabridged (v 1.1). Based on the *Random House Unabridged Dictionary*©, Random House, Inc., 2006. Available at: http://dictionary.reference.com/browse/neopagan.

separate from bodies; and (3) hypothesis holding that an immaterial force animates the universe.[356] Yet other traditions are pan-entheistic (belief that God is the universe, and yet more than the universe; God has an identity of his own separate from the universe), pantheistic (belief that God and the universe are identical) or duotheistic (belief that God is comprised of two deities, usually male and female counterparts; often called: "The God and The Goddess" or "The Lord and The Lady").

Pagans identify themselves in ways similar to more common faith traditions. For example, in the Christian faith, believers often refer to themselves as "Christian" and/or by a specific denomination, such as "Methodist." Similarly, in Paganism, devotees may identify themselves as Pagan (or Neo-Pagan to distinguish themselves from the pagans of early history) and/or by a specific tradition name, such as Wiccan. Beyond identifying a particular faith and path, a Pagan may also call himself/herself a Witch as a positive, affirmation of faith. Unfortunately, in common, modern-day parlance, the term "witch" often has a pejorative connotation. Historically, though, the word "witch" has not always had a negative connotation. For instance, it was a common practice in earlier times to refer to the village herbalist or midwife as either a "witch" or a "wise woman." As Reginald Scot says in his *Discoverie of Witchcraft*,[357] "At this day it is indifferent to say in the English tongue, 'she is a witch,' or 'she is a wise woman.'"

Furthermore, some individuals, many of whom have completed a great deal of self study and/or training, are identified as Priest or Priestess. This title may be one of self-bestowal or it may be received from another individual or group. For example, a member of a Gardnerian Wiccan Coven (coven is defined as a dedicated group of Wiccans who meet regularly to study, celebrate and worship) would go through a year and a day training to receive their "first degree" initiation. There are typically three degrees that may be attained. A third degree initiate, for example, may then start a coven.

Additionally, many Pagans have what is called a "magickal" name (Pagans sometimes spell magic as magick to differentiate their spiritual practice from slight of hand tricks). Magickal names are sacred and special, often known only to the individual or a select group. For some, their magickal names are never to be spoken aloud, only to be known by the gods. For others, it is a name of power, a name to be used during ritual observances. And for yet others, it may be adopted as their mundane, every day name. Some of these names may be preceded by the title Lady or Lord, which often must be earned within a particular tradition. Magickal names are also often comprised of the names of symbols, colors,

---

356 Definitions of animism cited from *American Heritage Dictionary*. Available at: http://dictionary. reference.com/browse/animism.

357 Scot, R. (1584). *The Discoverie of Witchcraft*. London. Quoted in: Newman, K. (1991). *Fashioning Femininity and English Renaissance Drama*. Chicago, IL: University of Chicago Press, 55. In the midst of an intense fervor of hatred and fear of witches perpetuated by the popes, Scot wrote to address the abuses of women suspected of being witches in sixteenth-century England; he made it a personal mission to "right the wrong." His book was widely read and exerted a strong influence on many, especially upon those who disagreed with him – principal among these was James Stuart, who attacked Scot in his 1597 *Demonology*; Stuart later became King James I of England and authorized the 1611 translation of the Bible commonly called the King James Bible. (Jeffers, S. 1989. *The Cultural Power of Occult Words: Occult Terminology in the Hebrew, Greek, Latin and English Bibles*, unpublished doctoral dissertation, 157–159.

plants, animals, and or deity names (e.g., Star, Bear, Lavender Moon, Persephone).

It is difficult to say that every Pagan believes "this or that." Paganism is a highly personal spiritual path. For some, it is a return to the Divine Feminine or Goddess Worship. For many, it is an acknowledgment that nature itself is Holy. Based on this understanding, Paganism is sometimes called "Nature-Based Religions." Margot Adler stated this succinctly in her book *Drawing Down the Moon.*[358]

> The world is holy. Nature is holy. The body is holy. Sexuality is holy. The mind is holy. The imagination is holy. You are holy. A spiritual path that is not stagnant ultimately leads one to the understanding of one's own divine nature. Thou art Goddess. Thou art God. Divinity is imminent in all Nature.
>
> It is as much within you as without.

Unfortunately, Paganism is often misunderstood by many in the general population, sometimes to the point of Pagans being treated unfairly because of their faith. It has been reported that Pagans have lost jobs, custody of children and been shunned by family when there faith is known. As a result of these and other forms of discrimination, some Pagans do not desire, often for fear of negative reprisal or personal safety, to publicize their faith. Hopefully, through education about Paganism, the public will become more aware and respectful of Paganism as a legitimate faith tradition among the many others in society.

According to the national organization Pagan Pride, in 1998 there were more than 450 000 self-identified Pagans in the United States. It is unknown what the worldwide number of Pagans (as defined in this chapter) might be. This lack of data is primarily due to there being no "worldwide" definition of Neo-Paganism.

Within Paganism, the most common tradition is Wicca,[359] in which the understanding of deity varies. For example, Gardnerian Wicca (popularized by Gerald Gardner in the 1950s) values balance between the male and female deities: both the God and the Goddess are worshipped. However, in Dianic Wicca, the focus is primarily upon the feminine aspect of deity. (The website www.witchvox.com, a well-respected online resource, lists 60 different traditions.) Wicca will be discussed in more detail shortly.

Wicca is a "folk" religion as opposed to an organized religion. It lacks many of the constructs of organized religions, such as a historical founder, set of sacred scriptures, single approach to liturgy, even a single creed.

Wicca is characterized by the view that nature itself is sacred and that time is more cyclical than linear. In its most popular form, it is duotheistic, although polytheistic forms are also common. It is seen as a religion of clergy with no laity, with each practitioner seen as a Priest or Priestess. Its rituals may be practiced anywhere (indoors or outdoors) because all places are seen as sacred. Individuals may practice alone as a "Solitary" (as a comparison, a Christian may not join a church) or in groups as with a Coven, which are typically no more than thirteen members.[360] While there are

---

358 Adler, M. (1986). *Drawing Down the Moon.* New York, NY: Penguin Books, preface ix.

359 Because of the large number of traditions and dynamic variations in beliefs, the authors have chosen to focus on Wicca for the purposes of this document.

360 A coven will most likely split and form another one

Christian churches with members in the dozens to members in the thousands, Pagan groups are inherently cellular and intimate (small). Larger groups may gather to publicly celebrate holidays or to participate in common rituals such as marriage or death. Basic practices are detailed shortly.

Basic Teachings

From the author's experience and study of Paganism, the following are the most broadly and commonly held tenets. However, it should be noted that not all Pagans follow all of these teachings.

- **All is Sacred.** Everything – all individuals, plants, animals, tools, items – is sacred and has inherent value and worth.
- **All is Connected.** A metaphor used to commonly understand this concept is a spider's web. Any movement or disturbance anywhere on the spider's web is felt throughout the whole web.
- **Harm None.** Simply put, one should live life in such a way that does not cause harm to another including oneself.
- **The Three-Fold Law.** Any action people take will come back to them three fold.
- **Magic.** This concept is akin to prayer, but often uses specific tools or techniques (*see* "Basic Practices" section) and may also be called, energy work, spell work or magick. Because of the concepts of "harm none" and the "three-fold law," Pagans typically only use magick for positive ends, such as healing, prosperity, and self actualization.
- **Immanent Divinity.** The divine, is not to be worshipped from afar. He/She/They reside within us and around us.

- **Personal Searching.** It is expected that individuals will either identify with a specific established tradition or develop their own personalized path. Personal responsibility is highly valued and promoted. Paganism and its many traditions are non-evangelical.
- **Common Symbols of Paganism:**[361]
  - *Pentacle*: Five-pointed star within a circle.

This symbol is often used as a symbol of protection. It also is widely recognized as representative of the elements: earth, air, fire, and water with the top most point representing spirit (a pentagram refers to the same star discussed earlier, without the surrounding circle).
  - *Triple Moon*: Three phases of the moon.

This symbol of the phases of the moon is used as a metaphor for the phases of life: waxing (youth), full (midlife), and waning (elder years).
  - *Triskele*: Triple spiral

---

if more than thirteen members become involved in one coven. Furthermore, an individual will likely only become a member of one coven at a time.

361 http://paganwiccan.about.com/od/bookof shadows/ig/Pagan-and-Wiccan-Symbols/. (accessed 22 Sept 2012).

This symbol of Death, Rebirth, and Life is also recognized as a triple representation of the Goddess, specifically a Wiccan symbol identifying the three main phases of a woman's life and fertility: *Maiden* (premenarche), *Mother*, and *Crone* (postmenopausal). These phases correspond with the triple moon symbol.

- **Correspondences**: Many Pagans believe that everything in the world has inherent attributes which help define its purpose and use. Plants, animals, crystals and stones, planets, deities, colors, times of day, and days of the week, just to name a few all have attributes. The concept of correspondences may be more easily understood through a discussion of the directions or "quarters."

- **Directions or "Quarters"**: How an individual associates with each quarter may be very personal. Many traditions have their own understanding of and correspondences for each direction. The example given here is from the Wiccan tradition. Because Wicca is so influential in American Paganism, many traditions practiced in America may have a similar understanding through different associated correspondences to those listed here. To illustrate one notable difference, some traditions such as the Druidic tradition do not honor the four directions. Instead, they honor Land, Sea, and Sky. Described in the table here are commonly held associations for each direction. For each direction, a list of correspondences follows: (other correspondences that could be listed are plants, animals, planets, deities, and so forth).

- **Wheel of the Year**: The natural cycle of the seasons, commemorated by the eight Sabbats (one of the eight major seasonal festivals that make up the Wheel of the Year), include the solstices, equinoxes and four additional festivals, sometimes referred to as the "cross-quarter days." The Wheel of the Year concept is based on the belief that the passing of time is a continuous cycle, like a wheel which turns and turns. The course of birth, life, decline, and death in human beings' lives is echoed in the change of the seasons in the natural world:
  - spring: birth, a time to begin new projects
  - summer: growth, a time dedicated to work toward attaining goals
  - autumn: harvest, a time to reap what has been sown
  - winter: death and rebirth, a time to reflect on the previous year and to gather resources for the following year.

- For spiritual holy days *see* "Special Days: Paganism" section.

Direction	Element	Personal Attribute	Ritual Tool	Time of Day	Season	Phase of Life
North	Earth	Body/Strength	Cauldron	Midnight	Winter	Death and Rebirth
East	Air	Mind/Intellect	Athame (ritual dagger)	Dawn	Spring	Birth and Youth
South	Fire	Spirit or Sexual self/ Passion	Wand	Noon	Summer	"Prime of life"
West	Water	Heart/Emotion	Chalice	Sunset	Autumn	Elder years

Basic Practices

- Individuals, groups and covens often have their own personal collections of liturgy. This liturgy may be kept in a book called a Book of Shadows.
- Rites of passage are honored and celebrated, including but not limited to: birth, puberty, pregnancy, menopause, aging, death. (Please see the sections "During Birth" and "During End of Life" for a few examples of types of rituals.)
- Life is experienced holistically (not split between mind and body or spirit and matter, for example).
- Ceremony and rituals are highly personal for an individual or group. They may be planned in detail with full liturgy or impromptu happenings filled with "divine inspiration."
- Tools: most tools have both practical and symbolic uses. For example, a cauldron is both a feminine symbol and a tool for cooking.
  - Cauldron: usually a cast iron pot or bowl, traditionally with three legs and a handle. Symbolically, it represents the womb of the mother goddess or a well of mysteries (it may be used to burn incense, cook food, contain fire or water).
  - Athame: usually a black hilted knife or small dagger. Symbolically, it represents all that is masculine.
  - Chalice: a cup, often stemmed. Symbolically, it represents all that is feminine.
  - Wand: a wooden stick, traditionally the length from one's elbow to one's longest finger; often made from oak, ash, willow, or apple, but could be made from any wood. Symbolically, it is used to concentrate the user's thoughts and energy.
  - Candles: used in a practical sense to provide light and may represent many things or be lit in honor of a particular deity, idea, desire or remembrance.
- Altar: An example of an altar arrangement is shown here. ("Lamp of Art" is an archaic term meaning "altar candle.")

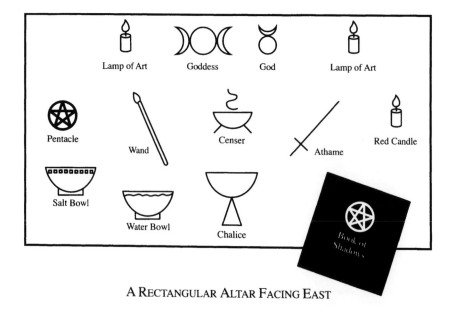

A RECTANGULAR ALTAR FACING EAST

- Symbols: *See* symbols listed earlier.
- Sacred items: Any object may be viewed (and therefore used) as sacred. Jewelry gemstones are favored items for magickal use. As indicated in the "correspondences," table gemstones are commonly understood to have their own properties. For example:
  - amber: protection, solar energy (fire)
  - amethyst: dreams, relieves stress, imagination and meditation
  - citrine: healing, increased physical energy, hope, encourages new beginnings
  - hematite: absorbing and grounding negative energy, balances energy
  - moonstone: lunar energy, psychic matters, clarity of thought (water)
  - obsidian: inner strength, protection (earth)
  - quartz: focusing energy for any purpose (air)
  - rose quartz: love, friendship, joy, self-healing
  - tiger eye: protection, balance, meditation

  (In the context of medical healing, a person may choose to wear or keep close by a gemstone(s) such as amber to protect from infection, citrine to boost their physical energy, amethyst to calm their worries and rose quartz to improve their own body's ability to self-heal.)
- Celebrate spiritual holy days as listed in "Special Days: Paganism" section.

Principles for Clinical Care
Dietary Issues

- There are no specific dietary rules associated with Paganism. Individuals identify their own dietary needs and/or preferences.

General Medical Beliefs

- There is no specific Pagan doctrine regarding medical beliefs or treatment.
- Individuals should be asked about their beliefs regarding the use of Western medical technology.
- Some Pagans may seek alternative therapies including but not limited to prayer, magick, energetic healing or reiki, herbalism, massage, and homeopathy. These therapies may be sought in conjunction with Western medical treatment or separately.
- Use of herbal treatments is fairly common among Pagans.

Specific Medical Issues

- **Abortion**: Individuals should be asked their own beliefs regarding abortion.
- **Advance Directives**: Individuals should be asked their own beliefs regarding use of advance directives in health care planning.
- **Birth Control**: Paganism does not have a specific position on birth control. It is a decision of the individual or couple.
- **Blood Transfusions**: Individuals should be asked their own beliefs regarding the use of blood products (e.g., blood transfusions).
- **Circumcision**: There is no Pagan doctrine regarding male circumcision. However, some Pagans may view male circumcision as mutilation. Female circumcision is considered to be mutilation and is not practiced.
- **In Vitro Fertilization**: Individuals should be asked their own beliefs regarding in vitro fertilization.
- **Stem Cell Research**: Individuals should be asked their own beliefs regarding stem cell research for therapeutic purposes.
- **Vaccinations**: There is no Pagan doctrine

regarding vaccinations. It is an individual decision.

- **Withholding/Withdrawing Life Support**: Individuals should be asked their own beliefs regarding withholding/withdrawing life support in medically futile cases.

Gender and Personal Issues

- There are no specific doctrines regarding gender, gender identity, or personal issues.
- All sexual orientations and gender identities are recognized and accepted among Pagans.
- It is up to each individual to identify preferences regarding gender of care provider.
- Modesty varies widely from person to person. Some Pagans are very modest while others are considerably less concerned about modesty issues.

Principles for Spiritual Care through the Cycles of Life
Concepts of Living and Dying for Spiritual support

- Life is a cycle.
- Death is a rite of passage.
- Many pagans believe in reincarnation or at least a very specific afterlife including but not limited to Summerland, Isle of the Blessed, Valhalla, and Heaven.
- Many pagans believe that the Wheel of the Year mirrors life experience for the cycle of birth to death.
- Because of this common belief in reincarnation and understanding of the Wheel of the Year as a symbol of their life cycle, death may not be feared but seen as a natural progression of the life cycle.

During Birth

- Ask the patient or family their preferences.
- There are no spiritual rules about medical interventions during the birthing process. A generalization can be made that Pagan women may be interested in having as natural a birth as possible.
- Celebrations and rituals vary from individual/group to individual/group for all cycles of life.
- A Blessingway ceremony may be held for the mother. It is celebration of her life and her (usually female) family's and friends' commitment to help her in whatever way she needs. The focus is on the mother to be and her needs and fears regarding her transition into motherhood. This ceremony is likely to be held prior to the birth and not in the hospital.
- A Wiccaning or other Blessing ceremony is held for the child once it is born. A Wiccaning is typically a naming ceremony for the infant and may be public or private. Whoever is present may be asked to express wishes they have for the child or to bring a symbolic gift to represent those wishes. The ceremony is primarily meant for the parents to present the child to the world. A God/dess Parent may be named at this time. A Wiccaning would likely not take place in a hospital; rather, the parents would host it once they were home and recovered from the birth. The following is a common blessing for a baby. The "waves" are a reference to the Goddess Brigid's sacred flame.

The Midwife's Blessing[362]
A small wave for your form

---

362 Oman, M. ed. (1997). *Prayers for Healing: 365 Blessings, Poems and Meditations from Around the World*. (prayer cited was written by Mahiri nic Neill). Berkley, CA: Conari Press, 142–143; also

A small wave for your voice
A small wave for your speech
A small wave for your means
A small wave for your generosity
A small wave for your appetite
A small wave for your wealth
A small wave for your life
A small wave for your health
Nine waves of grace upon you,
Waves of the Giver of Health.

(*This blessing could be performed in the hospital.*)

- As stated earlier, there is no Pagan doctrine regarding male circumcision. Some Pagans, however, may view male circumcision as mutilation. Female circumcision is considered to be mutilation and is not practiced.
- Pagan women may be interested in any of the following (it is important to ask about individual preferences):
  ○ natural birthing process
  ○ home birthing
  ○ minimal medical interventions
  ○ doula supported birth:

  A doula who accompanies a woman in labor mothers the mother, taking care of her emotional needs throughout childbirth. A doula also provides support and suggestions for partners that can enhance their experiences of birth. A postpartum doula continues that valuable emotional support and guidance,

helping a family make a smooth transition into new family dynamics.[363]

  ○ Using alternative pain control such as meditation, singing, or chanting
  ○ Breast-feeding.
- It is recommended that health care professionals ask the patient and family what priorities they have and how best they can support them during this time.
- If a patient has openly shared that they are Pagan with their health care provider, it would be sensitive of that practitioner to find out if the patient is a solitary practitioner (not associated with a group or coven) or if they would like an individual, such as a Priest or Priestess, or a group such as a spiritual community or coven, to be contacted on their behalf.
- In the case of fetal demise or death of a baby, there is no set Pagan ceremony or ritual. Health care professionals should ask patients how they might wish to spiritually recognize such an event.

During Illness

- The spiritual needs and desires of Pagan patients will vary greatly by individual.
- Ask the patient or family their preferences.
- Some Pagans may have a Priest or Priestess in their community with whom they may wish to speak or notify of their illness.
- Not all Pagans are open about their faith. Be aware that Pagan patients may not be from a Pagan family and may wish to keep their faith private.
- A Pagan patient may seem to have two "families": a "biological family" and a

available at: http://books.google.com/books?id=bN2AiDImffEC&pg=PA142&lpg=PA142&dq=%22a+small+wave+for+your+form%22&source=web&ots=qswxNTshzU&sig=zesR4UIk1t14k_FeC-hj-4zrqWE&hl=en#PPA142,M1. (accessed 22 Sept 2012).

363 Quote obtained from Doulas of North America (DONA International), available at: www.dona.org/mothers/index.php. (accessed 22 September 2012).

"chosen family," both of which should be treated with equal respect. The chosen family members are considered spiritual sisters, brothers, mothers, fathers, and so forth.

- If patients do indicate they are Pagan, never assume that their family is aware of their beliefs.
- Many Pagans associate with a particular deity in whom they find support in prayer; they worship using a small altar with symbols that represent their faith.
- Many Pagans believe in energetic healing such as reiki (a system of hands-on touching based on the belief that such touching by an experienced practitioner produces beneficial effects by strengthening and normalizing certain vital energy fields believed to exist within the body), therapeutic touch, laying on of hands, and so forth.
- A Pagan patient may wish to have a Priestess or Priest from their group or coven present.
- Always ask permission from patient or family before administering any type of spiritual care: counseling, prayer, and so forth.
- Pagan patients may not be comfortable discussing their faith with an "outsider."
- A Pagan patient may reject conversing with a hospital chaplain for fear of being evangelized.
- It is recommended that health care professionals ask the patient and family what priorities they have and how best they can support them during this time. For example, knowing if the patient is a "solitary" or if they would like an individual, such as a Priest or Priestess, or a group such as a spiritual community or coven, to be contacted on their behalf.

During End of Life

- Same considerations as those in the "During Illness" section.
- Be aware that the patient and patient's biological family may have very different spiritual ideas about the meaning of death.
- It may be important for Pagans to be as conscious as possible during the transition to death. For many, death is seen as a transition, not an ending and having conscious awareness of the transition may be valued.
- There is no Pagan doctrine regarding viewing of the body in the hospital. Ask patient or family preferences.
- It is recommended that health care professionals ask the patient and family what priorities they have and how best they can support them during this time. For example, knowing if the patient is a "solitary" or if they would like an individual, such as a Priest or Priestess, or a group such as a spiritual community or coven, to be contacted on their behalf.

Care of Body

- Ask family members for their preferences.
- Have a compassionate awareness for the possibility of a discrepancy between beliefs of the patient's biological and chosen family.
- Embalming and disposition are individual decisions.
- Ask the patient or family members regarding donation of the body for medical research.

Organ and Tissue Donation

- An individual decision; check with family concerning preferences.

Scriptures, Inspirational Readings, and Prayers

These readings are not associated with any particular point in the life cycle, illness, healing, or end-of-life process. They may be used at any time.

Circle Closing[364]

By the earth that is her body
And the grove that is his home
By the air of her breath
And the music of his song
By the fire of her bright spirit
And the heat of his passion
By the water of her living womb
And the dew of his tears
The circle is open but unbroken
May the peace of the Goddess go in
  our hearts
And the dance of the God enliven our
  days
Merry Meet, Merry Part and Merry
  Meet Again.

LITURGY

Charge of the Goddess

Listen to the words of the Great
  Mother, Who of old was called
  Artemis, Astarte, Dione, Melusine,
  Aphrodite, Cerridwen, Diana,
  Arionrhod, Brigid, and by many
  other names:
Whenever you have need of anything,
  once a month, and better it be when
  the moon is full, you shall assemble
  in some secret place and adore the
  spirit of Me Who is Queen of all the
  Wise.

You shall be free from slavery, and as
  a sign that you be free you shall be
  naked in your rites.
Sing, feast, dance, make music and
  love, all in My Presence, for Mine
  is the ecstasy of the spirit and Mine
  also is joy on earth.
For My law is love is unto all beings.
  Mine is the secret that opens the
  door of youth, and Mine is the cup
  of wine of life that is the cauldron of
  Cerridwen, that is the holy grail of
  immortality.
I give the knowledge of the spirit
  eternal, and beyond death I give
  peace and freedom and reunion with
  those that have gone before.
Nor do I demand aught of sacrifice,
  for behold, I am the Mother of all
  things and My love is poured out
  upon the earth.
Hear the words of the Star Goddess,
  the dust of Whose feet are the hosts
  of Heaven, whose body encircles the
  universe:
I Who am the beauty of the green
  earth and the white moon among
  the stars and the mysteries of the
  waters,
I call upon your soul to arise and
  come unto me.
For I am the soul of nature that gives
  life to the universe.
From Me all things proceed and unto
  Me they must return.
Let My worship be in the heart that
  rejoices, for behold,
all acts of love and pleasure are My
  rituals.
Let there be beauty and strength,
  power and compassion, honor and
  humility, mirth and reverence within
  you.

---

364 Provided by the author from memory; it has a long history from oral tradition in Paganism, the original author of which is unknown.

And you who seek to know Me, know that the seeking and yearning will avail you not, unless you know the Mystery: for if that which you seek, you find not within yourself, you will never find it without.

For behold, I have been with you from the beginning, and I am That which is attained at the end of desire.

—Traditional by Doreen Valiente, as adapted by Starhawk[365]

Special Days: Paganism

Dates of spiritual holy days listed here are for the northern hemisphere, as they are meant to correspond with the seasons. Please note that all holidays begin at sundown of the preceding date given.

November 1 *Samhain* – "SOW-in" marks autumn's end. This is widely recognized as the Pagan "New Year." It is a time to honor ancestors and those who have died in the preceding year.

On or near December 21 *Yule* – This is the winter solstice. On this longest night of the year, Pagans may celebrate by: extinguishing all lights as the sun sets the night before, sitting vigil and waiting for sunrise, welcoming the sun as it rises the following morning.

February 1 *Imbolg/Imbolc* – "IM-bolk" is the halfway point between the Winter Solstice and the Spring Equinox. It is widely recognized as a day dedicated to the Celtic Goddess Brigid, and recognizes the beginning of spring.

On or near March 21 *Ostara* – "Oh-STAR-ah" is the Spring Equinox. It is named for a maiden goddess of spring and is a celebration of new love and growth.

May 1 *Beltane/Bealtaine* – "BELL-tane" is also known as May Day. As weather warms and spring turns to summer, it is a time to celebrate the fertility of life. Many Pagans celebrate this by dancing the may poll.

On or near June 21 *Litha* – "LEE-thah" is the summer solstice, the longest day of the year; it is also known as midsummer.

August 1 *Lughnasadh/Lunasa* or *Lammas* – "LOO-nah-sah" or "LAH-mus" is the feast of the Celtic god Lugh and is the first "harvest" festival. It is the beginning of the harvest season, a time to celebrate the fruits of one's labor.

365 www.reclaiming.org/about/witchfaq/charge.html

On or near September 21 *Mabon* – "MAH-bun" is the autumn equinox and second harvest festival. Days are getting shorter as winter approaches. It is time to take stock of what has been accomplished and what yet still needs to be done before the reflective time of winter arrives.

Church of Scientology

*The true story of Scientology is simple, concise and direct. It is quickly
told: A philosopher develops a philosophy about life and death;*

People find it interesting; People find it works;

People pass it along to others; and it grows.[366]

Prepared by:
Church of Scientology International
Los Angeles, CA

History and Facts

Lafayette Ronald Hubbard, respectfully referred to as Ron or LRH, is the Founder of the Scientology religion. He was born on March 13, 1911 in Tilden, Nebraska, the son of naval commander Harry Ross Hubbard and Ledora May Hubbard. At 12 years of age, the inquisitive Ron had his first introduction to the principles of Freudian psychoanalysis through his friendship with US Navy Commander John C. Thompson, MD, whom he met on a 1923 sea voyage from the Pacific Coast to Washington, DC, and who took the inquisitive young man under his wing. In 1927, at the age of 16, young Ron took the first of his several trips across the Pacific Ocean during which time he began to study Far Eastern cultures. His time spent in the company of monks and Chinese elders proved an invaluable experience in his quest to find answers to the human dilemma. By the age of 19, long before the advent of commercial flight, Mr. Hubbard had traveled more than a quarter of a million miles, including voyages not only to China, but also to Japan, Guam, and the Philippines.

While attending George Washington University, Mr. Hubbard embarked on a personal search for answers to the questions about man's existence and spiritual

---

366 Hubbard L. R. (2007). *Scientology: A New Slant on Life.* Los Angeles, CA: Bridge Publications, 15.

potential. Ron left his university studies in 1932, determined that the answers he sought did not reside in the halls of academia. He continued his research, while funding it through a successful career writing for the pulp magazines and for Hollywood. His research, though, was interrupted by World War II, in which he served as a lieutenant (junior grade) in the US Navy. Applying the basic principles of Dianetics he developed in the closing months of the War, he aided other injured soldiers in the recovery process. By 1949, he had recovered from his own combat wounds and published his original thesis of Dianetics. The first full text on the subject, *Dianetics, the Modern Science of Mental Health*, released on May 9, 1950, has become the most successful self-help book ever published, selling over 21 million copies in 52 languages. (In 2006, *The Guinness Book of World Records* named L. Ron Hubbard the world's most widely translated author.)

Within a year and a half of the release of *Dianetics*, Mr. Hubbard embarked upon another journey of discovery – entering the realm of the human spirit. The outgrowth of this journey was the birth of the Scientology religion in 1952: a modern religion to give modern mankind a route to higher levels of awareness, understanding, and ability, memorialized in a lecture by Mr. Hubbard on March 3, 1952 entitled "Scientology: Milestone One." The first Church of Scientology was incorporated on February 18, 1954 by several students of Mr. Hubbard. In the following years, through his writings and lectures, Mr. Hubbard continued to make his discoveries available to those who sought answers. This resulted in a rapid expansion of Scientology churches around the world – in the United States, Canada, Australia, the United Kingdom, Europe,

and South Africa. On September 1, 1966, with Scientology established as a worldwide religion, Mr. Hubbard resigned his position as Executive Director of the Church and stepped down from all boards of all Church corporations in order to fully devote himself to research.

On January 24, 1986, having fully completed his research and with Scientology in broad application on five continents and in over 60 countries, L. Ron Hubbard departed this life. The legacy of his life's work continues in the religion he founded. Its principles are based wholly upon his research, 35 million words of writings and recorded lectures; the collection of these materials constitutes Scientology's scripture.

At this point, one might be tempted to ask several questions: "How is L. Ron Hubbard viewed by Scientologists as the founder of the religion? Is he considered a highly-exalted prophet like Moses, Buddha, Muhammad, Bahá'u'lláh or even considered divine as Jesus of Christianity?" The answer to those questions is that Scientologists do revere Mr. Hubbard and consider him to be mankind's greatest friend. However, he was simply a mere man, not a prophet or a divine being.

Now, in order to more fully understand Scientology and the succeeding sections, the following paragraphs about Mr. Hubbard's writings provide a basic foundation covering *Dianetics, the Modern Science of Mental Health* and the transition to the religion of Scientology, which is clearly delineated in an essay entitled *My Philosophy*.

Dianetics

L. Ron Hubbard's path to the founding of the Scientology religion began with certain discoveries he made in his research into the nature of man. He announced his findings in 1948 as "Dianetics," a word that means "through the soul" or what the spirit is doing to the body through the mind.

With Dianetics, Mr. Hubbard discovered a previously unknown and harmful part of the mind that contains recordings of past experiences of loss, pain, and unconsciousness in the form of mental image pictures. These incidents of spiritual trauma are recorded along with all other experiences of one's life in sequential order on what he termed the "time track." The painful incidents recorded on this time track exist below a person's level of awareness and collectively accumulate to make up what is called the "reactive mind," the source of all unwanted fears, emotions, as well as psychosomatic pains and illnesses – as distinct from the "analytical mind," that portion of the mind which a person uses to think, observes data, remember it and resolve problems.

Dianetics provides a method to address the reactive mind by uncovering this previously unknown spiritual trauma and erasing its harmful effects on an individual. When this occurs, one has achieved a new state of spiritual awareness called "Clear." On achieving the state of "Clear" one's basic and fundamental personality, artistry, individual character, inherent goodness, and decency are all restored.

Scientology

The breakthrough from Dianetics to Scientology came in the autumn of 1951, after Mr. Hubbard observed many people practicing Dianetics' techniques and found a commonality of experience and phenomena which were of a profoundly spiritual nature – contact with past life experiences. Mr. Hubbard emphasized in his work that man IS a spiritual being, who has a mind and a body.

Awareness of the human spirit has existed as a universal ingredient of almost every religion in every culture. However, words such as "spirit" and "soul" were encumbered by centuries of misunderstanding the interpretations of these terms. Mr. Hubbard felt that a new word was needed to clarify the human spiritual nature. Therefore, he adopted the Greek letter *theta* (θ), which he had assigned in 1950 to represent the transcendent "life force." By adding an "n," the word *thetan* was "coined" as the term used to describe the spiritual essence of humankind.

My Philosophy

L. Ron Hubbard 1965[367]

The subject of philosophy is very ancient. The word means: "The love, study or pursuit of wisdom, or of knowledge of things and their causes, whether theoretical or practical."

All we know of science or of religion comes from philosophy. It lies behind and above all other knowledge we have or use …

The first principle of my own philosophy is that wisdom is meant for anyone who wishes to reach for it. It is the servant of the commoner and king alike and should never be regarded with awe …

The second principle of my own philosophy is that it must be capable of being applied.

Learning locked in mildewed books is of little use to anyone and therefore of no value unless it can be used.

The third principle is that any philosophic knowledge is only valuable if it is true or if it works.

These three principles are so strange to

---

367 Compiled by staff of the Church of Scientology International. (1998). *What is Scientology?* Los Angeles, CA: Bridge Publications, 720.

the field of philosophy, that I have given my philosophy a name: SCIENTOLOGY. This means only "knowing how to know."

… man likes to be happy and well. He likes to be able to understand things, and he knows his route to freedom lies through knowledge.

Therefore, for 15 years I have had mankind knocking on my door. It has not mattered where I have lived or how remote, since I first published a book on the subject my life has no longer been my own.

I like to help others and count it as my greatest pleasure in life to see a person free himself of the shadows which darken his days.

These shadows look so thick to him and weigh him down so that when he finds they are shadows and that he can see through them, walk through them and be again in the sun, he is enormously delighted. And I am afraid I am just as delighted as he is.

… If things were a little better known and understood, we would all lead happier lives.

And there is a way to know them and there is a way to freedom.

The old must give way to the new, falsehood must become exposed by truth, and truth, though fought, always in the end prevails.

In one form or another, all of the world's religious traditions offer the hope of spiritual freedom – a condition free of material limitations and suffering. Scientology offers a very practical approach to attaining this spiritual aim. Of this, L. Ron Hubbard wrote,

For countless ages a goal of religion has been the salvage of the human spirit. Man has tried by many practices to find the pathway to salvation. He has held the imperishable hope that someday in some way he would be free.

Mr. Hubbard continued, "And here, after these ages of grief and suffering, through terrible wars and catastrophe, the hope still lives – and with that hope, accomplishment."[368] Thus, while the hope for such freedom comes from ancient sources, what Scientology is doing to bring about that freedom is modern. And the technologies with which it can bring about a new state of being in man are likewise new.

In the wider arena, through the spiritual salvation of the individual, Scientology seeks the ultimate transformation – a civilization without insanity, without criminals and without war, where the able can prosper and honest beings can have rights, and where man is free to rise to greater heights. By 2010, there were over 8500 Scientology churches, missions, related organizations, groups, and activities spanning the globe, ministering to millions of people in 165 countries in over 50 languages, with approximately one third of that number in the United States. And these numbers continue to rise.

Basic Teachings

Even though Scientology was born in the West, and its beliefs are expressed in the technological language of the late twentieth century, Scientology owes a debt to some of the Eastern faiths of antiquity. For example, in the Vedas (the sacred scriptures of Hinduism), one finds a statement on the distinctions among spirit, mind and body as well as the concept of a Creator or Supreme Being (Hymn of Creation, Riga Veda X.129, Naasdeeya Sooktam). Scientology's

---

368 Hubbard, L. (1965). *The Golden Dawn*. East Grinstead, England: Church of Scientology. No page numbers.

understanding of *thetan* is consistent with the Hindu belief of *atman* (Sanskrit, translated as "soul") which is eternal.

Similarly, Mr. Hubbard embraced the Buddhist concepts that a person can achieve personal enlightenment through one's own efforts; that right conduct is essential to higher states of existence; and that the true self does not hold such emotions as greed or hatred. The Buddhist concept of rebirth is very similar to the Scientology belief in past and future lives. Thus, Scientologists consider themselves greatly indebted to Buddhism.

What distinguishes Scientology from these and other earlier faith traditions, though, is the employment of a precise and modern technology for applying those ancient, but timeless concepts to contemporary life. This attention to application is a central tenet of Scientology.

The Creed of the Church of Scientology
We of the Church believe:

That all men of whatever race, color or creed were created with equal rights;

That all men have inalienable rights to their own religious practices and their performance;

That all men have inalienable rights to their own lives;

That all men have inalienable rights to their sanity;

That all men have inalienable rights to their own defense;

That all men have inalienable rights to conceive, choose, assist or support their own organizations, churches and governments;

That all men have inalienable rights to think freely, to talk freely, to write freely their own opinions and to counter or utter or write upon the opinions of others;

That all men have inalienable rights to the creation of their own kind;

That the souls of men have the rights of men;

That the study of the mind and the healing of mentally caused ills should not be alienated from religion or condoned in nonreligious fields;

And that no agency less than God has the power to suspend or set aside these rights, overtly or covertly.

And we of the Church believe:

That man is basically good; that he is seeking to survive;

That his survival depends upon himself and upon his fellows and his attainment of brotherhood with the universe.

And we of the Church believe that the laws of God forbid man:

To destroy his own kind; to destroy the sanity of another;

To destroy or enslave another's soul;

To destroy or reduce the survival of one's companions or one's group.

And we of the Church believe:

that the spirit can be saved and that the spirit alone may save or heal the body.[369]

- Scientology's religious doctrine includes certain fundamental truths. Prime among them is that man is a spiritual being whose existence spans more than one life and

---

369 Hubbard. *Scientology: A New Slant on Life*, 23.

who is endowed with abilities well beyond those which he normally considers he possesses. He is not only able to solve his own problems, accomplish his goals and gain lasting happiness, but also to achieve new states of spiritual awareness he may never have dreamed possible.

- Scientology holds that man is basically good, and that his spiritual salvation depends upon himself, his relationships with fellow human beings and his attainment of brotherhood with the universe. In that regard, Scientology is a religious philosophy in the most profound sense of the word, for it is concerned with no less than the full rehabilitation of man's innate spiritual self – his capabilities, his awareness, and his certainty of his own immortality.
- People come to their own understanding of the divine through the study of Scientology writings and the process of auditing (*see* "Basic Practices" section for description of auditing).
- Spiritual salvation as understood in Scientology as addressing one's transgressions against his fellows, taking responsibility for them, and creating a future where one works in harmony with one's fellows and all.
- The ultimate goal of the Scientology religion is to help people: achieve complete certainty of their spiritual existences, their relationship to the Supreme Being and their own role in eternity.

Basic Practices

- The religious practices of auditing and training are by far the most significant in Scientology. They are the *sine qua non* of Scientology, for they light the path to higher states of awareness and ability and,

eventually, to spiritual enlightenment. The essence of Scientology lies in these distinctive methods by which its principles can be applied to the betterment of individual lives.

○ *Auditing*: The central religious practice of Scientology is auditing (from Latin, *audire*, "to listen"), which is a precise form of spiritual counseling between a Scientology minister and a parishioner. Scientology ministers are of either gender. They complete studies to become a minister and a formal ordination. Those studies include study of the great religions of the world. In auditing, the minister, or *auditor* ("one who listens") asks the parishioner a series of specific questions in the area of spiritual travail being addressed in that particular session. Once the auditor locates the area of spiritual trauma, he will ask further specific questions or give directions needed to help the parishioner address and come to grips with that incident, experience, or area of life.

○ *Training*: There is no part of life that Scientology training fails to address – from the seemingly mundane to those issues of ultimate concern. Studying Scientology principles will enable people to answer many questions they have about themselves, their fellow human beings, and the universe. Training is thus a path of personal revelation and an indispensable part of an individual's progress to enlightenment. Scientology training consists of intensive study of the discoveries and fundamental truths contained in Scientology scripture. The goal of training is that people will utilize what they learn and contribute to making this a better world. Training is generally conducted in a Scientology course room, located in every Mission and Church of Scientology. However, the Church offers many "extension" courses as well, which are performed from home, with the individual mailing in the lessons to the Church for review. Scientologists also study L. Ron Hubbard's books and lectures outside a formal course room setting and may welcome the opportunity to do so during their convalescence.

- Churches of Scientology hold congregational services to celebrate religious holidays, perform rites of passage (e.g., birth, christenings, ordinations, marriages, funerals) as well as acknowledge other significant dates and events.
  - Scientologists celebrate birthdays and New Year's Day.
  - Even though not Christian, Scientologists who have grown up in predominant Christian countries generally celebrate the Christmas holiday because its message of peace on earth and goodwill toward all, just as Scientologists raised in other cultural traditions will respect the religious holidays of those traditions.
  - Scientologists who convert from another faith will often continue to celebrate the days that are meaningful to them from the faith traditions in which they were raised, both out of respect for their religious heritage and because the ceremonies and traditions have personal meaning for them. This does not lessen their adherence to Scientology as their primary religious expression.
  - Scientologists also have their own special days, which include major events in the Church's history. One of these is October 7, the anniversary of the formation of the International Association

of Scientologists; another is the second Sunday in September, known as Auditor's Day on which all auditors are honored for their work. May 9, the date marking the publication of *Dianetics*, is another special day of celebration. Scientologists also celebrate L. Ron Hubbard's birthday on March 13. On all of these days, Scientologists will usually gather at their Church or a rented hall, where recent accomplishments for the year are reviewed and goals set for the future. L. Ron Hubbard's birthday celebration also includes a party with music and the sharing of a birthday cake.

- **Observances of Holidays**: To commemorate important dates in its history, the Church of Scientology observes holidays in all parts of the world through the course of the year. The most significant are celebrated internationally, with events videoed and then shown locally at all Scientology churches and missions around the world. In those cities where the local church building cannot accommodate the thousands of parishioners attending the event, suitable auditoriums are rented. Major events are important to every Scientologist, whether in Africa, America, Asia, Australia, or Europe, as they provide a special spirit of unity. The major Scientology events feature briefings by senior ecclesiastical leaders on such subjects as the introduction of L. Ron Hubbard's works into new nations or sectors of society, the outstanding accomplishments of individual Scientologists and reviews of worldwide expansion. Events also feature releases of new Scientology books, materials, courses and news regarding the activities of social betterment programs – all cause for celebration. Although highly dignified affairs, Scientology events are also joyous. Other notable events, such as the founding or anniversary of the founding of the church in a particular country or a city, may be locally observed. Members of the Church of Scientology also observe traditional religious holidays such as Christmas. Local holidays, such as the United States Independence Day and French Bastille Day are not singled out, although Scientologists celebrate those occasions in their own countries according to custom.

- **Church Ceremonies**: Scientology ministers perform the same types of ceremonies and services that pastors, rabbis, and priests of other religions perform. These include Sunday morning services, weddings, naming ceremonies for newborns, as well as funeral rites to mark the passing of their fellow human beings. An ordained minister conducts a Sunday morning church service, which would begin with a welcome from the minister, followed by a time of congregants greeting one another, a sermon taken from *The Background, Ministry, Ceremonies & Sermons of the Scientology Religion*, and a closing prayer.

- **Church Ministers**: Scientology ministers are of good moral character, have trained as Scientology auditors, have graduated from the Scientology Minister's Course and have been duly ordained in a Scientology Church (pastors and chaplains). The Scientology Minister's Course includes a study of the great religions of the world. All Scientology auditors are required to become ordained ministers. Each Scientology Church has a chaplain who helps people in times of need. For instance, the chaplain may help

a couple experiencing marital discord, help a parent deal with a troubled child or any other problem for which parishioners would turn to their chaplain for help. In addition to ordained ministers, Scientology has a program known as Volunteer Ministers. Anyone can become a Scientology Volunteer Minister regardless of religious affiliation. A person studies the *Scientology Handbook* to learn basic Scientology principles which they can use to assist people who need help in their lives. The idea of Volunteer Ministers was actually borrowed from the basic pattern of the "barefoot doctor of China" who would administer help to alleviate the troubles of man. He was not highly trained, but he was the only means of assistance available to many people. Scientology Volunteer Ministers help comfort and assist those in need in their local communities as well as in disaster relief.

- **Contributing to the Community**: The Church of Scientology and its members are committed to rectifying societal ills: in the local neighborhood, the nation, and in the world as a whole. The tools employed are those acquired from a study of L. Ron Hubbard's works, including his drug rehabilitation technology, his effective study methods (called "study technology" which includes clarification of terminology through use of dictionaries, demonstration of various concepts with small objects, and learning a subject on a gradient – taking things one step at a time – so one builds greater and greater understanding), his essays on safeguarding the environment and, perhaps most important, the deep compassion for others that pervades everything he wrote. Scientologists are expected to give back to the community. They work on literacy, antidrug, prisoner reform, and human rights campaigns. They are especially expected to act as Volunteer Ministers in their local communities and often travel great distances to help in disaster relief efforts. In response to both natural and man-made disasters, Volunteer Ministers work hand in hand with the Red Cross and other volunteer groups bringing relief to people around the world.

- **Sharing the Faith or Beliefs of Scientology**: Scientologists consider that L. Ron Hubbard's teachings and writings are useful to people in all walks of life. Thus, Scientologists will invite others (with no pressure or coercive efforts to convert) to read a book by Hubbard to learn about Scientology. There are numerous books used as basic texts, including *Scientology: A New Slant on Life*; *Scientology: The Fundamentals of Thought* (Bridge Publications, Inc., 2007), and *The Creation of Human Ability* (Bridge Publications, Inc., 2007). In answer to inquiries about Scientology, most Scientologists will answer briefly, and then give a book so that people can come to their own understanding.

Principles for Clinical Care
Dietary Issues

- Scientologists have no dietary restrictions with respect to religious beliefs.
- Scientologists recognize the importance of nutrition and exercise in one's overall health.
- Since the practice of auditing addresses the spirit, a person undergoing auditing is not allowed to ingest alcohol for at least 24 hours before receiving auditing. For

this reason, most Scientologists drink very little alcohol, if at all.

General Medical Beliefs

- Scientology teaches that a contributing factor to injury and illness is predisposition of a person's spiritual condition. They (i.e., injury and illness) are precipitated as a manifestation of a person's current spiritual condition. And they are prolonged by any failure to fully address the spiritual condition. The causes of the predisposition, precipitation, and prolongation of injury and illness are addressed with assists. Assists help individuals heal by facilitating removal of the reasons for precipitating and prolonging the condition and lessening the predisposition to further injury or continuing illness. (For discussion of assists, see "During Illness" section.)

- Scientologists recognize there are three parts to a person: the spirit, mind, and body. Scientologists recognize the need to address all three of these for full recovery. To that end, Scientologists welcome competent medical care from nonpsychiatric-oriented medical doctors, naturopaths, orthomolecular specialists, and other specialists in the medical field.

- Scientologists appreciate proper medical care and healing professionals. This includes medication when needed. A Scientologist will likely ask for the most natural means of healing to be tried first. For example, a person found to have high cholesterol would likely want to try diet changes and exercise before using medication. A Scientologist would discuss the options with their doctor and work out the best course of action.

- Scientologists would expect a medical professional to try the least invasive, most life-affirming methods to treat illness before turning to surgery or more radical treatments.

- Scientologists believe that communication is very important; a nurse or doctor will find Scientologists open to speaking about their conditions, reviewing best options, and being very involved and engaged in their recovery and healing.

- Scientologists would expect a medical practitioner to explain to them every step of a medical procedure, and would usually want the meanings of medical terms explained to them in lay terminology. They would very much expect to be part of the decision-making process of their medical treatment.

- Scientologists affirm the validity of traditional Western medical procedures in the treatment of illness and disease.

- Scientology teaches against the consumption of any type of mind-altering drug. These include both illegal drugs (peyote, marijuana, cocaine, etc.) and legal drugs used to treat so-called psychiatric "disorders." Drugs such as modern antidepressants (selective serotonin reuptake inhibitors), benzodiazepenes, serotonin-norepinephrine reuptake inhibitors, both older and more modern antipsychotics, any of the classes of drugs used to treat attention deficit hyperactivity disorder including methamphetine, and more modern drugs for so-called hyperactivity are not acceptable forms of treatment for any Scientologist.

- Scientologists do not accept interventions from the field of psychiatry. The Church provides its own counselors to address any underlying spiritual distress the person may be experiencing.

- Scientologists do understand that people can have mental and emotional difficulties

to the degree that they may become a danger to themselves or others. In such circumstances Scientologists would likely agree to a mild soporific to help a person calm down. They would expect a full, searching physical examination to discover the underlying physical cause for a person exhibiting mental difficulties that do not dissipate with food, rest, and supportive help. Again, full consultation with family or loved ones of the of the afflicted individual would be appropriate.

Specific Medical Issues

- **Abortion**: The Church of Scientology does not mandate a position on abortion. This is an individual's personal choice and Scientology parishioners are totally free to decide for themselves. Scientologists are not advised or encouraged, however, to use abortion as a means of birth control. As described in *Dianetics: The Modern Science of Mental Health*[370], even attempted abortions are traumatic physically and spiritually to an unborn child, as well as to the mother. Abortion is therefore rare among Scientologists, who recognize that even an unborn fetus may already be occupied by a spiritual being. In some instances, however, abortion might be a recourse owing to health concerns for the mother or other personal factors. The Church never advocates abortion to Church staff or to parishioners.

- **Advance Directives**: A Scientologist will often have signed an advance directive making his or her wishes known, especially with regard to no psychiatric diagnosis or "treatment." If not, those

---

370 Hubbard L. Dianetics: The Modern Science of Mental Health. Commerce City: Bridge Publications; 2007.

closest to the patient will be able to carry out the patient's wishes.

- **Birth Control**: The Church of Scientology does not mandate a position on birth control. It is an individual's personal choice and Scientology parishioners are totally free to decide for themselves. In Scientology, procreation and the rearing of children is one of the Eight Dynamics of existence. Couples are free to decide the size of their own family and Scientologists do so in accord with their determination as to the greatest good across their dynamics.

- **Blood Transfusions**: Scientology has no restrictions regarding blood transfusions, surgery, anesthesia, first aid for broken bones or accidents, or the curing of disease with routine and necessary medical treatments.

- **Circumcision**: The Church has no position on circumcision. It is an individual decision for cultural, not religious, reasons.

- **In Vitro Fertilization**: The Church has no official position on in vitro fertilization; it is an individual decision.

- **Stem Cell Research**: The Church has no official position on stem cell research for therapeutic purposes; it is an individual decision.

- **Vaccinations**: The Church has no official statement on vaccinations, but sees the value of them in enhancing community health; it is an individual decision.

- **Withholding/Withdrawing Life Support**: Scientology has no fixed dogma or teachings regarding extending life with physical means. It is an individual decision. Scientologists would appreciate being kept as comfortable as possible at end of life.

Gender and Personal Issues

- Scientology as a religious movement has no prescriptions or proscriptions with respect to gender and personal issues.

- Scientologists have no class or racial distinctions, and cultural differences are accepted as long as they do not conflict with the truths discovered by L. Ron Hubbard.

Principles for Spiritual Care through the Cycles of Life

Concepts of Living and Dying for Spiritual Support

- Scientology teaches that a person is an immortal soul. A person has lived through many lifetimes and will live through many more.

- Scientologists do not see illness or death as punishment.

- Scientologists do not fear death because death is not the final state of human existence; it is a transition to a future human life.

- Scientologists understand that a body does not live forever; knowledge of this can lessen the traumatic effect of death. However, as with all people, the loss of a loved one is a traumatic experience and Scientologist family members will benefit from the care and comfort of a compassionate hospital chaplain or nurse if a trained Scientologist counselor is not immediately available. Hospital personnel should not be shy about offering comfort regardless of difference in religious preference.

During Birth

- There are no Scientology teachings proscribing natural childbirth or caesarian section.

- A basic Scientology teaching is the expectation that a baby's birth be performed in as quiet and calm an atmosphere in the delivery room (whether at home or in a hospital) as possible. This teaching is about respecting the mother, and others being supportive, calm and as quiet as possible around her during childbirth.
- A Scientologist would usually speak to a baby from birth with a welcoming, loving attitude. Often a parent will tell the baby where they are, what has just happened, explain to the child how delighted the adults are that the child has joined their family. This could include telling the child its name and telling the child who the other people in the room are. An understanding of the fact that a *thetan* has been through many lives, and may have very recently experienced death before assuming this new life, makes it only logical that a newborn would be welcomed in this way.
- Breast-feeding is a mother's choice.
- A new mother will benefit from assists (*see* "During Illness" section). These will help her recover more quickly. An example of an assist for the mother of newborn would be to have the mother look around the room and notice something she has. The direction (command) would be: "Look around here and find something you have." This could be done for about an hour the first day and 2 hours the following day. The assist could be repeated daily as the new mother desires. Such an assist can help the mother more quickly overcome the trauma of childbirth, ease discomfort, and speed recovery by focusing her attention from the pain she experienced in the childbirth process into the present environment.
- There are no special clinical rituals for a fetal demise in the Scientology religion. The parents would discuss the arrangements with their doctor and minister.
- As stated earlier, the Church has no position on circumcision. It is an individual decision for cultural, not religious, reasons.

During Illness

Scientologists welcome spiritual aid and counseling from a Scientology minister, family, or friend. Because Scientologists view that the relieving of any spiritual trauma is essential to a full and swift physical recovery, friends, family, or Scientology clergy will visit Scientologists to give them "assists."

An "assist" is an action to alleviate spiritual/emotional discomfort in concert with appropriate medical care and, thus, help a person recover more rapidly from an accident, illness, or upset (i.e., relational problem). Assists usually take the form of a series of questions asked or instructions given.

An assist in no way intrudes upon the role of medicine. An assist is not a substitute for medical treatment and does not attempt to cure injuries requiring medical treatment but is complementary to it.

Probably the most widely used assist is called a **Touch Assist**. This can be readily used in a clinical setting to help someone recover from an illness or injury. The purpose of the touch assist is to reestablish communication with injured or ill body parts. This is done by repetitively touching the ill or injured person's body and putting the person into communication with the body. The procedure can be applied by anyone. The details of a touch assist include the following eight steps:

1.   Administer first aid that may be needed

before you begin the assist. For example, if the person has a bleeding wound it should be dressed as the first action.

2. Have the person sit down or lie down – whatever position will be more comfortable for the person.

3. Instruct the person that you are going to be doing a Touch Assist and explain briefly the procedure: relate the command "Feel my finger"; ensure the person understands it; tell the person to let you know when he has performed the command.

4. Give the command "Feel my finger," then touch a point, using moderate finger pressure. (Do *not* touch and then give the command; that is the incorrect sequence. Touch with only *one* finger. If you use two fingers the person could be confused about which one he was supposed to feel.)

5. Acknowledge the person's response to the touch by saying "Thank you" or "OK" or "Good," and so forth.

6. Continue giving the command, touching and acknowledging when the person has indicated he has fulfilled the command.

7. The assist is continued until there are noticeable improvements in the person's condition from what he says or how he looks. The way to determine these improvements is called *indicators*. *Indicators* are conditions or circumstances arising during an assist which "indicate" whether the assist is accomplishing or not accomplishing its purpose. When a bad condition improves, that is a good *indicator*. A Touch Assist is continued until the person being helped has *good indicators*.

8. When this occurs, tell the person, "End of assist."

The method for performing a Touch Assist is described thusly. The affected area is approached with the finger and the finger is pulled back. This is repeated with varying degrees of closeness to and distance from the affected area. The goal is ultimately to actually approach and touch the affected area and pull the finger back to its farthest distance from the affected area.

In performing the assist, one attempts to follow the nerve channels of the body, which include the spine, the limbs, and the various relay points like the elbows, the wrists, the back sides of the knees, and the fingertips as touch points as well. The goal of this intervention is to restore the "communication wave flow" through the body, which was impeded as a result of the injury or illness, to enhance one's overall sense of well-being. No matter what part of the body is being aided by the assist, the areas touched should include the extremities (hands and feet) and the spine.

Furthermore, the touching must be balanced to include both sides of the body. For example, when the person's right big toe is touched, the left big toe should be touched; when a point a few inches to one side of the person's spine is touched, a spot the same distance from the spine on the opposite side is touched.

In addition to addressing the left and right sides of the body, the front and back sides must also be addressed. In other words, if attention was given to the front of the body, attention must also be given to the back.

The same principle applies in giving an assist to a particular body part. For instance, one might be addressing an injury on the front of the right leg. The Touch Assist would include the front of the right leg and the back of the left leg, in addition to the usual actions of touching the extremities and spine.

A Touch Assist may need to be given daily to achieve a result. One Touch Assist might result in only a small improvement or none at all. A second Touch Assist on the following day might result in more improvement. A third Touch Assist on the next day might result in eradicating the pain completely or at least making it bearable. On the other hand, it could take numerous days of performing Touch Assists before achieving the desired results. The number of Touch Assists that can be performed is unlimited.

Another assist that is often utilized with patients who have problems with internal organs is called the **Body Communication Process**. (A "process" is defined as an exact series of directions or sequence of actions taken to accomplish a desired result.) The Body Communication Process is used when a person has been chronically out of communication with his body, such as after an illness or injury, or when the person has been bed-ridden for a long period of time.

The Body Communication Process may be done only after necessary medical attention or other necessary assists have been done. The purpose of this process is to enable the *thetan* to reestablish communication with the body. The process includes seven steps:

1. The individual lies on his back on a couch, bed or cot. Doing this assist on the clothed body with shoes removed gives satisfactory results. Any constricting articles such as neckties or tight belts should be removed or loosened. It is not necessary to remove any clothing except for heavy or bulky garments. Where more than one session (session is the period of time during which the processing occurs) of this process is given, the body position may be varied to advantage by having the person lie face downward during alternate sessions.

2. Use the command "Feel my hands" (or "Feel my hand" on the occasion where only one hand is applied).

3. Explain the purpose of this process to the person and tell him briefly what you are going to do.

4. Have the person close his eyes. Then place your hands on the individual's shoulders with a firm but gentle grip, using an agreed-upon firmness, and give the command.

5. When the person replies, acknowledge him using: "Thank-you," "Alright," "Good," "OK," "Fine," or similar words.

6. Place your hands in different positions on the body, giving the command and acknowledging the person's response. Touch the chest, front of chest, sides of chest, both sides of the abdomen at the waist, then one hand going around the abdomen in a clockwise direction (clockwise because this is the direction of flow of the large bowel). Continue with both hands on the small of the back, one on each side and lifting firmly; one hand placed over each hip with firmer pressure on these bonier parts, then down one leg to the knee with both hands and down the other leg to the knee with both hands, then back to the other leg and down over the calf, the lower calf, the ankle, the foot and the toes and down the other leg from the knee to the toes. Then work upward in a flow toward the shoulders, down each arm and out to the fingers, both hands behind the neck, one on each side, sides of the face, forehead

and back of the head, sides of the head, then away toward the extremities of the body. An infinite variety of placing of the hands is available avoiding, of course, the genital areas or buttocks in both sexes and a woman's breasts. The process proceeds up and down the body toward the extremities.

7. The process is continued until the person has a good change, a cognition (a cognition is a new realization about life. It is a "What do you know, I ..." statement; something a person suddenly understands or feels) and very good indicators (an indicator is a condition or circumstance arising during a process which "indicates" – points out or shows – whether the process is going well or badly. For example, the person receiving the process looking brighter or looking more cheerful would be a good indicator.) At this point the assist, may be ended. Tell the person, "End of assist."

The Body Communication Process assist should not be continued past a cognition and very good indicators. However, it can be repeated as often as needed.

The person giving assists would usually speak to the nurse on duty and arrange assist times with the nurse or doctor while a patient is in a hospital. Numerous assists can be given throughout the day. (Note, these assists are simple to learn and if no trained Scientology minister is available, hospital personnel are welcome to learn how. Instruction is available online at www.volunteerministers.org.)

- Scientologists welcome visits and conversations from a minister of any faith. While they would appreciate caring words from such a person, they would obviously not want someone to try to convert them to another religion. A Scientologist, though, would be open to a discussion about religion and how most religions hold many fundamental beliefs in common.

- A basic tenet of Dianetics and Scientology is the need for silence if possible during actual moments of pain or unconsciousness, and certainly a quiet and calm environment around the ill or injured.

- A Scientologist is likely to ask many questions and want to have everything that is being done explained to them – both what and why. A basic teaching of Scientology is that communication is a key component to understanding.

During End of Life

- At end of life, a Scientologist will want to be told what is happening. Even a person in a coma can be addressed, telling them the day of the week, where they are, giving them information on what is happening. There are also assists that can be given to a person in a coma.

- Scientologists appreciate factual information about the body's condition in order to gain an understanding of exactly what is occurring with the body. A physician may find a Scientologist asking seemingly endless questions; taking a few minutes to explain what is happening will be greatly appreciated.

- Scientologists welcome spiritual aid and counseling from a Scientology minister.

- Scientologists would take measures to ensure that all their worldly affairs were put into good order before death. They will appreciate any help to put their personal affairs (e.g., business, family, financial) in order that others are not burdened with these issues.

- An ordained Scientology minister or

Scientology volunteer minister can provide assists to help terminally ill patients who might feel overwhelmed at the thought of losing their friends and their families.

- Scientologists will often be more concerned about their loved ones, friends, work colleagues than with themselves at the time of their departing because they know that those around them will grieve their loss. So, they will be pleased that anyone who wants to say goodbye has the chance to do so.
- Scientologists will want to address any unresolved issues with family or others before departing this life.
- A person coming to the end of life would want to have those who care for them close by, supporting them through the process of leaving the body.
- A memorial service is usually performed in a Scientology chapel, with friends and family attending to give the person a proper goodbye and wish them well on their future journey. A typical service would conform to this model: people would be sitting in chairs or pews; music would play before and after the service. Often, friends or family will say a few words about the person's life before the funeral message. The service concludes with the formal funeral message and the opportunity for those attending to say their goodbyes to the deceased.
- Above all, Scientologists would appreciate support and encouragement at a time of loss.

Care of the Body

- Scientologists usually chose cremation for disposition of the body.

- Scientologists would be agreeable to a medical or legal need for an autopsy.
- Scientologists would usually be agreeable to donating their bodies for medical research; it is an individual decision.
- Scientologists would not usually be interested in viewing the deceased's body. The physical shell is not the person. The *thetan* (spirit/soul) leaves the body at death.
- There are no special religious rituals associated with preparing a body for cremation.
- Disposal of the final remains after cremation would be as directed by the family.

Organ and Tissue Donation

- There are no specific teachings regarding organ and tissue donation. It is an individual decision and should be discussed with the family. It may be preferable for a chaplain and/or nurse who are trained designated requesters to be consulted for assistance.

Scriptures, Inspirational Readings, and Prayers

Rather than readings, there are numerous Scientology assists that can be given to a person who is ill. Assists can be learned by anyone, and can do much to relieve the stress and speed the healing of an ill person. There are assists that can be used for a person in a coma, for a person who is upset that their body is doing badly, and many others.

For information on numerous types of assists, consult pages 193–229 of *The Scientology Handbook* (Los Angeles, CA: Bridge Publications).

Special Days: Scientology

To commemorate important dates in its history, the Church of Scientology observes holidays in all parts of the world through the course of the year. The most significant are celebrated internationally, with events videoed and then shown locally at all Scientology churches and missions around the world. In those cities where the local church building cannot accommodate the thousands of parishioners attending the event, suitable auditoriums are rented. Major events are important to every Scientologist, whether in Africa, America, Asia, Australia, or Europe, as they provide a special spirit of unity.

The major Scientology events feature briefings by senior ecclesiastical leaders on such subjects as the introduction of L. Ron Hubbard's works into new nations or sectors of society, the outstanding accomplishments of individual Scientologists and reviews of worldwide expansion. Events also feature releases of new Scientology books, materials, courses and news regarding the activities of social betterment programs – all cause for celebration. Although highly dignified affairs, Scientology events are also joyous.

Other notable events, such as the founding or anniversary of the founding of the church in a particular country or a city, may be locally observed. Members of the Church of Scientology also observe traditional religious holidays such as Christmas. Local holidays, such as the United States Independence Day and French Bastille Day are not singled out, although Scientologists celebrate those occasions in their own countries according to custom.

The following are international holidays celebrated by Scientologists.

March 13 *L. Ron Hubbard's Birthday* – The birthday of the Founder of Dianetics and Scientology, March 13, 1911, is commemorated each year with a major celebration honoring L. Ron Hubbard's achievements and his continuing contributions to mankind. Outstanding churches and missions are recognized for service to their parishioners and communities during the previous year.

May 9 *Anniversary of Dianetics* – The annual international celebration on this day salutes the publication of *Dianetics: The Modern Science of Mental Health* on May 9, 1950. It is the occasion when Scientologists and community leaders from around the world acknowledge the contributions Dianetics has made to the betterment of individuals and society at large and the daily miracles that occur through its widespread application.

June 6 *Freewinds Maiden Voyage Anniversary* – On this date in 1988, the Sea Organization Motor Vessel *Freewinds* began her maiden voyage. Scientologists convene aboard the *Freewinds* each year for a week of special briefings and acknowledgments of their work in bringing a greater understanding of Scientology to others and helping improve conditions through Scientology.

Second Sunday in September *Auditor's Day* – On this day auditors are acknowledged for their skill and dedication. Top auditors from around the world are recognized.

October 7 *International Association of Scientologists (IAS) Anniversary* – Members of the IAS gather each year at Saint Hill, former home of L. Ron Hubbard, in England to commemorate the founding of the IAS in 1984 and to rededicate themselves to its aims. The annual IAS freedom awards are presented and annual convention of IAS delegates is held.

December 31 *New Year's Eve* – This event welcomes in the new year with a review of accomplishments of the previous 12 months and a look forward to plans for further reach into new areas of society with L. Ron Hubbard's technology. Stellar accomplishments of Scientology parishioners helping others gain the benefits of Scientology training and auditing are acknowledged.

Secularism

Not religious, sacred or spiritual.[371]

Prepared by:
Michael Irwin, MD, MPH
Former Medical Director of the United Nations
Founder of the Secular Medical Forum of the United Kingdom
Surrey, England
michael-hk.irwin@virgin.net

History and Facts

Scepticism about religious beliefs dates back many centuries for as Lucretius, a Roman poet, noted over 2000 years ago, "Religions are equally sublime to the ignorant, useful to the politician, and ridiculous to the philosopher."[372]

It was in the sixteenth century, however, that atheism – or a disbelief in gods – first began to be publicly voiced. For example, in 1542, Francisco Vimercati, at the University of Padua in Italy, declared that matter was eternal without beginning or end, and that everything which exists had a natural cause and there was no personal immortality.

Early in the seventeenth century, a Frenchman, Pierre Charron published *De la Sagesse* (*Concerning Wisdom*), which noted that

all religions have this in common, that they are an outrage to common sense ... all religions, without exception, share the same characteristics – all discover and publicize miracles, sacred mysteries, prophets, festivals, articles of faith and beliefs necessary for salvation, each pretending to be better and truer than the others.[373]

During this century, *De la Sagesse* was successfully reprinted many times.

In the eighteenth century, a bestseller was *Le Traite des Trois Imposteurs* (*Treatise on Three Impostors*), written by a Dutchman, Jan Vroesen; the imposters to which the author made reference were Moses, Christ, and Muhammad, and this book stressed that "ignorance and fear have given birth to superstition, have created the gods and, assisted by the impostures of rulers, have transformed laws that are actually human into inviolable divine decrees."[374] During this century also, especially in the university

---

371 Quote from *The Concise Oxford Dictionary*, 10th edition, London: Oxford University Press; 2001.
372 Huberman, J. (2007). *The Quotable Atheist*. New York, Ny: Nation Books, 192.

373 The quote in the text is an English translation from *De la Sagesse* cited by Ludovic Kennedy in his book *All in the Mind: A Farewell to God*, (1999); London: Hodder & Stoughton, 167.
374 Ibid, 169. The quote here was taken from a review

towns of Europe, many were beginning to question the debatable doctrine that "God" had made the world in 7 days and later on had sent his only son to Earth to preach the redemption of sinners and by his sacrificial death had saved us from ourselves.

The principal Founding Fathers of the United States of America were essentially secularists. Thomas Jefferson believed that "Christianity is the most perverted system that ever shone on man"; Benjamin Franklin thought that "lighthouses are more useful than churches"; and James Madison noted that "the fruits of Christianity" are "pride and indolence in the clergy" and "ignorance and servility in the laity." In 1797, John Adams (by then president) signed a treaty which began: "As the Government of the United States of America is not, in any sense, founded on the Christian religion."[375]

The word "secularism" (from the Latin *saecularis*, which means "of this world") was coined only in the 1850s, in England, by George Holyoake, a leading Freethinker of his day, who noted, "Secularism is the province of the real, the known, the useful, and the affirmative: it is the practical side of skepticism."[376]

Then, in 1859, came Charles Darwin's *The Origin of Species*, which rocked the boat of Christian orthodoxy more alarmingly than anything which had been said or written previously. "Organized" secularism, though, is relatively recent. For example, the National Secular Society in the United Kingdom was only founded in 1866 by Charles Bradlaugh, who was a fierce supporter of birth control (which at that time was almost unmentionable). Bradlaugh was a republican, who wanted the courtesy titles given to the children of noblemen to be abolished; he was a radical Member of Parliament, who was not allowed to take his seat in the House of Commons for 6 years because of his known atheism and convoluted legal arguments over taking the necessary oath of allegiance to Queen Victoria, which ended with the words "So help me, God."

In the twentieth century, France and Turkey officially separated religion from the state, becoming "secular states," while the United States gradually became, perhaps, the most religious country in Christendom, as well as a land of religious pluralism.

The "history" given here can be equally useful for introducing agnosticism, atheism, humanism, or secularism. All of these world views stress that this life is the only one of which we have any definite knowledge, and therefore all human effort should be focused wholly toward its improvement. All agree that supernaturalism is based upon ignorance, and generally is opposed to progress. All emphasize that morality is social in origin and application, and should definitely not based on a "faith book," such as the Bible or the Qur'an.

It is also important to mention that "religious" people can have secularist views; an example is the belief in the separation of religion and the state. Furthermore, "secularists" can have religious views; an example of this is some kind of belief in an afterlife.

of Vroesen's book by Professor Silvia Berti and cited in Kennedy's book.

375 Dawkins, R. (2006). *The God Delusion*. London: Bantam Press, 40, 43. All of the "Founding Fathers'" quotes in this paragraph were taken from this source.

376 Holyoake, G. (1896). *English Secularism*. Chicago, IL: Open Court Publishing Company. The quote was publicized earlier in the January 19, 1853, of the *Reasoner* as cited in Edward Royle, *Victorian Infidels* (1974); Manchester: Manchester University Press, 150.

Basic Teachings

- Secularism is mainly concerned with the complete separation of religion and the state, and especially the abolition of all privileges granted to religious organizations.
- Secularism does not try to suppress or interfere with religion; in spite of what religious opponents might say, it is not a "promoter of atheism"; it simply wants to create a society where religion and all other areas of society are kept separate.
- A secularist's vision of society is one in which religion knows where it belongs: which is in its places of worship and in believers' homes; it should play no part in government, in education, in the health care professions, or in the organization of that society.

Basic Practices

- Secularists support all types of good causes – donating to the Red Cross, involvement in various activities to "save the planet" – to name a few.
- Secularists live life to the fullest from appreciating good drama, music, and art to enjoying the wonders of the world ranging from excitement of witnessing a beautiful sunset or the fascination of going on African safari to see animals in their natural environment.

Principles for Clinical Care
Dietary Issues

- Secularism does not concern itself with specific dietary problems, although some secularists may be vegetarian, for example, for other reasons.

General Medical Beliefs

- Secularism is opposed to religious influences in all the health care professions where these may affect the manner in which health care is provided.
- Secularists believe that all health care professionals who invoke conscientious objection to avoid what is normally required of their profession, must always refer their patients seeking the specific services to which they object to others in the same profession who do not have such personal difficulties, as quickly as possible.
- Secularists are naturally not opposed to physicians, nurses, and all other health care professionals holding religious views, which, at times, may even inspire them; but these personal opinions must not influence how these professionals care for their patients.
- Secularism does not accept that "divine interventions" can occur to influence treatment, and certainly does not believe in any way that "spiritual beliefs" play any part in medical treatment regimens.
- Secularists are strong in their view that all health services relating to HIV/AIDS and sexually transmitted infections must not be subjected to the influence of religious organizations or faith-based motivation. Such services include prevention (provision of barrier contraception and instruction in their proper use), health promotion and education (counseling on reducing the risk of infection), support for those infected with HIV/AIDS and sexually transmitted infections, testing and treatment. It is important to stress that secularists believe that there is no real evidence that abstinence-only programs are effective (these are certainly irrelevant to the large proportion of people in the

world at risk today). It is vital for children and young adults to be given adequate information to enable them to engage in safe sexual relationships. Sex education must explore the wide diversity of human relationships and must give correct information about sexual health, responsibility and choice (it is most unfortunate that certain religious influences still oppose meaningful sex education in schools).

- Secularism strongly believes that physician-assisted dying should be legally possible for the terminally ill.

Specific Medical Issues

- **Abortion**: Secularism strongly supports the right of women to have legal and safe abortions. It is imperative that there is no return to the times when illegal backstreet abortions (with complications such as hemorrhage, secondary infection, perforation of the uterus, and death of the mother) occurred. Women's lives must not be controlled by religious influences. On a "life and death issue," such as performing an abortion, secularists generally agree that "conscientious objections" can be permitted for physicians, providing that they refer the woman making the request without delay to another medical colleague.
- **Advance Directives**: Secularists fully support the use of advance directives and believe that all health care professionals should set an example and complete one; these documents could, at some future date, be extremely important for the family, friends, physicians, and nurses looking after each of us.
- **Birth Control**: Secularists fully support all practical methods of birth control – it is simply a matter of personal choice.
- **Blood Transfusions**: Secularism has no

restrictions on blood transfusions and has no problem with medications which may contain certain ingredients.

- **Circumcision**: Secularists generally believe that the removal of a child's foreskin, for nonmedical reasons, should never be performed. In fact, they would usually agree that it is the duty of health care professionals to educate parents against such ritual procedures. Likewise, secularists strongly deplore female genital mutilation which can cause so much pain and permanent suffering.
- **In Vitro Fertilization**: Secularism fully supports in vitro fertilization.
- **Stem Cell Research**: Secularism supports stem cell research for therapeutic purposes and believes it must be properly financed and supported, especially as the possible benefits for treating certain diseases seem, at present, to be excellent.
- **Vaccinations**: Secularism has no restrictions on and fully supports vaccinations.
- **Withholding/Withdrawing Life Support**: Secularism agrees that withholding or withdrawing life-measures should be possible in medically futile situations.

Gender and Personal Issues

- In general, secularism sees no specific problems in this area, except perhaps individual preferences (e.g., an elderly female patient may not wish to be bathed by a male attendant).

Principles for Spiritual Care through the Cycles of Life
Concepts of Living and Dying for Spiritual Support

- Because secularists have generally focused on what can be seen in this small corner of the universe, they usually have no expectations of what will happen when they die. But, they are fairly certain that nothing will survive their deaths except their immediate descendants, and relatives and friends remembering what they have done during their lives.

- Many Secularists hold the opinion that those who believe in an "afterlife" sometimes have trouble coping with death, especially if they believe they might experience the fear of "God" on the day of judgment (perhaps even of "hell," which used to be that "great abyss of terrible flames"?). This prospect of an afterlife can produce thoughts of guilt, sin, and punishment, which are not attractive prospects.

- Whether one is religious or not, death can be a blessed escape from the burdens of old age; similarly, if one is suffering from a prolonged illness, it is a merciful release for the one who dies and also for those close to that person who have provided terminal care.

- Many secularists, however, will be honest with themselves and state the obvious that nobody on Earth today can be 100% certain of what happens upon death; hopefully, especially if dying at an advanced age, they will welcome the opportunity to find out. However, if there is an afterlife, they will discover that it is an even stranger adventure than being born and, therefore, perhaps something to be welcomed.

- Throughout their lives, secularists will derive pleasure of a purpose in life from helping others, enjoying what the world offers and making the world, what they believe to be, a better place.

- One aspect of hope is for other secular-

ists to continue improving what has been achieved.

During Birth

- The usual secularist (except those who might have a religious belief as well) will have no special views about birth, apart, perhaps, from enjoying the excitement and wonderment of becoming a parent.

- One specific issue might be the matter of circumcision. As stated earlier, Secularists generally believe that the removal of a child's foreskin, for nonmedical reasons, should never be performed. In fact, they would usually agree that it is the duty of health care professionals to educate parents against such ritual procedures. Likewise, secularists strongly deplore female genital mutilation which can cause so much pain and permanent suffering.

- With respect to "blessings" and "naming ceremonies," secularists dislike the expression "Catholic child" or "Muslim child." Instead, one should say "a child of Catholic parents" or "the child of Muslim parents" because children are much too young to know how they really feel about such issues.

- In the case of fetal demise or death of an infant, secularists would welcome compassionate, supportive care; they would not want "words of comfort" to include religious expressions, idioms, or quotes from holy books.

During Illness

- Secularists, when ill, simply want health care professionals to provide the best possible care, without letting any personal views based on religious beliefs prevent this. They will be content to rely on the support of relatives and friends to help them through their illness.

- If a secularist has a religious belief, then the appropriate religious support also might be helpful.

During End of Life

- Many secularists, and religious people as well, support physician-assisted suicide and voluntary euthanasia, with adequate safeguards, for competent terminally ill adults.
- Health care providers should offer compassionate care.
- Secularists support referrals to palliative care and hospice when appropriate.
- Non-religious secularists would welcome reassurance that everything will be done to keep them comfortable through this final stage of life, with the least possible degree of "fuss." Intended expressions of support like "you will be going to a better place" or "you will see God soon" would not be appreciated.

Care of the Body

- In death, there are no special requirements to be observed as to how everything is to be handled for secularists without any specific religious belief.
- Respect for the body is to be expected, and general comfort is to be provided to relatives and close friends.

- Some secularists will wish to be buried, and others will prefer to be cremated; there is nothing in secularism that prescribes which is to be followed.
- There are no restrictions regarding autopsy; it is a matter of individual choice.
- There are no restrictions regarding donation of the body for medical research purposes; it is a matter of individual choice.

Organ and Tissue Donation

- Organ and tissue donation are matters for an individual secularist to personally decide.

Scriptures, Inspirational Readings, and Prayers

- The reading of any scriptures/devotional materials and/or reciting of any prayers are up to the individual to perhaps indicate before dying or for the secularist family to decide after someone has died.
- Readings from the writings of past and present Freethinkers might be selected if a funeral is held. These include Albert Einstein, Stephen Jay Gould, Julian Huxley, Bertram Russell, Carl Sagan, George Bernard Shaw, Peter Ustinov, or selections from secularist journals such as the *Freethinker* (a UK publication).

Shintoism

When on the way to the Shrines one does not feel like an ordinary
person any longer but as though reborn in another world.[377]

Prepared by:
William R. Lindsey, PhD
Member/Faculty, Center for East Asian Studies
Associate Professor of Religious Studies
The University of Kansas Department of Religious
  Studies
Lawrence, KS

Reviewed and approved by:
Akira Naito, MD, PhD
Research Fellow, Department of Immunology
Chelsea and Westminster Hospital
Imperial College Healthcare NHS Trust
London, England

History and Facts

Shinto is a bold hue in the composition of religions – Buddhism, new religions, Christianity, and Confucian ethics – coloring Japan. Unlike these religions, however, Shinto is unique. It claims no person as its founder; nor does it possess a creed or set of central teachings; nor is it structured on lines of ecclesial authority. What Shinto claims, however, is to make manifest a native and timeless faith that is coterminous with the divine genesis of Japan, at once ancient and contemporary, and centered on the worship and celebration of *kami* (神). The two Chinese characters comprising the term Shinto (神道) mean the "*kami* way." But what is *kami*, and what is the *kami* way? A well-known expression among the Japanese is a good place to start: *yaoyorozu no kami ari*. Although this literally means "there are eight million *kami*," the expression actually points not to a specific number but rather to the sheer number of phenomena considered to be *kami*. Typically translated as "gods," *kami* is better understood if left untranslated.

Generically, *kami* means sacred power or numinous quality; in common and devotional usage, it refers to particular beings (supernatural, and even human and animal) and objects empowered by this quality that inspire in people a range of emotions and affections such as awe, reverence, fear, hope, and love. A classic definition of the faith states:

> *kami* signifies, in the first place, the deities of heaven and earth. ... It is hardly necessary to say it includes human beings. It also includes such objects as birds, beasts, trees, plants, seas, mountains and so forth. In ancient usage, anything whatsoever which

377 Sadler, A. L. trans. (1940). *The Ise Daijingu Sankeiki or Diary of a Pilgrim to Ise.* Tokyo, Japan: Zaidan Hojin Meiji Seitoku Kinen Gakkai. As reprinted in Earhart, H. Byron. (1974). *Religion in the Japanese Experience: Sources and Interpretations.* Encino, CA: Dickenson Publishing Company, 25.

was outside the ordinary, which possessed superior power, or which was awe-inspiring was called *kami*.[378]

Shinto posits the power of *kami* – a vitalistic power to create, to sustain and rejuvenate, to make one marvel – to reside potentially anywhere: in heaven and on earth; in deities, in people with extraordinary talents and gifts, and in the wonders of nature.

The most casual traveler to Japan is a frequent witness to symbolic expressions of this power. One conspicuous symbol is a rope, often interspersed with hanging white paper streamers, looped around an object such as a special tree or an unusually large stone. This signifies the object as possessing *kami* power and/or acting as the abode or alighting place of a deity possessing such power. Similarly, Shinto shrines and their grounds, marked off by the distinctive gateway called a *torii* that divides the sacred precincts of shrines from the mundane world outside, are potent loci of *kami* power. The "*kami* way," then, is human participation in this power through acts of worship, festival, and prayer. Much of this participation is tied to seasonal, communal and lifecourse celebrations. When this participation is undertaken with a sincere heart and mind – typically expressed through physical acts of purification – one may draw near to a *kami* and seek the deity's beneficence.

Throughout much of Shinto's traceable institutional history, Buddhism (which entered Japan in the sixth century and carried with it the prestige and intellectual weight of continental Asia) tended to dominate the native religion ritually, doctrinally, and institutionally. For centuries, the worship of *kami* and the worship of buddhas coexisted in a variety of combinatory relationships, with Buddhism in the privileged position. A prevailing conceptual expression of this relationship linked the buddhas and *kami* together as two faces of sacred reality. The *kami* were understood to be the worldly, phenomenal reality of the higher, numinous reality of the buddhas. Complex institutional arrangements also existed. Elaborate temple-shrine complexes, for example, were constructed by political elites throughout the country, creating cultic sites that tied political power to local spiritual power centers. At such sites, the power of Buddhist divinities and *kami* were actively worshipped in common "as twin elements in a system that was completely mixed."[379] Most Japanese during this time did not and could not distinguish between worshipping *kami* and worshipping buddhas.

In 1868, however, a new government seeking to modernize Japanese society as rapidly as possible displaced the ancient, moribund rule by a string of military strongmen called shoguns and, over the next several years, injected profound changes into society. One such change was severing this centuries-old combinatory relationship. As deemed appropriate to the modern spirit, Shinto and Buddhism were officially separated into two distinct, autonomous traditions. However, "Shinto" stood as less a singularly recognized tradition than a helpful term adapted to categorize several varieties and purposes of *kami* worship.

---

378 This definition comes from the eighteenth-century philologist Motoori Norinaga (1730–1801). See de Bary, W. T., D. Keene, G. Tanabe, et al., eds. (2001). *Sources of Japanese Tradition*. Vol. 1. 2nd ed. New York, NY: Columbia University Press, 18.

379 Teeuwen, M. and F. Rambelli. eds. (2003). Introduction to *Buddhas and Kami in Japan*: Honji Suijaku *as a Combinatory Paradigm*. London: Routledge and Courzon, 3.

"State Shinto," for example, anchored the nationalistic ideology of the emperor as a living *kami* and Japan as a sacred nation from the late nineteenth century until American occupation forces disestablished it in 1945. "Folk Shinto" came to embrace any number of deep-rooted, localized forms of *kami* worship, many of which are tied to the seasonal rhythms and economic concerns of agricultural and fishing villages. The rapid urbanization of Japan in the latter half of the twentieth century has made the future of Folk Shinto tenuous since much of it is linked to a diminishing rural way of life.

More germane for the purpose of this chapter, though, is "Shrine Shinto," which refers to the worship of deities within thousands of established shrines located throughout Japan. Many of these shrines comprise a network of local branch shrines tied to large, well-known shrines visited by worshippers from around the country. This network is the commonest form of Shinto Japanese encounter when practicing the *kami* way. Most of the deities enshrined and celebrated in Shrine Shinto are limited to a mere handful of *kami*. Approximately one third of shrines in Japan, for example, are dedicated to Inari, the deity of harvest, fertility, health, and wealth. In addition, "Shinto" has also been used to categorize new, revelatory, sectarian religious movements that arose in the nineteenth and twentieth centuries and incorporated in varying degrees aspects of *kami* worship into their theology, liturgy, and healing. These movements are commonly termed "new religions" in both scholarly and popular writings. Several of them have made missionary inroads in countries outside Japan, including the United States. Since the discussion here primarily concentrates on Shrine Shinto, the use of "Shinto" from this point will refer to this pervasive form of the religion. In any reference to a Shinto new religion, the faith's formal name will be used so as to avoid confusion with Shrine Shinto.

Interestingly, although Japanese emigrated in large numbers in the twentieth century to countries such as the United States and Brazil, Shinto has not journeyed well past the borders of Japan. There are few Shinto shrines outside of Japan. To most Japanese Americans, Shinto is as "foreign" as it is to an American of non-Japanese descent. To most Japanese, however, the practice of Shinto and the religio-cultural assumptions underlying it are considered a natural extension of being Japanese. In this respect, Shinto is the "ground bass of ... [Japanese] religion: functional, affirmative, this-worldly."[380] Considering the significant number of Japanese citizens living, working, and studying overseas – particularly in the United States – awareness of Shinto is desirable because it is one key in understanding how Japanese define and act on their sense of ultimate concern and meaningfulness in life.

Basic Teachings

- Shinto possesses no creed or central teachings.
- From a Shinto perspective, it possesses an ancient and enduring faith in the primordial power of the native *kami*.
- The lack of a controlling ecclesial authority has produced a decentralized environment where priests act as primary interpreters of the *kami* to which their shrines are dedicated. Since this decentralized environment also extends to the laity, priestly

---

380 Bellah, Robert N. (1970). *Beyond Belief*. New York, NY: Harper & Row, 126.

and lay views concerning *kami* are often not in agreement. Lay devotees bring their own interpretations of a shrine's *kami* – the deity's sacred story, its incarnate forms, its efficaciousness, its purpose in their lives – into their devotion and prayers. Some see this lack of ecclesial authority and authoritative teachings as a structural weakness of Shinto, but in the absence of a single authority there emerge in Shinto multiple individual "shintos" by which individual devotees – priest and lay alike – may come to know and worship *kami*.

- Outside of fixed events such as shrine festivals, Shinto does not hold regular services of worship in the manner of many western religions. Rather, the majority of people visiting shrines do so throughout the calendar year, often without seeing a priest, in order to bring their needs and prayers directly to the *kami* in simple but sincere forms of worship. What holds Shinto together as a unity of multiple "shintos" is the practicing of faith in *kami* rather than the teaching about *kami*. Examples of this practice are described in the next section. Nevertheless, there are commonly held cultural beliefs that have deeply informed the practice of Shinto.

- **Life is Pure and Good**: This is foundational to all beliefs. Since the vitalistic power of *kami* empowers all environments (divine, human, and natural), closeness and harmony, as opposed to distance and estrangement, characterize human life in its relationships with deities and nature. Shinto rejects any notion of a fall or original sin, of a tragic chasm separating human and divine. Instead, Shinto asserts that life is inherently good and pure, and death, though an unavoidable and unfortunate component of life, is inherently polluted.

- **Death is Pollution**: This fundamental outlook is related in the creation story of Japan found in the *Kojiki* (古事記) and *Nihongi* (日本紀), which are collections of sacred myths compiled in the eighth century and held in high esteem in Shinto. In the story, the Japanese islands and all natural phenomena are created through the sexual energy of two *kami*, Izanagi and his consort Izanami. After giving birth to fire and suffering terrible burns, Izanami dies and enters the underworld. Izanagi, missing and desiring her, enters the underworld to bring her back, but upon seeing her decomposing body, he shockingly realizes the incompatibility of life and death. He escapes the underworld, closes off its entrance from the world of the living, and purifies his body in a stream, washing away the impurities of death. Life and death and their opposing valuations captured in the creation myth also express Shinto's sensitivity to broad notions of purity and pollution. Although death is polluting, the pollution of death is not permanent. Funeral and post-funeral rites, which for most Japanese come under the ritual purview of Buddhism, are designed to move the souls of the recently dead from a polluted state of confusion and disorientation to a purified and stable ontological state of being family ancestors. This ritual process typically extends 49 days after death.

- **Purity and Pollution**: The former is associated with states or forces of life, production, creation, strength, and health, while the latter indicates states or forces of death, decline, decomposition, weakness, and illness. This sensitivity underlies the Japanese tendency to demarcate between inner and outer, where inner is pure and outer polluted. Thus, the custom of removing one's shoes when entering a house is not simply one of cultural courtesy but a way to avoid tracking in dirt, both literal and figurative, from the outside. Similarly, having children wash their hands and gargle after outside activity is common among mothers and kindergarten teachers. Much of the practice of Shinto and *kami* worship is an explicitly religious expression of these general concerns and activities. It is geared toward promoting and prolonging states of purity to enhance individual and communal life in all realms of endeavors from business prosperity to personal health, while overcoming or avoiding the polluting affairs of life in the world. In terms of rituals on the lifecourse, Shinto and Buddhism have developed over the centuries a division of sacred labor divided on the life/purity-death/pollution scheme. Shinto is responsible for the life-affirming stages such as birth, coming of age, and marriage. Buddhism takes responsibility for death and post-death stages such as funerals and periodic memorial services. Accordingly, Shinto's ideals and practices play a more prominent role in the promotion and preservation of health, but they diminish considerably once death is imminent, giving way to Buddhism to deal ritually with the demise of the body and the maintenance of the soul.

Basic Practices

- Shinto is preeminently a religion of practice. One is less a confessor of Shinto than a doer of Shinto. People enact their faith in the power of *kami* to grant life-enhancing benefits (e.g., protect health and home, promote prosperity, and bind familial and community ties) in a number of culturally and ritually prescribed ways. A few are described here. These are more typical of lay participation in the power of *kami* than they are of priestly participation. Although Japanese partake in one or more of these practices anytime they visit a shrine, special times in the calendar set aside for celebrating the *kami* are extremely popular occasions for visiting shrines to seek the blessings for oneself and family. Although the number and variety of these special times are immense, notable examples are the New Year (January 1), the 7-5-3 Festival (for the celebration and protection of children aged 3, 5, and 7 years on November 15), and festival days unique to each *kami* such as the popular Hatsuuma Festival in early February, which is a celebration at all shrines throughout the country dedicated to the *kami* Inari.

- **Priests**: Many priests serving shrines professionally prepared for their vocation at one of two Shinto universities, Kokugakuin University and Kogakkan University. Although these private universities are open to all and provide numerous fields of study, their departments of Shinto Studies uniquely define them. These departments offer courses in Shinto institutional and intellectual history, ritual, and worship, and even field work involving religious asceticism. In a Shinto Studies department, the typical student is a young college-aged man, 18–22 years old, training to take over his father's position as priest at a home shrine that has been passed down through the family for generations. Other men serve large, national shrines with a number of clergy on the payroll. Although there are female priests, the vast majority are males.

- **Purification**: Before approaching *kami*, some manner of purification, typically by water, is necessary. For most laity, this is done by simply washing one's hands and rinsing one's mouth (reminiscent of children washing their hands and gargling) at a water font located on shrine grounds. Others, particularly those involved in intense faith relations with a *kami*, may choose to undergo more vigorous and complex purification such as standing under a waterfall or immersing oneself in the ocean. Priests also undergo elaborate purification that may include water rites, sexual abstinence and food taboos. This purification and the authority of their office allows priests, as opposed to the laity, to draw close to the power of *kami* by entering the holiest recesses of the shrine where the sacred object (typically a mirror) representing the *kami* is located.

- **Drawing Lots**: Some visitors to Shinto shrines participate in the power of *kami* by purchasing and drawing fortune lots called *o-mikuji* (御神籤). These are strips of paper on which are printed one's general fortune along with short, specific statements concerning a series of life categories ranging from illness and pregnancy to academic and business endeavors. The fortunes are tied to a special tree within the shrine compound. To outsiders and skeptics, the practice of *o-mikuji* may be nothing more than a frivolous waste of time and money. To many Japanese, however, it is a way of participating in the beneficial power of *kami* in making one attentive to the possibilities and potential challenges that lie ahead in one's life.

- **Amulets**: Purchasing amulets for a particular benefit – traffic safety, safe pregnancy, family happiness and such – is another common activity at Shinto shrines. Some shrines are especially famed for a specific benefit like the popular Suitengû Shrine in Tokyo that is noted for helping women to conceive children and give safe births. Unlike fortunes, amulets are taken from shrines and attached to the objects to which the benefit is directed such as a car (traffic safety), a pregnant woman's clothing or purse (safe pregnancy), or within the home (family happiness). Through the amulet, the shrine's *kami* power becomes intensely transposed to the needs of the person.

- **Petitioning**: This is common to virtually all Shinto shrines, large and small, famed and obscure alike. When a person petitions the *kami* of a shrine, she usually first purifies herself with water (typically available through a fountain on shrine grounds) by rinsing her hands and/or mouth, rings a bell attached to the front of the shrine notifying the *kami* of her presence, and then bows and claps her hands twice or three times before offering a silent and sincere request. In addition, she may write her petition on a small wooden votive tablet called *ema* (絵馬) and hang it on a board in the shrine compound that is filled with other tablets on which are written numerous requests to the *kami*. These "letters to the gods" are written in a ritualized manner turning on the phrase "so that."[381] "So that my grandmother remains in good health throughout the year." "So that my father returns safely from his trip." Concerns of personal and familial health are a dominant theme, and as the uniform use of "so that" indicates the faith orientation toward disease and ill-health

---

381 The phrase "letters to the gods" comes from Ian Reader's study of *ema* in Reader, Ian. (1991). Letters to the gods: the form and meaning of *ema*. *Japanese Journal of Religious Studies*, 18(1), 23–50.

is usually prevention. An important twist on this kind of petitioning is that of cutting oneself off from a troubling situation or a poor state of health. Known as *en-kiri* (縁切り), which means connection-cutting, this type of petition acknowledges the person is already in a situation where he is connected to a personal, social, or physical affliction from which he hopes to cut himself off through the power of *kami*. Here, the faith orientation toward sickness is intervention. At the priestly level, petitions to the *kami* are definitive of formal worship and expressed through stylized reading of ritual prayers called *norito* (祝詞). *Norito* comprise both ancient examples preserved through the ages and recognized universally by Shinto shrines as well as contemporary works penned by individual priests for specific worship occasions. Ancient or new, these prayers are written in classical, rather than modern, Japanese and dramatically intoned. Consequently, they are difficult for most Japanese to understand when they hear them in a formal ceremony. Like the pre-Vatican II Latin mass and the Sanskrit hymns of the *Rig Veda*, the power of *norito* is that of "[b]eautiful, correct words, intoned with reverence and awe [to] bring about good influences."[382]

Principles for Clinical Care
Dietary Issues

- Few Japanese are vegetarian or follow any explicit dietary laws. Many are aware that the Japanese on average have the longest life spans, and they give credit to a diet in which fish, soy products and vegetables are stressed. A good diet, balanced among food groups, includes rice and is eaten in moderation. Rice in particular, most notably highly polished white rice, is seen as an active promoter of health and vigor. Rice has deep cultural roots in Japanese identity. It is not simply the staple food of the Japanese, but a core symbol of the Japanese. The origins of rice cultivation are linked in mythological sources to *kami*. In addition, since the color and sheen of polished rice symbolizes purity, it and its fermented liquid cousin, sake, are the most common items offered to *kami* during formal worship in shrines. As a staple of Japanese hospital fare, white rice is more than a filling starch. It is a subtle sign to patients that they are putting something pure and wholesome into their bodies, and by doing so they can anticipate a return to full health.

- Food is a customary gift to bring to hospital patients in Japanese culture. Reflecting a latent Shinto concern on purity as indicative of health, the emphasis is on fresh, high-quality (and necessarily expensive) items such as fine fruits.

- Supplements to a normal diet (or in response to a poor diet of too much fat and alcohol) such as herbal mixtures, powdered kale juice, and small doses of highly concentrated vitamin and mineral drinks are popular and readily available in stores. Recently, awareness of the importance of dietary fiber has stimulated the creation and marketing of various high fiber food supplements. (Constipation is consistently a topic of worry among Japanese, particularly women, and is seen as an indicator of the state of overall, day-to-day health.) These supplements, meant to "cleanse" the body of hurtful elements like excess alcohol and hardened feces,

---

382 Nelson, John K. (1996). *A Year in the Life of a Shinto Shrine.* Seattle: University of Washington Press, 40.

parallel Shinto ideas of purging pollutants in order to regain a purified state.

General Medical Beliefs

- Since Shinto has no central ecclesial authority, it is institutionally unable to advocate medical beliefs. Japanese familial and cultural beliefs are more influential, but they tend to be broadly informed by Shinto values attaching religious importance on states of purity that are expressed through concerns of bodily health and vigor and the elimination of "pollutants."

- Medical care should be highly competent and administered compassionately and attentively. A recent Japanese neologism based on English pronunciation, *doku hara* (ドクハラ), which is short for "doctor harassment," expresses a sense among some patients, particularly women, that some physicians treat their concerns not only lightly but at times with insulting disdain that is humiliating.

- Most people practicing Shinto understand illness is caused by a number of factors such as viral and bacterial infections, genetic abnormalities and environmental factors.

- If a chronic ailment persists and seems to be resistant to treatment, a person may interpret the cause as being a vengeful spirit, an angry ancestor, or some kind of disruption in the harmony of this world and the spirit world. He may contact a priest or shamanistic healer for spiritual consultation and purification or exorcism.

- Other chronic conditions (dizziness, susceptibility to cold, arthritis) that do not respond well to direct medical treatment may be interiorized by a person, interpreted as a condition unique to his identity as a person, and thus tolerated. It also is a means by which he may seek sympathy from others as well as offer it himself to those suffering from a similar complaint.

- In Shinto new religions, medical treatment is allowed and sought, but it is believed only to cure the symptoms and not the root cause of the illness. The root of all illness in Shinto new religions lies with the heart-mind, or the self, of the believer being out of harmony with the vital energy of the universe. This lack of harmony causes disruption in social relations and in the somatic body. In Kurozumikyô, for example, illness is caused when a person's self or *kokoro* (心) has become dark and out of harmony with the bright, vital force animating the universe called *yôki* (陽気). This debilitating condition of the *kokoro* is brought on by the person failing to cultivate the *kokoro* through one's moral bearing and social relationships with other people. Pastoral counseling and healing intervention – blowing and rubbing hands on the afflicted part of the body by a fellow faith member whose *kokoro* is bright and strong – are necessary to overcome this debilitation, restore the inherent brightness of the person's *kokoro*, and reorient the person.

- Acupuncture and moxa cauterization, while not related to Shinto per se, are very popular treatments used in addition to modern medicine among the Japanese.

Specific Medical Issues

- **Abortion**: Abortion is legally and readily available in Japan. Because most religious organizations, including Shinto, do not actively press their views on abortion within the body politic, abortion does not produce the level of religious and political rancor in Japan as compared to the United States.

- **Advance Directives**: Advance directives ought to be discussed with family members first. Family is the key mediator between medical staff and patient when end-of-life issues arise. A common belief among Japanese is that a patient's spirits must be kept high, even when he has entered the terminal stage of an illness. Direct discussions with a patient concerning death are seen to sap hope and serve only to bring death more swiftly. Although this custom of deflecting to family direct discussions about death between a terminally ill patient and his medical staff may be seen as a type of denial in the west, it reflects Shinto values of embracing both life and the centrality of the family in the life of each individual.
- **Birth Control**: Although ancient myths concerning *kami* are often rich in fertility motifs and symbols, and a number of Shinto's contemporary ritual practices such as the distribution of amulets to women for uneventful and safe pregnancies point to fecundity as a religious value, there is no institutional position on birth control, including the pill, which Japan legalized in 1999.
- **Blood Transfusions**: Blood transfusions present no ethical or religious qualms for those practicing Shinto.
- **Circumcision**: Infant circumcision is rarely practiced inside Japan, and it is unlikely that Japanese parents residing in the United States would request or desire it.
- **In Vitro Fertilization**: Fertility treatment is generally acceptable, even desirable given the discomfort many Japanese feel toward adoption outside of "blood ties."
- **Stem Cell Research**: Shinto is a very decentralized religion with no guiding canonical or ecclesial authority. Therefore, stem cell research is neither endorsed nor unendorsed by traditional teachings; it is an individual's or family's decision. However, there are some religious groups in Japan, notably the Shinto-derived new religion Ômoto-kyô, which actively oppose stem cell research, as well as abortion and capital punishment.
- **Vaccinations**: Vaccination is not religiously problematic for those practicing Shinto.
- **Withholding/Withdrawing Life Support**: End-of-life decisions ought to be first discussed with the family rather than with the patient directly, unless the patient expresses her own opinion first.

Gender and Personal Issues

- Although males have dominated the field of medicine in Japan, recently the number of female MDs has increased. Accordingly with this increase, women have greater choice in selecting physicians based on gender than they have had in the past. The notion of doctor harassment arises in part from the double hierarchy of male/physician–female/patient, and may encourage some women to seek a female doctor in the belief that it will encourage more open and respectful communication.
- In the specialty of obstetrics and gynecology, there is a growing preference for female practitioners. However, this is only a personal preference, not a religious demand. Many women hold no preference and seek only attentive and compassionate care.
- Mothers more than fathers are highly involved in their children's basic health maintenance.

Principles for Spiritual Care through the Cycles of Life

Concepts for Living and Dying for Spiritual Support

- Shinto interprets death as pollution and evil. Institutionally and ritually, it largely eschews matters of death, handing it over to Buddhism, some new religions, and Christianity.
- Systematic views of life after death do not exist among most Japanese, but there is a belief, backed by Buddhist death and memorial ritual, that ties to one's family continue after death through the new ontological identity of an ancestor.
- Shinto is not naïve about or indifferent to death. It accepts death as a natural though unfortunate aspect of life, as the death of Izanami – who dies in the midst of giving birth – represents.
- Rather than focus on death, Shinto unabashedly focuses on life. By largely avoiding death, it does not take death frivolously but rather takes life seriously. Death surely comes to all, but before that singular moment arrives there is a life to live. How well one accepts that singular moment of death is dependent on how one lives countless moments of life. What matters is that one has lived a life in full appreciation of the blessings (*on*, 恩) bestowed upon one by *kami*, parents, teachers, friends, coworkers, and others. Returning these blessings (*hô on*, 報恩) in one's actions in relationship with *kami* and others defines a harmonious, morally grounded, well-lived life.

During Birth

- Birth is an ambivalent event. It is an absolutely joyous occasion, an extension of the family, and yet one couched in concern for the newborn and mother's health, both of whom are assumed to be in a highly vulnerable state due to bodily weakness and exhaustion brought on by 9 months of pregnancy and the physical trial of birth. In Shinto, this ambivalence is expressed through the purity/pollution scheme. Because of bodily vulnerability and blood loss, the mother and infant are in an unavoidably polluted state. The passage of time is necessary in order for the polluted state of mother and child to diminish. This respect for the power of time after the birth event is translated back into the contemporary medical scene whereby a new mother will spend a week or more in a hospital even after experiencing a medically "uneventful" pregnancy and birth.
- Many women choose to wear a belly wrap called *hara obi* (腹帯) from approximately the fifth month after conception until birth. This is believed to keep the fetus warm and maintain its position in the womb. Amulets for safe birth may also be worn.
- After the passage of approximately thirty days from birth, the infant is taken to the shrine in the locality of his or her home to be formally introduced to the *kami* and receive the deity's protection. Often the infant's grandmother, rather than the mother who is still considered to be in a weakened state, will accompany the baby to the shrine along with other members of the family. This is a time when familial ties are intensified and celebrated in presence of the *kami*. It is also the child's first experience in a series of life-affirming rites of passage closely tied to Shinto. If the infant is a boy, the priest paints in red the ideogram for "big" (大) on the forehead. If a girl, the priest paints "small" (小). Red is the celebratory color

symbolizing life and good health. In this spirit, the priest attempts to induce from the baby a loud cry when he smears the wet, crimson coat on the sensitive skin. The cry allows the *kami* to hear the voice of its newest charge, while also signaling the baby's overall health and vigor.

- Fertility treatment is generally acceptable, even desirable given the discomfort many Japanese feel toward adoption outside of "blood ties."

- Fetal demise brought on by either miscarriage or abortion can be an emotionally trying event. A belief that some Japanese use to interpret fetal demise and mitigate feelings of loss or guilt holds that the soul of a dead fetus returns to a watery, unformed realm of origins from which it came to await another chance for birth. Here, fetal death is interpreted not as a permanent end to life but a sending back and delaying of life. Although Buddhism and several new religions have developed ritual services for memorializing fetuses, Shinto has largely avoided participation in this ritual marketing due to its association with death.

- In case of fetal demise, it is perhaps best to use clinical and pastoral language that refrains from speaking of loss as permanent and instead implies loss as temporary and even recoverable at a later time. A counselor should listen attentively to the language a Japanese patient uses in expressing her feelings about fetal loss and adopt it as a template for any necessary counseling. While the notion of temporary loss suggests the logic of fetal rebirth, it does not imply reincarnation and karmic destiny as understood in orthodox Buddhist thought. A counselor should refrain from applying "textbook" Buddhist ideas to the experience of loss, and, again, listen carefully to the patient and adapt to her language.

During Illness

- Shinto priests are shrine ritualists, so they rarely act in the role of pastoral counselor to the ill in a hospital setting. Still, Shinto embraces the Japanese cultural value placing great importance on family members taking an active role in caring for loved ones who are ill.

- If a patient is a member of a Shinto new religion, she is likely to seek ritual healing that channels positive, life-sustaining energy (e.g., rubbing hands on the body, blowing on the body, facing one's palm to the body) by a fellow layperson or a clergy member if possible.

- Many people who practice Shinto are respectful and open to other religions' insights, and have some passing familiarity with Christianity in particular. A few may practice both Shinto and Christianity. Still, religious literature and counseling that is overtly Christian or Western in its assumptions may be confusing and frustrating for a patient who is not Christian.

- Counseling should stress the love and prayers of family and friends in Japan and abroad, which helps the patient acknowledge his own place in a harmonious web of meaningful human relationships.

- Gifts of pajamas and bedding are common so the patient may feel as comfortable as possible. These gifts suggest the core Shinto theme of cleanliness and purity to help overcome the polluted state of the ill body.

- Japanese are very sensitive to gifts or objects brought into the hospital room that bode ill or well for recovery. Potted plants are considered poor gifts because their roots suggest a rooted, long-term hospital stay. Roses and carnations are generally acceptable, but white flowers, particularly chrysanthemums, are to be avoided because of their association with death and funerals. It is best to inquire from the patient or family member about personal likes before buying a gift.

- Japan is an intensely gift-giving society. Medical staff may be offered gifts from the family and patient. These should be accepted in the spirit in which they are offered.
- Photographs of family, friends, life in Japan, along with letters and cards of support decorating a hospital room are likely to be comforting to a patient.
- If the patient is diagnosed with cancer or a life threatening condition, the family rather than the patient should be consulted beforehand, unless the patient expresses his opinion first.

During End of Life

- If the patient has entered a terminal stage, it is best to inform the family first rather than the patient directly. Generally, consultation with the family on how best to inform the patient is preferable. Similarly, end-of-life care and advance directives ought to be broached with the family rather than the patient. However, if the patient expresses his opinion first concerning his own care, then it is best to consult directly with him.
- Upon death, family connections to the deceased will continue through periodic Buddhist memorial rites for a number of years. These rites, plus the day-to-day interaction surviving family members may have with the deceased at home in front of the family Buddhist altar, indicate the strength of family identity. Accordingly, family members ought to

have maximum time with the terminally ill to affirm ties and review their life together as a family.

- Up until recently, most people died at home in Japan. Now, most terminally ill patients die in hospitals. Hospice care may be an acceptable choice if available, particularly if the dying person is not the mother for it is she who will likely carry the burden of home care.
- Hospice care in Japan does not take place in the home but in institutions typically linked to hospitals. A Japanese family needs to understand all the options available in American style hospice care.
- If hospice care is unavailable or undesirable, an emotionally supportive environment should be encouraged so the family feels free to be with and support the dying patient for long periods of time. For mature and adult children in the case of a dying parent, this is not only emotionally satisfying but culturally affirmative of the values of filial piety.
- Once death occurs, the family should receive support in answering questions concerning the death of the loved one and in planning for funerary arrangements. Typical of such questions are: How did death occur medically and did the person suffer at the end? In Japanese culture such questions are meant to put both the family and medical staff at ease in acknowledging the "failure" of medical care, in other words, that death proved to be a natural course that medical care ultimately could not reverse. For the family, a description of the cause of death and reassurance that there was little or no suffering involved helps members cope with grief and contributes to an individual narrative of the deceased. For the medical staff, answers to such questions act as

professional assurances to them and the family that the patient received the best care possible.

- Having some time with the body of the deceased is the rule in Japanese hospitals. Typically, a body is transported to a small room in the basement of the hospital where family members may spend private, final – often emotion-filled – moments with their loved one prior to the public funeral. A funeral may very likely entail the transportation of the body to Japan for a Buddhist (or in a few cases Christian) ceremony and cremation. Funeral and cremation customarily occur on the same day.

Care of Body

- Almost all Japanese are cremated after death, whether they are Buddhist, Christian, or members of new religions. This may well be the preference for a family living outside of Japan, though the family should be consulted ahead of time.
- American cremation differs from Japanese cremation and the family should be made aware of the difference before making a decision. Unlike American cremation where the body is reduced completely to ashes and tiny bone fragments, Japanese cremation creates fewer ashes and larger bone pieces. These bones are central to funeral rites. The family transfers the bones to the urn by picking them up in anatomical order and placing them in the container, ideally from legs to skull bones. At the very least, it is important that a large piece of the skull tops the bones and ashes. In this way, the family "builds" the person anew in preparation for the deceased's new identity and status as an ancestor.
- As cremation supposes, securing the body

is important. Assumed but unconfirmed death such as suspected drowning is an event that likely requires counseling.

- Embalming is not traditional. Washing and displaying the body in a coffin prior to cremation are, however, traditional steps in funerary rites. The growth of the corporate funeral industry in Japan has weakened some of these steps that historically were in the hands of family and the local Buddhist priest.
- The deceased is memorialized in a photograph, displayed at funeral and memorial services, as well as on the family Buddhist altar.
- If either the family or medical staff requests an autopsy, then it should be done as efficiently and respectfully as possible.
- Donation of the body for medical research is in most cases simply not addressed. However, a family may be open to the possibility if the patient has made it clear that she desires her body be donated for research purposes. The family should be allowed to broach the subject first rather than a medical professional.

Organ and Tissue Donation

- Organ and tissue donation is an extremely controversial subject among Japanese. Until Japan's Diet passed the Organ Transplant Law in 1997, Japanese seeking organ transplants had to take prohibitively expensive medical sojourns, typically to the United States, for treatment. The 1997 law recognized the concept of brain death and thus the legality of procuring organs and tissue. Many Japanese, including some physicians and religious leaders, are uncomfortable with this definition. It goes against traditional interpretations of death measured in the stopping of organ functions, cessation of blood circulation, and the accompanying loss of bodily warmth. Also, many see organ procurement as an act disrespectful to the body. Shinto, given its lack of ecclesial authority, has no single position. Some Shinto new religions, most notably Ômotokyô, vigorously oppose organ donation. Tenrikyô, one of the oldest and most established of the Shinto new religions, teaches the body is a unique gift from the deity *Kami* the Parent. Its nationally reputable hospital in Nara, however, applied and received government permission to be an organ transplant center. This is indicative of the depth of ambivalence concerning brain death and organ donation among Japanese.

- Great care should be taken in broaching the subject with a family facing the imminent death of a loved one. Attending physicians should be discreet in asking for the family's opinion directly. Japanese in a foreign culture could feel under pressure to accede to the wishes of an authority figure (the physician) in a land they may not completely understand at a time when they are grieving. It may be best to follow the lead of most Japanese intensive care unit physicians and leave it up to the family to initiate dialogue concerning organ donation, which the family likely will not do. In Japanese culture, silence is often an answer. If the subject has to be discussed from a legal perspective, it may be preferable for a chaplain and/or nurse who are trained designated requesters to be consulted for assistance.

Scriptures, Inspirational Readings, and Prayers

- Shinto does not have canonical scriptures in the manner of "revealed" religions.

Shinto is a religion of prayer and petition rather than a religion of the book. For many laity, the prayers to the *kami* are sincere, silent words spoken from the heart in front of a shrine, or they are simple, written requests upon wooden *ema* to be dedicated to the *kami* in order to receive divine beneficence. For priests conducting formal worship, the prayers to the *kami* are intoned *norito* written in classical Japanese. An abridged and adapted version of one of the oldest *norito*, which is still invoked in one form or another today, is provided here. The Shinto new religion Kurozumikyô, for example, has adopted it as part of its healing rituals. This prayer was originally intoned twice each year at the imperial court – at the end of the sixth and twelfth months – to purify the entire country of evils and pollutions each half-year brought on by disease, pestilence, divine judgment, and the immoral and improper actions of the people. It follows a narrative where all the sins and misdeeds are collected and taken away through the benevolent actions of the *kami*, leaving the land and its people once again in a pure state.

From: *The Great Exorcism of the Last Day of the Sixth Month*

The various sins perpetrated and
  committed
By the heavenly increasing people to
  come into existence
In this land which the Emperor is to
  rule tranquilly as a peaceful land:

First the heavenly sins:
Breaking down the ridges,
Covering up the ditches,
Releasing the irrigation sluices,
Double planting,

Setting up stakes,
Skinning alive, skinning backwards,
Such sins are called heavenly sins.

The earthly sins:
Cutting living flesh, cutting dead
flesh,
Leprosy, skin excrescences,
The sin of violating one's own mother,
The sin of violating one's own child,
The woes from creeping insects,
The woes from deities on high,
The woes from birds on high,
Many such sins will appear.

[When the kami of the heavens and
earth receive the petition of the
great court priest]
Then, beginning with the court of the
Emperor, Sovereign Grandchild of
the kami,
In the land of the four quarters under
the heavens,
Each and every sin will be gone.

As a result of the exorcism and
purification,
There will be no sins left.
They will be taken to the great ocean
by the kami called Se-ori-tu-hime,
When she thus takes them,
They will be swallowed in a gulp by
the kami called Haya-aki-tu-hime,
When she thus swallows them with a
gulp,
The kami called Ibuki-do-nusi will
blow them away with his breath to
the Underworld,
When he blows them away,
The kami called Haya-sasura-hime
will wander off and lose them.

When she loses them,
Beginning with the many officials
serving in the Emperor's court,
In the four quarters under the
heavens,
Beginning from today,
Each and every sin will be gone.[383]

Special Days: Shinto

Note: Since Shinto is highly decentralized, many festivals are specific to only a single shrine or a particular *kami*. Throughout the year there are hundreds of festivals, large and small, sponsored by shrines individually or collectively in worship of *kami* tied to the locality and/or history of each shrine. Therefore this list is not exhaustive but rather reflects only major days of celebration in which most Shinto shrines participate.

January 1 *New Year's Day* – Not only marks the beginning of the New Year but also, as such, carries Shinto ideals of renewal and purity. Shinto shrines are bustling with worshippers on this day and for

---

383 Abridged and adapted from Philippi, D. L. trans. (1990). *Norito: A Translation of the Ancient Japanese Ritual Prayers*. Princeton, NJ: Princeton University Press, 45–48.

several days after as people pray to *kami* for health and happiness for the coming year.

Second Monday in January *Adult Day* – A celebration of all young people who have turned 20 years of age in the previous year. Twenty marks the age of legal adulthood in Japan.

February 11 *National Foundation Day* – Celebrates the establishment of the nation in 660 BCE by the legendary emperor Jimmu, as described in Shinto mythology. Although this is an important day in the Shinto calendar, given the religion's close identity with the nation, for most Japanese it is significant only because it affords them a day off from work as one of Japan's national holidays.

July 7 *Tanabata* – Sometimes called the Star Festival as it marks the meeting of the stars Vega and Altair in the Milky Way. It celebrates the personification of these stars as the weaving maiden and the cow herder who can only meet once a year to share their love. People, particularly children, write their wishes on colorful strips of paper and hang them from bamboo branches. Some areas of Japan celebrate Tanabata (literally, seventh night) in August, which is the traditional seventh month of the lunar calendar, which Japan abandoned in the nineteenth century as part of its modernization program.

November 15 *Seven-Five-Three Festival* – In premodern Japan this festival was a means to gain protection for children at the critical ages of 3, 5, and 7 years by *kami* to avert sickness and death. In modern Japan parents may still seek the blessings of *kami*, but it is more a time to celebrate one's children by dressing them in fine clothes, visiting a shrine, and taking pictures.

December 31 *New Year's Eve* – On this day people clean their homes in anticipation of the New Year and its promise of newness, freshness, and purity. Many also head to Shinto shrines to welcome the New Year at midnight.

Glossary of Shinto Terms

ema: Votive wooden plaques upon which people write their prayers to the *kami*. They dedicate the *ema* to the *kami* by hanging them within the grounds of the shrine.

en-kiri: Meaning "cutting ties," this is a genre of request one makes to a *kami* in order to cut oneself away from negative and detrimental situations such as ill-health or an unhappy human relationship.

hara obi: A "belly wrap" many pregnant Japanese women wear to keep the fetus warm and in position in the womb. They are sometimes purchased at Shinto shrines whose *kami* are reputed to offer safe and easy delivery.

hô on: "To return blessings." The proper response to favors one has received from *kami*, parents, teachers, and others is an attitude of gratitude. Shinto stresses this attitude in all people in order to cultivate the values of loyalty, dedication, and humility (*see* entry for *on*).

kami: Typically translated as "gods" but means more precisely sacred power or numinous quality. Any being (heavenly or earthly), animal, or natural phenomenon exhibiting this power or quality is a *kami*.

Kojiki: Produced in 712 and also known in English as *Record of Ancient Matters*, this text and the *Nihon shoki* comprise the earliest collection of Shinto mythology.

kokoro: Incorporating both English meanings of mind and heart, this is an ubiquitous concept in Shinto new religions. As mind-heart it means an individual's cognitive and emotive "self." Cultivation of spiritual power, healthy bodies and social relationships requires each person's self to harmonize with the positive vital energy of the universe. New religions claim efficacious techniques that can direct the harmonization between the self and the universe.

Nihon shoki: Produced in 720 and also known in English as *Chronicles of Japan*, this text and the *Kojiki* comprise the earliest collection of Shinto mythology.

norito: Formal written prayers composed by Shinto priests in classical Japanese and intoned during formal ritual worship of *kami*. *Norito* comprise both ancient examples still in ritual use and ones newly penned.

o-mikuji: Written fortunes obtained at Shinto shrines that spell out possibilities toward one's health, prosperity, work and educational success, love, and social relationships.

on: "Blessings" or "favors." Shinto recognizes each person is brought into being and made socially whole by a number of blessings received from *kami*, parents, teachers, and so forth, throughout life. *On* stresses the ties that bind each person to *kami*, family, community, and work.

yôki: Positive and vital force animating the universe. In Shinto new religions vulnerability to disease is due to the *kokoro* of an individual being out of harmony with this pure and rejuvenating force. Such disharmony is typically caused by a lack of moral rectitude, poor faith, and self-centered behavior that disrupts one's relationship with people and with *kami* (*see* entry for *kokoro*).

Sikhism

God is One, the only truth, the creator, the fearless, without enmity,
the omnipresent, the unborn, the indivisible,
who can be achieved by His own grace.[384]

Prepared by:

Gurinder Singh, MD, MHA
Clinical Professor of Ophthalmology, The University of
  Missouri-Kansas City
Kansas City, MO
Clinical Professor of Ophthalmology, The Kansas
  University Medical Center
Kansas City, KS;
Malika G Singh
The University of Missouri-Kansas City School of
  Medicine
Kansas City, MO;
Karta Purkh Singh Khalsa
Sikh Representative on Greater Kansas City Interfaith
  Council
Kansas City, MO

Reviewed and approved by:

William R. Lindsey, PhD
Associate Professor of Religious Studies
Member/Faculty, Center for East Asian Studies
The University of Kansas Department of Religious
  Studies
Lawrence, KS

History and Facts

The word "sikh" means "learner" or "disciple" and is the term used to denote adherents of the religious tradition begun by Guru Nanak Dev (1469–1539), the first of ten human gurus (God-filled spiritual leaders). Guru Nanak was raised in a Hindu family in the Punjab region of northwestern India, which had a strong Muslim presence. Early on he experienced both the religious insights of Hinduism and Islam.

One morning at the age of 30, he was bathing in a river and underwent a powerful religious experience where he came into the presence of God, was enlightened, and became a guru (one who leads his followers from darkness or ignorance to light, spiritual elevation). This experience of the true God led him to assert that God was not exclusive to Hinduism or Islam. Guru Nanak then traveled extensively for twelve years to many places including Haridwar, Kurukshetra, and Varanasi (holy sites of Hinduism), Mecca and Medina (holy sites of Islam) and, according to some beliefs, to Jerusalem (holy site of Christianity and Judaism). He also visited Baghdad – a small

---

384 The quote represents the essence of Sikh philosophy as summarized in the first verse of the *Sri Guru Granth Sahib*; it is also called the *Mool Mantra* or the basic formula. Sikh tradition credits Guru Nanak Dev as the author of the *Mool Mantra*.

shrine was erected commemorating the event and it still stands today. A primary reason for his journeys was to understand various religions, especially, Hinduism, Islam, Buddhism, Jainism and, according to tradition, Christianity and Judaism, and over and above promote Oneness of God (*Ik Oankaar*) in this world. As a result of his travels, he accepted the teachings of other religions that agreed with his philosophy and spoke against what he perceived as misguided beliefs, superstitions, and ritualism of his time. In principle, Guru Nanak sought to rise above the Hindu and Muslim teachings of his day by devotion simply to God. He regarded no religion or people superior to others, and each human being a creation of the same God and being equal. As a result, he rejected the caste system of his time and the subjugation of women as well.

A human guru is a profoundly spiritually gifted soul, who drives away the darkness of ignorance and ego by teaching enlightenment that is found in knowing the word of God. A human guru exemplifies in his own life the unifying relationship with God; that He is the divine truth, the Original Guru, eternal, self-existent, all-creative, omnipresent, and full of grace. Nearing his death, Guru Nanak sought to preserve the active presence of a guru in the nascent Sikh community by selecting a spiritually accomplished disciple named *Lehna* to succeed him upon his death. Guru Nanak renamed him *Angad* ("ang," which means "part of me" while the "ad" means first or primal). This name suggests the spiritual continuity of the human gurus in teaching the word of God. This continuity of the gurus has sometimes been described to be like a single flame that can be transferred from torch to torch, each torch casting away the darkness

with the same light. This does not mean that the ten human gurus were mere copies of each other, for each guru contributed significantly and uniquely to the Sikh community and faith.

The second guru, Guru Angad Dev, developed *Gurmukhi*, a distinctive script for the Punjabi language allowing access to the sacred writings of Guru Nanak and his successors. Heretofore the sacred literatures had been under the control of a priestly class who knew Sanskrit and could misinterpret verses to their own advantage. The third guru, Guru Amar Das, began the Sikh tradition of feeding the hungry by means of *langar* kitchens, which continues to this day. Royalty sat equally with beggars and were served the same food prepared by Sikh devotees. The fourth guru, Guru Ram Das, founded the holy city of Amritsar and the famous "Golden Temple" (the Vatican for Sikhs) on water on the site of an ancient healing spring. The fifth guru, Guru Arjan Dev, compiled the Sikh teachings into a book form, called the *Adi Granth*. He was martyred for keeping Guru Nanak's faith alive. The sixth guru, Guru Hargobind Rai, was the first to establish a civil as well as a martial authority for Sikhs. The seventh and eighth "Nanaks," Har Rai and Har Krishan, established diplomatic relations with India's mogul emperors and lead the Sikh community to a full status among India's myriad spiritual groups. The ninth guru, Guru Teg Bahadur, stood against the forced conversion of Kashmiri Hindus and was sacrificed/beheaded by the Moghul emperor Aurangzeb.

The tenth guru, Guru Gobind Singh, founded the *Khalsa Panth* (Sikh brotherhood) and the five *Kakaar* (the five religious symbols). Of great importance to the development of the Sikh faith, Guru Gobind

Singh in 1699 also proclaimed that the line of human gurus would end with him and from that point on the scriptures, the *Sri Guru Granth Sahib*, would be the ever-living guru who would guide the community throughout its future generations. He added the teachings of the ninth guru, Guru Teg Bahadur, to the sacred text of *Adi Granth*, thereby compiling the present day holy book, *Sri Guru Granth Sahib*. Guru Gobind Singh was the first to bow to this immortal guru, the *Sri Guru Granth Sahib*, which is written in prose that not only preserves the writings of the human gurus but also includes Hindu, Muslim, *Bhagat*, and *Sufi* texts. These voluminous scriptures contain 1430 pages in several languages, but written in *Gurmukhi* script. These scriptures are not stories of how humans were created, but a compilation of teachings concerning the means by which the mind and soul can progress to higher spiritual and moral levels. The text is compiled in 31 *ragas* (ways of singing). Therefore, the teachings can be read or sung.

The early fifteenth century witnessed descent of tyranny and oppression over peace-loving Hinduism in India by Islamic invaders from Afghanistan. Guru Nanak took to his pen and teachings to challenge the onslaught of Babar on the defenseless and helpless Hindus. While Guru Nanak spoke against Islam, he also rejected the ritualism of his own birth-religion of Hinduism. Guru Arjan Dev accepted his sacrifice to defend the religion of the Hindus from the cruelty of Islam. Similarly, when Guru Teg Bahadur was beheaded in defense of Hinduism, not his own religion of Sikhism, but the onslaught of Aurangzeb's sword continued, Guru Gobind Singh rose to face the challenge by reorganizing and galvanizing his people to form an army. He infused and injected the sense of bravery into a demoralized and cowardly

nation by creating *Khalsa* in April of 1699. Guru Gobind Singh, born as Gobind Rai, in a special ceremony, celebrating *Baisakhi*, converted/baptized five of his disciples/followers, *Panj Pyare*, to *Khalsa* and gave them *Singh* (meaning Lion) as their last name. He bowed to these *Panj Pyare* and accepted baptism from them and changed his own name to Guru Gobind Singh. He wanted to dispel the caste system by discarding and rejecting the last names based on the castes and adopting *Singh* (meaning Lion) and *Kaur* (meaning Princess) as last names for men and women, respectively. All men of Sikh faith are named *Singh* and all women are named *Kaur*. With time, the old last names have made inroads into Sikhism, and a many use *Singh* and *Kaur* as their middle names.

The basis of Sikhism is monotheism, the same theme as first accepted by Hinduism (by naming God as *Braham*; not to be confused with *Brahma*) and later by Abraham and incorporated into Judaism, Christianity, and Islam. Islamic monotheism arrived in India through earlier Muslim conquests; Guru Nanak was instrumental in reinforcing monotheism in the Indian subcontinent, and in introducing a unique concept that God could be achieved by directly praying to Him, without an intermediary. This concept challenged the role of priests and pundits in a major way. Because of this rigorous adherence to belief in one God, Sikhs use no images or idols in worship, as do Hindus. Furthermore, Sikhs do not proselytize for converts or advocate for holy pilgrimages, as do Muslims. Sikhism is a separate and distinct revelation by Guru Nanak, its first prophet.

The human body and every living object is the physical manifestations of the creator God on this earth; this concept is the core element and fundamental principle of Sikhism. Sikhs believe that God lives within the soul, and the purpose of this life is to discover/realize God within this human body, but egoism overpowers the mind and inculcates all other vices that keep people detached from, or unaware of, God. Reunion with the creator God is the purpose of life for Sikhs. The path to reunion with God is unconditional devotion to Him by "killing one's ego." To "die while yet alive" is the purpose of every Sikh. The only way this reunion can be achieved is through the medium of prayer and meditation in solitaire or in "the company of the holy" or *Saadh Sangat* (Sikh term for congregation) as a means of direct access to God. The reunion with the creator can be achieved through direct access to God; one does not have to go through an intermediary. There is no priestly class in Sikhism though there are "*granthis*" who physically care for the sacred scriptures and "*ragis*" that form "*jathas*" to lead the congregation in singing Sikh hymns. Therefore, in conjunction with prayer, reunion with God can be achieved by confronting and fighting against the worldly forces and vices that caused the separation of the soul from God.

Unlike some faith traditions that advocate a withdrawal from society and an ascetic lifestyle for this special type of closeness with God, Sikhs disavow the validity of asceticism and promulgate the importance of loyalty and devotion to normal family living as a householder. Indeed, Guru Nanak was married and had two sons. His religious awakening did not lead him to abandon family and household obligations in order to seek an ascetic lifestyle. However, people have to detach themselves from the five moral evils that arise from the ego and worldly desires: (1) lust (*kaam*), (2) anger (*krodh*), (3) greed (*lobh*), (4) love and

attachment (*moh*), and (5) pride (*ahankaar*). In this sense, the Sikh tradition of living out one's faith in the midst of living in the world of family, work, and secular society makes dedication to God even more challenging.

At the present time, there are approximately 23 million Sikhs around the world. This makes it the fifth-largest organized faith tradition behind Christianity, Islam, Hinduism, and Buddhism. About 2 per cent of India's population is Sikh with perhaps more than half a million in the United States. While most in the United States are "cradle" Sikhs (immigrants or children of immigrants), some came to the faith through Yogi Bhajan, who brought the Sikh teachings to the West. American (i.e., Western) converts practice *Kundalini Yoga* as a way to deepen the practice of their adopted faith, but this is not practiced by the mainstream Sikhs. *Sindhi* Sikhs are followers of Guru Nanak and *Sri Guru Granth Sahib*, who attend Gurdwara and Sikh ceremonies but do not keep *Five Kakaars* recommended by Guru Gobind Singh.

Basic Teachings

- Sikh concepts/stages of spiritual evolution:
  - *Manmukh* – A person who is controlled by 'mind' and is self-centered, only thinking about her/himself and the material world around her/him and is totally oblivious to God.
  - *Sikh* – A person who believes in one Immortal Being, ten gurus, from Guru Nanak to Guru Gobind Singh, the *Sri Guru Granth Sahib*, the utterances and teachings of the ten gurus, and who does not owe allegiance to any other religion.
  - *Khalsa* – A person who has shed her/

his ego and truly honors the memory of Guru Gobind Singh through actions and deeds as cited in the *Reht Maryada* (Official Sikh Code of Conduct) and by the baptism bequeathed by the tenth guru.

- *Gurmukh* – A person who has achieved *mukti* (salvation) and is totally God-centered. (Such a person is not necessarily a Sikh. Sikhism recognizes that individuals of other faiths may also be completely God-centered and free of self-centeredness.)

- Sikh philosophy, summarized in the first verse of the *Sri Guru Granth Sahib*, is called the *Mool Mantra* or the basic formula.
  - God is One whose names and qualities are infinite.
  - He is the creator of the universe and cosmos.
  - He is the only truth, the supreme truth.
  - He is the only immortal.
  - He is without fear or enmity.
  - He is omnipresent, pervading the universe.
  - He is unborn and undying, never to be born.
  - His grace enables all to achieve union with Him.
  - All may worship Him.

- Four key concepts of Sikhism are reflected by the Sikh symbol which is displayed on the *Nishan Sahib*, the saffron triangular flag which flies outside Sikh *Gurdwaras* (literally, "guru's door" but commonly understood as Sikh Temples). In the center of the symbol (formed from four weapons), there is a double-edged sword, a *Khanda*, representing knowledge of divinity. Surrounding the *Khanda* is a circular medieval weapon called a *Chakkar* symbolizing the unity of divinity. On either side are crossed daggers (*Kirpaans*) representing *Miri* and *Piri*, symbolizing spiritual and temporal power. Summary of the Four Key Concepts:

1. Knowledge of divinity
2. Unity of divinity
3. Spiritual power
4. Temporal power.

- Sikhs believe in reincarnation, which is the transmission of the soul from one body to another until the soul is liberated from the cycle of birth and death. However, the point of being a Sikh is to become liberated through devotion and good acts in this lifetime so one can dispel ego and open up oneself totally to being united with God at death, instead of being reborn in another body, either human or nonhuman, which some might consider a spiritual setback or even punishment for not living up to the moral standards of Sikh faith.

- Sikhism requires that one's work be morally upright, one's meditation faithful, and one's wealth shared with others.

- Since all are children of God, all are obligated to defend the helpless.

- Basic Sikh philosophy of life: the "five vices" to be avoided are pride, anger, greed, attachment, and lust; and the "five weapons" against them are contentment, charity, kindness, positive attitude, and humility.

- Because of the equality of men and women, either may be the *granthi* (reader of the scriptures) in communal worship.

Basic Practices

- Each and every major event of life starts as well as ends with a prayer to God. This prayer, called *Ardaas*, constitutes naming all of the eleven gurus, remembering the martyr, seeking permission and support to do something and, afterward, thanking God for the achievements. The day starts with an *Ardaas* and ends with an *Ardaas*.

- Living in family units is an important part of the Sikh faith, with sons continuing to live in their parents' homes after marriage. In old age, parents live with their son/s. Daughters live with their in-laws after marriage.
- Sikhs are encouraged to give 10% of their net earnings to charity.
- Sikhs do not use tobacco, alcohol, other intoxicants, illicit drugs, or gamble.
- Sikhs begin each day with washing and prayers.
- The *Kakaars* – Following baptism, a Sikh is called a *Khalsa*, the pure one, and wears the *Kakaars*, the five religious symbols more commonly known as the "Five Ks" all the time.
    1. *Kes* (*kesh*) – Uncut hair: Hair is considered a gift from God. Leaving it uncut represents spirituality and obedience to God. In order to keep the uncut hair neat, a turban is worn by males and a scarf by females. The headdress is a symbol of honor and should be highly respected.
    2. *Kangha* – Small wooden comb: The comb, which is used to groom the hair, also represents cleanliness.
    3. *Kara* – Steel bracelet: The *Kara* is a carry-over from the days when rings were worn on the head and arms as armor in battle. It is worn by most Sikhs and on the right wrist. According to the modern interpretation, the *Kara* can represent self-restraint and connectedness to God. The circular shape is symbolic of eternity, and the iron is symbolic of strength.
    4. *Kirpaan* – Symbolic short sword: The sword was used as a tool for self-defense purposes; it was never to be used to threaten or participate in any aggressive act. Sikhs are peace loving and the *Kirpaan* is a symbol of defending truth and justice. Presently, *Kirpaan* brooches are often worn instead of useable swords.
    5. *Kachhehra* – White undergarment knickers: The knickers represent purity of moral character and modesty.

Note: The Five Ks are not intended to foster superiority over non-Khalsa Sikhs or non-Sikhs. Such a fostering is antithetical to the ideals of the Sikh faith. They are meant to keep Sikhs who join the ranks of the Khalsa united in the pursuit of the aims and ideals of the Gurus. Adherence to the Five Ks is a requirement of the Sikh faith; the wearing of the kara is almost universal among all Sikhs.

- Sikhs remember and meditate upon *Waheguru* (pronounced wah-HEY-gur-oo), the name of God, throughout the day.
- Sikhs rise in the *Amrit Vela* (hours before dawn) to bathe, worship and meditate upon God, sing from and read the Holy Scriptures (*Sri Guru Granth Sahib*) or the collection of writings by Guru Nanak called the *Adi Granth*.
- Communal worship is important and traditionally held in a *gurdwara*, but services can be held anywhere the *Sri Guru Granth Sahib* (sacred text) is present. In the presence of *Sri Guru Granth Sahib* and in the *gurdwara*'s worship space, shoes are not worn, heads must be covered and men and women sit separately on the carpeted floor. Tobacco, tobacco products, and alcoholic products are forbidden. In the *gurdwara*'s kitchen, the *langar*, the communal vegetarian meal, is

prepared. Traditionally, men and women eat together by sitting on the floor as a way to demonstrate equality. Communal worship days are often chosen on the basis of the more accepted day of worship dominant in a particular culture; in the United States Sikhs worship on Sunday. The *gurdwara* is open every day for worship and prayers to everyone. People of other faith traditions are welcome and treated with equality, respect, and dignity. One can find shelter and food, for short terms needs, in the *gurdwara*.

- *Gurpurbs* are festivals marking the birth or death of a guru. The most commonly celebrated festivals are: Guru Nanak's birthday in November; Guru Gobind Singh's birthday in January; and Guru Arjan Dev's martyrdom day in June. Additionally, *Bandhi Chhor Diwas* is observed by Sikhs to commemorate the release of the sixth guru from prison, and *Baisakhi* (or *Vaisakhi*) is a harvest festival that commemorates the founding of the *Khalsa Panth*, the Sikh brotherhood by Guru Gobind Singh in 1699.

- Sikhs strive to serve all humanity (without regard for religious affiliation), particularly in defense of the helpless and marginalized. Ninth guru, Guru Teg Bahadur offered himself as a 'sacrifice' to protect and defend the weak and meek Kashmiri Hindus, and was beheaded in Delhi by the forces of Aurangzeb. Some scholars go to the extent of saying that without the protection of Sikhs, Hinduism might have been wiped off from this earth by Islam.

- Sikhs respect and actively work to defend all spiritual paths and religious traditions as tenaciously as their own.

- Sikhs have traditionally valued and honored women in contrast to the majority culture throughout the centuries. A famous ancient quotation by Guru Hargobind signifying the high value of women is "Woman is the conscience of Man." According to Guru Nanak, woman is the mother of kings and emperors. Therefore, how could she in any way be inferior to man? Even though the structure of Sikhism is patriarchal by contemporary standards, women have equal social status.

- Sikhs greet each other with folded hands, a head bow and say "*Sat Sri Akal*" (literal meaning: The Creator is the only Truth). *Sat Sri Akal* is the only method of greeting at the time of meeting, of departure, of happiness, of sorrow, and so forth. Sometimes people greet each other especially at religious gatherings by saying "*Waheguru ji ka Khalsa, Waheguru ji ki fateh*"(literal meaning: This *Khalsa* – person – belongs to the Guru, and Victorious is the Guru).

- Sikhs place a high value upon sharing food and eating and doing acts of service together.

- Rules of conduct include:
  ○ Life of honesty
  ○ Life of truth
  ○ Life of restraint
  ○ Life of householder (i.e., family oriented)
  ○ Life of piety (i.e., spiritual, moral, ethical lifestyle)

  Truth is the highest virtue, but higher still is the truthful living.[385]

- Truthful living includes
  ○ earning an honest living (*kirat karni*)

---

385 Quote handed down by oral tradition, attributed to Guru Nanak Dev.

○ meditation in God's name (*Naam japna*)

○ sharing the fruits of one's labor with the needy and avoiding exploiting the labor of others (*wand chhakna*).

Principles for Clinical Care
Dietary Issues

- Sikhs are often lacto-vegetarians (no meats), although some have dispensed with this tradition. In Punjab, though, Sikhs will eat goat or chicken as often as once a week. However, meat is not an essential or even an important part of a meal. It is never served as part of *Langar* (the food cooked and served in Gurdwara). The only formal ruling on meat is that Sikhs are forbidden to eat meat that has been sacrificed in a religious ceremony to God (e.g., *zabiha* or *halal* meat prepared in the Islamic tradition). Those who have accepted/taken *amrit* (the vows of the *Khalsa*) are committed to eating the lacto-vegetarian diet.
- The family may wish to share *prasad* (holy food which has been blessed during a religious ceremony) with the patient.
- Sikhs do not observe ritual fasts.

General Medical Beliefs

- Assisted suicide and euthanasia are not encouraged. Termination of life in any form is against the principles of Sikhism.

Specific Medical Issues

- **Abortion**: Abortion is not encouraged except for medical reasons because sanctity of life is an important principle of the Sikh faith.
- **Advance Directives**: Patients are encouraged to complete health care directives and medical durable power of attorney.

- **Birth Control**: There is no clear-cut ruling on this issue, but termination of life is immoral and not approved of.
- **Blood Transfusions**: Blood transfusions are allowed.
- **Circumcision**: Circumcision is not practiced as a part of the faith. Parents may request circumcision.
- **In Vitro Fertilization**: In vitro fertilization is a medical procedure, a mutual agreement reached between doctor and patient. There are no religious implications for Sikhs. However, artificial reproduction is only allowed within a marriage between a husband and a wife.
- **Stem Cell Research**: It is acceptable to use genetic engineering (e.g., stem cell research) to cure a disease. Stem cell research is a scientific, not religious issue. Human cloning is not acceptable.
- **Vaccinations**: Sikhs believe that health care is a real responsibility for the householder. It is also very much a personal choice as to vaccinations. Each choice must be viewed in light of what is healthy for each individual.
- **Withholding/Withdrawing Life Support**: Keeping a patient on artificial life support for a prolonged period of time in a vegetative state is not encouraged.

Note: Medical issues are modern day developments and no formal ruling is found in Sri Guru Granth Sahib, the holy book. To the best of my knowledge, there are no subsequent rulings on these issues (G. Singh).

Gender and Personal Issues

- Women enjoy equal social status, if not superior, to men. Guru Nanak challenged the prevalent inferior status of women in Hindu and Islamic cultures by questioning how a woman could be inferior to a man if she is the one who gives birth to the kings and saints and is a mother of a new life.

- In Sikh culture, men embrace each other as demonstration of happiness, and women do the same. However, embracing or even touching a person of the opposite gender is unaccepted. That is why most Sikhs fold their hands and say *Sat Sri Akal* (God is the Only Truth) to greet a person of the opposite gender instead of shaking hands. Sikhs will often prefer for medical personnel to be of the same sex as the patient. This is especially true for those of Indian heritage. If this is not possible, provide a chaperone of the same gender. This is more important in the case of female patients, and at childbirth.
- Females may insist upon covering their bodies with something more than a hospital gown, especially during examinations.
- The male adult elder is traditionally the spokesperson for the family; therefore, questions should be directed to him.
- Respect for modesty and privacy is important. Limit unnecessary touching and respect the patient's personal space.
- Always consult the patient and/or family before removing any hair on any part of the patient's body, both male and female.
- Sikhs wish to keep their hair covered with cloth, scarf, turban, or paper caps even when going in for surgical procedures.
- Cleanliness is a very important part of Sikh life. The patient should be allowed to bathe daily unless medically prohibited. Hair, including male facial hair, should be shampooed and conditioned as needed and combed by nursing staff. Hair may be allowed to dry naturally, with towel or with use of a hair dryer.
- Sikhs wash their bodies with water after using bathroom facilities. The use of toilet

paper is gradually becoming an accepted practice for cleaning oneself. Making water easily accessible to Sikh patients, though, in some sort of washbasin, would be an expression of understanding. Wet wipes can also be used.

Note: There is no formal ruling of the faith on the present-day life care options and medical beliefs and procedures in Sikhism. These listed have simply evolved with time, are personal decisions and are not governed by the teachings of Sikhism.

Principles for Spiritual Care through the Cycles of Life
Concepts of Living and Dying for Spiritual Support

- Life is not the beginning or the end. Life is a moment in the journey back to the Creator.
- All aspects of human life are opportunities for reunion with God.
- The physical body is perishable, but the soul is eternal, yearning for reunion with God.
- The goal for all of life is liberation from the cycle of life and death and reunion with God.
- Human life is a divine gift, and the *mukti* (liberation from the cycle of life and death), thereby; termination of life (bodily death) is a returning back to the Divine Source from which life originally came.
- Suffering is the result of *karma*, and it releases one from the negative acts of this or previous lifetimes. Therefore, it has meaning and must be endured with a steady faith in God.
- Dying and death is an opportunity to reexamine and reaffirm one's faith and acceptance of the will of God.

During Birth

- Some women will prefer female physicians and nursing personnel.
- Circumcision is not practiced as a part of the faith. Parents may request circumcision.
- Some mothers may want to save the umbilical cord from the placenta as a sacred remembrance of the motherly connection with the baby that was carried and nurtured in the womb for 9 months.
- Traditionally, mother and child are not separated for the first 40 days of the child's life except in medically necessary circumstances.
- An infant may be required to wear the religious symbols: the *Kakaar*. Most Sikhs, though, will only put the *Kara* on the infant's right wrist and dispense with the other four symbols.
- The naming practice involves opening the Holy Scriptures at random and taking the first letter of that page. A name is chosen using that letter. There is not a set period of time for the naming of the child.
- Males take the name *Singh*, which means Lion, and women take the name *Kaur*, which means Princess. This practice originated in order to remove names that indicated attachment to a particular caste. These gender specific designations may be used as a last or middle name and can be a method of identification that an individual is of the Sikh faith.
- In Western countries, many female Sikhs are adopting the name of "Singh" as a legal surname (for immigration, tax purposes, social security number, etc.)
- Contact priest or *granthi* for birth rituals.

During Illness

- Playing devotional music or listening to hymns from the *Sri Guru Granth Sahib* can provide spiritual support. The hymns and chants are called *Kirtan* and the recitations are called *Paath*. Sikhs may request an audiotape of *Kirtan* to be played at their bedsides.
- It is culturally and religiously important to visit the sick. Family and friends will tend to visit in groups. Please be patient with them.
- Visitors will often bring flowers.
- It is important not to interrupt prayers for routine care.
- A prayer room for Sikhs or an interfaith space would be meaningful. The space should be carpeted and quiet.
- If possible, establish a relationship with the local *gurdwara* (Sikh Temple) and a *granthi* (reader of scriptures) as resources. Scriptures are recited in the original languages. Thus, there is the need to request someone fluent in the language of scripture from the Sikh Temple.
- Many Sikhs will place pictures of Guru Nanak (the first guru) and Guru Gobind Singh (the tenth guru) by the bedside of the ill. They do not worship the pictures in any way, but are spiritually strengthened as they recall the greatness and spiritual devotion of these holy individuals.
- Sikhs may consider illness to be the will of God. They also believe that they have a role in the return to health, and this includes receiving medical treatment.
- The items of the *Kakaar*, such as the wooden comb or steel bracelet, should be kept close to the patient. The headdress should be respected, and if it needs to be removed, it should be given to the family. If this is not possible, it should be placed with the patient's belongings, but it should not be placed with the shoes because this would be considered disrespectful. Sikh patients may wish to keep

their head covered with an alternative covering after they have removed their headdress. A scarf or handkerchief can be used if it is large enough to be tied behind the head comfortably.

- If the patient and family are recent immigrants from Punjab or another country, it may be necessary to arrange for an interpreter. Take appropriate time to explain tests, procedures, and side effects with appropriate family members.
- Encourage the patient to complete a health care directive and medical durable power of attorney.
- Encourage the patient to complete an estate plan.

During End of Life

- Health care providers should contact the temple (gurdwara), the patient's relatives, the priest (addressed as Bhai Ji, Bhai Sahib, or Granthi Sahib) and the reader of the scriptures (granthi) when death is imminent for spiritual support through chanting, singing, and recitation of scriptures.
- Reciting and repeating Waheguru, Waheguru, Satnaam, Satnaam gives spiritual support and comfort at end of life. Health care professionals can facilitate this act of compassion.
- Remind the patient to concentrate on God and Guru.
- Remind the patient not to be afraid, but to trust in God's will and in Guru's power and protection.
- Presence of the priest is especially meaningful to family when patient is critically ill or dying.
- Family and/or friends should contact the temple and the priest when patient dies for last rites and funeral arrangements.
- Family may share prasad (sacred meal)

after the patient's death and may begin reciting (paath) or singing (kirtan).

- Touching the feet of the deceased by the family and friends is a gesture of respect to the deceased. Health care professionals can also touch the feet as a sign that they respect the deceased.
- Immediate family members, especially women, will often weep loudly as an expression of grief at the time of death.

Care of the Body

- Allow the family and priest to follow Sikh traditions for preparing the body for the funeral if requested. This would include: washing the body with fresh yogurt to eliminate any extraneous bacteria; dressing the body with fresh clothes, along with the appropriate positioning of the Kakaars with the body; covering the body with a, preferably unused, white cloth; and wrapping a saffron turban or scarf around the head. Chaplain or nurse should be consulted for assistance.
- Cremation is the only means of disposition of the body. The chaplain or nurse and the funeral home director should be consulted for assistance.
- Embalming is prohibited.
- The body should be transported to the funeral home as soon as possible, unless the family is waiting for a close relative to arrive to view the body. A chaplain or nurse should be consulted for assistance.
- The Kakaar (religious objects) should remain with the body.
- Cutting of the hair is forbidden before or after death.
- Autopsy is permitted if legally required and if it might benefit others.
- Organ donation for medical purposes/ research is an individual decision. A chaplain or nurse should be consulted

for assistance. Advance planning for such donations is required by most receiving organizations. Last-minute donations are usually not acceptable.

Organ and Tissue Donation

• Organ and tissue donation is permitted and is an individual decision. A chaplain and/or nurse who are trained designated requesters should be consulted for assistance.

Scriptures, Inspirational Writings, and Prayers

• Reciting and repeating *Waheguru, Waheguru, Satnaam, Satnaam* gives spiritual support and comfort at end of life. This act of compassion can be facilitated by health care professionals.
• Sikh patients may find comfort in texts from the *Sri Guru Granth Sahib*, subtitled as *Japji Sahib* and *Sukhmani Sahib*. Individuals can select those that would be of comfort to them.

THE TEN GURUS

1. Guru Nanak Dev (1469–1539)
2. Guru Angad Dev (1504–1552)
3. Guru Amar Das (1479–1574)
4. Guru Ram Das (1534–1581)
5. Guru Arjan Dev (1563–1606)
6. Guru Hargobind Rai (1595–1644)
7. Guru Har Rai (1630–1661)
8. Guru Har Krishan (1656–1664)
9. Guru Teg Bahadur (1621–1675)
10. Guru Gobind (Rai) Singh (1666–1708)

Further Reading

Cunningham, J. D. *History of the Sikhs*. Dehli, India: Rupa; 2007.

Duggal, K. S. (1988). *Philosophy and Faith of Sikhism*. Honesdale, PA: Himalayan Institute Press.

Gordon, J. J. H. *The Sikhs*. Patiala, India: Languages Department, Punjabi University. Delhi, India: Punjab National Press; 1970.

Joshi, L. M. (1969). *Sikhism*. Patiala, India: Punjabi University. New Delhi, India: Pauls Press.

McLeod, H. (1997). *Sikhism*. New Delhi, India: Yoda Press. Available at: www.amazon.com/Sikhism-Hew-McLeod/dp/0140252606#reader_0140252606.

Payne, C. H. (1970). *A Short History of the Sikhs*. Patiala, India: Languages Department, Punjabi University. Jullundur City, India: Swan Printing Press.

Singh, K. (2006). *The Illustrated History of the Sikhs*. New Delhi, India: Oxford University Press.

Singh, K. (2004). *A History of the Sikhs*. Vols. 1–2. 2nd ed. New Delhi, India: Oxford University Press.

Singh, P. (1999). *The Sikhs*. India: Random House.

Takhar, O. K. (2005). *Sikh Identity: An Exploration of Groups Among Sikhs*, Burlington, VT: Ashgate Publishing.

Teece, G. *Sikhism: Religion in Focus*. Mankato, MN. Black Rabbit Books; 2004

http://en.wikipedia.org/wiki/Sikhism

www.allaboutsikhs.com

Special Days: Sikhism

January 4 *Guru Gobind Singh's Birthday*

April 13 *Baisakhi* (Birthday of the *Khalsa* and beginning of harvest festival)

During first week of June *Guru Arjan Dev's Martyrdom day*

First full moon night in November *Guru Nanak Dev's Birthday*

Diwali, Lohri, Basant-Panchami, Christmas, New Year's Day, and so forth, are other special days Sikhs commonly celebrate with other religions and festivals.

Glossary of Sikh Terms

Adi Granth: The holy book Sri Guru Granth Sahib, compiled by Guru Arjan Dev (the fifth guru) in 1603–1604), and does not have the teachings of Guru Teg Bahadur (the ninth guru). Also know as Kartarpuri Biir.

ahankaar: Pride and ego; the first and primal vice that brings the person to his or her downfall.

Akal Purkh: The immortal being – Almighty, the God.

Amrit: 'Nectar of immortality'; sweetened initiation water used during Sikh initiation/baptism.

Amrit Vela: The Pure and Pious time, just before dawn, to pray to God.

Angad: (*Ang*: part, *Ad*: primal) – The primal part of the body; name given to the second Guru by Guru Nanak.

Ardaas: The Khalsa or Sikh prayer, a formal prayer recited at the beginning and the conclusion of most Sikh rituals.

Baisakhi (or *Vaisakhi*): A harvest festival that commemorates the founding of the *Khalsa Panth*, the Sikh brotherhood by Guru Gobind Singh in April of 1699.

Bandhi Chhor Diwas: The celebration day observed by Sikhs to commemorate the release of the sixth guru from prison, along with 51 Hindu kings who held onto Guru's coat to be released from the prison.

Bhai Ji or *Sahib*: "Brother"; title given to the piety, the priest in a Sikh *gurdwara*.

Bhagat: The contributor to Sri Guru Granth Sahib who was not one of the Gurus (e.g., Kabir, Namdev, Trilochan).

Braham: The One, the Almighty, The Creator who created this universe.

Brahma: Braham's assignee or representative responsible for creating new life in the universe.

Chakkar: A circle, representing the life/universe; symbolizing the unity of divinity; a heavy metallic ring worn on head to protect from enemy sword.

Five Ks: Five items, each beginning with the initial "K," which Sikhs of the Khalsa must wear. The five are Kes, Kangha, Kachhehra, Kirpaan, and Kara.

Granthi: Custodian of a *gurdwara*; who recites from the holy book, *Sri Guru Granth Sahib*.

gurdwara: Sikh temple (literal meaning: Guru's door).

Gurmukh: A person who listens to Guru, has achieved *mukti* (salvation), and is totally God-centered.

Gurmukhi: A distinctive script for the Punjabi language.

Gurpurb: "Guru's day," festivals marking the birth or death of a guru.

guru: (*Gu*: darkness and *Ru*: light) A teacher who leads his followers from darkness to light or from ignorance to spiritual elevation.

halal: The meat obtained/prepared by bleeding the animal to death, while reciting verses from the Koran (holy book of Islam).

Harimandir Sahib: The holiest shrine for the Sikhs, as Vatican is for the Christians, located in Amritsar, gilded with gold, and therefore also called the "Golden Temple" (*Hari*: God, *mandir*: temple; God's temple).

Ik Oankaar: One God, the creator is one, the One Being.

Japji Sahib: The very first subsection of Guru Nanak's teachings in *Sri Guru Granth Sahib*.

jatha: A group of Sikhs.

kaam: Lust; one of the five vices of human beings.

kachhehra: A pair of breeches, knickers, which must not extend below the knees, and must be worn all the time, worn as one of the Five Ks or *Kakaars*.

Kakaars: The five items, starting with the initial K, to be worn all the time by a Sikh/Khalsa.

kangha: Wooden comb, worn as one of the Five Ks or *Kakaars*.

kara: Iron wrist ring, worn as one of the Five Ks or *Kakaars*.

karma: The destiny, fate of an individual, generated in accordance with the deeds performed in one's present and past existences.

Kaur: "Princess"; the last name of a Sikh female, now getting more and more to be the middle name.

kes: (Kesh) Uncut hair, worn as one of the Five Ks or *Kakaars*.

Khalsa: The religious order established by Guru Gobind Singh in 1699; the person belonging to that order; the pure/pious one.

Khanda: Two-edged sword; Khalsa or Sikh symbol comprising a vertical two-edged sword over a quoit with two crossed *kirpaans* below the quoit; representing knowledge of divinity.

kirat karni: To earn an honest living.

kirpaan: Sword or poniard, worn as one of the Five Ks or Kakaars, only for self-defense.

kirtan: Singing of hymns from *Sri Guru Granth Sahib*.

krodh: Anger; one of the five vices of human being.

langar: The kitchen attached to every Gurdwara from which food is served to all regardless of caste and creed; the meal served from such a kitchen.

Lehna: The original name of the second Guru, Guru Angad Dev.

lobh: Greed; one of the five vices of human being.

manmukh: A person who is controlled by 'mind' and is self-centered.

Miri-Piri: Doctrine that the Guru possesses temporal (*Miri*) as well as spiritual authority (*Piri*).

moh: Love and attachment toward family and material world; one of the five vices of human being.

Mool Mantra: "The basic formula"; the summarized description of the Almighty, God, given by Guru Nanak.

mukti: Liberation from the cycle of rebirth; control over one's vices.

Naam: A summary term expressing the total being of *Akal Purkh*.

Naam japana: To recite the divine Name of *Akal Purkh*.

Nishan Sahib: The saffron triangular flag, Sikh flag, which flies outside Sikh *Gurdwara*.

paath: A reading from the Sikh scriptures.

Panj Pyare: The "Cherished Five" or "Five Beloved," the first five Sikhs to be initiated as members of the Khalsa by Guru Gobind Singh in April 1699; five Sikhs in good standing chosen to represent the community.

Panth: The Sikh community; a "path" or "way"; system of religious belief or practice.

prasad: Sacramentally offered sweetened food/pudding, usually at the end of the Sikh ceremony; God's grace.

Ragas: The musical/recital ways of singing the hymns. Sri Guru Granth Sahib is compiled into a total of 31 ragas.

ragi: The singers of holy hymns; who do *kirtan* from *Sri Guru Granth Sahib*.

Reht Maryada: Official Sikh Code of Conduct.

Saadh Sangat: The company of the "Holy," the Sikh congregation.

Satnaam: His name "Naam" is the only Truth.

Sat Sri Akal: "God is the Only Truth"; the Sikh greetings to young or old, male or female, while meeting or departing, usually said with folded hands and bowed head.

Sindhi: People from the Sindh province in India and Pakistan.

Singh: "Lion"; the last name given to male Sikhs by Guru Gobind Singh to infuse/inject sense of bravery, and to discard the caste system among Sikhs by dropping the occupational last names.

Sri Guru Granth Sahib: The holy book compiled by Guru Arjan Dev but finished by Guru Gobind Singh (the tenth guru) by adding the teachings of Guru Teg Bahadur.

Sufi: A member of one of the Muslim mystical orders.

Sukhmani Sahib: "The Treasure of Happiness/Pleasures"; a subsection of teachings of Guru Arjan Dev in the holy book *Sri Guru Granth Sahib*.

Waheguru: "Praise to the Guru"; modern Sikh name for God.

Waheguru ji ka Khalsa, Waheguru ji ki fateh: Sikh greetings meaning "Khalsa belongs to the Guru, and victory to the Guru."

wand chhakna: To share the earned living/food.

zabiha: The meat prepared in the Islamic tradition.

Spiritualism

As the sunflower turns its face toward the light of the sun, so Spiritualism turns the face of humanity toward the light of truth.[386]

Prepared by:
The Reverend Lelia E. Cutler, NST, CM
President, National Spiritualist Association of
** Churches, Inc.**
National Headquarters
Lily Dale, NY

Reviewed and approved by:
Robert A. Nash, MD, FAAN;
The Reverend Sharon Snowman, NST, CM, CH
Secretary, National Spiritualist Association of Churches
Lily Dale, NY

History and Facts

The publication of the 1847 book *The Principles of Nature*, by Andrew Jackson Davis, was a precursor to what is called Modern Spiritualism. Davis made the astonishing claim that the "spirit" of Emanuel Swedenborg had dictated the book which discussed the evolution of the world, culture and religion. Then, on March 31, 1848, Margaret Fox and her daughters, Catherine (Katie) age 9, and Margaretta Fox (Maggie), age 11, stated that, through "telegraphic rapping" in their home at Hydesville, New York, near Rochester, they had established communication with the spirit of murdered peddler Charles B. Rosna. As a result of these girls' experience and their mother's help, communication with spirit commenced. The religion of Modern American Spiritualism points to this day in 1848 as its beginning. The first public demonstration took place November 14,

1849 in Corinthian Hall, Rochester, New York, and started the spread of Spiritualism across the United States, as well as to the shores of Europe, Australia, Africa, and eventually around the world.

Spiritualism's roots date from antiquity. Ancient Spiritualism prevailed in all countries and spirit communication was the basis of many ancient religious belief systems. However, these traditions incorporated within their structures the belief that spiritual phenomena occurred due to miraculous intervention, superstitions, use of magic, or mystical events. The following discussion in this paragraph serves to validate this point. Professor Boscowen, a noted archaeologist, stated in his *Records of the Monments*:

> In dreams and visions the primitive Akkadians, the people of ancient Akad, a region in north Babylonia, about the years 2800 BC to 11 BC, saw the shadowy forms of the departed human beings, which led them

---

386 Quote is the motto of Spiritualism, available from the website www.nsac.org/history.php.

to regard these forms as still existing in some dark, far distant subterranean place.[387]

In the Egyptian *Book of the Dead*, one finds the theory of the soul and its transmigration; sun worship impressed the minds of the Egyptians of a spiritual universe, and they practiced healing at the temple in Alexandria. The Persians also believed in an afterlife and in the harmony of all souls with God. The Greeks, as well, had a belief in future life that spirit can be recognized when it appears; they also had a belief in guides and the doctrine of reincarnation. The Orientals, likewise, believed in immortality, reincarnation, salvation by one's development and acceptance of responsibilities, ancestral worship, karma, and preexistence. Similarly, the Nordics believed in communication with spirit, that death does not bring instant knowledge and death does not transform one's character. Not unlike the other traditions mentioned, the Hebrews believed in communication with spirits and God. And in ancient times, Christians taught immortality and mediumship, along with the idea of a physical body and a spiritual body.[388]

Spiritualism is defined as the science, philosophy, and religion of continuous life, based upon the demonstrated fact of communication, by means of mediumship, with those who live in the spirit world. It has a goal of satisfying one's logic, mind, and heart. Spiritualism gives a person the key that can be used to find the answers to life's many and difficult questions. It provides the knowledge that, by using prayer and meditation, people can become more aware of their responsibilities to themselves and to others. Through this inner awareness and guidance received through spirit communications, a person can take the necessary actions to improve his or her own life and contribute to the improved welfare of the entire human race.

Spiritualism is a common-sense religion, accepts all truths and endeavors to prove the validity of those truths. The many truths are found in nature, in other religions, in science, in philosophy, in Divine Law and are received through spirit communication. A major premise of Spiritualism is that humans are spiritual beings, an indivisible part of the Divine. God is the Spirit within each individual waiting to be consciously accepted and activated. Thus, one of the desires of Spiritualism is to awaken this internal spirit and enable individuals to move beyond the five senses to a higher level of awareness.

Some of the pioneers of Spiritualism include Professor Robert Hare (1781–1858), a professor of chemistry at the University of Pennsylvania and one of the best-known men of science in America at the time. Some of his investigations are discussed in one of his books, *Experimental Investigation of the Spiritual Man*. Nathaniel Potter Tallmadge (1795–1864), a United States Senator from Wisconsin, was one of 13 000 Spiritualists on a memorial petition asking Congress to appoint a select committee that investigated the claim of possible communication with the so-called dead. Robert Dale Owen (1801–1875) served in the Indiana Legislature and was responsible for introducing the bill that organized the Smithsonian Institute; he promoted Spiritualism as part of his book *Footfalls on*

---

387 William St. Chad Boscawen cited in Colville, W. (1906). *Universal Spiritualism*. New York, NY: R. F. Fenno and Company, 297.

388 Colville. *Universal Spiritualism*, 295–303. The overview of the different religions' beliefs came from this source.

the Boundaries of Another World.

Horace Greeley (1811–1872), an American journalist and political leader, was named the Abraham Lincoln of Modern Spiritualism; he became the sponsor of the Fox sisters when they stayed in New York City. Professor Joseph Rhodes Buchanan (1814–1899) coined the term "psychometry" after an intense study of the "soul-of-things." Judge John Worth Edmonds (1816–1874) was instrumental in forming the New York Circle in 1851, and is the author of *Spiritualism*, volumes I and II, and *Appeal to the Public*. Professor J. S. Loveland (1818–?) was the author of the first American book on Spiritualism, *Esoteric Truths of Spiritualism.*

Cora L. V. Richmond (1840–1923), known as the "silver-tongued orator," attended the first convention for the National Spiritualist Association in 1893 and became the vice-president of the organization. Thomas Grimshaw (1866–1938) became superintendent of the Bureau of Education for the Morris Pratt Institute and, with the Honorable Mark A. Barwise of Maine, prepared the first *General Correspondence Course* on Spiritualism. There are many more pioneers in Spiritualism, and references can be found in: the compilation titled "Pioneers of Spiritualism," volumes I–V, written by Audra Cutlip; *Modern American Spiritualism* by Emma Hardinge Britten; along with others listed in the recommended reading in the Morris Pratt Course.

The National Spiritualist Association of Churches (NSAC) publishes a *Spiritualist Manual* which is on the podium of all NSAC Spiritualist churches. Most Spiritualist organizations publish their own manual and it is used in lieu of a "holy" scripture. However, all Spiritualists revere and use other scriptures, including the Christian Bible. A listing of all references is contained in the *Spiritualist Manual.*

The NSAC has approximately 100 auxiliaries in the United States. There are many other Spiritualist associations in the United States, and a listing of churches can be found online (www.nsac-churches.org/cssa convention/Churches.html). Some of the larger and more active Spiritualist organizations would include the International General Assembly of Spiritualists headquartered in California, United Metaphysical Churches headquartered in Roanoke, Virginia, American Federation of Spiritualists headquartered in Massachusetts, and the Bridge of Light headquartered in Texas. When groups break off from a national organization, they often go independent, and there are numerous independent groups.

Spiritualism has spread around the world. The International Spiritualist Federation (ISF, a fraternal Spiritualist group founded in 1923) lists liaisons in Australia, Austria and Hungary, Belgium, Canada, England, Finland, France, Iceland, Netherlands, New Zealand, Scotland, Sweden, Switzerland, and the United States. There are also members from Brazil, Chile, and other South American countries.

The Spiritualist National Union (SNU), founded on October 18, 1901, with its headquarters in England, is one of the largest Spiritualist organizations existing in the world today. The Arthur Findlay College, located in Stanstead, England, is known as the world's foremost college for the advancement of Spiritualism and Psychic Sciences. Stansted Hall, built in 1871, was bequeathed to the SNU by J. Arthur Findlay, MBE, JP, a former Honorary President of the Union. Spiritualists from around the world study there.

The SNU has seven principles:

1. The Fatherhood of God
2. The Brotherhood of Man
3. The Communion of Spirits and the Ministry of Angels
4. The continuous existence of the human soul
5. Personal responsibility
6. Compensation and retribution hereafter for all the good and evil deeds done on earth
7. Eternal progress open to every human soul.

(These seven principles of the SNU, created by Emma Hardinge Britten, differ from those used in the United States by the NSAC; *see* "Basic Teachings" section. However, the services and practices of the two organizations are similar in content.)

Spiritualist organizations in other parts of the world have adopted the same principles as the SNU or the NSAC, and some have changed or modified the principles to fit their own belief system.

Spiritualists come from every walk of life – bankers, builders, nurses, teachers, bookkeepers, sales clerks, electricians, and so forth. Spiritualism is the key that sets humanity free: free to live and grow in the physical through love and law; free because life is continuous, the spirit never dies. "There is no death, there are no dead."

Basic Teachings

- Spiritualism is a *science* because it investigates, analyzes, and classifies facts and manifestations demonstrated from the spirit side of life.
- Spiritualism is a *philosophy* because it studies the laws of nature both on the "seen and unseen" sides of life and bases

its conclusions upon observation. It accepts statements of observed facts of past ages, and conclusions drawn therefrom, when sustained by reason and by results of observed facts of the present day.

- Spiritualism is a *religion* because it strives to understand and to comply with the physical, mental, and spiritual laws of nature, which are in essence the laws of God.
- The purpose of the organized movement of spiritualism as represented by the National Spiritualist Association of Churches may be stated in part as follows:
  - To teach the truths and principles expressed in the *Declaration of Principles* and in the definitions of a spiritualist, a medium, and a healer.
  - To teach and proclaim the science, philosophy and religion of modern Spiritualism.
  - To encourage lectures on all subjects pertaining to the spiritual and secular welfare of humanity.
  - To protest against every attempt to compel humanity to worship God in any particular or prescribed manner.
  - To advocate and promote spiritual healing.
  - To protect and encourage spiritual teachers and mediums in all laudable efforts in giving evidence of proof to humanity of a continued intercourse and relationship between the living and the so-called dead.
  - To encourage every person who holds present spiritual beliefs to always be open to restatement of those beliefs as future thought and investigation reveal understanding of new truths; thereby, leaving every individual free to follow the dictates of reason and conscience in spiritual matters.

- Foundational beliefs of the faith are contained in nine *Declaration of Principles*[389] in their original form with explanations of each principle by Joseph P. Whitwell, third president of the National Spiritualist Association of Churches, Inc., who served in the early to mid-twentieth century.

1. *We believe in Infinite Intelligence.* By this, Spiritualists express belief in a supreme Impersonal Power; called by some, God, by others, Spirit, and by Spiritualists, Infinite Intelligence. Infinite Intelligence pervades and controls the universe, is without shape or form and is impersonal, omnipresent, and omnipotent.

2. *We believe that the phenomena of nature, both physical and spiritual, are the expression of Infinite Intelligence.* In this manner, Spiritualists express belief in the immanence of Spirit and that all forms of life are manifestations of Spirit or Infinite Intelligence, and thus, all are children of God.

3. *We affirm that a correct understanding of such expression and living in accordance therewith constitute true religion.* A correct understanding of the laws of nature on the physical, mental, and spiritual planes of life and living in accordance with them will allow for realization of the highest aspirations of the soul, which is the correct function of true religion.

4. *We affirm that the existence and personal identity of the individual*

continue after the change called death. Life here and hereafter is all one life whose continuity of consciousness is unbroken by that mere change in form whose process we call death.

5. *We affirm that communication with the so-called dead is a fact, scientifically proven by the phenomena of Spiritualism.* Spirit communication has been experienced throughout history and is amply recorded in both sacred and profane literature of all ages. Spiritualism accepts and recognizes these manifestations and interprets them in the understanding and light of natural law.

6. *We believe that the highest morality is contained in the Golden Rule: "Do unto others as you would have them do unto you."* This precept points the way to harmony, peace, and happiness. Wherever tried, it has proven successful; and when fully understood and practiced it will bring peace and happiness to all of humanity.

7. *We affirm the moral responsibility of the individual and that we make our own happiness or unhappiness as we obey or disobey nature's physical and spiritual laws.* Individuals are responsible for the welfare of the world in which they live. If people are to obtain heaven upon earth, they must learn to make that heaven, for themselves and for others. Individuals are responsible for their own spiritual growth and welfare. Errors and wrongdoing must be outgrown and overcome. Virtue and love of good must take their place. Spiritual growth and advancement must be attained by aspiration and personal striving. Individuals must bear their

---

389 These principles were adopted in the following manner: Principles 1–6 adopted in Chicago, IL, 1899; Principles 7–8 adopted in Rochester, NY, 1909; Principle 9 adopted in St. Louis, MO, 1944; Principle 9 revised in Oklahoma City, OK, 1983; Principle 9 revised in Westfield, NJ, 1998; Principle 8 revised in Rochester, NY, 2001; and Principle 6 revised in Ronkonkoma, NY, 2004.

own burdens in overcoming wrong doings and replace them with right actions.

8. *We affirm that the doorway to reformation is never closed against any soul here or hereafter.* Spiritualists discard the teachings of eternal damnation and accept the thought of the continuity of life beyond death. They accept no such teaching as "hell fire," but Spiritualism does teach that transgression of natural law and wrong-doing will necessarily bring remorse and suffering which can only be relieved by the individual's own efforts, if not in this life, then in the hereafter.

9. *We affirm that the precepts of prophecy and healing are divine attributes proven through mediumship.* Spiritualists affirm their belief in and acceptance of the truth that prophecy, mediumship, and healing are not unique, but are universal, everlasting and have been witnessed and observed in all ages.

- A simplified form of the *Declaration of Principles* (as follows) is used by the Children's Progressive Lyceum.

  1. We believe in God.
  2. We believe that God is expressed through all Nature.
  3. True religion is living in obedience to Nature's Laws.
  4. We never die.
  5. Spiritualism proves that we can talk with people in the Spirit World.
  6. Be kind, do good, and others will do likewise.
  7. We bring unhappiness to ourselves by the errors we make, and we will be happy if we obey the laws of life.
  8. Every day is a new beginning.

9. Prophecy and healing are expressions of God.

- Definitions of a *spiritualist*, a *medium*, and a *healer*:
  - A *Spiritualist* is one who believes, as the basis of his or her religion, in the communication between the physical and the spirit world by means of mediumship; it is also one who endeavors to mold his or her character and conduct in accordance with the highest teachings derived from such communication. To become a Spiritualist, a person shows interest, desire, and willingness to attend membership classes, usually one night a week for six weeks.
  - A *Medium* is one who is sensitive to "vibrations" from the spirit world. Through him/her, intelligences in that world are able to convey messages and produce the phenomena of Spiritualism prophecy which consists of: clairvoyance, clairaudience, gift of tongues, laying on of hands, healing, visions, trance, apports, revelations, raps, levitation, automatic and independent writing and painting, photography, materialization, psychometry, direct and independent voice, and any other manifestation which proves the continuity of life.
  - A *Spiritualist Healer* is one who, either through his or her own inherent powers or through mediumship, is able to impart vital, curative force to pathologic conditions. To become a healer, a person must be a member of the organization and take the required courses.
- Training for work as a healer, medium, minister, or National Spiritualist Teacher requires completion of the 30 lesson Educational Course on Modern Spiritualism as administered by the

Morris Pratt Institute (or equivalent course of study through the Center for Spiritualist Studies or college level courses of study). Completion of the course takes an average of 2½ years. If a person desires to become ordained through the NSAC, they must first take the Morris Pratt Study Course or equivalent courses through the Center for Spiritualist Studies. They must also attend the two-week Pastoral Skills Seminar, which is an intensive course in the skills and abilities used as a minister in the religion of Spiritualism (or any other religion's seminary training). The practice received in this two-week intensive includes counseling techniques, lecturing pointers, visitation "do's and don'ts," and what is expected of a person serving Spiritualism as an ordained minister. If individuals wish to obtain their commission as a healer, this path is separate from the course for a minister, but includes a lot of the same study. There are certain lessons in the Morris Pratt Course required for the healing certificate, and there is a requirement for affidavits from persons receiving healing, stating it was received in accordance with the definition of a Spiritualist Healer. Acceptance of affidavits for a healing commission includes wording to the fact that a pathologic condition was healed or improved substantially during the healing. If one decides to obtain certification as a medium, the requirements are similar in that certain lessons in the Morris Pratt Study Course must be completed, and affidavits must be obtained showing identification of spirit through mediumship which is identifiable by the recipient of the message. The National Spiritualist Teacher's degree is also a separate credential obtained through completion of the

MPI course or equivalent studies, completion of the Pastoral Skills seminar, and an extensive exam, both written and oral with the National Board. These credentials may be obtained individually, or a person may decide to obtain all of the certifications available. Many students often take the ordination and NST exams at the same time since they include some of the same information.)

- **Spiritualism teaches:**
  - personal responsibility
  - people do not have souls, but are souls and have a body
  - people are spiritual beings, even though in the physical world
  - what people sow on earth, they reap in the afterlife
  - the spark of divinity dwells in all
  - no need to fear death because it is a "portal" to the spirit world
  - comfort for the bereaved through knowledge of continuous life.
- The inhabitants of the spirit world, under proper conditions, have the power to return to this world and manifest themselves in various ways: from a mental suggestion to a visual appearance. All people are spiritual beings, evolved from the lower forms of life, through the period of consciousness, to the state of the higher moral and spiritual faculties; these faculties survive unaffected by the decomposition of the physical body. Spiritual happiness does not depend upon belief or creed, but upon character. The universe is an aggregation of forces and matter, which always moves and acts in the same manner under the same conditions and is not capriciously governed.
- The whole duty of humanity consists in taking the first steps in the attainment of knowledge and in gradually developing

character and nature to harmonize with the fully unfolded spiritual state. This duty encompasses the entirety of one's conduct: mentally, morally, and spiritually.

Basic Practices

- Spiritual education is a most important preparation for spiritual progress, which leads to happiness in the present and the hereafter. For the spiritual evolution of people's souls, they must practice self-control, self-reliance, as well as reliance upon the instructions of their teachers. If people know what they believe, then under trials, tests, and sorrowful conditions, they will be at peace in their faith and in the wisdom and protective power of their faithful but invisible friends.

- Spiritual healing is recognized by many sacred texts, including the Christian New Testament, and is a tenet of ancient and modern religions. A spiritual healer possesses a gift, or talent, for passing healing energy from spiritual forces to recipients. This energy helps to bring about relief, cure, and healing of both mental and physical conditions.

- Modes of spiritual healing include:
  - *Contact Healing* – In contact healing, the physical contact assists the healer transfer curative energy to the recipient. The healer's hand or hands are placed upon the recipient's head, shoulders or both, becoming a conduit through which this energy flows. Many contact healers place one hand upon the recipient's forehead and another upon the back of the neck. Contact with the head and shoulders is sufficient for the purpose of healing.
  - *Absent Healing* – This is a curative power sent to someone at a distance

through prayer. Positive prayer creates a bond with Infinite Intelligence and healing spirit entities. Prayer is a mighty force. When linked with energy from the spirit realms, it expands to embrace the positive, eliminates the negative and helps perfect health to manifest itself. Without this help, the healer is powerless to relieve the recipient's condition. The NSAC Prayer for Spiritual Healing (*see* "Scriptures, Inspirational Readings, and Prayers" section) is offered on behalf of the recipient. Absent healing works even if the individual does not know healing is being sent
  - *Magnetic Healing* – A superabundance of magnetic energy within the physical being of some people helps to facilitate the ready transference of the extra healing energy to others.

- Normal church services are held on Sundays and include the following components: Opening, hymn, invocation, reading of the Declaration of Principles, healing service, special music selection, lecture, offering, announcements, hymn to raise vibration for message service, message service, benediction, and closing hymn. The healing service may include a healing hymn, a meditation, and the laying on of hands healing, and may take place in the middle of the worship service or just before the worship service. Services are also held on Wednesday evenings and may be special services of just messages or a healing service, or they may follow the normal order of worship.

- Individuals desiring to join the church are expected to attend worship services for approximately six months, complete an application on the NSAC approved form, be approved by the board of directors of the church; they are then extended the "right hand of fellowship" during a worship service. The right hand of fellowship includes a prayer for the candidate, a list of questions which require an affirmative answer, and a closing prayer, followed by the singing of *Blest Be the Tie* and an invitation to the congregation to welcome the new member following the service.

- People are encouraged to take classes on meditation, developing mediumship, healing, public speaking and platform decorum, history of Spiritualism, comparative religion, and other subjects as requested. Home circles are encouraged and are the basic learning tools for mediumship and meditation.
- All Spiritualists are encouraged to participate in community activities, and most churches keep a food pantry for those in need.
- Spiritualists do not proselytize but hold discussion groups for anyone interested in the religion and philosophy of life.

Principles for Clinical Care
Dietary Issues

- Spiritualism has no dietary restrictions. Based on the concept of personal responsibility, Spiritualists believe that they must practice healthy eating and exercise habits to take care of the body which is the residence of the divine spark. It is important to take care of the temple (body) to ensure progressive living until death.

General Medical Beliefs

- Spiritual healing, recognized in many religions, has been a principle of Spiritualism since its beginning. Evidence is growing in the medical community of the importance of spiritual healing in the well-being of patients.

- A Spiritualist healer works with the spirit, mind, emotions, and the body of the recipient. A Spiritualist healer is aware that when stress is removed from the mind and emotions, the body will respond naturally. This brings about holistic healing in the patient.
- A Spiritualist healer is one who, either through his or her own innate power or through mediumship, is able to transmit curative energies to the physical conditions of others. The results of spiritual healing are produced in several ways:
  - by spiritual influences working through the body of the medium to transmit curative energies to the diseased parts of the recipient's body
  - by spiritual influences enlightening the mind of the medium so that the cause, nature, and seat of the disease in the recipient is made known to the medium
  - by the application of absent healing treatments whereby spiritual beings combine their own healing energies with the energies of the medium and cause them to be absorbed by the system of the recipient.
- Spiritualist healers acknowledge the importance of the medical community and work in cooperation with it at all times.
- Spiritualism recognizes that the medical community is an instrument of healing of the Infinite.
- Spiritualism's counseling guidelines for spiritual healing and physical cure are:
  - Strengthening one's innate healing ability by sitting regularly in meditation and by practicing a healthy lifestyle.
  - Believing in the body's ability to generate its own healing energy. Thought is the basis of all actions. Thoughts have an impact on every cell for either health

or disease. Anger, fear, hatred, jealousy, and despair depress vital energy. Faith, hope, happiness, and kindness stimulate essential life forces and promote healing.

- ○ Practicing affirmations and daily saying the NSAC Healing Prayer.
- ○ Placing one's feet flat on the floor and hands laying open on the lap when sitting for healing; this creates a positive flow of energy.
- ○ Remembering that healing is a *complementary* therapy, *not* an alternative therapy.
- ○ Seeing a licensed healing professional if one has not done so and to never give up taking either medication or the health care professional's advice.
- Spiritual healers should not make medical diagnoses or provide psychological counseling unless specifically licensed to do so.
- Spiritual healers should not recommend drugs or a specific type of treatment, manipulate the recipient's body, or use/sell any product (including herbs or crystals) in giving a healing.

Specific Medical Issues

- **Abortion**: Spiritualism stands on the premise that the individual is responsible for her own happiness regarding abortion. It is not the prerogative of organized religion to mandate what constitutes happiness to an individual. It is the individual's right to make an informed choice in the matter as she alone would be responsible for her actions. This statement does not say Spiritualism is pro-choice; it states the faith is in favor of informed choice.
- **Advance Directives**: Spiritualism affirms life and death with dignity. It also affirms the right of each individual, by the use of advance directives, to determine the extent to which the medical community or family may interfere with the treatment of a terminal or irreversible condition. Spiritualists are obligated to follow the law.
- **Birth Control**: As stated under Abortion, Spiritualism stands on the premise that the individual is responsible for their own happiness regarding children. It is not the prerogative of organized religion to mandate what constitutes happiness to an individual. It is the individual's right to make an informed choice in the matter of having children, and any means to encourage or discourage the birth process.
- **Blood Transfusions**: Spiritualism has no specific directive relating to blood transfusions. It is an individual choice.
- **Circumcision**: Spiritualism has no specific directive relating to circumcision. It is an individual choice.
- **In Vitro Fertilization**: Spiritualism has no specific directive relating to in vitro fertilization. It is an individual choice.
- **Stem Cell Research**: Spiritualism supports all life-saving research.
- **Vaccinations**: Spiritualism has no specific directive relating to vaccinations, only to encourage healthy bodies and support for the medical community.
- **Withholding/Withdrawing Life Support**: Spiritualism believes in life and death with dignity. Withdrawing/withholding life support in medically futile cases does not violate the teachings of faith.

Gender and Personal Issues

- There are no gender or personal issues in the practice of Spiritualism. Any issues in this area would be individual choice.

Principles for Spiritual Care through the Cycles of Life

Concepts of Living and Dying for Spiritual Support

- Every soul will progress through the ages to heights, sublime and glorious, where God is Love and Love is God.
- Death is not the cessation of life, but simply a change of condition.
- Death is viewed as part of life and not a punishment.
- Those who have passed on are conscious not asleep.
- There is communion between the living and the dead.
- God's message to mortals is "There is no death ... That all who have passed on still live and there is hope in the life beyond for the most negative."
- Spiritualism teaches that the soul is eternal.
- Children and other persons who die before they have reached full stature grow to full stature in the spirit world; they are able, by the exercise of will power, to make their appearance, in size and form, as it was at the time of their passing. These laws apply also to the baby who dies physically unborn.
- The purpose of life in the spirit world is to unfold the mental, moral, and spiritual faculties; to study the works of nature, to help perverse and undeveloped spirits out of their low condition, to minister to earth's children (either through influence directly exerted or through the instrumentality of mediums), to enjoy the fellowship of kindred minds, and to share the sweetness of pure love; in short, to complete the individualization of the human soul.

During Birth

- After the birth of a child, Spiritualism has a "Naming Ceremony" in which the parents and God-parents participate. In "naming" the child, the minister uses flowers to sprinkle over the child instead of water; special poems or songs may also be used as part of the ceremony. Anyone can perform this ceremony, but it is recommended that a minister be included as this can be termed a legal ceremony.
- Fetal demise or death of a baby is handled like the death of any other person, with the decisions made by the parents of the child.

During Illness

- The patient or family may request a visit from a minister or commissioned healer.
- The religious needs and desires of the patient will vary greatly by individual; some like a healer to be present, some like a prayer session, and some just need the presence of a member of the clergy. The minister should always ask the patient and/or the family about appropriate times for visitation and inquire about any special needs.
- The family should freely contact a minister or member of the church board whenever a member is hospitalized or needs an in-home visit.
- Healing is a primary focus of the Spiritualist religion, and its clergy and commissioned healers willingly visit patients.
- Some patients will welcome a visit by a minister, healer, volunteer, or chaplain, while others may see it as intrusive. The patient's wishes should be respected.

During End of Life

- Patient/family may request visit from a minister or commissioned healer.
- Patients may appreciate a gentle touch, a visit, or a prayer.
- When visiting a patient nearing death, the minister will often talk to them of those in the spirit world who are waiting to assist them in the transition. The patient may talk of seeing their parents or loved ones around them, and the minister adds support to these images. Knowing that loved ones in Spirit draw near when the death experience is imminent is a comfort to the patient.

Care of the Body

- The family of the deceased generally makes funeral and burial arrangements in consultation with their minister and the funeral home in charge of the burial.
- If the body is to be buried, a viewing is usually held the day before the actual funeral and committal services.
- If the body is cremated, the family may decide to have a memorial service at the convenience of the family members.
- In Spiritualism, the "clay body" is committed to Mother Earth when buried, and is scattered with appropriate services when cremated.
- If the individual wishes for their body to be donated for medical research, that is a personal choice. There is no restriction or directive concerning donation in the Spiritualist belief.
- If an autopsy is required, there is no restriction in Spiritualism.

Organ and Tissue Donation

- Organ and tissue donation is a personal decision for each individual.

Scriptures, Inspirational Readings, and Prayers

- There are no prescribed prayers for use in Spiritualism other than the Healing Prayer.
- The prayer for Spiritual Healing is recited at all worship services in Spiritualism and also repeated, whenever needed, to help an individual with healing. The children's version of the Healing Prayer is used in the Children's Progressive Lyceum meetings.
- It is also appropriate and encouraged for patients or family to simply pray spontaneously. This would also apply in times of grief and loss.

CHILDREN'S HEALING PRAYER

I ask God's Healing Power to make
  me whole and well.
I know that I work with God,
  through my thoughts and actions to
  make this happen.
I ask God's Healing Power to heal
  other people near and far away,
I trust that God will answer this
  healing prayer.

PRAYER FOR SPIRITUAL HEALING

I ask the great unseen healing force
  to remove all obstructions from my
  mind and body and to restore me to
  perfect health.
I ask this in all sincerity and honesty
  and I will do my part.
I ask this great unseen healing force
  to help both present and absent
  ones who are in need of help and to
  restore them to perfect health.
I put my trust in the love and power
  of God.

SAMPLE FUNERAL SERVICE FOR ADULT

Selected Poem

Address

The question propounded by Job, "If a man die shall he live again?" has been asked by countless millions. It has been an absorbing thought down through the ages and even today, the question remains unanswered to many. Some persons still assert that the death of the body ends all, but the consensus is that there is a celestial as well as terrestrial life. There are places in that heavenly realm inhabited by intelligent, spiritual beings, who once lived on earth in mortal form as we now live.

Jesus said: "In my Father's house are many mansions"; it certainly is logical to conclude that mansions in the skies, like mansions on earth, are intended to be occupied. It also seems reasonable to believe that the spirits of humanity, retaining their mental and soul attributes, as well as their individuality, pass on to live in homes or mansions suited to their various spiritual conditions. Such indeed is the conviction of modern investigators, and we have reason to believe that many of the learned ancients held similar opinions.

We have learned that good spirits often come to our sides to prompt us to do right and to protect us against snares and negative influences. We have learned that life in the spiritual spheres is just as natural as this life: that there are schools to educate and develop the young and the old, conservatories of music, assemblies of the wise and employments for all. We have learned that it is the privilege of the spirit, as it becomes purer and holier, to pass to higher abodes, better suited to its advanced condition; but above all, we have learned that the bond of mutual love between departed spirit and mortal is never severed and that loving spirits often forego their privileges and wait in lower spheres until their loved ones have left the body, that they may, hand in hand with them, climb the spiritual heights.

Further comments, followed by eulogy, music, and prayers.

Committal

The one you love is not here. The Spirit of our departed (brother or sister) dwells no more in this discarded body. This mortal form has served its purpose; tenderly and reverently we now commit it to the care of Mother Earth, in the sure knowledge that (his or her) life continues. Amen.

SAMPLE FUNERAL SERVICE FOR CHILD

Selected Poem

Address

One of the distinguished preachers of this country, the Rev. Minot J. Savage, once said: "But we say, the little one's life was incomplete. He had only sat down to the feast when he was snatched away. He was a bud that had no time to bloom. But who gathers a bouquet and does not think the buds the finest part? The bud is as perfect as the flower. And, were it not, can it not blossom in any conservatory but ours?"

"And shall heaven have no children in it? Must none but gray hairs pass through the gates? Or shall not, rather, glad, gleesome children, with flowing hair and merry eyes go with laughter through its doorways?"

Further comments, followed by eulogy, music and prayers.

Committal

The one you love is not here. The Spirit of our departed (brother or sister) dwells no more in this discarded body. This mortal form has served its purpose; tenderly and reverently we now commit it to the care of Mother Earth, in the sure knowledge that (his or her) life continues. Amen.

SAMPLE POEMS

There is no Death

There is no death! The soul lives on
for aye,
'Tis but a changing to another sphere,
E'en though the body passes back to
earth
The soul lives on, in spirit life, as
here;
It will expand, and thrive, and ever
grow,
And still retain its influences o'er
those left on earth, until they, too,
shall go
To join those who have merely gone
before.
There is no death! 'Tis but a higher
growth,
The soul continues to another scene
Devoid of all encumbrances of earth –
Shorn of all pain and suffering so
keen;
And while we'll miss its daily
presence here,
And from its sweet companionship
are torn,
We will be blessed, inspired and
comforted
By its o'er shadowing love, in heaven
born.
There is no death! 'Tis but a change
of form,
Enabling the soul to reach its own,

and there expanding with each cycle
made
As it ascends near to the heavenly
throne;
Our life on earth is but a transient
stay,
As onward to a future life we tread,
And, having gained experience of
earth,
We then pass on with those the world
calls dead.
There is no death! For life can never
die,
Life is as potent as the truth itself, It
lives forever, through eternity;
And when, in turn, the summons
comes to us
To pass unto the land that lies
beyond,
We should not sorrow, but should
even rejoice
That we've gained our freedom from
earth's bond.

—Author unknown

Away

I cannot say, and I will not say that he
is dead. He is just away!
With a cheery smile and wave of the
hand,
He has wandered into an unknown
land.
And left us dreaming how very fair
It needs must be, since he lingers
there.

And you – O you, who the wildest
yearn
For the old-time steps and the glad
return –
Think of him faring on, as dear

In the love of there as the love of
  here.
Think of him still as the same, I say,
He is not dead – he is just away

  —James Whitcomb Riley[390]

Special Days: Spiritualism

January 25 *Founders Day* – Celebrating the founding of the NSAC Lyceum.

March 31 *Anniversary of the birth of Modern American Spiritualism in Hydesville, New York.*

Fourth Sunday in March *Gratitude Day* – A special offering is taken in NSAC Spiritualist churches for donation to the Spiritualist Benevolent Society, which provides stipends to retired workers who are in need.

Easter Celebration of the continuity of life as demonstrated by the resurrection of Jesus of Nazareth; celebration of new birth in nature.

August 11 *Birthday of Andrew Jackson Davis* – Andrew Jackson Davies was known as the Poughkeepsie Seer, and the Father of Spiritualism; he founded the Spiritualism Lyceum as seen in a vision for the education of children into Spiritualism and the study of God and nature.

Fourth Sunday in September Special collections are taken in NSAC churches for the benefit of the General Fund Endowment Fund of the NSAC for the promulgation of Spiritualism.

September 27 *Anniversary of the founding of the National Spiritualist Association of Churches in 1893 in Chicago, Illinois.*

November 1 *Anniversary of the registration of Spiritualism as practiced by the NSAC as a separate denomination of religion with the United States Government;* registered for a period of 1000 years.

Christmas Celebrate the birth of Jesus of Nazareth, master teacher, healer, and medium; celebrate the season of Love.

---

390 *Collier Complete Works of James Whitcomb Riley.*
  (1916). Vol. 4. New York, NY: Harper and Brothers,
  1000; available at: www.jameswhitcombriley.com.

Glossary of Spiritualist Terms

absent healing: The administration of the healing energies directly from the universal source or through the direction of a spirit doctor to patients without them (i.e., patients) having any direct contact with a healer or medium.

apport: The dematerialization and transporting of an object from one place to another; an apparent penetration of matter by matter.

astral body: Etheric body or double; an exact replica of the physical body, however nonphysical; the means of out-of-the-body experiences (OOBEs).

aura: Field of energy surrounding and emanating from a physical being, place, or thing; an emanation surrounding human beings, chiefly encircling the head and proceeding from the nervous system; a permanent radiation around the human body.

automatic writing: Flow of intelligent writing produced without conscious control or by one in a disassociated state of conscious being.

cataleptic clairvoyance: Occurs when the body is in a trance state, resembling sleep, induced by hypnotic power. When in this state, the spirit leaves the body and is able, at its own will or the suggestion of the hypnotist, to travel to remote places and to see clearly what is transpiring in the places it visits and to observe spiritual as well as material things in its environment.

clairaudience: Clear hearing; power of hearing sounds removed from the natural hearing conditions or environment; parapsychology refers to it as extrasensory information received as sound.

clairsentience: Clear capacity for sensing or feeling; an awareness of general sensing as distinguished from visual and auditory modes.

clairvoyance: Literally means "clear seeing"; in Spiritualism, it has a technical meaning and refers to psychic sight. Clairvoyance may be either subjective or objective. It is often difficult, if not altogether impossible, for even the clairvoyant to distinguish between the two.

contact healing: Direction of the universal energy forces of healing by touch (i.e., laying on of hands).

direct voice: Type of phenomena whereby a voice without a visible source is clearly heard; in spiritualistic circles, believed to be transmitted through ectoplasm extended from the medium or sitters.

ectoplasm: Invisible chemical component of living matter in the physical body; capable of appearing in vapor-like forms; responsible for all physical phenomena.

etheric body: Counterpart or double body of substance relative to the physical body that continues its existence after cessation (death) of activity of the physical body.

inspirational speaking: A form of mediumship in which the medium is not rendered wholly unconscious. In this phase, the spirit does not thoroughly control the nerve center through which the organs of speech are manipulated. Sometimes, inspirational speakers are influenced in the same speech by several spirit intelligences, and thus the speech itself will be a combination of the thought of the speaker and the influencing spirits.

laying on of hands: General expression found in spiritual literature that denotes the performance of spiritual or psychic healing; the healer often places a hand on the person or lightly touches the diseased area.

levitation: Raising of any physical object into the air without use of any visible means or agency; term frequently used in a restricted sense and often refers to the raising of the human body.

magnetic healing: Ability of an individual to direct or impart curative forces, energy, or vitality to another individual, thus rejuvenating them; considered non-spiritual in nature because the energies involved do not originate from a spiritual source; however, there can be a blending of magnetic and spiritual healing, though not clearly distinguishable.

materialization: Phenomenon related to physical mediumship; temporary appearance of forms or objects in various degrees of solid states: human forms, distinguishable faces, and physical characteristics; some psychics claim materialization of coins and buttons, and so forth.

meditation: A kind of conscious, deliberate mental process of deep and continued reflection on a subject with the ultimate goal being enlightenment.

medium: One whose organism is sensitive to vibrations from the Spirit World and through whose instrumentality, intelligences in that world is able to convey messages and produce the phenomena of Spiritualism.

objective clairvoyance: Psychic power or function of objectively seeing spiritual beings, objects, and things. A few persons are born with this power; in some it is developed, and in others it has but a casual quickening. One clairvoyant may see objectively spiritual things which to another may be invisible, because of the degree of difference in the intensity of the power.

psychic: As a noun, it is a word synonymous with the term sensitive and sometimes interchangeable with the term medium; as an adjective, describes paranormal character of abilities and events occurring outside the known physical laws and principles.

psychic photography: Supernormal ability to produce images on a photographic plate; often times taken by camera and film under normal conditions but after developed found to have both living and ethereal figures represented.

psychometry: Paranormal ability of a psychic or medium by which historical data is obtained on an object, usually by touching or handling it.

raps: Sounds of tapping, knocking, or striking; in physical form of mediumship believed to be produced by ectoplasmic rods; sounds produced by etheric/spirit beings.

Spiritualist: One who believes, as the basis of his or her religion, in the communication between this and the Spirit World by means of mediumship, and who endeavors to mould his or her character and conduct in accordance with the highest teachings derived from such communication.

Spiritualist healer: One who, either through inherent powers or through mediumship, is able to impart vital, curative forces to pathologic conditions.

subjective clairvoyance: Psychic condition that enables a medium to view pictures and images which are seen as visions by the medium without the aid of the physical eye. These pictures and images may be of the things spiritual or material, past or present, remote or near, hidden or uncovered, or they may have their existence simply in the conception or imagination of the spirit communicating them.

telepathic clairvoyance: Subjective perception in picture form of thought transmitted from a distance.

trance: An induced or spontaneous sleep-like condition or an altered state of consciousness.

trance-control clairvoyance: Psychic state under which the control of the physical body of the medium is assumed by a spirit of intelligence and the consciousness of the medium is, for the time being, dethroned. In this case, the controlling spirit is really the clairvoyant, who simply uses the medium's body as a means of communicating what the spirit sees.

visions: Although this word has several

connotations, it is used in the spiritual or religious sense to denote an apparition, or something that is seen by a means using other than ordinary sight.

X-ray clairvoyance: Form of clairvoyance which partakes of the characteristics of the X-ray, and seems to be objective. The clairvoyant who possesses this power is able to see physical objects through intervening physical matter, can perceive the internal parts of the human body, diagnose disease, and observe the operations of healing and decay.

Sufism

*Come, come, whoever you are, Wanderer, worshipper, lover
of leaving. Ours is not a caravan of despair.*

Even if you have broken your vows a thousand times, It doesn't matter

Come, come yet again, come.

Rumi

Prepared by:
Ruth Batina VanDam-Hinds, MEd, MA, LPC
Cherag, Swope Park Health Services
Kansas City, MO
batina323@yahoo.com

History and Facts

First, a word of warning: this chapter is not written in a scholarly fashion, as that is not a good picture of the true spirit of Sufism. This is written for the busy practitioner who doesn't mind if the reading is a little bit light.

I spoke with two Zoroastrian leaders, one in the Chicago area and one in Anaheim, California, who both told me that Sufism, a mystical path, began with Zoroaster in the ancient Indo-Iranian culture that traveled out of Central Asia some millenia ago. It was unclear to me what this date might have been. My Sufi teacher (or Murshid), Khabir Kitz, told me that Zoroaster means someone who brings light and that there may have been more than one.

I also read the book *Kebzeh* by Murat Yagan who states that the village he came from in the Caucasus Mountains by the name of Kebzeh has had a mystical,

spiritual, and also a social tradition that goes back 26 000 years. Interestingly, this is about when the Mayans say there was a major change in the world.

And of course, it is well known that prior to literacy, there were cultures who worshipped the Divine as a feminine being in a mystical way. In fact, there is at least one Doctor of Medicine who wrote a book about how once people became literate, the Divine became perceived as male due to the switch from dominant right brain to dominant left brain activity that had taken place due to writing.

Some Sufi orders feel that they emerged from early Moslem leaders who were mystics and approached the Divine through the heart rather than having to analyze everything ad infinitum. Some of these orders include Nashqabandi and Bektasi, Some say that Sufism started with Jelalluddin Rumi in the twelfth century. He was an Islamic teacher of law in Konya, Turkey. His family had escaped Afghanistan due to Ghengis Khan's spreading empire.

Unknown to Rumi, as well as most of the people conquered by this generation of Mongols, Ghengis Khan was also a mystic who was open to his people's worshipping the Divine in the way that was best for them. He himself found the Divine in nature and so he had a very close and abiding relationship with the creator and creation and only attacked cities after they killed his ambassadors.

After Rumi's family escaped to Turkey and Rumi was busy teaching law, along came a poor bedraggled looking man by the name of Shems who was from Tabriz in Persia. He knew that Rumi was the person that the Divine (called Allah in Islamic cultures whether a Moslem or not) meant for him to find. He immediately started teaching Rumi both with spoken words and on a spirit level with the Divine as the medium through which their hearts connected and communicated.

Shems did some shocking things such as throwing an important text, written by Jelalludin's father, into a well. He was trying to teach that we can only truly be one with the Divine through our hearts. This kind of behavior as well as other things Shems did, such as seeming to Rumi's students to monopolize their beloved teacher, engendered animosity and jealousy in Rumi's students. Shems disappeared after guiding Rumi on the path of being full of the light of the Divine. It is unclear whether he died or something else happened. In any case he'd done what he'd set out to do.

Around this time, Francis of Assisi appeared, not yet a saint. It is unclear whether he turned to his mystical communion with God before or after getting to know Rumi. However, all that is needed to confirm the connection between these two is to stay at a retreat center provided by a Franciscan Monastery in eastern Missouri. The similarities between Francis and Jelallaudin are clear when one knows the history of both, including that they were contemporaries and knew each other.

This path from Rumi is the path I'm most familiar with. The Mevlevis who grew immediately out of Rumi's teachings, is where the turn used by "whirling" Dervishes, or Sufis, had its start. This branch still exists in many countries. Some Mevlevis are Moslem and some are not. Rumi had come to understand that all religious traditions can lead to the Divine each in their own way with some basic similarities in belief.

The tradition that first made its way to the West grew out of the Chisti lineage found in India, very honoring of Christ's teachings as the name hints. Hazrat Inayat Khan (Hazrat is a term denoting love and respect for the person) grew up in India as a Moslem Sufi who was living in a largely Hindu country. Due in part to the Mongolian (Mogul) Khans and their descendants, as well as the diversity of religions in the country, there was more acceptance of a variety of religious traditions that are seen as leading to the Divine. Inayat learned wisdom from his family and Sufi teachers.

When Inayat Khan first started to learn from his Murshid, he wanted to write down what his teacher was saying. When he got out his writing tools, his teacher stopped teaching as this is to be a path of the heart, not the head. When he wanted to tell and ask, his teacher put a finger to his lips, teaching silence.

As a young, gifted musician, his teacher told Inayat that he was to go to the West to bring Sufism in a way that made sense and was appealing in its simplicity in the West.

Inayat spent time in the United States, Europe, and Russia. He met his wife in the United States. She already had some of the same ideas for healing that he'd been taught and they were very compatible. However, the United States was not compatible with them as Inayat, although an Aryan, had brown skin and his wife, who was European American, had much lighter skin.

Before they left, he had some students who were able to carry on with helping other spiritual people to catch a deeper view of the numinous nature of the Divine so that they could allow the light of the Divine to shine through them and so help others to catch the truth, wisdom, love, joy, and peace which can only come from a heartfelt sense of the Divine in us.

Inayat Khan and his family lived in Europe, including Russia, meeting such people as Carl Jung, and heads of state, as his magnetic suffusion of light lit others and helped many to see that God is love in all its many forms.

Inayat Khan, a member of the royalty of India, due to being descended from Mongol/Mogol Khans, was seen by many as being a king due to his wisdom and bearing. He certainly was, as is the ideal king, generous and giving of his time and the light of his wisdom. He drew on the wisdom of Rumi's teaching that all paths to the Divine that are spiritual and filled with light, love, harmony and beauty, are sacred.

At this point, he broke from the requirement of many Moslems, that one must be a Moslem to be a Sufi as seen by some other Sufi orders. This changed Sufi path is sometimes called Universal Sufism. It is important to note here that some other Sufi lineages/traditions don't agree with this acceptance of other paths into the teachings of Sufism.

There are many Sufi teachers who caught the spirit of what Rumi, Chisti, and Inayat Khan were trying to get across. One is Samuel L. Lewis, and others include Inayat's other mureeds, or students, and his sons, Vilayat and Hidayat, who have led in the Sufi path, as well as his daughters Noor-un-Nisa and Khair-un-Nisa.

Basic Teachings

I said, My heart wants a kiss from You.
You say: "The price of a kiss is Life."
My heart came up beside me and said:
"It's a cheap down payment."

—Rumi

The easiest way to describe the basic teachings of Western or "Universal" Sufism is to quote the "Ten Sufi Thoughts." Please note that these are *thoughts*, not beliefs.

Ten Sufi Thoughts

There are ten principal Sufi thoughts that comprise all the important subjects with which the inner life of man is concerned.

1. There is one God, the Eternal, the Only Being; none else exists save God.
2. There is one Master, the Guiding Spirit of all souls, who constantly leads all followers toward the light.
3. There is one Holy Book, the sacred manuscript of nature, which truly enlightens all readers.
4. There is one Religion, the unswerving progress in the right direction toward the ideal, which fulfills the life's purpose of every soul.
5. There is one Law, the law of Reciprocity, which can be observed by a selfless

conscience together with a sense of awakened justice.

6. There is one human Family, the Brotherhood and Sisterhood which unites the children of earth indiscriminately in the Parenthood of God.

7. There is one Moral Principle, the love which springs forth from self-denial, and blooms in deeds of beneficence.

8. There is one Object of Praise, the beauty which uplifts the heart of its worshipper through all aspects from the seen to the unseen.

9. There is one Truth, the true knowledge of our being within and without which is the essence of all wisdom.

10. There is one Path, the annihilation of the false ego in the real, which raises the mortal to immortality and in which resides all perfection.

Another important thought is that Hazrat Inayat Khan is not to be worshipped and his words are not to be considered as sacred scripture. It is not to be a cult of personality, by Inayat's own words. Therefore, many Sufis wisely do not wish to have or be gurus, but do willingly learn from their teachers, which includes everyone and everything they meet.

A twelfth thought is that someday we will reunite with the Beloved (Divine Oneness).

Basic Practices

Understanding makes the trouble of life lighter to bear.

Discussion is for those who say, "What I say is right and what you say is wrong." A sage never says such a thing.

—Inayat Khan

- These two quotes, seemingly oxymoronic, point out that understanding comes from the Divine within one's heart and soul rather than with argument.

- There are some other basic practices which Hazrat Inayat Khan brought to the West. These show evidence that he brought a well-rounded view of the Divine garnered from the "People of the Book" (Jewish, Christian, and Islamic people), Hinduism, Buddhism, Zoroastrianism as well as Divine Feminine and Divine Nature centered traditions. These became more well known in the United States through his student, Murshid Sam, or Samuel L. Lewis. Not only did Murshid Sam wake up the hippie generation to the idea that God is Love, but also spent many years learning from spiritual teachers in Asia so that he could be full of love himself.

- Breath is considered to be an important healing tool. The slow breaths used by mothers giving birth in this country are considered to help one to stay in balance, especially if the in breath is through the nose.

- Another basic practice is meditation. Meditation is more a listening or receiving practice than a giving or asking attitude. There are so many ways to meditate. Some people lie down flat with a timer set and no music, others sit, eyes open or not, so they don't fall asleep, some have soothing music in the background, and some are standing and moving in a group sometimes verbalizing in words or sounds. And there's always the laughing meditation where one laughs for 45 minutes without stopping.

- There are also practices that help one to be less *self*-conscious which are more advanced and a Sufi teacher would be needed for these.

- It may be important to note here that a cherag may help patients of any faith tradition. The task of the cherag is to be a bearer of the light of the Divine (much as other religions ask of their devotees) without casting a shadow of criticism, complaint, negativity, and so forth.

Principles for Clinical Care

Our thoughts have prepared for us the happiness or unhappiness we experience.

—Inayat Khan

There are probably as many ways to look at this for Sufis as there are religions and other spiritual traditions in the world. If the patient has a home base religion, it is important to know what the principles are for that particular religion. That may be the first step or a later step depending on the individual.

Dietary Issues

O wondrous creatures,
by what strange miracle do you
so often not smile?

—Hafiz

- The only dietary issues are those which the individual Sufi or Dervish brings from their base religion or from health issues.
- For Sufis, diet runs the gamut and is more closely related to the individual's personal religious beliefs, dietary inclinations, and any health issues, the last of which should be known by medical staff. Some Sufis follow Kosher laws, some follow Hilal laws, some are simple vegetarians, while others are vegans. And there are those who consider humans to be omnivores who need both animal and plant nutrients, some who stay away from particular foods and some who will eat anything.

- The underlying principle is that our bodies are the temple of the Divine. In order to fully connect with the Divine, whatever name we use, it is important to be in good health. Good health means that we can have blissful experiences while still remaining sober enough to be safe.
- Because of the preventive dietary practices of most Sufis (preventing disease and dis-ease), dietary issues have to do with an openness to using a variety of healing foods. People are encouraged to eat nutritious food, eat more plant material than animal, and *maybe* to fast before prayer and other spiritual activities.
- But these are not rules and, some would say, are simply sensible.

General Medical Beliefs

Health is an orderly condition caused by the regular working of the mechanism of the physical body.

—Inayat Khan

- Again, the medical beliefs of Sufis vary widely depending on the person's base religious tradition.
- Some religions want to say that if one is sick, it is due to karma, or due to past experiences that still linger with something to be learned. Others say that disease is caused by sin and that the sick person needs to, "get right with God/the Lord." Still others say that disease is caused by dis-ease and that it's important to release stress and give up the burdens that keep bringing us down.
- These all seem pretty similar to a Sufi.

And at the base of this is connecting with the Divine. Prayer is asking for help and Meditation is listening. Sufis do both and many do more of one than the other. Both are important, and the phrase, "Thy will be done," is an intrinsic part of the process. We tend to be very aware that life is a journey and that we do not know what is on it, only that we want to learn from life's lessons (which are often painful) so we don't have to repeat that lesson.

- It may not be wise to tell patients this, but certainly they can be asked if they have experienced something like this before and wonder aloud why this keeps happening to them.

- Because the Inayati Sufi Lineage (from Hazrat Inayat Khan) has a healing service that is performed regularly, it will probably help you, the reader, to know something about this. Again these vary depending on members, but there are certain basics.

- Part of the process entails cleansing ourselves of any disease, so it's important to be fairly well when participating. Since this is a mystical practice (i.e., unexplainable), it is important for providers to be free of dis-ease as well so this is not passed on in any way.

- The invocation of Sufi Inayat Khan is used: *Toward the One, the perfection of love, harmony and beauty, the only being. The only being. Unite us with all the illuminated souls that form the embodiment of the Master, the Spirit of Guidance.*

- Cleansing breaths are used while imagining that any unwanted sludge is washed away. There is an awareness that the world, including our health, is quite often manifested from the thoughts we have. So if we expect to have a bad day, we probably will, and if we focus on heart attacks at a young

age, we may very well have that manifest in our own bodies. For more information on this, the book *Mental Purification and Healing: Volume IV of The Sufi Message* volumes, by Hazrat Inayat Khan, is very useful. *The Book of Sufi Healing* by Shaykh Hakim Moinuddin Chishti may add some additional information that may or may not work for your Sufi patient.

- The prayer *Nayaz* is spoken: *Beloved Lord, Almighty God, through the rays of the sun, through the waves of the air, through the all-pervading Life in space, purify and revivify me and I pray, heal my body heart and soul.* It is difficult to send untainted healing energy to others when our own inner being is full of disease/dis-ease.

- Then, as each name from the list of people who have asked for healing is read, the participants visualize that name written out while thinking *ya shaffee, ya kaffee (O remedy, O healer)* and while sending healing energy from the Divine and through us to the sick person. The list is comprised only of names of people who have asked for this. Following this we do a similar meditation/prayer for all those whose names have not been mentioned but who also need healing.

- The service is concluded with the prayer Khatum, a blueprint for healing in and of itself:

O Thou who art the perfection of love
  harmony and beauty, the Lord of
  Heaven and Earth
Open our hearts that we may hear thy
  voice which constantly comes from
  within,
Disclose to us Thy Divine Light,
  which is hidden in our souls,
that we may know and understand
  life better.

Most merciful and compassionate
  God,
Give us Thy great goodness;
Teach us Thy loving forgiveness;
Raise us above the distinctions and
  differences
which divide;
Send us the Peace of thy Divine
  Spirit,
And unite us all in Thy Perfect Being.
Amen.

Otherwise, medical beliefs vary according to the individual, as stated earlier.

Specific Medical Issues

I felt in need of a great pilgrimage, so I sat still for three days and God came to me.

—Kabir

- **Abortion**: Abortion is not covered in Sufi teachings except that every soul is a part of God, but no dogma about when the soul enters the body. The decision is left to the individual.
- **Advance Directives**: These are not covered in Sufi teachings except for a consideration of others as well as seeing our bodies as a place where the Divine resides. The decision is left to the individual.
- **Birth Control**: Birth control is individually chosen or not. The best birth control is control of self and will so that what is best for the couple and the community is the path chosen. There is neither sanction nor encouragement, but an underlying respect for all of creation as part of the Divine. The decision is left to the individual.
- **Blood Transfusions**: Blood transfusions are not covered in Sufi teachings. The decision is left to the individual.

- **Circumcision**: Circumcision is not specifically covered in Sufi teachings. The decision is left to the individual or family.
- **In Vitro Fertilization**: In vitro fertilization is not covered in Sufi teachings. The decision is left to the individual.
- **Stem Cell Research**: Stem cell research is not covered in Sufi teachings except for a consideration of others as well as seeing our bodies as a place where the Divine resides. The decision is left to the individual.
- **Vaccinations**: Vaccinations are not covered in Sufi teachings. The decision is left to the individual.
- **Withholding/Withdrawing Life Support**: This is not covered in Sufi teachings except for a consideration of others as well as seeing our bodies as a place where the Divine resides. The decision is left to the individual.

Psychiatric issues can be more complicated or less complicated depending on the provider and the patient. Part of the Sufi path is the movement toward Divine Personality. It is important that the Sufi patient have a basic hold on reality. It is also absolutely necessary that the patient feel respected as a child of or part of the Divine.

Surgery can be difficult for anyone. Before surgery, it is best if the surgeon and nurses meditate on/pray for the healing of their patient, including imagery of what that means in the body. This can be done in the way most comfortable and familiar to the provider.

There are also a number of specific practices that are for specific problems. One example is doing the sun walk when fighting a chest disease such as breast cancer. This is an activity that really needs to be seen and caught rather than taught in words alone to replicate its effect, and this is best done with a Sufi teacher or healer.

In addition, it is good if the ill Sufi contacts a healing conductor who will make sure his or her name is on the healing list if the patient wishes and so that the healer may visit.

Gender and Personal Issues

Live with dignity, women, live with dignity, men.

Few things will more enhance our beauty as much.

—Rabbia

- As for gender and personal issues related to Sufism, these would again be as much on a continuum as with humanity as a whole. Some Sufi women are very much into women's rights while others have gone through that and have let the Divine take care of that and other possible inequities.
- Because Sufism is a tradition that is immersed in love and light, people who are drawn to it are often those who have been treated badly by life in one or more ways. Quite often there has been some type of victimization in the past and so they are attracted to such a loving and accepting group.
- These people are also people who want to connect in a loving way with the Divine, other people and all of creation. Sometimes they have eschewed the intellectual, combative world which is more traditional in the West and possibly even are not still working in that environment.
- As we grow in Sufism, these no longer hold power over us. And since you won't know where this person is in their growth, it is best to be gentle, not denigrating of the patient's beliefs, lifestyle, or

peacefulness, even subtly. Sufis tend to be well educated, intelligent people who are able to see cynicism and patronizing behavior and then your ability to help them will be diminished.

Principles for Spiritual Care through the Cycles of Life
Concepts of Living and Dying for Spiritual Support

To treat every human being as a shrine of God is to fulfill all religion.

—Inayat Khan

- For Sufis, the cycles of life include pre-birth and post-death of the corporeal body. Life is not confined by how our senses perceive it.
- Because Sufis believe that the Divine is in all beings, things, and actions, it is important to start a new life with as much love for the precious new being that will emerge as both parents, especially the mother, are able to give. This would include loving thoughts of the child no matter how conceived. This will be felt by the unborn child and will bring a more loving and peaceful being into the world.

During Birth

When the soul is born on earth, its first expression is to cry. It finds itself in a new place which is not familiar to it. It finds itself in captivity.

—Inayat Khan

- Birth must also be a loving experience with loving family, friends, hospital staff, and so forth, surrounding the new mother and child with the light of wisdom, love, joy, peace, acceptance, and a warm regard for both. If the hospital staff expects bad things of the mother and/or newborn, they may manifest.

- This is not to say that lies and platitudes are a good idea. The mother and child are part of the Divine as much as anyone in the room.
- There's a wonderful Sufi song, "I see God in you, I see God in you, I see God everywhere," which is sung while dancing: turn to a partner, pull together with eyes locking, and go past to the next to repeat, then turn a full circle in place while singing the third phrase, and repeat. I was singing the song on a drive home after visiting my sweetheart one time and got out at a rest area still singing. As I walked singing to the restroom door, a mouse raced in and out under the crack of the door until it figured out which way to go. I laughed as it did this and sang to the mouse.
- It is important to keep this feeling about mother and child and between mother and child throughout *life*. It makes for a very happy life if we see that we are all part of the Divine and worthy of love.

During Illness

[O]ne can be too sensitive to germs, one can exaggerate the idea of germs, making the idea more than the reality.

—Inayat Khan

- Illness quite often occurs when it is not possible to continue this feeling and there is disharmony in our lives. Sometimes we can almost feel that we are out of step with where our lives should be. Instead of continuing doing things the same way and expecting different results, it is important to step out of the dance of life, refresh ourselves, and take another step in learning what our manifestation in creation is. Only then does it make sense to get back to expecting harmony.

- There is so much more that could be said about living life, and much of it has already been said. One more example is how Dances of Universal Peace work for me. Sometimes when we're in the circle moving and singing to the Divine, someone next to me is overly forceful with movements. I have learned that rather than teach that person the right way to do the dance by rigidly enforcing what I want, I imagine my muscles becoming soft as warm butter. After learning *and using* this, my shoulders and arms have lost their tendency to end up in pain from stressors in many places.

During End of Life

Death is a change that comes through the inability of the body to hold what we call the soul.

—Inayat Khan

- For Sufis, the date of one's death is the date of their Urs, or wedding with the Beloved, the day when the beings of light that we are have stepped out of our temporary holders (bodies) and become fully one with the Divine. It can be truly rapturous.
- As a hospice volunteer, I've read soothing passages to the person from their sacred scriptures and sung loving, accepting songs in English. Some of this may be related to the need of most people in the process of moving on to complete unfinished business which needs resolution prior to departure.

Before my mother died, my husband and

I made a "Travel poster for Heaven." My mother, always a fundamentalist Christian, was showing signs of reluctance to die (strange since she'd known for a long time that she would go to Heaven), although it was clearly going to be soon. I went to visit my mother with the poster and had a half hour alone with her while she slept. I'd put up the poster on the wall where we could both see it. When she closed her eyes in sleep, I held one hand toward it and hovered the other above her head. I visualized that the hovering hand was actually supporting her on her back and the right hand was holding her right arm as we advanced down the path in the picture. I saw things in the picture then that I couldn't see after this walk. The idea was to take a day trip to Heaven. We were about halfway down the path (in my visualization) when my mother opened her eyes and asked me why my hand was on her back. My physical hand was still hovering above her head. This kind of help is such a blessing to those who are dying as well as to those who will stay in this world after they go on.

After my mother's death, many experiences have taught me of the beauty and harmony in all of creation, that bad/difficult events seem to stop happening when I've learned the lesson from them, and that there is a basic goodness in everyone. Sometimes the goodness is so veiled from the view of the self and others, that it is hard to believe it's there. Yet it is. As with most Sufis and some professionals, the knowledge is that the transition from a living body that holds the soul or spirit, to the soul's remembering and reclaiming its existence as a being of light is full of wonder and delight. I still miss my mother sometimes although it's been nearly 6 years since her passing. But I also remember several miracles surrounding her death that are similar to the story told here.

Care of the Body

Toward the One, the perfection of love, harmony and beauty, the Only Being. United with all the illuminated souls who form the embodiment of the Master, the Spirit of Guidance.

—Inayat Khan

When there is an acknowledgement that the life has left the body, this may not always be so easy to see. The Dali Lama, in *Advice on Dying*, talks about how some very spiritual monks "die" and yet their bodies do not start to decay for days or weeks. I recently spoke with a Sufi Healing Conductor in Kansas City who said that when her old cat died recently, his body didn't start to decay for 2–3 days. He remained soft and warm. She let her other "four-leggeds" be around the body to allow them to say good-bye and grieve in their own ways.

Yet, again, it depends on the base religion. Some religions do cremation while at least one feels that this desecrates the element fire. One leaves bodies on window ledges of a tower for the crows to recycle. Some Sufis simply want a memorial service and try to give funeral money to the poor to sustain them.

So it is individual.

Organ and Tissue Donation

[I]n reality, the greatest ethic or moral that one can learn in life is friendliness, which culminates in generosity.

—Inayat Khan

Often, Sufis just plan funerals and memorial services in the usual way. But there is a generosity to Sufis that sometimes inspires them to request organ donation and/or for the body to be used for scientific research after their passing.

Scriptures, Inspirational Readings, and Prayers

> I have learned so much from God
> That I can no longer
> Call
> Myself
>
> A Christian, a Hindu, a Muslim,
> A Buddhist, a Jew.
>
> The Truth has shared so much of
>   Itself
> With me
>
> That I can no longer call myself
> A man, a woman, an angel,
> Or even pure
> Soul.
>
> Love has
> Befriended Hafiz so completely
> It has turned to ash
> And freed
> Me
>
> Of every concept and image
> My mind has ever known.
>
> — Hafiz

This poem by the Sufi poet Hafiz is pretty descriptive of the spirituality of Sufis. As mentioned, scriptures can come from any religion and some Sufis believe that Nature is the sacred manuscript on which the Divine has written all necessary messages.

True Sufism does not have dogmatic beliefs or rules the breaking of which is considered sin, separating one from the Divine.

The Ten Sufi Thoughts are a good source of how Sufis might live their lives. And in the tradition of which I am a part, influenced as it is by Eastern religions (Christianity is one of these), Jesus' admonition to love God with all your heart, soul, and mind and to love your neighbor as yourself seems to be a good bedrock on which to build one's life, and may sum up the aforementioned ten thoughts mentioned.

It seems strange to list special days, specific writings and such things that are more typical of organized religions. However, to be fair to you, the reader, some favorite resources are translations of Hafiz's poetry by Daniel Ladinsky, translations of Rumi's poetry by Coleman Barks, writings by Hazrat Inayat Khan, also called Sufi Inayat Khan. *Bowl of Saki* and *Sufi Teachings* may be good books to start with. The book *Love Poems from God*, translated and compiled by Daniel Ladinsky, is a favorite for me. It includes the poetry of saints from various traditions, including Christianity. Also, Vilayat Khan, Inayat's son, has written and spoken extensively on the connection between Sufism and science.

It is clear from reading these translations that Barks and Ladinsky use modern images to express what the poets are saying. This makes a lot of sense since most of us don't speak the original languages or properly understand all the nuances from the cultural influences of the time.

There are books that say one must be a Moslem/Muslim in order to be a Sufi. Actually, many Moslems think of Sufis as heretics, so this does not always work.

Many Sufis do celebrate Rumi's Urs as a joyful commemoration of his life as well as the Urs of other wise and helpful teachers. All other days are celebrated by Sufis as holy days as well. It's also wise to find out what the Sufi's religious tradition might be and look in the appropriate chapter of this book for their holidays.

There is a service which Cherags, Sufi ministers, conduct called variously Service of Universal Peace and Universal Worship Service. This is done more or less formally depending on the Cherag conducting it and the situation.

Generally, six to eight spiritual/religious traditions are represented both by a candle (representing the light it has brought to the world) and a text with sacred, or at least wise words from that tradition. There is generally a topic which instructs the passages chosen.

Sometimes a kind of unformed version is used in which individuals or groups choose passages followed by some prayers and an illuminating, unifying message of how all the passages are addressing the same thing in slightly different ways. This is especially useful since life is multifaceted.

There are also often (and this is where it gets good for people who don't like to sit through the service) dances which are done corresponding with the specific religions and the passages. These are called Dances of Universal Peace.

An example, with the theme of love from the Christian tradition might be one sung to a 1960s folk tune in which the words are, "Love, love, love, love, The Gospel in one word is love. Love your neighbor as yourself, love, love, love." The same tune is used for the words, "Spirit of peace, to your cause we give our strength, that love may reign and war may cease, mir, miru mir." (Mir means peace and miru is Russian for the concept of peace on earth.)

There are six concentrations in the Inayati Sufi orders that are paths to the aims of Sufis. The Ziraat part has to do with valuing and meditating on the Divine in nature. The Service of Universal Peace is something like a worship service. The Healing order with conductor concentrates on healing for the people whose names are on the list each week, and who have requested this. Dances of Universal Peace are to introduce people to Sufism and allow them to participate on whatever level they wish. Zikr is a way to remember the Divine with prayer, chanting, song, and dance. Words can be silent, whispered, or verbalized aloud. The Esoteric School is for those who have been initiated as a Sufi and wish to learn more deeply about this path. Underlying all is the movement toward brotherhood and sisterhood among the human family.

In summary, the word Sufi, related to the Greek word for wisdom, has been in use for hundreds of years. Sufis value wisdom above simple knowledge of facts and so approach the Divine through a heart full of love. Because of this, Sufis are more interested in the heart of the person than in the outward appearance.

Sufis often have a strong belief in the power and desire of the Divine to heal those who suffer. An intrinsic part of this is the belief that the Divine is in everything in creation and that all of creation is part of the Divine.

Because of being able to see God in everyone and everything, and because of the desire to be in harmony with the Divine in all of creation, Sufis tend to be truly peaceful. When we are not, our bodies suffer. One of the main teachers in the United States, Murshid Sam, said that he would like to see a peace demonstration that demonstrated peace. I have now seen some. It is important to remember that the more we breed peace, the less dis-ease and disease will be in the world.

Because, as Hazrat Inayat Khan says, "Illness is an inharmony," it is important to be at peace and thus harmonious for the health of ourselves, the world, and creation.

May the blessings of God rest upon you,
May God's peace abide with you,
May God's presence,
Illuminate your heart,
Now and Forevermore.

Websites with additional information:
http://ruhaniat.org/
www.sufiorder.org/
www.sufimovement.org/
http://shiningheartcommunity.org/

Taoism

The Way of Harmony with Universal Nature[391]

Prepared by:
Peter. F. Cunneen, MATCM
Taoist Mentor, Integral Way Society
Geneva, Switzerland

Reviewed and approved by:
Donald D. Davis, PhD
Professor of Psychology and Asian Studies, Old
** Dominion University**
Norfolk, VA

History and Facts

Taoism emerged from the experience of the ancient Chinese people living with and observing nature around them and within them. Its first formal writings came from the Warring States period approximately 2500 years ago, and it sprouted into folk-religious forms during the Han dynasty 500 years later and continues today in philosophical, religious, and various spiritual-esoteric traditions. Its principal ideas, constructs, and teachings have been part of the fundamental way of life for the Chinese people, even as other religious traditions have immigrated into or emerged over the centuries (e.g., Buddhism, Confucianism) and have greatly influenced the traditional Chinese arts, medicine, and physical sciences. The central tenets emphasize the authority of the natural spiritual reality of the universe, the potential spiritual development of all people and the self-responsibility of people in achieving their spiritual evolution or de-evolution.

Thus, there is no central external authority setting rules concerning medical or other issues over the more formalized folk-religious Taoist sects, nor over the more esoteric spiritual traditions because it is recognized that true authority of life is one's own developed inner consciousness.

Basic Teachings

The Basic Taoist teachings are a major underpinning of all the classical Chinese arts and sciences, leading to the development of traditional Chinese medicine, acupuncture, *feng shui* (geomancy), Chinese astrology, the fine arts, the physical arts of *Tai Ji* and *qi gong*, many of the physical sciences (early alchemy and chemistry, astronomy, and many ancient technological achievements), and other subjects.

- **Subtle Universal Natural Law** – *Calamities and blessings do not come through any definite, distinguishable door; it is the person who invites them.*[392]

---

391 Quote provided by P. F. Cunneen, author of this chapter.

392 Ni, H. (1991). *The Key to Good Fortune.* Los Angeles, CA: SevenStar Communications, 2.

Taoists believe that the universe has a subtle responsiveness. They see every action gives birth to a complementary reaction, that the environment of one's mind, the condition of one's body or the state of one's political system or economy invites certain types of growth and development and hinders others. This is the basis of Taoist moral systems, not that certain thoughts and actions are considered "right" or "wrong" but that they foster constructive or destructive subtle energy patterns. While the accumulated lifetime of behavior colors the soul influencing the life beyond, Taoism also believes in an immediate reciprocal response. Thus, virtuous behavior brings its own reward of a heavenly life, while immorality brings people down into a living hell. Taoists value living a simple and natural life, de-emphasizing, but not ignoring their desires, rather keeping to only what is needed, being conservative with their energy to allow generosity through selfless service to others. Based on this understanding, Taoists believe that people can have some influence to create health, wealth, and happiness to shape their destiny by cultivating the right physical, mental, and spiritual conditions.

• **Tao**

Tao is the Subtle Origin and primal energy of the universe. We recognize the Subtle Origin of the universe as the mysterious mother of existence and non-existence. The universe is naturally so. It was neither created nor designed. Even though there is no personified creator, Tao, the primal energy which exercises and develops itself, brings forth all the manifestations of the universe. The universe can be comprehended by the human mind without creating a personified God. The original energy becomes the law of its manifestation. Everything manifested and un-manifested is a spontaneous expression of the nature of the Subtle Origin; no intentional design is needed.[393]

Tao, the subtle reality of the universe cannot be described. That which can be described in words is merely a conception of the mind. Although names and descriptions have been applied to it, the subtle reality is beyond the description.[394]

This suggests that only by integration with one's spiritual nature can one be in touch with the inner depth of reality and True Nature. The mind is a useful, but limited tool as it works by separating itself from that which it observes. Thus, reality is divided between the observer and that which is observed, giving birth to a dualistic nature. This dualism is therefore a creation, and not the original nature of life. For humans to function separated from their original integral nature, rooted only in this dualistic nature is the source of human ills and immorality. Thus, the ultimate goal is to unite with Tao, the True Nature and become an integral being with a nondualistic nature.

• *Yin/Yang* – The ancient Taoist perspective is that the universe emerged from an unimaginable unity that gives birth to all things. All things born of this oneness have their relative, contrasting, and complementary natures, or *yin* and *yang* aspects. The manifested universe of *yin* and *yang* obey natural laws that can be

---

393 Ni, H. trans. (1979). *The Taoist Inner View of the Universe and the Immortal Realm*. Los Angeles, CA: SevenStar Communications, introduction.

394 Ni, H. trans. (1979). *The Complete Works of Lao Tzu, Tao Teh Ching & Hua Hu Ching, Tao Teh Ching*. Los Angeles, CA: SevenStar Communications, 7.

seen in every aspect of life, whether in the movement of the cosmos or in the life of the cell. It is like a magnet. To create a complete circuit one needs a north and south pole which attract each other and complete each other. This results in the *Tai Ji* principle, the maintenance of a dynamic equilibrium of opposites. As an overly strong action in any one direction invites a strong reverse response (like two north ends of the magnet repelling one another), the moderation of harshness and the cultivation of gentleness can be applied to smooth the path of life. Thus, the recognition of the hidden opposite in any situation fosters a broader perspective on what might be considered "good" or "bad" fortune. This has led to an appreciation of how aggressive or violent energy sows the seeds of its own demise, whereas gentleness and quietude tend to produce less stress, less wear and tear, thus promoting endurance and longevity.

- *Qi* – (*Chi*) is the vital, unseen force animating all movement, change, and activity. It is the *qi* that acts as the invisible web that allows for the subtle communication, responsiveness, and unity of nature. Thus, human beings, while born into the relative sphere of *yin* and *yang*, have the potential to unite with the unlimited sphere of oneness – Tao, the mother of all things. By understanding the natural pattern of unceasing changes in *yin* and *yang*, and cultivating their *qi*, people can learn to harmonize with nature. In harmonizing with nature, Taoist practitioners seek balance as the basis of their physical, emotional, and mental health, and promote calmness as a foundation for the development of spirit. The unimpeded flow of *qi* is considered the basis of health and harmony while the blockage

of *qi* is the basis of disease, a sight for pain, inflammation, pathogenic growth, and disharmony. The balance, flow, and harmony of *qi* are fundamental to many traditional Chinese cultural, artistic, and scientific achievements and attributable to the broad influence of Taoist philosophy.

- **Three Treasures** – A key to Chinese medical practice as well as Taoist cultivation is an understanding of the "three treasures" at the core of human life. They are: the *jing*, the physical essence or seed; the *qi* or vital energy; and the *shen*, the innermost guide or spirit. These different levels are interdependent, so the health of the physical being is a basic first step in spiritual development and any true spiritual development will have evident positive influence on the health of the body and mind. The holistic understanding of medical phenomena comes naturally from this line of thinking. Any overly strong, hidden, or enduring emotional experience is considered to have the potential to cause disease as it affects the spirit-mind and can scatter or obstruct the flow of *qi*. The conservation of *jing*, the storing, balancing and smooth flow of *qi* and the peacefulness of *shen* are considered fundamental for a healthy life. The refinement of the more gross physical aspects into the more subtle spiritual aspects is the direction of Taoist esoteric development. The goal of this transformative process, called "Internal Alchemy," is the complete spiritualization of one's being, producing a timeless experience of life. Someone who achieves this is referred to, in Taoist metaphorical language, as an "Immortal."

- *Wu-Wei* – *Wu-Wei*, sometimes translated as "non-doing," is the principle of living a nondualistic life. Thus, nothing is done beyond what is needed. Nothing is done to excess. When completed with a task, one immediately withdraws. One does not hold favorites, nor force others to accept one way against another. What this means is that one does not go beyond one's natural ability, extend where there is not a counterbalancing receptivity, nor exhaust oneself. One tends to live simply, keeping to what one needs and neglecting extraneous desires. One's thoughts, words, movements, and life become more seemingly effortless, smooth, and unhurried, as they tend to move in harmony with and are thus supported by other natural forces and the environment. The outward sign of the union of Tao is this harmonious action of *wu-wei*. Sages who live life in this way experience their life and emotions lightly, like mild changes in the weather, without ever obscuring the blue sky and brightly shining heavens beyond.

Basic Practices

Most of Taoist practice is for achieving balance and harmony both within oneself and between oneself and the surrounding social and natural environment. In this way, the adept strengthens his or her physical health as the foundation for their mental and spiritual development. Total integral development of mind, body, and spirit is stressed because it is recognized that the same dynamic patterns of change at one level reflect on all other levels of life. Thus, feeling emotionally stuck might be partly relieved with regular physical movement. This is because *qi* flowing on one level of reality (the body) will tend to induce its flow in all other aspects (mind and emotions). Thus, an imbalance originating from

one level of life may manifest as an imbalance or disease in another area. This idea of different levels of reality having mutual influence and operating in parallel with the same natural dynamics or obeying the same universal laws is basic to Taoist thinking. In this way, every single individual is said to be a microcosm of the universe, with all the basic constituent parts available for complete development. But, this development depends on what one does and thus the need for practice and self-cultivation.

There is a multitude of practices, all having to do with the cultivation of the three treasures of life: (1) *qi* (vitality), (2) *jing* (essence), and (3) *shen* (spirit). Some practices will emphasize one or more of these three, but generally all are addressed in varying degrees. Any constructive activity performed with physical composure, mental clarity, and sincerity can become a practice and have spiritual value. This includes sitting, standing, walking, gentle movement (exercise), sleeping, and recitations. The most basic practice is to live in harmony with nature, adjusting one's routine with the daily and seasonal changes. Rising with the morning sun (the *yang* aspect of the day) and resting when it sets establishes a basic pattern of simplicity, respect, and confluence with natural forces. It is also a way to conserve energy as the sunlight literally supports the *yang* active aspect of life, while the *yin* with its relative coolness, darkness, and quietude that exists at night allows for more of the *yin* nature – contemplation, rest, and internal recuperation – to flourish. The study of changes in the external and internal nature is the subject of one pillar of Taoist thought, the *I Ching* or Book of Changes.

- *Qi Gong* – One of the oldest health traditions in China are physical practices generally referred to as *qi gong*, energy work, or *nei gong*, internal (energy) work. These include sets of gentle physical movements, meditations, postures with or without specific internal energy guidance. Some of these qi *gong* exercises are more physical and support the healthy foundation of life. They work with movements that stretch, tone, and adjust the energies of the muscles, tendons, and bones, dissolve emotional blockages or address specific health problems by adjusting the energies of the different organ systems of the body. Taoist movement practices are gentle, slow, circular, fluid in rhythmic conjunction with the breath and practiced with a balanced focus and internal poise. Thus, they foster the smooth flow of *qi*, gentleness of mind and spirit, and sensitivity to allow one's natural form to emerge. *Tai Ji Chuan* (same as *Tai Ji*) is a practice that reflects these attributes. It arose from the *qi gong* and martial arts traditions and today exists in either more relatively martial arts or health-oriented forms. There are also more spiritually oriented *qi gong* movements and meditations practiced with a subtle, internal focus.

- **Daily Life and the Emotions** – For a traditional Taoist, emotions are natural, but are not emphasized. Emotions do not exist except that they live in and influence the physical body in some way. They are seen as useful in motivating action, but are hidden causes of disease (physical, mental, or spiritual imbalance) if unchecked, exaggerated, or stockpiled. Thus, to practice a natural gentle flow of emotions in response to life's changes is healthy, but more is not encouraged. Physical movement that understands energy flow can dissolve the tensions arising from these undue emotional influences. Regular

practice of the gentle movement arts of *Tai Ji* and *qi gong* is considered one way to dissolve stressful emotional buildup and encourage a fluid internal disposition. With a relatively harmonious and peaceful emotional state, the emergence of a deepened connection with the source of wisdom may be attained.

- ***Teh*, The Way of Virtue** – Taoist spiritual practice also includes the practice and realization of virtue (*teh*). The *Tao Teh Ching* (The Virtuous Way, Way of Virtue) describes how focusing on what is essential and reducing what is nonessential leads one to a more direct and creative life where the ego and its emotional excesses are diminished and one's inherent integrated nature emerges. This purified internal nature reflects the positive aspect of the universal nature. Living with one's inherent nature is considered natural virtue and anything that goes against this is considered inherently nonvirtuous. Thus, while there are no given commandments of what is good or evil, it is understood that all immoral behaviors damage the individual and possibly others in that they disturb the harmony with the universal spiritual nature and its inherent respect and kindness. One aspect of spiritual cultivation is self-reflection, supported by quiet meditation, to reveal the ways in which people have fostered or abused the virtuous harmony within themselves or others.

- **Invocations** – Invocations are short spiritual writings recited for purification and refinement of mind and spirit. Based on the ancient teaching, *thinking is louder than thunder*, they are read with sincerity and clear-mindedness to cause a response from the divine realm of existence. This follows the universal subtle law of energy correspondence whereby similar energy levels respond to one other.

- **Talismans** – Energy takes many forms. Talismans are visual representations or short writings that carry a positive intent or spiritual symbol. They are placed in particular places in the home, workspace, place of self-cultivation, or worn on the person. The value of a talisman is found both in the process of creation and later usage. (The classical Chinese discipline of practicing calligraphy is an art with spiritual overtones related to this practice.) When spiritually developed people extend their minds into a particular image, a subtle power is created that can be used for healing or other related purposes.

- **Shrine** – Some individuals will want to establish a small shrine while a patient at a health care facility. This may consist of various pictures, spiritual books, objects, or symbols that have spiritual significance for that person and which provides them with physical reminders and a place of focus to reconnect with the divine energy supporting all life. Generally, a shrine also includes symbols of the three levels of life – *earthly* physical nature, *human* nature, and the *heavenly* spiritual sphere. The shrine may include reminders of natural elements (fire, metal, water, wood, and earth) – incense (fire) in metal holder (metal), bowl of water (water), plant (wood) in soil (earth) – which symbolize the integral nature of life within each person and all of life.

- **Rituals** – There are rituals that can be done by individuals or groups for self-alignment or harmonization with the natural energies of the environment. For instance, the energies of the earth have a natural biorhythm, being particularly strong at the four points of the solar calendar – spring and autumn equinox, summer and winter solstice. Taking advantage of or adjusting to the natural energy that one lives with is considered a fundamental Taoist practice. It is like knowing how to "ride the waves of life," taking the support of positive natural forces and minimizing the negative effects of destructive ones. These rituals might involve group meditations, recitations or invocations, and so forth. However, individual practices coupled with living a virtuous, daily life are considered fundamental for Taoists; group rituals are generally of secondary importance.

Principles for Clinical Care
Dietary Issues

- There are no dietary restrictions. All substances are evaluated as to their positive quality (inherent *qi*) seeking some usage as a food, medicine, or other productive purpose. For instance, some plants would be very bitter tasting and unpalatable but are useful as a medicine for their detoxifying properties with infectious disease. The overall quality of a potential food is evaluated the same way a traditional physician evaluates his or her patients – a constitution based on genetics and upbringing. Thus, foods naturally cultivated in good soil will receive a richer supply of nutritive support. Animals raised where they have an active lifestyle and eat a suitable, healthy diet will be healthier (better *qi*) and thus be more valuable as a potential source of food. Foods that are produced with modern industrial methods, overly processed and denatured in preparation are considered to have less positive human value because of their loss of natural vitality (*qi*).

- Healthy eating is based on the concept of a simple, natural, balanced diet. Excessive desire and emotions are seen as related to and encouraged by an excessive diet of any kind. Therefore, eating too much or eating overly rich food, very spicy food, artificial food, stimulants, or an absolutely strict asceticism would all be considered ways of harming oneself.

- The idea of food quality and one's relationship with the earth for spiritual and physical nourishment is inherent Taoist thought given in a public address given by Hua-Ching Ni: *When I eat, it is the pure, positive energy that is my true nourishment.* This refers to the pure, positive energy of people's minds and of their foods. The respect and thankfulness that flows from a calm mind is considered the best way to approach food and life. The fact that people quiet themselves to receive what is available for nourishment prepares them physiologically for optimal digestion and absorption of foods. Being picky and judgmental about foods creates nervous tension that disturbs optimal digestion. Instead of choosing foods that merely stimulate the senses, one must remember it is the inner quality of the foods that offers the true value.

- The health properties of food and the use of food-therapy were subjects of professional health care study even in ancient China. The relationship of the effects of specific herbs and foods were studied and understood so that a physician of traditional Chinese medicine (based on Taoist thought) might equally give his patients a prescription of herbs and an adjustment in diet for dealing with their particular complaints.

- What constitutes a healthy, balanced diet varies depending on one's constitution, gender, occupational needs, age, and specific health condition. For instance, certain foods are more difficult to digest and should be minimized with those with poor gastrointestinal function. Other foods are necessary to build blood or have special properties to boost the immune system, and so forth. Eventually, this depends on a proper medical analysis. But there are some general rules. For instance, one of the ancient ideas is to classify substances into a temperature gauge. Warming substances would raise body temperature and metabolism, activate more movement, and tend to create dryness. Cooling foods would lower body temperature, quiet activity, and tend to create fluids. Balance is the key. Thus, in summertime, more cooling and moistening foods such as many fruits and vegetables; water-based, lighter cooking methods; more raw and juiced foods and less rich, greasy food; less meat; and less overall substance would be generally recommended. In the winter, more cooked food, longer cooking methods, more roots and seeds, more animal products, dried foods, and less raw or juiced foods would be considered appropriate.

General Medical Beliefs

- Health and illness are considered relative terms because the concept of health has broader implications beyond the mere physical form and the absence of any identifiable disease. True health suggests a balanced integration and healthy development of the body, mind, and spirit.

- Some diseases would be considered purely a physical problem, others to have a mental-emotional cause and still others a spiritual basis. While health is the goal and a reflection of an enlightened one, illness could be the result of circumstances totally beyond one's control or there could be much that one has contributed to the deterioration of one's health. Taoists would attempt to prevent the occurrence of disease through their practice to treat arising problems early in their progression and to address the root cause of the condition whenever possible.

- Taoists believe that not all diseases can be cured by physical medicine alone, and in fact some do not require any medicine at all if the true source of the condition can be addressed (i.e., for those that originate in the mind and spirit).

- The basic tenets of traditional Chinese medicine, the use of acupuncture to influence the flow of qi and balance of *yin* and *yang*, are an outgrowth of Taoist belief and practice. Many major contributors to this medical system from ancient times have been renowned Taoist sages (as well as academics, Buddhist monks, folk healers, etc).

- In choosing medical treatments, Taoists would more likely want less intervention, more conservative treatment, and more natural methods. Traditionally, herbal medicines would be the chief medical remedy as well as acupuncture, dietary therapies including fasting, specialized *qi gong*, meditation, or invocation depending on the circumstances of the individual and the specific nature of the malady. Today, Taoists may rely more on western medicine, traditional methods, or a combined approach. How particular individuals decide what they wish to do at any particular time is left up to their understanding and is not dictated by any common religious decree or strict doctrine.

- The quality of the healing environment, the positive intention and harmonious interplay of the physicians, and other subtle factors (even astrological) are also considered important influences on health care in addition to the actual medical methods employed.

- **Organ Transplantation**: The internal organs are considered to be the center of the entire integral physiological systems that have physical and spiritual dimensions. Therefore, the idea of organ transplantation is like welcoming another member to one's individual spiritual family, a challenging task at any level. This means that a Taoist would be cautious about being an organ/tissue recipient.

- **Preventive Medicine**: A major precept in Taoist health care would be to take care of problems when they are new and when they are small. Taking care of women before pregnancy and during child-rearing while placing a priority on pediatric care and preventive medicine is seen as a way to boost the overall health of society. Waiting until bad habits are formed and health problems have developed is creating a much more difficult situation to treat.

Specific Medical Issues

- **Abortion**: Abortion would not be considered lightly, but only upon deep reflection as to the relative harm to the mother, baby, and their future life prospects. It is also important to avoid inviting people into the world (conception) without reasonable love and support.

- **Advance Directives**: Taoists should be recommended to make advance directives on acute care/end-of-life issues as they may have a variety of personal choices, but may want control over their death.

- **Birth Control**: It is a decision of the individual or couple.
- **Blood Transfusions**: Large-scale blood transfusions are problematic in how they impact the spiritual reality of an individual because the recipient is taking on some of the spiritual residue of the donor.
- **Circumcision**: Taoists may choose to circumcise their infant sons for cultural, not religious, reasons; it is an individual decision.
- **In Vitro Fertilization**: Assisted reproductive techniques (e.g., in vitro fertilization) may introduce various external energies to the couple in the form of the medical personnel handling the procedures or borrowed egg or sperm. Thus, spiritual qualities beyond the ones of the couple making the harmonization become involved in the process that is essential for the formation of life. This creates a more complex, risky, and challenging situation. The individuals make their own decisions; some people are comfortable with risk and challenges, but no one should proceed unprepared as if everything is perfectly normal.
- **Stem Cell Research**: Stem cells as undifferentiated cells seem to be physical matter most connected to what the Taoists call Pre-Heaven stage of existence, the undifferentiated oneness or spiritual unity that exists before birth, before things split into *yin*, *yang*, and all the myriad complexities. As this stage of existence has ultimate creativity and ultimate potential for application, the enthusiasm is understandable. On the other hand, without a true holistic perspective, many seeming advances of modern medicine do not lead to the bearing of the hoped-for happy fruit. Where there is the most excitement and potential, the more reflection must be utilized.
- **Vaccinations**: The Taoist practical worldview welcomes any medicine that can prevent disease as long as its total effect is benign or positive on general health.

  Practicing Taoists should be open to the use of vaccines as long as they feel confident there are no hidden negative effects. The discovery of the process of vaccination is generally accredited to Edward Jenner at the turn of the eighteenth century, but his work was based on ancient Chinese therapies for smallpox that recognized some of the principles now current (a Taoist doctor named Ge Hong, third century AD).
- **Withholding/Withdrawing Life Support**: Withholding/withdrawing life support in medically futile cases is supported in Taoism.

Gender and Personal Issues
- In Taoism, men and women are understood as equally valuable members of the human family. If anything, Taoist health care priorities favor women and children, as they are the source and future of society.
- Modern life is seen to be too heavily *yang* or rough and masculine in its current form; supporting women and the *yin* or feminine principle aids in healing this societal imbalance. In fact, if anything, Taoist philosophical and spiritual thought favors the gentler path of the feminine principle. One example often cited is the image of water, yielding on the outside, but strong at the center, soft, yet able to wear away stone.

Principles for Spiritual Care through the Cycles of Life

Concepts of Living and Dying for Spiritual Support

- Death is considered a natural process whereby the higher elements of the soul, the *Hun*, extricates itself from the lower aspects, the *Po*, which seeks to cling to the physical level of life. What is referred to as death is merely one half of the journey. If one has led one's life resulting in a greater refinement and purification of spirit, the higher soul has a chance to ascend; otherwise the heavy qualities of the lower soul carry one down. In either case, it is a continuation of the journey in a different, nonphysical form. Life, the integration of spirit with a physical body, offers the opportunity of movement and change. Death, a purely spiritual dimension, offers the opportunity of rest. When the time for death arrives, it is appropriate to wrap up one's earthly affairs, release all attachments, and open oneself up for a spiritual journey.

  If I enjoy a good life and have many things to give, it is Heavenly virtue displaying its benevolence through me. If I have little and undergo many difficulties, it is the Heavenly Realm building me stronger.[395]

During Birth

- The time of conception is seen as when the combined subtle quality of the couple attracts an individual soul of harmonious subtle quality that merges with the parents' physical essence (seed and egg) to form a unique human being.

- As the type of soul attracted is dependent on the quality of the couple's energy, the health of the parents leading up to conception is an opportunity to engender the best possible consequence of happy and healthy offspring.

- It is advised to avoid sexual activity for the purposes of conception when there is anger, intoxication, or discord between the couple or in upsetting or frightening circumstances, such as a thunderstorm. This is because these will all disaffect the peaceful quality of the couple and thus disturb the responsiveness of the soul.

- General advice during pregnancy is for the mother to foster externally what she is busy fostering internally – creative nurturing. Thus, giving free reign to creative interests, spending time in nature, relaxing, and nurturing new growth is encouraged. As the mother is the baby's first environment, the attempt is to create a relatively stress-free condition in the mother's life.

- Nearing delivery, it is advised for the mother to avoid images of cutting, bleeding, or anything that might startle or frighten her. At delivery, natural methods may be preferred.

- The mother may ask to keep the placenta. The dried placenta is utilized in natural Chinese medicine in soup, tea, or remade in tablet form as a tonic, especially used for recovery after childbirth and other times of exhaustion.

- During the postpartum period, traditionally the mother receives help from the family making her feel like she doesn't have to get out of bed for a month nor resume her normal duties for 6 months. Many health problems are considered

---

395 Ni, H. (1984). *Workbook for Spiritual Development of All People*: Los Angeles, CA: SevenStar Communications, 163.

to have started for women who have not fully recovered their strength from their pregnancy and delivery.

- There are no rituals for birth that would take place in a hospital. Of utmost importance is to take care of the mother and baby.
- If a baby dies in the hospital, there is nothing special for Taoists that is different from anyone else who experiences such an unfortunate time. Kindness, understanding, and compassion for the family would be helpful.

During Illness

- Self-reflection is valued to consider one's contribution to one's current health condition and how changes in mental attitudes, emotional excesses, and poor lifestyle or diet could be utilized to establish a positive internal healing environment. A balanced attitude that seeks positive growth from whatever life presents is what is valued.
- Special meditation, invocation, or other methods may be utilized to help in health restoration. The individual may practice these alone or with an intermediary who has special experience or skill. For instance, someone suffering from bronchial asthma may have considerable phlegm and fluids accumulating in their lungs. A particular *qi gong* meditation would focus the mind on this area of the body, silently intoning a specific tonal vibration that gently dissolves blockages in the lungs and relaxes the constricted passageways. Later, a visualization coordinated with the breath would give a specific colored image of energy being drawn into the lung tissues, strengthening the lung function and restoring their vitality emerging from disease.

Other special movements would be used to boost the immune system, relax the nervous system, tone the digestive system, and so forth.

- In the context of illness, astrological considerations and/or a consultation of the *I Ching* may be considered by the patient for guidance and support in coping with their specific situation.
- The key issue in extending help is sincerity of mind and a positive directed purpose.

During End of Life

- Rather than dying from a tortured illness or violence, in extreme pain or distress, achieving a natural, peaceful death is considered an achievement for a Taoist.
- Death is considered a natural process whereby the higher elements of the soul extricate themselves from the lower aspects that seek to cling to the physical level of life. This process may achieve varying degrees of success and may take varying amounts of time – from a single instant up to 7 days – depending on the spiritual development of the individual. The most spiritually advanced individuals know when it is the right time to die and may even prepare others for their passing. These patients would prefer to leave the earth in quietude and without the stress of heroic life-saving methods to interrupt the subtle process of the soul untying the cords of life.
- Respecting the wishes of those who wish to die in peaceful, familiar surroundings and who may not want the body disturbed for some short period of a few hours to a few days after death would be consistent with the highest level of Taoist esoteric belief.
- The practice of "Untying the Spirits" can

aid anyone in the time of passage fostering transcendence and detachment. This requires someone of special spiritual training (a Taoist mentor, coach, monk, or *qi gong* master might be knowledgeable in such matters) to perform.

- There are no absolutes, but medications that would alter consciousness would not be generally welcomed except in short-term, temporary conditions. Maintaining quiet awareness during the Earthly transition has spiritual value.
- Life support measures that continue physical life, but compromise the natural integral nature of life, are not considered to have positive value. Thus, extending life support in medically futile cases is not supported.

Care of the Body

- Autopsy, if performed for some positive purpose, is acceptable.
- The physical remains have no special value.
- Disposition of the body (cremation, burial) is an individual decision.
- Donation of the body for medical research is an individual decision.
- There are no prescribed rituals for preparation of the body after death in a clinical setting.

Organ and Tissue Donation

- Organ/tissue donation is an individual choice; Taoists may be less likely to offer their individual organs for donation because they believe in the integral nature of the body and do not consider their organs as purely mechanical parts that can be "plugged in and out." As for the body, once the soul has left, there is really no particular value given to the physical remains. Thus, Taoists would be less likely to be living donors, but might be open to donating their body for others if people find this beneficial. It may be preferable for a chaplain and/or nurse who are trained designated requesters to be consulted for assistance.

Scriptures, Inspirational Readings, and Prayers

- *Tao Teh Ching* and *Hua Hu Ching* by Lao Tzu, *I Ching*, *Bao Po Zi* by Ge Hong, as well the writings of Chuang Tzu, Hui Nan Tzu and the compilations of the Taoist Canon are considered the fundamental texts, various English sources.
- The following invocation may be used during times of illness or to heal a broken heart. Recite three times, silently or aloud. It is your sincerity that carries the healing power. You may specifically visualize your illness being completely healed, with a full restoration to health and wholeness.

READING DURING ILLNESS

Invocation for Health and Longevity[396]

I am strong; the sky is clear.

I am strong; the earth is stable.

I am strong; people are at peace with one another.

I am supported by the harmony of all three spheres.

All of my spiritual elements return to me.

All of my spiritual guardians accompany me.

The yin and yang of my life being are well integrated.

My life root is firm.

---

396 Ni, H. (1990). *Power of Natural Healing*. Los Angeles, CA: SevenStar Communications, 129–130.

As I follow the path of revitalization,
my mind and emotions become
wholesomely active.
The Goddess of my heart nourishes
my life abundantly.
Internal qi (energy) enhances my
spiritual growth,
and all obstacles dissolve before me.
The channels of my life energy are
balanced.
My natural healing power
contributes to a long and happy life,
so that my virtuous fulfillment in the
world can be accomplished.
By following the subtle law and
integral way of life, I draw ever
closer to the divine realm of the
Subtle Origin.

READING FOR END-OF-LIFE PROCESS

At the end of life, a Taoist is engaged in purifying and simplifying existence, gathering subtle spiritual energy and untying the knots of physical attachment becoming completely unaffected by the world in keeping to the wholeness of being.

The Subtle Body of Tao[397]

The true source is beyond description.
Pure law is formless and unspeakable.
Though appearing as two,
in essence there is only one.
For want of a better word,
the ancients called it Tao.

This primal mystery is the Mother of
all.
All phenomena proceed from it.
All phenomena journey back to it.

---

397 Ni. *The Taoist Inner View of the Universe and the
Immortal Realm*, 132–133.

Through phenomena, we also return
to the great mystery.

Existing – yet not existing.
Doing nothing – yet leaving nothing
undone.
While remaining eternally free,
it masters all through selfless activity.

Although Tao is one,
the spirits are many.
Residing in the true heaven of
sublime energy,
they are pure reflections of Tao.
Through them, the great oneness can
be known.

Their lives are subtle and deep.
They appear to be born with and
without form.
Self-formed and self-denying,
they are the most mysterious of all
beings.

For a long time we are trapped
in this earthly net of life.
We lose ourselves behind a soiled veil
and appear separated from the truth.

Through enlightenment by the spirits,
the way of release is known.
In no time, the veil is lifted,
and we are free of all bondage.

When we receive the power of the
true source,
we are free and never lose the way.
Centuries of guilt are washed away
and the accumulated evil of many
lives is cleansed.

The influence of pure law is
everywhere.

Our body is the shrine where we worship it.
Our light and it's light merge into one.
In this way, no part of reality is missed.

If you see only life and death,
you will become confused and misdirected.
If you accept one thing and reject another,
you will isolate yourself.

If you think the calculating mind can know Tao,
you are far indeed from the ultimate truth.
With a pure heart and clear mind only,
can one regain the power of Tao.

Without regarding this as being the only truth,
we worship the subtle body of Tao.
From the beginning, Tao serves us,
and in return, we humbly serve the Tao.

The uncountable stars have their number.
The unfathomable seas have their limit.
The void can be captured and the wind tied,
but the subtle body of Tao is beyond all knowing.

O mystery of mysteries, heart of hearts,
you are the most revered of all.
Dwelling in the depth of the deep,
you are the universal essence of all.

Special Days: Taoism

Special days of Tao are those that have a special high energy of their own nature rather than commemorations of historical past individuals, ideas or events. All of these days are considered to be opportunities for greater success with personal cultivation as the energy is stronger, more open and sensitive at this time. Except for the New Year, it is particularly considered a good time to cultivate forgiveness and cleansing. For the other energy days, I have given the energy for the northern hemisphere; the southern hemisphere is reversed.

January 26 *New Year's Day* – This day marks the beginning of a new energy phase or influence in the 60-year cycle of the traditional Chinese calendar. This cycle represents the influences on human and worldly affairs of the changing heavenly (ten stems) and earthly (12 branches represented by the animal figures) influences. Thus, each year brings different special qualities following the astrological calendar. It also corresponds to the beginning of spring in the Chinese calendar. To be harmonious with this new energy by wearing something new, gathering in groups, and celebrate the rebirth of *yang* energy in the universe forms the general guidance of the day.

March 20 *Spring equinox* – This day is considered the high point of the energy of spring, represented by the Wood Elemental Phase, an energy of warm, rising, creative, active *yang*.

June 21 *Summer solstice* – This day is considered the high point of the energy of summer, represented by the Fire Elemental Phase, an energy of heat, brightness, and outward expansion of *yang*. The earth receives the most amount of sunlight as this is the longest day of the year.

September 22 *Autumn equinox* – This day is considered the high point of the energy of autumn, represented by the Metal Elemental Phase, an energy of cool, downward, reflective, inward *yin*.

December 21 *Winter solstice* – This day is considered the high point of the energy of winter, represented by the Water Elemental Phase, an energy of dark, hidden, cold *yin*. The earth receives the least amount of sunlight as this is the shortest day of the year.

Glossary of Taoist Terms

feng shui: Literally meaning wind and water, *feng shui* is ancient Chinese geomancy. *Feng shui* is the art and science of understanding and harmonizing with the effects of natural environmental forces to make adjustments to maximize their positive effects. Much as Chinese acupuncture is the art of adjusting and harmonizing the internal energies or environment of the body, *feng shui* works with the external energies. This may include the placement of the contents of a room to facilitate traffic flow or of crops to make use of the sun, water, and shade conditions in agriculture. Some schools of *feng shui* also look at the arrangements of cosmic forces and their effects on the people and places they inhabit. *Feng shui* is a discipline with guidelines that are compatible with many techniques of agricultural planning and many of the new green technologies. Space, weather, astrology, psychology, and pseudo-geomagnetism are basic components of *feng shui*. Proponents claim that *feng shui* has an effect on health, wealth, and personal relationships.

hun/po: The ancient Chinese considered people to be an accumulation of various spiritual entities united together. The *hun* is a part of the soul that has potential beyond the physical body while the *po* is the part of the soul that only exists within human form. In human beings, the *hun* is related to psychic and psychological faculty of vision, imagination, and clear direction endowing the ability to discern their path, stay clear in their direction, imagine possibilities, and move forward toward their goals. The *po* are the animating agents of life processes that take place beyond people's conscious awareness and control. They are closely related to the autonomic nervous system, the sensory receptors, especially the primitive touch responses of the skin, the interior sense receptors of the visceral organs and the primal animal instincts. At death, the *hun* and *po* separate: the *po*, or ghostly aspect clinging to the body; and the *hun*, if developed, having the potential for transformation to a continued spiritual life beyond

jing: Chinese word for "essence," specifically kidney essence. Along with *qi* and shen, it is considered one of the "Three Treasures of Traditional Chinese Medicine" (TCM). *Jing* is stored in the kidneys and is considered as the physical seed of one's body, related to the reproductive essence and potential. It is yin in nature, which means it nourishes and fuels the body. As such, it is an important concept in the internal martial arts. *Jing* is related to one's inherited traits and genetic disposition (similar to DNA).

nei gong: any of a set of Chinese breathing and meditation disciplines associated with Taoism and especially the Chinese martial arts. *Nei gong* (*nei*, internal; *gong*, work or skill) practice is the so-called "soft or internal style" Chinese martial arts rather than external forms which work with the outward body structure (joints, muscles). *Nei gong* exercises involve cultivating physical stillness and or conscious (deliberate) movement, designed to produce relaxation or releasing of tension combined with many specialized breathing techniques. In martial arts, the fundamental purpose of this process is to develop a high level of coordination, concentration, and technical skill that is known as neijin. Otherwise, the ultimate purpose of this practice is for the individual to become at one with heaven or the *Tao*.

Qi (chee): a fundamental concept of traditional Chinese culture. *Qi* is believed to be part of everything that exists, as a "vital force" or "primal energy." It is frequently translated as "energy flow" or "breath of life." *Qi* is said to

exist in many different inter-transformable states, as in a solid, liquid or gas. Thoughts would thus be said to be a manifestation of the *Qi* of the mind and movements of the *Qi* of the body. Therefore, *Qi* expresses the inherent ability of something to function, a holistic concept, rather than only a narrow, finite type of substance. Of course, there are many states of *Qi* that are not visible or audible as in radio waves, microparticles, ideas, and so forth.

Qi gong: a generic modern term for any number of Chinese-originated exercise systems that involve coordination of mental focus, breath, and movement. *Qi* most closely translates as energy, while *gong* means work applied to a discipline or the resultant skill attained. Thus, *qigong* means energy work. It is mostly practiced for health maintenance or health restoration purposes, but there are also some who practice it professionally as a therapeutic intervention aligned with traditional Chinese medicine. Various forms of traditional *qigong* are also widely taught in conjunction with Chinese martial arts. There are a multitude of *qigong* practices, some more physically expansive, some more internal and meditative, with effects ranging from physical health, mental-emotional clarity and balance, and spiritual development. A considerable amount of modern Chinese research has suggested benefits for a number of illnesses, including high blood pressure, arthritis, ulcers, tuberculosis and heart disease, among others.

shen: a keyword in Chinese philosophy, Chinese religion, and Traditional Chinese Medicine. *Shen* is the most subtle or spiritual aspect of someone or something. Applied to a person, it is said to be the innermost guiding force of life, including the "soul" and its two aspects, *hun* (spiritual soul) and *po* (physical soul) as well as consciousness, will, and intellect. It may also be applied to spiritual energies not tied to the physical sphere or whenever discussing the level of what exists as the utmost subtle nature of any phenomena. The Oxford English Dictionary (2nd ed.) defines *shen* thusly: "In Chinese philosophy: a god, person of supernatural power, or the spirit of a dead person."

Tai Ji Chuan: Chinese movement art with martial and health applications that uses softness to overcome hardness. When practiced regularly, *Tai Ji Chuan* reduces stress and improves health. The foundation of *Tai Ji* skill, the regular practice of a very slow movement form consisting of a flowing sequence of movements that gently exercises the muscles and joints, regulates the blood, and calms the mind. Suitable for people of all ages and level of fitness, this exercise system requires no special equipment and can be easily integrated into one's daily life. *Tai Ji Chuan* (*tai ji* – the supreme ultimate or infinity, *chuan* – boxing) is an exercise crafted on the interflowing principles of *yin* and *yang*. The practice of *Tai Ji Chuan* thus directly trains one to master these life principles both externally and internally. *Tai Ji* may be used to refer to any harmonious system realizing the balance of *yin* and *yang* as seen in the *TaiJitu* or *Yin/Yang* symbol.

Tao/Dao: often translated as "The way of nature." The concept of Tao suggests an underlying inherent universal oneness which gives birth to constant change. These changes all occur within the relative sphere of *yin* and *yang* or complementary, opposing forces. This brings a dynamic balance and order to the universe even as all phenomena shift and evolve from being into nonbeing, potential into actual, substance into energy. *Tao* is everflowing, the source of all power and transformation. It manifests itself through all cycles and transitions: the change of seasons, cycles of life, shifts of power, time, and

so forth. *Tao* is the subtle universal law of Nature. For a follower of *Tao*, this model of the universe is at the same time seen as a model for governing one's life or any system. To be rooted in the deep unity of nature, while allowing for adaptation and creativity with the superficial changes is to foster sustainability and endurance. The symbol of the *Tao*, called the Taijitu, is of interwoven black and white halves of a circle, representing *yin* and *yang*, each balancing and giving birth to the other. Simply stated, *Tao* is the way and order of the universe.

teh: Key concept in Chinese philosophy, usually translated "inherent character; inner power; integrity"; or "moral character; natural virtue." In the *Tao Teh Ching*, (Classic of the Way and its Virtue), the singular primal text of philosophical Taoism, *teh* is described as the natural manifestation of a life in harmony with *Tao*. The implication of this is there is an inherent or self-evident moral nature, consistent with the underlying principles of the universe.

wu-wei: The practice of *wu-wei* and the efficacy of *wei-wu-wei* are fundamental tenets in Chinese thought and have been mostly emphasized by the Taoist school. The aim of *wu-wei* is to achieve a state of harmony or union with the Tao. As a result, individuals align their efforts with natural forces so that their results are gained with more ease and less friction. This gives the idea of the "gentle overcoming the hard" or in martial arts obtaining an irresistible form of "soft and invisible" power. This power is born of acting with the poise of a calm and unified disposition, without the extra force of emotion or desire, creating a state wherein things seemingly happen of their own accord. This can be compared to an athlete when things slow down and they feel "in the zone." This concept emerges from the understanding of *yin* and *yang* (where any action will have a corresponding reaction) in which one seeks to moderate extremes and not under or over-react to passing phenomena, but hit the bull's eye in life.

yin/yang: The concept of *yin* and *yang* polarity describes two primal, opposing but complementary forces to be found in all phenomena of the universe. This concept is at the cornerstone of most branches of Chinese philosophy, as well as traditional Chinese medicine. *Yin*, meaning literally the shady side of a slope, is the dark, dense, receptive, contracting, downward-seeking, consuming, feminine aspect. *Yang*, literally meaning the sunny side of a slope, is the bright, light, active, expanding, upward-seeking, producing, masculine aspect. *Yin* and *yang* are descriptions of complementary opposites and never as absolutes. Nothing is considered 100% *yin* or 100% *yang*, but some composite of varying amounts. While seemingly opposite, they are never apart. They function in a complementary fashion much like people's left and right legs cooperate to achieve walking. Thus, substance cannot exist without function, inhale without exhale, up without down and so on. Understanding this relativity in all phenomena, one seeks the balancing point or middle way in life.

Unitarian Universalism

We need not think alike to love alike.[398]

Prepared by:
The Reverend Kathy Riegelman, Chaplain
Saint Joseph Medical Center
Kansas City, MO

Reviewed and approved by:
The Reverend Rob Eller-Isaacs
President, Unitarian Universalist Ministers Association
Co-minister, Unity Church-Unitarian
St. Paul, MN

History and Facts

During the first three centuries of the Common Era, there was a plethora of Christian writings reflecting diversity of beliefs about the church, salvation, the person of Jesus, among other things. One dispute was whether Jesus was God, one with the Father in the Trinity, coeternal and of the same substance. Those who disagreed with this view may have considered Jesus in some other sense divine or simply as a teacher commissioned by God. Such views were later sometimes called "unitarian" to distinguish them from the official "trinitarian" teaching of the Church. Unitarianism held that God is one person while Trinitarians held that God was one in three mutually indwelling persons. Another early teaching was that a merciful God would not condemn anyone to eternal damnation, a view termed "universalist."

However, when Christianity became the favored religion of the Roman Empire in the fourth century under Emperor Constantine, a series of councils attempted to standardize Christian teachings, and trinitarianism was made official. But dissenting views persisted and developed.

In the sixteenth century, unitarian ideas were part of a growing dissent. A book called *On the Errors of the Trinity* by Spaniard Michael Servetus was circulated throughout Europe, but in Geneva he was burned at the stake as a heretic in 1553. The "liberal wing" of the Protestant Reformation took hold in the remote mountains of Transylvania in Eastern Europe where Unitarian congregations were first established. The first edict of religious toleration in history was declared in 1568 during the reign of Transylvanian John Sigismund, the first and only Unitarian king. Sigismund's court preacher, Frances David, had argued that individuals should be allowed theological liberty; he said, "We need not think alike to love alike." In Poland, Laelius Socinus and his nephew Faustus Socinus developed Unitarian views that flourished until they were suppressed

---

398 Fewkes, R. (1993). From "God is One," a responsive reading adapted from Francis David, a sixteenth-century Unitarian, by the Reverend Richard Fewkes in the Unitarian Universalist hymnal, *Singing the Living Tradition*. Boston, MA: Beacon Press, number 566 (no page number).

in 1638. The idea of individual choice of religious belief threatened both governments and ecclesiastical establishments.

Although unitarian beliefs have their roots in Eastern Europe, these same religious ideas began to emerge in England in the seventeenth century. In 1791, scientist and Unitarian minister Joseph Priestley had his laboratory burned and was "hounded" out of England. He subsequently moved to the United States where he established Unitarian churches in the Philadelphia area. But North American Unitarianism emerged largely from within the religious establishment of New England Puritanism. Each town was required to establish a congregationally independent church that followed Calvinist doctrines. Initially, these congregational churches offered no religious choices for their parishioners, but over time the strict doctrines of "original sin" and "predestination" were questioned.

By the mid-1700s, though, a group of evangelicals were calling for the revival of Puritan orthodoxy. They asserted their belief in humanity's eternal bondage to sin. Those who opposed the revival, believing in free human will and the loving benevolence of God, eventually became Unitarian. During the first 4 decades of the nineteenth century, hundreds of congregational churches fought over ideas about sin and salvation, and especially over the doctrine of the Trinity. In 1819, Unitarian minister William Ellery Channing's sermon, "Unitarian Christianity," gave the Unitarians a strong platform upon which to build. Six years later, the American Unitarian Association was organized in Boston, Massachusetts. Many congregations declared themselves Unitarian. Ralph Waldo Emerson's 1838 Harvard "Divinity School Address" intensified an expansive development of the faith by placing intuition above tradition.

Universalism (distinct from Unitarianism) was a more evangelical faith than Unitarianism. After officially organizing in 1793, the Universalists spread their faith across the eastern United States and Canada. Its initial development in America occurred along the Atlantic seaboard. The earliest preachers of the gospel of universal salvation appeared in what were later called the Middle Atlantic and Southern states. By 1781, Elhanan Winchester had organized a Philadelphia congregation of Universal Baptists. Among its members was Benjamin Rush, the famous physician and signer of the Declaration of Independence. At about the same time in the rural interior sections of New England, a small number of itinerant preachers, among them Caleb Rich, began to disbelieve the strict Calvinist doctrines of eternal punishment and preached universal salvation. They discovered from their biblical studies the new revelation of God's loving redemption of all. John Murray, an English preacher who immigrated to the American continent in 1770, helped lead the first Universalist church in Gloucester, Massachusetts, in the effort to separate church and state.

From its beginnings, Universalism challenged its members to reach out and embrace people whom society often marginalized. The Gloucester church included a freed slave among its charter members, and the Universalists became the first American denomination to ordain women to the ministry, beginning in 1863 with Olympia Brown. Hosea Ballou became the denomination's greatest leader during the nineteenth century, and he and his followers, including Nathaniel Stacy, led the way in spreading their faith.

Other preachers followed the advice of Universalist publisher Horace Greeley and ventured west. One such person was Unitarian Thomas Starr King (whom Lincoln credited with saving California for the Union) described the difference between Unitarians and Universalists this way: "Universalists believe that God is too good to damn people, and the Unitarians believe that people are too good to be damned by God."[399] Lincoln also borrowed from Unitarian minister Theodore Parker the phrase, "of all the people, by all the people, for all the people," which indicates the broad sympathies within both Unitarian and Universalist movements. The Universalists believed in a God who embraced everyone, and this eventually became central to their belief that lasting truth is found in all religions, and that dignity and worth is innate to all people regardless of sex, color, race, or class. As early as the 1830s, both groups were studying and promulgating texts from world religions other than Christianity. In 1900, Unitarians were the major force in the creation of what is now the International Association for Religious Freedom, the first international interfaith organization. By the beginning of the twentieth century, humanists within both traditions advocated that people could be religious without believing in God. No one person, no one religion, can embrace all religious truths.

Growing out of an inclusive theology was a lasting impetus in both denominations to create a more just society. Both Unitarians and Universalists became active participants in many social justice movements in the nineteenth and twentieth centuries. Parker was a prominent abolitionist, defending

fugitive slaves and offering support to American abolitionist John Brown. Other reformers included Universalists such as Charles Spear who called for prison reform, and Clara Barton who went from Civil War "angel of the battlefield" to become the founder of the American Red Cross. Unitarians such as Dorothea Dix fought to "break the chains" of people incarcerated in mental hospitals, and Samuel Gridley Howe started schools for the blind.

As other denominations softened their own theologies, Unitarian and Universalist memberships declined. By the middle of the twentieth century, Unitarians and Universalists thought they could have a stronger religious voice if they merged, and they did so in 1961, forming the "Unitarian Universalist Association of Congregations," of which about 1000 exist with perhaps 250000 actual members. Many Unitarian Universalists became active in the civil rights movement. James Reeb, a Unitarian Universalist minister, was murdered in Selma, Alabama, after he and 20% of the denomination's ministers responded to Martin Luther King Jr.'s call to march for justice.

Today, Unitarian Universalists continue to work for greater racial and cultural diversity. In 1977, a women and religion resolution was passed by the Association, and since then, the denomination has responded to the feminist challenge to change sexist structures and language, especially with the publication of an inclusive hymnal. The denomination has affirmed the rights of bisexuals, gays, lesbians, and transgendered persons, including ordaining and placing gay and lesbian clergy in its congregations; in 1996 same-sex marriage was affirmed.

All these efforts reflect a modern understanding of universal salvation.

---

399 Frothingham, R. (1865). *A Tribute to Thomas Starr King*. Boston, MA: Ticknor & Fields, 121.

The denomination's history has carried it from liberal Christian views about Jesus and human nature to a rich pluralism that includes theist and atheist, agnostic and humanist, pagan, Christian, Jew and Buddhist, and other perspectives. Grounded in its history and with an eye to the future, Unitarian Universalism continues to evolve and unfold.[400]

Basic Teachings

- With its historical roots in the Christian tradition, Unitarian Universalism is a liberal religion (i.e., a religion that keeps an open mind to the religious questions with which people have struggled in all times and places).
- Unitarian Universalists believe that personal experience, conscience, and reason should be the final sources of authority in religion, and that in the end, religious authority lies not in a book or person or institution, but in one's self, and that the free exchange of ideas in the local congregation can support, assist, and refine one's faith.
- Unitarian Universalists are "non-creedal"; members are not required to subscribe to a creed.
- Unitarian Universalists are governed by "Congregational Polity." In other words, each congregation is self-governing. Authority and responsibility for the affairs of the congregation are vested in the membership of the congregation, not in the denomination, the clergy, or a synod. Each congregation may assign certain powers to an elected board of trustees.

Only local congregations have the power to ordain.

- As within a single congregation, a variety of theological perspectives can be found; so, within the denomination, there exists a wide variety of approaches to worship: from high-church liturgy at King's Chapel in Boston to informal discussion-group or lecture formats sometimes found in "fellowships" (congregations without clergy) to a typical mainstream white Protestant service.
- While each individual and each congregation may, in the freedom of the spirit, vary from others, common values are reflected in the "Unitarian Universalist Association Principles and Purposes." However, individuals do not have to subscribe to the contents of this document for church membership.

The **Unitarian Universalist Principles and Purposes** contains the following:

We, the member congregations of the Unitarian Universalist Association, covenant to affirm and promote:
- The inherent worth and dignity of every person.
- Justice, equity and compassion in human relations.
- Acceptance of one another and encouragement to spiritual growth in our congregations.
- A free and responsible search for truth and meaning.
- The right of conscience and the use of the democratic process within our congregations and in society at large.
- The goal of world community with peace, liberty, and justice for all.
- Respect for the interdependent web of all existence of which we are a part.

---

400 Material on the history of Unitarian Universalism is adapted from Rev. Mark W. Harris, *Unitarian Universalist Origins: Our Historic Faith* (Boston, MA: Unitarian Universalist Association).

The living tradition which we share draws from many sources:

- Direct experience of that transcending mystery and wonder, affirmed in all cultures, which moves us to a renewal of the spirit and openness to the forces which create and uphold life.
- Words and deeds of prophetic women and men which challenge us to confront powers and structures of evil with justice, compassion, and the transforming power of love.
- Wisdom from the world's religions which inspires us in our ethical and spiritual life;
- Jewish and Christian teachings which call us to respond to God's love by loving our neighbors as ourselves.
- Humanist teachings which counsel us to heed the guidance of reason and the results of science, and warn us against idolatries of the mind and spirit.
- Spiritual teachings of earth-centered traditions which celebrate the sacred circle of life and instruct us to live in harmony with the rhythms of nature.

Grateful for the religious pluralism which enriches and ennobles our faith, we are inspired to deepen our understanding and expand our vision. As free congregations we enter into this covenant, promising to one another our mutual trust and support.

Basic Practices

Religious practice within Unitarian Universalism is as diverse as its membership. Religious practices will be particular to each person's theology. Those caring for the patient need to ask the patient what practices are most helpful and meaningful during hospitalization.

- **Prayer or meditation**: Some Unitarian Universalists are comfortable with the word "prayer." Others are more comfortable with meditation or simply conversation or shared silence. Chaplains or other caregivers offering prayer should ask the patient what practice is most meaningful. Many Unitarian Universalists have some discomfort with the word "God." Other acceptable invocations may include Spirit of Life, Spirit of Love, Spirit of Hope, Healing Spirit, Source of All, Eternal Mystery, Great Mystery of Life, and Eternal Spirit of the Universe.
- **Service**: Many Unitarian Universalists engage in social justice work as religious practice. Some understand social justice as a "religious obligation."[401] As individuals, congregations, and an association, Unitarian Universalists are committed to a wide variety of social causes: women's issues; equal rights for gay, lesbian, bisexual, and transgender persons; well-being for children; racial justice; economic equality; education; health care; food production and distribution; human rights; environmental issues; freedom of choice for women; immigration; gun control; homelessness; and nonviolent resolution of world conflict.
- **Life-long learning**: Most Unitarian Universalists are well educated and value learning on many levels. The values of reason, creativity, and the development of each individual's theology are lived out through reading and study from many genres and disciplines, including the sacred texts of the world's religions. The Reverend Lisa Doege writes:

---

401 Schulz, W. ed. (1993). *The Unitarian Universalist Pocket Guide*. 2nd ed. Boston, MA: Skinner House Books, 5.

[O]ur lack of a single authoritative scripture or authoritative law or authoritative ecclesiastical body calls us to do the demanding, often subtle, at times confusing, at times exhilarating work of examining each text or idea as it comes to us. ... We must have the insight to discern our beliefs, the courage to declare them, and the humility to abandon them, no matter how cherished or long held, if we come to know them as false or harmful.[402]

- **Communing with nature**: Many Unitarian Universalists find the Sacred in nature. Connection with nature can be achieved through walks, gardening, vacations, and social justice projects.
- Ritual observance in Unitarian Universalist worship is relatively rare. Many of the rituals Unitarian Universalists practice are drawn from its Judeo-Christian roots. A few congregations practice Holy Communion, gather for a Tenebrae service on Good Friday, offer a Seder meal at Passover, and/or light the Menorah during Hanukkah.
- The following three rituals are specifically Unitarian Universalist. The first involves the symbol of the Unitarian Universalist faith: the flaming chalice ritual, common to most congregations as one of the opening elements of worship. Another is the Flower Communion ritual, developed by Norman Chapek, derived from the faith's Eastern European roots. A final example is the Water Communion, a gathering ritual often practiced in the early fall. These rituals have endless variations.
  - *Lighting of the chalice*: A typical chalice-lighting might begin with a person early in a worship service igniting a flame in a chalice-like vessel with words about the meaning of the occasion for that person or the congregation. Some congregations may use a regular statement all may say together. Sometimes a song, such as "Rise Up O Flame," may be sung. The flaming chalice recalls the burning at the stake of Jan Hus in 1415 for, and among other things, taking the then clergy-only communion chalice to the laity.
  - *Flower communion*: At an appropriate Sunday in spring, congregants bring flowers to the gathering and leave with flowers others have brought, symbolizing the importance of our diverse community and the beauty we bring to one another.
  - *Water communion*: Waters collected from summer travels are brought to a fall Sunday gathering and poured into a common vessel, with each person relating the place, circumstance, and meaning from which the water was derived. This ritual emphasized the importance of coming together as a worshipping community.
  - Many Unitarian Universalist congregations have lay pastoral care teams who are responsible for visiting the sick, providing meals, transportation, child care, and so forth.
  - Cultural differences among Unitarian Universalists are not a major issue. Many Unitarian Universalist congregations are taking steps to increase the cultural, ethnic, and socioeconomic diversity among their members. Currently, most Unitarian Universalist congregations are comprised of middle to upper-middle class, well-educated

---

402 Doege, L. (2000). By what authority? (sermon, First Unitarian Church, South Bend, IN, September 24, 2000).

European Americans. Theological diversity is more typical than cultural diversity.

Principles for Clinical Care
Dietary Issues

- There are no particular dietary restrictions for Unitarian Universalists. "Ethical eating," a growing trend among Unitarian Universalists, is a response to the seventh principle, which calls Unitarian Universalists to respect and care for the environment. Ethical eating may be variously interpreted from favoring organically grown foods, "free-range" food over animals raised in confinement, foods that are produced as directly as possible from the earth (eating cereals as opposed to eating cattle which have eaten cereals), to vegetarianism, to modesty of intake with awareness of those in the world with poor nutrition, to unmodified crops (genetically original), to food produced by those benefiting from fair labor practices.[403]

General Medical Beliefs

- Most Unitarian Universalists have no restrictions on medical treatments/interventions.
- Most Unitarian Universalist patients want to be fully informed about their treatment and included as a partner in their health care.
- Hospice care is acceptable and is often encouraged, allowing patients to be in their homes, surrounded by loved ones at the time of death.

Specific Medical Issues

- **Abortion**: Most Unitarian Universalists are pro-choice; thus, abortion is acceptable. In 1977, the General Assembly of the Unitarian Universalist Association passed the General Resolution, "Abortion," which "affirm[s] the right of each woman to make decisions concerning her own body and future."[404] The resolution continues by affirming the need to provide safe and legal abortions for women of all means. While most Unitarian Universalists are pro-choice, they also understand that "[t]he pro-life/pro-choice debate rarely acknowledges the critical point that nobody is in favor of abortion: Women have abortions because of complicated and competing realities in their lives."[405]
- **Advance Directives**: In 1978, the General Assembly of the Unitarian Universalist Association passed a General Resolution on the Legality of Living Wills. This resolution affirms that the Unitarian Universalist "heritage of religious freedom extends into the nature of life and destiny."[406] The resolution also recognizes that advances in medical technology mean that life can be artificially extended. This resolution "affirms and defends the right of each person to sign a legally binding Living Will."[407] This strong

---

403 Material on ethical eating is drawn from Amy Hassinger, "Eating ethically," *UU World*, 2007, 21(1), 28–34.

404 Unitarian Universalist Association. Abortion. 1977 General Resolution, August 24, 2011. Available at: www.uua.org/socialjustice/socialjustice/statements/20250.shtml (accessed 2 September 2012).

405 Sinkford, W. (2005). Real moral values, *UU World*, Volume XIX (2): 7.

406 Unitarian Universalist Association. Legality of Living Wills. 1978 Resolution, August 24, 2011, www.uua.org/socialjustice/socialjustice/statements/20279.shtml (accessed 2 September 2012).

407 Unitarian Universalist Association, Legality of Living Wills, 1978 Resolution.

emphasis on individual religious freedom and recognition of the natural cycle of life and death means that Unitarian Universalists strongly believe in being proactive regarding health care. Many will have completed their advance directive and named a Durable Power of Attorney for Health Care Decisions.

- **Birth Control**: Unitarian Universalists support the use of birth control for many reasons, including the need for population control, the right of women to have control of their own bodies, and respect for feminist theologies and social ethics.[408]
- **Blood Transfusions**: There are no restrictions on the use of blood products.
- **Circumcision**: Circumcision is a personal or family decision, usually without religious significance.
- **In Vitro Fertilization**: Infertile couples are supported by the community and encouraged to pursue fertilization treatments. Homosexual couples often use in vitro fertilization as a method to have biological children. The community supports the efforts of all couples, whether heterosexual or homosexual, in family planning.
- **Stem Cell Research**: Stem cell therapies are accepted by Unitarian Universalists because scientific data supports stem cell therapies as a viable treatment for many degenerative and debilitating diseases. This view is consistent with the importance of the intellect and scientific data in guiding health care decisions. Unitarian Universalists believe the choice of stem cell therapies should be available for those

who want them. It is then up to the individual, whether as Unitarian Universalists or as members of other faith traditions, to decide what treatments are morally acceptable.[409]

- **Vaccinations**: Most Unitarian Universalists understand immunizations to be an important component of overall health care. Individual choice and family values guide the decision whether or not to be immunized. As with other health care issues, Unitarian Universalists want to be fully informed of the benefits and risks of immunizations. A General Resolution on a National Health Act adopted by the Unitarian Universalist Association in 1971 is consistent with the Unitarian Universalist focus on social justice and availability of health care for all. The resolution states the following in regard to immunizations: "To make certain that … [p]ediatric care, inclusive of all immunizations necessary, be made available to every child."[410]
- **Withholding/Withdrawing Life Support**: Unitarian Universalists do not believe in prolonging life, particularly if there is not an acceptable quality of life. The first principle, which affirms "that human life has dignity"[411] guides

---

408 Unitarian Universalist Association of Congregations. Reproductive Choices. 1998 General Resolution. Last updated March 19, 2012. Available at: www.uua.org/socialjustice/issues/reproductive/reproductivehealth/24042.shtml (accessed 2 September 2012).

409 More information on specific aspects of stem cell research as supported by the Unitarian Universalist Association may be found at the following: Unitarian Universalist Association. Pass the Stem Cell Research Enhancement Act, 2006 Action of immediate Witness. Last updated August 24, 2011. Available at: www.uua.org/socialjustice/social justice/statements/8064.shtml.

410 Unitarian Universalist Association. National Health Plan, 1971 General Resolution. Last updated August 24, 2011. Available at: www.uua.org/socialjustice/socialjustice/statements/19770.shtml. (accessed 2 September 2012).

411 Unitarian Universalist Association of Congregations. The Right to Die with Dignity. 1998 General Resolution. Last updated March 19,

decisions about end-of-life care. Many Unitarian Universalists view the compromise of dignity as a violation of the first principle. Therefore, withholding and/or withdrawing life support is acceptable. Most Unitarian Universalists want a "natural" death.

Gender and Personal Issues

- There are no particular gender, modesty, or privacy issues of the Unitarian Universalist religion. All health care issues should be guided by the first principle, which calls us to affirm the inherent worth and dignity of every person.

Principles for Spiritual Care through the Cycles of Life
Concepts of Living and Dying for Spiritual Support

- Unitarian Universalists have no one belief about life after death. A wide variety of beliefs regarding the afterlife include: belief in Heaven, belief in reincarnation, and the belief that there is no afterlife at all. Many find comfort in the strength of community. Unitarian Universalist beliefs on immortality often are centered around the belief that the values and goodness of each person who dies becomes a part of the lives of those who love the deceased. Unitarian Universalism as a religious tradition is primarily directed toward this life, and not on what happens after death.
- Unitarian Universalism's focus on social justice means that individuals find comfort in knowing they have made a difference in the world. Leaving a legacy of making the world a better place and knowing that others will continue their work is important.
- Suffering is seen as inherent in the human condition. Illness is not a punishment. When looking for explanations for suffering, many Unitarian Universalists will look for answers consistent with scientific knowledge. For example, heart disease is known to be both hereditary and dependent on one's lifestyle.

During Birth

- Baptism is not generally practiced among Unitarian Universalists.
- Parents often choose to have their child "Dedicated" at some time early in the child's life. The dedication is a rite of passage that connects the child to the congregation by affirming the congregation's support of both the child and his or her parent/s. The dedication commonly takes place in the context of a worship service in the church, however, parents may choose to have a private child dedication outside of the context of worship.[412]
- In the case of a fetal demise, the parents may be comfortable with a naming and/or blessing ceremony. The ceremony should respect the parents' beliefs and spiritual practices. Either the parents' minister or a hospital chaplain could perform a blessing ceremony, although there are no restrictions against a layperson performing a naming or blessing ceremony.
- As stated earlier, circumcision is a personal or family decision, usually without religious significance.

2012. Available at: www.uua.org/statements/statements/14486.shtml (accessed 15 October 2012).

412 For material appropriate for a child's Dedication, see Edward Searl, *Bless This Child: A Treasury of Poems, Quotations, and Readings to Celebrate Birth* (Boston, MA: Skinner House Books: 2006).

During Illness

- The senior minister or ministry team of the congregation should, with the patient's permission, be notified of her or his hospitalization or health crisis.
- The minister, or the designated pastoral care provider, will typically make visits to the sick and/or coordinate care based in the congregation.
- The value of community carries into times of illness for Unitarian Universalists. Family and friends should be allowed to visit as appropriate, based both on the patient's condition and specific health condition (e.g., if a patient needs rest, it is important to limit visitors). A patient's "family" may be both biological and/or by choice.
- Those caring for Unitarian Universalists should feel free to ask the patient and/or family what is meaningful and appropriate for the patient, including whether a patient is comfortable with prayer. Many Unitarian Universalists meditate or pray and will accept prayer from a caring person. Prayers should be respectful of the individual's theology, particularly in reference to whether the patient is a theist or an atheist.
- When offering readings or scripture, consider the individual's beliefs and preferences. While reading a Psalm may be comforting for one Unitarian Universalist patient, another may find more meaning in a reading from the *Tao Te Ching*. The chaplain or others caring for the patient may find guidance by asking the patient if they have any "wisdom words" that are particularly meaningful at times of illness or difficulty. Many Unitarian Universalists have poems or passages from scripture or literature that guide and ground them during times of difficulty.

- Special attention needs to be given to gay and lesbian couples; a patient's partner needs to be treated with the same respect as the spouse of a heterosexual couple. Many same-sex couples have named their partners as their Durable Power of Attorney for Health Care Decisions.
- Spiritual care providers need to be sensitive to the patient's individual theology, beliefs, and practices. Most Unitarian Universalists are comfortable answering questions regarding their faith. The following are typical questions a chaplain or other spiritual care provider can ask.
  - What are your sources of spiritual support?
  - Is the word "God" meaningful for you?
  - Is prayer or meditation something you find helpful?
  - Are there any spiritual practices that would be helpful for you at this time?
  - Is there a spiritual leader you would like to visit you?
  - Is there scripture, poetry or literature that would be helpful?
  - Are there reading materials, audio or video tapes, and so forth, that you would find helpful?
  - Do you have requests or instructions for me or others on the staff that would enhance the spiritual care you desire?

During End of Life

- Most Unitarian Universalists want a "natural" death. "[D]eath [is not viewed] as something unnatural, but as a natural passage – like birth, one of the hinges upon which life turns."[413]
- The value of community contributes to

---

413 Buehrens, J. and F. Church. (1989). *Our Chosen Faith: An Introduction to Unitarian Universalism*, Boston, MA: Beacon Press, 15–16.

meaning at end of life. Family and friends should be allowed to visit as appropriate, based both on the patient's condition and specific health condition (e.g., if a patient needs rest, it is important to limit visitors). A patient's "family" may be both biological and/or by choice.

- Those caring for Unitarian Universalists should feel free to ask the patient and/or family what is meaningful and appropriate for the patient, including whether a patient is comfortable with prayer. Many Unitarian Universalists meditate or pray and will accept prayer from a caring person. Prayers should be respectful of the individual's theology, particularly in reference to whether the patient is a theist or an atheist.

- When offering readings or scripture, consider the individual's beliefs and preferences. While reading a Psalm may be comforting for one Unitarian Universalist patient, another may find more meaning in a reading from the *Tao Te Ching*. The chaplain or others caring for the patient may find guidance by asking the patient if they have any "wisdom words" that are particularly meaningful at times of illness or difficulty. Many Unitarian Universalists have poems or passages from scripture or literature that guide and ground them during times of difficulty.

- Many Unitarian Universalists will have completed Advance Directives for Health Care Decisions. Their wishes contained in theses documents should be honored.

Care of the Body

- There are no special needs regarding care of the body after death.

- The body of the deceased should be treated with respect and dignity. Family and friends should be allowed the option

to be with the deceased, to view the body and say their final goodbyes. This is especially important because cremation is the preferred means of disposition of the body for many Unitarian Universalists.

- Most Unitarian Universalists would agree to an autopsy if one were recommended or if there was uncertainty about the cause of death.

- Some Unitarian Universalists would consider donation of the body for medical research.

- The Memorial Service, which is scheduled at a time in the future that is convenient for family and friends, is often referred to as a Celebration of Life. The Memorial Service does not have to be officiated by ordained clergy. The service often includes readings, music, a eulogy (often prepared and delivered by a family member or close friend), and a time for those in attendance to share stories and memories of the deceased.[414]

Organ and Tissue Donation

- Organ and tissue donation is a personal choice for Unitarian Universalists. Many Unitarian Universalists are in favor of organ and tissue donation, especially because the opportunity to help others aligns with the ethical living and justice-seeking aspects of Unitarian Universalism. It may be preferable for a

---

414 For materials appropriate for memorial services for Unitarian Universalists, see Edward Searl, *In Memoriam: A Guide to Modern Funerals and Memorial Services*, 2nd ed. (Boston, MA: Skinner House Books, 2000); Edward Searl, ed., *Beyond Absence: A Treasury of Poems, Quotations, and Readings on Death and Remembrance*, (Boston: Skinner House Books, 2006); and Carl Seaburg, ed., *Great Occasions: Readings for the Celebration of Birth, Coming-of-Age, Marriage, and Death*, (Boston, MA: Skinner House Books, 1998).

chaplain and/or nurse who are trained designated requesters to be consulted for assistance.

Scriptures, Inspirational Readings, and Prayers

"We consider bibles and religions divine – I do not say they are not divine; I say they have all grown out of you, and may grow out of you still; it is not they who give the life – it is you who give the life." These lines of Whitman sum up in a succinct and beautiful way, the Unitarian Universalist attitude toward scripture ... [T]he totality of religious impulse is simply too vast to be narrowed down to a single text, even one as rich and varied as the Bible, or any other holy scripture.[415]

- Scripture, as this quote implies, is a very inclusive term for Unitarian Universalists. While many traditions define scripture as the religious texts specific to their particular faith, Unitarian Universalism's understanding of scripture is guided by the theological diversity that is inherent in the tradition. As noted earlier, the faith draws inspiration from many sources: direct experience, words and deeds of prophetic women and men, wisdom from the world's religions, Jewish, Christian, and Humanist teachings, and the teachings of earth-centered traditions. Sources of scripture include the sacred texts of all the world's religions, poetry, and literature.
- Poets who are popular among Unitarian Universalists and whose poetry is often incorporated into worship services

include Robert Bly, e. e. cummings, Emily Dickinson, T. S. Eliot, Kabir, Denise Levertov, Pablo Neruda, Kathleen Norris, Mary Oliver, Adrienne Rich, Ranier Maria Rilke, Theodore Roethke, Jellaladin Rumi, May Sarton, Rabindranath Tagore, and Walt Whitman.

- Others whose poetry or literature may bring comfort or inspiration to Unitarian Universalists include Maya Angelou, Wendell Berry, William Blake, Annie Dillard, Ralph Waldo Emerson, Kahlil Gibran, Thich Nhat Hanh, Langston Hughes, John Keats, Martin Luther King Jr., Lao Tsu, Marge Piercy, Carl Seaburg, Starhawk, Henry David Thoreau, Pierre Teilhard de Chardin, Lord Alfred Tennyson, Howard Thurman, and William Butler Yeats.
- For a comprehensive selection of readings, see the anthology of readings included in the Unitarian Universalist Hymnal: *Singing the Living Tradition*.[416] The prayers, meditations, readings, and hymns included here are selected from *Singing the Living Tradition*, with page numbers cited.

---

415 Doege, L. (2000) By what authority? (sermon, First Unitarian Church, South Bend, IN, September 24, 2000).

416 For additional readings see the following collections of meditations, readings, and poetry: Kathleen Montgomery, ed., *100 Meditations: Selections from Unitarian Universalist Meditation Manuals*, (Boston, MA: Skinner House Books, 2000), Patricia Frevert, ed., *What We Share: Collected Meditations*, vol. 2, (Boston, MA: Skinner House Books, 2002), Patricia Frevert, ed., *All The Gifts of Life: Collected Meditations*, vol. 3, (Boston, MA: Skinner House Books, 2002), Margared L. Beard, ed., *Listening For Our Song: Collected Meditations*, vol. 4, (Boston, MA: Skinner House Books, 2002), and Mary Bernard, ed., *Singing In The Night: Collected Meditations*, vol. 5, (Boston, MA: Skinner House Books, 2004).

SELECTED UNITARIAN UNIVERSALIST
PRAYERS AND MEDITATIONS

#483 The Peace of Wild Things

When despair for the world grows in
me and I wake in the night at the least
sound in fear of what my life and my
children's lives may be, I go and lie
down where the wood drake rests in
his beauty on the water, and the great
heron feeds.

I come into the peace of wild
things who do not tax their lives with
forethought of grief. I come into the
presence of still water. And I feel
above me the day-blind stars waiting
with their light. For a time I rest in
the grace of the world, and am free.

—Wendell Berry

#498 The Moments of High Resolve

In the quietness of this place,
   surrounded by the all-pervading
   Presence of God, my heart
   whispers:
Keep fresh before me the moments of
   my High Resolve, that in good times
   or in tempests,
I may not forget that to which my life
   is committed.
Keep fresh before me the moments of
   my high resolve.

—Howard Thurman

#505 Let Us Be At Peace

Let us be at peace with our bodies
   and our minds.
Let us return to ourselves and become
   wholly ourselves.

Let us be aware of the source of
   being, common to us all and to all
   living things.
Evoking the presence of the Great
   Compassion, let us fill our hearts
   with our own compassion – toward
   ourselves and towards all living
   beings.
Let us pray that we ourselves cease
   to be the cause of suffering to each
   other.
With humility, with awareness of
   the existence of life, and of the
   sufferings that are going on around
   us, let us practice the establishment
   of peace in our hearts and on earth.

—Thich Nhat Hahn

#524 Earth Mother, Star Mother

Earth mother, star mother,
You who are called by a thousand
   names,
May all remember we are cells in
   your body and dance together.
You are grain and the loaf that
   sustains us each day,
And as you are patient with our
   struggles to learn
So shall we be patient with ourselves
   and each other.
We are radiant light and sacred dark
   – the balance –
You are the embrace that heartens
And the freedom beyond fear.
Within you we are born, we grow,
   live, and die –
You bring us around the circle to
   rebirth,
Within us you dance forever

—Starhawk

#515 We Lift Our Hearts in Thanks

For the sun and the dawn which we
did not create;
For the moon and the evening which
we did not make;
For food which we plant but cannot
grow;
For friends and loved ones we have
not earned and cannot buy;
For this gathered company which
welcomes us as we are,
from wherever we have come;
For all free churches that keep us
human and encourage us in our
quest
for beauty, truth and love;
For all things which come to us as
gifts of being from sources beyond
ourselves;
Gifts of life and love and friendship;
We lift our hearts in thanks this day.

—Richard M. Fewkes

#681 Deep Peace

Deep peace of the running wave to
you.
Deep peace of the flowing air to you.
Deep peace of the quiet earth to you.
Deep peace of the shining stars to
you.
Deep peace of the infinite peace to
you.

—Adapted from Gaelic Runes

SELECTED UNITARIAN UNIVERSALIST POEMS

#490 Wild Geese

You do not have to be good.
You do not have to walk on your
knees.
for a hundred miles through the
desert repenting.
You only have to let the soft animal of
your body
love what it loves.
Tell me about despair, yours, and I
will tell you mine.
Meanwhile, the world goes on.
Meanwhile the sun and the clear
pebbles of the rain
are moving across landscapes,
over the prairies and deep trees,
the mountains and the rivers.
Meanwhile the wild geese, high in the
clean blue air
are heading home again.
Whoever you are, no matter how
lonely,
the world offers itself to your
imagination,
calls to you like the wild geese, harsh
and exciting –
over and over announcing your place
in the family of things.

—Mary Oliver

#504 i thank You God

i thank You God for most this
amazing
day: for the leaping greenly spirits of
trees
and a blue true dream of sky; and for
everything
which is natural which is infinite
which is yes
(i who have died am alive again today,
and this is the sun's birthday; this is
the birth

day of life and love and wings: and of
  the gay
great happening illimitably earth)
how should tasting touching hearing
  seeing
breathing any – lifted from the no
of all nothing – human merely being
doubt unimaginable You?
(now the ears of my ears awake and
now the eyes of my eyes are opened)

        —e. e. cummings

#525 Web
Intricate and untraceable weaving
  and interweaving,
dark strand with light:
Designed, beyond all spiderly
  contrivance, to link, not to
  entrap:
Elation, grief, joy, contrition,
  entwined; shaking, changing,
  forever
forming, transforming:
All praise, all praise to the great web.

        —Denise Levertov

#529 The Stream of Life
The same stream of life that runs
  through my veins night and day
runs through the world and dances in
  rhythmic measures.
It is the same life that shoots in joy
  through the dust of the earth
in numberless blades of grass and
  breaks into tumultuous waves of
  leaves and flowers.
It is the same life that is rocked in the
  ocean-cradle of birth and of death,
  in ebb and in flow.

I feel my limbs are made glorious by
  the touch of this world of life.
And my pride is from the life-throb
  of ages dancing in my blood this
  moment.

        —Rabindranath Tagore

SELECTED UNITARIAN UNIVERSALIST READINGS

#419 Look to this Day
Look to this day!
For it is life, the very life of life.
In its brief course lie all the verities
  and realities of your existence.
The bliss of growth, the glory of
  action, the splendor of beauty;
For yesterday is but a dream, and
  tomorrow is only a vision;
But today, well-lived, makes every
  yesterday a dream of happiness
And every tomorrow a vision of
  hope.
Look well therefore to this day.

        —Kalidasa

#468 We Need One Another
We need one another when we would
  be comforted.
We need one another when we are in
  trouble and afraid.
We need one another when we are in
  despair, in temptation,
and need to be recalled to our best
  selves again.
We need one another when we would
  accomplish some great purpose,
and cannot do it alone.
We need one another in the hour of
  success,

when we look for someone to share
our triumphs.
We need one another in the hour of
defeat,
when with encouragement we might
endure, and stand again.
We need one another when we come
to die,
and would have gentle hands prepare
us for the journey.
All our lives we are in need, and
others are in need of us.

—George E. Odell

#447 At Times Our Own Light Goes Out

At times our own light goes out and
is rekindled by a spark from another
person. Each of us had cause to think
with deep gratitude of those who have
lighted the flame within us.

—Albert Schweitzer

#637 A Litany of Atonement

For remaining silent when a single
voice would have made a difference
We forgive ourselves and each other;
we begin again in love.
For each time that our fears have
made us rigid and inaccessible
We forgive ourselves and each other;
we begin again in love.
For each time that we have struck out
in anger without just cause
We forgive ourselves and each other;
we begin again in love.
For each time that our greed has
blinded us to the needs of others
We forgive ourselves and each other;
we begin again in love.

For the selfishness which sets us apart
and alone
We forgive ourselves and each other;
we begin again in love.
For falling short of the admonitions of
the spirit
We forgive ourselves and each other;
we begin again in love.
For losing sight of our unity
We forgive ourselves and each other;
we begin again in love.
For those and for so many acts both
evident and subtle
which have fueled the illusion of
separateness
We forgive ourselves and each other;
we begin again in love.

—Robert Eller-Isaacs

#527 Immortality

It is eternity now.
I am in the midst of it.
It is about me, in the sunshine;
I am in it, as the butterfly in the
light-laden air.
Nothing has to come,
It is now.
Now is eternity,
Now is the immortal life.

—Richard Jeffries

#646 The Larger Circle

We clasp the hands of those that go
before us,
and the hands of those who come
after us.
We enter the little circle of each
other's arms and the larger circle of
lovers,

Whose hands are joined in a dance,
and the larger circle of all creatures,
Passing in and out of life, who move
also in a dance,
to a music so subtle and vast that no
ear hears it except in fragments.

—Wendell Berry

#698 Take Courage
Take courage friends.
The way is often hard, the path is
never clear, and the stakes are very
high.
Take courage.
For deep down, there is another
truth: you are not alone.

—Wayne B. Arnason

#721 We Remember Them
In the rising of the sun and in its
going down,
we remember them.
In the blowing of the wind and in the
chill of winter,
we remember them.
In the opening of the buds and in the
rebirth of spring,
we remember them.
In the blueness of the sky and in the
warmth of summer,
we remember them.

In the rustling of leaves and in the
beauty of autumn,
we remember them.
In the beginning of the year and when
it ends,
we remember them.
When we are weary and in need of
strength,
we remember them.
When we are lost and sick at heart,
we remember them.
When we have joys we yearn to
share,
we remember them.
So long as we live, they too shall live,
for they are now a
part of us, as we remember them.

—Roland B. Gittelsohn (adapted)

SELECTED UNITARIAN UNIVERSALIST
HYMN

#123 Spirit of Life
Spirit of Life, come unto me.
Sing in my heart all the stirrings of
compassion.
Blow in the wind, rise in the sea;
move in the hand, giving live the
shape of justice.
Roots hold me close; wings set me
free; Spirit of life, come to me, come
to me.

—Words and music by Carolyn
McDade

Vodou and Afro-Atlantic Religions

Onor e respé.

Honor and Respect.[417]

Prepared by:
Dowoti Désir
Founder, Durban Declaration and Programme of Action Watch Group
Haitian Vodou Priest, Scholar, and Human Rights Activist
New York, NY

History and Facts

In the Americas, African slaves were found in colonial America, Ayiti (Haiti), Brazil, Cuba, the Dominican Republic, Guadalupe, Jamaica, Martinique, Puerto Rico, Trinidad and Tobago, as well as other places. These along with their descendant communities and among West and Central Africans, practiced a religious tradition that prevails in spite of numerous attempts to discredit and vilify it. The religion of the Africans in these various places is called Vodou. However, it also came to be known as *Candomble, Lukumi, Macumba, Obeah, Arara, Sango, Palo Majumbe,* and *Santeria* in varying locales. These *orisa*-based (*orisa* refers to spiritual beings) traditions are often collectively known as "The Religion" and acknowledged as forms of Afro-Atlantic Spirituality. The specific elements of each tradition vary with the geographic and historic framework of each country or region

their fundamental core however, remains the same.

Vodou has historically been defined as a dance to the sacred spirit. From the heartland and western arm of Africa, Vodou (also spelled Voudou) is an indigenous religion, discipline, and philosophy that provided its practitioners with a comprehensive order for recognizing and utilizing the healing properties of the natural world. It encompasses the lessons of the known and unknown universe and acknowledges the lives, contributions, and continued presence of the dead.[418] Etymologically, Vodou is derived from the roots "vo" and "dou/dun" which mean "to draw sacred water; create a metaphysical opening; borne of divine oracle; and to value peace." Philosophically, Vodou instructs practitioners to consider their individual situations and places in the universe, maintain balanced or objective

---

417 The quote, provided by Dowoti Désir, author of this chapter, is a traditional Haitan salutation.

418 The foundation of the author's remarks applies to all Afro-Atlantic or *orisa*-based religions, but the bulk of the content presented is from the perspective of a *Voudouysan* – a Vodou practitioner and specifically that of an *Asogwe* or high priest.

awareness (*konesans*) as they navigate through the known, unknown, and unknowable spaces of life.

Vodou is a system of beliefs many West and Central Africans developed to create a place of orientation through ritual, song, dance, entering states of grace or trance, and knowledge of the natural world that bridges communities of the living with the community or inhabitants of *Ginen* (the ancestral homeland, the realm of the ancestors). Vodou also aids in tying the lives of Africans from the Motherland to the Americas. However, in much of the Americas, some African-based traditions have taken on the appearance of or have been integrated with certain branches of Christianity. In Haiti in particular, sacred rites are integrated with Roman Catholicism for a variety of reasons (e.g., the humanity of the Africans was not recognized unless they converted to Christianity). Furthermore, Vodou has created allegiances with and incorporated the spiritual elements of indigenous Arawak, Caribe, and other peoples into its tradition, along with components of European paganism and Free Masonry. Thus, Haitian Vodou and much of the religions of the Afro-Atlantic are the products of many traditions.

Vodou is neither ancestor-worship nor is it animism in the conventional sense, but a discipline that seeks the ecological relationship between humanity and *Bondje* (God). It teaches one to seek balance and harmony between the forces dynamic and inert as they are aligned with the four moments of the sun (its placements at sunrise, noon, sunset, and night) and its movements in the universe (i.e., two solstices and two equinoxes). Similarly, the phases of human development: birth, adolescence, maturity, and death echo the same phenomena. As individuals move through life following their own natural rituals, they must recognize their own growth and energy are tied into the cosmos and are a part of its rhythms. This helps determine the most propitious time to act and to heal.

Thus, Vodou asks its adherents to honor and respect life in the world as they find it as well as to honor and respect those kinship lineages and ancestral forces that came before them. This knowledge of personal history ensures two things: (1) one's predecessors never die as long as their names are recognized and cited, but instead have simply made a transition into another realm like the moon ascending from the horizon, and (2) an understanding that people's current lives are the accumulation and the summation of the many lives that came before them.

Furthermore, the religions of the Afro-Atlantic are neither monotheist nor polytheist per se. The divine presents itself to the mortal world by way of more accessible beings that may have direct relations to the supplicant (e.g., in ancestors). The divine may also be understood as a guardian or guide, analogous to that of a saint or prophet in other world religions. The latter are also deemed forces of nature, the most enlightened spiritual entities. Among Vodou practitioners, these spiritual beings are known as *lwa* (in the language of Fon) and *orisa* (in the language of Yoruba).

The *lwa* and the *orisa* are not unlike humans. The relationship one has with a spirit is both contractual and reciprocal. Devotees of the Religion understand that in order to secure a favor of a spirit, they must not only pray for it, but be prepared to offer something in exchange for what is received. Thus, the world exists on a scale of pluses and minuses (i.e., in order to maintain balance in the world, individuals must give back something if they are taking something). Each spirit also has its own likes and dislikes, and requires certain things (e.g., various foods or libations) to maintain and mark their presence in the world such as foods or libation.

Aligned in a highly evolved, deeply codified world with specific colors, libations, mathematical principles, musical rhythms, dances, and so forth, with which they are individually associated, the spirits are readily known by their devotees. The names of these spirits, though, may vary with geographic location, linguistic, and demographic settlements of Africans on the continent and the Diaspora.[419] Furthermore, some spirit beings have acquired greater importance with the trauma and aftermath of the Middle Passage (the triangular route that Europeans and white Americans created among three key regions – African, American, and the Caribbean – to exchange enslaved African lives and labor for goods and raw materials). Other spirits and deities have fallen into states of obscurity, although yet they generally remain recognizable among initiates cross-culturally.

In Vodou and its sister religions, God – the Good God – (*Bondje, Olumudare, Yahwe*, among her/his many names) is evident in such daily acts as the rising of the sun and as mysterious as in the lives of creatures resident in the cracks and crevices of trees. The seen, the unseen, and the actions of humans sharing the world are manifestations of *Bondje* in action. God has many faces; his or her divine presence resides in all creatures. This concept is the basis for the Haitian salutation, *"onor e respé"* (i.e., honor and respect). To honor and respect manifestations of life; humanity; one's health and well being; the environment; death and the *lwa*. Furthermore, God is not an abstract entity. *Bondje*, prevails literally in the movements of one's life through the presence of spiritual intermediaries manifest as *lwa* or *orisa*. *Bondje* is not only omnipresent but also omnipotent. Because of this, humans should be careful to not lightly invoke God. To dare to conjure God is less about one's humility as much as it speaks to the navigation and protocol within a complex structure of Vodou and other Afro-Atlantic religions.

For example, Vodou devotees speak first to their ancestors when help for some situation is needed; common sense is used when exercising recommendations made through their interventions. With the guidance of *Manbo* and *Hougan Asogwe* (female and male priest reflectively) offerings are made to *orisa* and to the *lwa*. After going through the work of offerings and prayer without resolution of the situation, God is approached. This not unlike the process people apply in their secular lives when confronted with a problem at work, for example. A person working in the mailroom does not go directly to the CEO with his or her concerns, but rather to mailroom manager. The problem may well find itself ultimately in the CEO's office to be solved, but not without working its way through the organizational management structure. Therefore, why would mortal beings even consider speaking directly to *Bondje* ("The CEO of CEOs") first, instead of working within the prescribed religious structure, beginning with applying life lessons from one's ancestors?

Outside of Africa, Haiti, and other places where Vodou is not commonplace, it is

---

419 The various places to which Africans and their descendants have been forced to flee involuntarily is known as the African Diaspora.

often misunderstood and subject to abuse. For example, important sacred and social constructs, such as the existence of zombies, have been misrepresented and the word is used in a derogatory manner. In reality, the term "zombie" means the "breath of God"; a zombie is a spirit that purportedly revives a dead person. Another example of abuse and misunderstanding of Vodou relates to what are commonly called "voodoo dolls." These items are depicted as cloth figures with pins or other sharp objects protruding though them to bring about harm to some unsuspecting soul. Such dolls are never used in this manner in Haiti or by Haitian people anywhere. On the contrary, dolls are filled with healing medicines, often tied to trees to whisper their respective owners' prayers to the wind, the sun, moon, earth, and sea. Unfortunately, misunderstandings such as these have resulted in mistrust among those who think of Vodou as superstition, witchcraft, and Devil worship and other culturally insensitive terms. Dishonoring Vodou and its 30 million plus adherents has created political and social ruptures among not only whites and blacks, Westerners and non-Westerners, but also within the African-descendant community itself. This is unfortunate and contrary to the belief system of Vodou which is based in unity and healing.

Basic Teachings

- Vodou's key tenets espouse egalitarianism, liberty, democracy, gender equality, unity, collective action, and self-sufficiency as practitioners honor and respect those who came before them, those who share this realm of existence with them and do their best to recognize the sacred Earth that nurtures them.

- All Vodou priests and many servers of the *lwa* as well as other members of the *orisa* family are essentially amateur botanists, as knowledge of leaves, barks, roots, and herbs is needed to create medicine.
- Divination is an important aspect of *orisa*-based cultures.
- Maintaining balance and order are central tenets of Haitian Vodou.
- Energy is neither created nor destroyed; initiates must, therefore, be mindful of the impact in the world of all they do regardless of scale or level of importance of such actions.
- Community plays a formidable role in shaping the character of an individual. Community also plays an important role in healing by providing a needed support mechanism.

Basic Practices

- Vodou and other *orisa*-based religions encourage lifelong spiritual development through: learning the various stories associated with the *lwa* and *orisa*; studying divination; making regular offerings based on annual readings. (Readings are sessions presided over by senior priests or diviners to determine the specific spiritual, personal, or communal goals that must be met by the collective.)
- Vodou ceremonies (*dans*) are held in temples called *hounfours*. The *hounfours* are sacred spaces. They are architecturally divided into the *peristyle*, the public space of where the *sosyete* (congregation) gathers, and the chambers of the *lwa* known as the *djevo* (a private, enclosed space where healing rites, both spiritual and physical occur). Baths, teas, the application of plants or oils to wounds or areas of stress and pain (some of which could

later be self-administered) tend to happen in the *djevo*. A distinctive physical characteristic of every *hounfour* is the *poto mitan* (a center pole that is both a line of separation and an umbilical between the terrestrial and celestial worlds). It is the means by which Spirit transfers itself from the heavens into ritual space of its servants – humanity.

- Ceremonies begin in the evening when opening prayers are recited. Drums mark the start of all ceremonies as priests salute Spirit, each other and the congregation. Generally, all the major *lwa* are greeted individually with a series of songs, specific drum rhythms, their particular salutations, and preferred libations in specified order.

- The Vodou calendar is lunar based. Thus ordinarily there would be no particular day of the week for scheduled worship. However, given the demands of contemporary, urban life, Saturday as a matter of convenience is often the night selected for hosting ceremonies. In other Afro-Atlantic communities, Sunday afternoon is preferred. Every day, though, is considered sacred and ceremonies may be performed on any given day.

- The *Manbo* or *Hougan* is a healer of the physical, mental, emotional, and spiritual self. Furthermore, priests in this community are not unlike spiritual leaders in other faith communities who play the role of mediator, educator, and sometime arbiter in communal affairs.

- To become a priest, one must be called by Spirit in a dream or, on occasion, in ceremonial circumstances. Several years of training in prayer, song, herbal medicines, divinations, dance, drumming, and other sacred arts are required. A rite of passage demanding isolation of the individual from all persons except other priests and the wearing of white clothing (symbolizing neutrality and rebirth) is de rigueur. The length of this symbolic rebirth varies with each specific tradition; generally speaking, however, it is 1 year.

Principles for Clinical Care
Dietary Issues

- The religions themselves vary in their approach to diets. Individuals should be consulted for any food taboos and their duration.

- In Vodou, the first 40 days of initiation into priesthood in particular have a number of dietary restrictions. Certain foods, which cannot be disclosed, are forbidden from being consumed during that time. None of the food restrictions, though, would have any adverse effects in medical situations.

- In *Lukumi* and other traditions such as *Candomble* or *Arara*, individuals have eating restrictions often lasting throughout the lifespan. These dietary restrictions vary with each individual and are determined during divination. Highly idiosyncratic, dietary restrictions vary with the spiritual guardian guiding their lives.

General Medical Beliefs

- Vodou is a tradition of healing.

- All servants of the *lwa* are taught to honor and respect human life and the earth they inhabit.

- The Earth, the retainer of all secrets, will be called on by Vodou practitioners to fortify the body and mind especially, in times of crises.

- In Vodou, the human body is a vessel, and the *lwa*, medicine for the spirit. Trance and possession mark entry of Spirit beings. This state of grace can be manifest in appearance as convulsions, incoherence, apoplexy, or aphasia.

- Homeopathic remedies are the choice for many Vodou practitioners and other Afro-Atlantic religious practitioners.
- Health care providers should take care to learn what, if any, natural medicines are being administered by *Dokte fwe* "Leaf Doctors" (botanists or healers with profound knowledge of botany) or *Hougan* and *Manbo* (formally initiated male and female priests respectively) or *bwisol* (priests whose spiritual powers are recognized but not formally initiated).
- If health care providers are not openminded toward Vodou patients' beliefs, this could very well put them at risk physically, spiritually, and psychologically as important revelations will not be made which could impact diagnosis and treatment.
- Health care providers may encounter resistance from Vodou practitioners, not to the use of pharmaceutical medications per se, but to their administration because of a potential lack of trust for the non-Vodou health care personnel as the history of medical abuse against African descendants is well documented.

Specific Medical Issues

- **Abortion**: Abortions are not prohibited. Midwives or specially trained initiates are permitted to oversee abortions and attend to extraordinary births (e.g., those involving defects or more than one baby).
- **Advance Directives**: These should be discussed with the patience and family.
- **Birth**: Umbilical cords and placenta should be offered to family after a child is born.

- **Blood Transfusions**: Often a source of discomfort because of blood-borne diseases, this should be discussed with the patient and family.
- **Circumcision**: Circumcision is very common after birth, although the family should be consulted.
- **In Vitro Fertilization**: This is an issue that the African-descendant community of immigrants has not addressed. Families and individuals should be consulted individually concerning their preferences.
- **Stem Cell Research**: This is an issue that the African-descendant community of immigrants has not addressed. Families and individuals should be consulted individually concerning their preferences if this is a viable and economically feasible option.
- **Vaccinations**: Attitudes are generally open and receptive to vaccinations. However, the purpose, effect, and longevity of the vaccination should be clearly explained.
- **Withholding/Withdrawing Life Support**: This is an issue that the African-descendant community of immigrants has not addressed as a whole. Families and individuals should be consulted individually concerning their preferences.

Gender and Personal Issues

- Vodou is a community-based culture in which matters that benefit the collective entity hold more weight than individual needs and concerns; all efforts are made to support every member of the community as much as possible.
- Men and women are considered equal in the Vodou society. Men do not have more authority than women. However, within the household away from the *hounfour* men often assume the role of decision

making. The *Hougan* or *Manbo*, however, have final say of the domains under their influence.

- The eldest child in the family has the right to state, and even override, the decisions of siblings concerning treatment of parents in medical emergencies.

Principles for Spiritual Care through the Cycles of Life

Concepts of Living and Dying for Spiritual Support

- Honor and respect the land and the life it brings forth, for the earth is sacred.
- Honor and respect all those who cross your path.
- Life is sacred, as is death.
- Do not fail to fulfill your own destiny or abuse the ability you have for shaping the destiny of another human being.
- Dying is not a fearful transition for the *lwa* are with devotees during their most vulnerable periods: entering life and egressing toward death.
- Before entering the world of the living, individuals have already negotiated a contract for existence with *Bondje*. They willfully decide what role they expect to play in life and determine a set of objectives to realize it. Should old age not meet us as planned, illness or accidents intercede on the path, people must live out the remainder of their lives knowing that they have done all that they could and can do to honor the arrangements previously made.
- If people are fortunate and have not only received but have given and shared love, furthered goodness, enabled acts of healing and justice, then they can be assured that they will be remembered and positive actions emulated. Behaviours that bring chaos and disequilibrium in the world

will not go unnoticed and will impact someone in their circle at some point in time.

- When possible, music should be played to aid the healing and transition processes.

During Birth

- When children are born, the umbilical cord of that child is buried under a tree. This may be conducted with or without the assistance of a Vodou priest. Trees are metaphorical umbilical cords between heaven and earth. Thus the child symbolically remains connected to the heavens as they are rooted to live on earth.
- Children born with their placentas intact are considered hosting a gift for divination or clairvoyance.
- Children born with peppercorn hair are not permitted to have their locks shorn until they themselves request it as these children are considered the children of specific spirits.
- The matriarch and patriarch of the family must be permitted to see the newborn child, no matter what the circumstances of the child or mother.
- Health care professionals might enable families to recite songs and/or prayer after fetal demise or death of a baby.
- The Vodou community shows support to family during birth with visits, preparing homemade meals, and by providing medicinal plants for cleaning the birth canal.
- Divination rites, and naming ceremonies maybe conducted by priests as part of birthing ceremonies.

During Illness

- If an individual believes that illness is the result of the ill will of another, then a priest should be consulted.

- If a mental health disorder is suspected, the health care worker should come to a mutual agreement for allowing the priest and patient to conduct work together providing no one's life is at risk. Together, the *Manbo* or *Hougan* and health care provider should agree to simultaneously consult with a social worker or social service agency and, if necessary, with a psychologist. A distinction should be made between spiritual disease and mental disorder.

- A sense of community especially among elderly and first generation immigrant practioners is critical to bringing about the emotional and mental state of being that facilitates healing.

- If there are health care workers familiar with the culture, country, or language of a patient, he or she should be encouraged to visit or speak with the patient even if they are not themselves health care professionals such as a cleric, orderly, or janitor.

- Allowances for medicinal herbs, plants, or other organic material in the patient's room or bedside should be made.

During End of Life

- The creation of small altars on a window sill, small table or shelf with photos, a candle, flowers, fragrance, or other meaningful elements should be allowed for those toward the end of life.

- The option of hospice care at home should be offered to a family; among the older generation of Vodou practitioners, dying at home or a place like home is associated with having led a good life.

- Upon making the transition below the sacred waters of *Ginen*, the mythic homeland and the realm of the ancestors, certain organic materials from the deceased must be collected such as hair and nail clippings. When collected, they are kept in special urns or jars. These matters are not the concern of the health care professional, but the community of priests and senior initiates. Members of the spiritual community must be given access to the deceased in a secure, private space.

- Hands of the grieving should be washed immediately following the funeral before anything or anyone else comes in physical contact with the deceased member's family, for purification, but also to clarify the separate worlds of the living from the dead. Water is a symbolic mirror and barrier between the world above and that below.

- The soul, the *Gwo Bon-zanj*, is believed to make final passage to the afterlife ten days after the body's consciousness (the *Ti Bonzanj*) has expired with the body. Ideally, autopsies and burials should be completed by then.

- Within 3 months of dying, some personal effects must be burned to further release the transitioned soul from the material or mortal world.

- One year and 1 day, but no later than 1 year and 3 months after transition, a "*rele mo' umba dlo*" (a ritual calling the dead from below the waters) must be conducted by a *Manbo Asogwe* or *Hougan Asogwe*.

- Health care providers should not make any judgments or offer opinion on the course of one's life or reason for illness or death other than scientific or medical reasons.

- The community, including priests and other initiates who in effect are family, should be allowed and encouraged to visit those terminally ill and otherwise.

Care of the Body

- Family members might want to view the body in the hospital. The deceased must look as natural or normal as he or she did in life, without tubes, taping, and so forth.
- Generally, one is buried at the base of the family home or on family land when in the countryside because the foundation of one's well-being is family and community. Cemeteries are used for the internment of the dead in cities and abroad.
- Cremation, while unusual, is currently being considered as an option in the community at large. Although how that process impacts one's *Asé* must still be addressed by the elders and priest of the communities.
- All efforts to minimize damage to the body of the deceased should be taken.
- The purpose of an autopsy should be clearly explained to the bereaved family.
- Requesting donation of the body for medical research would be an offense and is not recommended unless there are truly extraordinary circumstances (e.g., death due to an extremely rare disease).

Organ and Tissue Donation

- Throughout the Afro-Atlantic, the vital organs of animals used in sacrificial rites are separated from other parts of the offering and treated carefully. Known as *Asé*, the manifestation of life, what to do with them among humans within the context of organ donation has not been discussed within the *orisa*-based community. This area requires further research and discussion, particularly among a community of African descendants who suffer from severe shortages of kidney, heart, and liver donations.
- To donate would be an individual decision.

Scriptures, Inspirational Readings, and Prayers

- Vodou and the Afro-Atlantic traditions are not text-based religions but, rather, those of action (i.e., song and dance), and they remain largely oral traditions. With recent scholarship among the *Lukumi* and *Santeria* community for instance, certain prayers are documented. In Vodou, prayers are often only partially documented. Vodou's prayers and songs are memorized and would never be fully disclosed to those outside the tradition. A devotee would be familiar with its songs and prayers. As Vodou has synthetic properties, it is not unusual for its adherents to cite any number of prayers found in the Roman Catholic faith. A French text or Bible would be acceptable as well as tapes, DVDs, and CDs of recorded devotional music and Vodou prayers, songs or chants.

Special Days: Voudou

The Vodou calendar is based on an agrarian and lunar cycle. While there are small rituals performed every day, special days for the *lwa* (spirits) are acknowledged throughout the year with Vodou ceremonies occurring in Haiti and her Diaspora. In the larger *orisa* community, the calendar dates vary for their spirits, even as they overlap with the community of Vodouysan or Vodou practitioners.

January 1 *Ayisyen or Haitian Independence Day* – This is also *Jou de lwa* (the Day of All *Lwa*) on which special prayers and ceremonies are held. All the *lwa* are praised and their special role in Haiti's independence is celebrated.

March 16 *Danballah Wedo* – The great pythons, the most senior of the *lwa* are celebrated on this day. He (Damballah) and his mate, *AyidaWedo*, hold the universe together with love and wisdom. Coincident with the coming of spring, they are forces of objectivity and coolness of being. This day signifies the joining of the male and female principle in people's lives.

May 1 The *lwa* Kouzen Zaka and Azaka (male and female, respectively) are honored throughout the month celebrating the season of life. As the *lwas* of agriculture, they tie to community to the land and its labor and are associated with prosperity and wealth. It is a time for giving thanks for and enjoying the bounties of hard work and well being. It is also a time for meditation and long term planning.

July 7 *Ogun* – The force of justice, lightening, and thunder is honored on this day. His path can be both one of virtuous order or utter destruction. Ogun forges the infrastructure that guides people's lives. He paves the paths individuals take, and on his day, people are to be clear, just and unfailing in the decisions they make. Ogun teaches about honor and respect. He speaks to the failure and virtue of strength, diplomacy and good governance. This is a time for critical self-examination.

September 8 *Erzuli Danto* – The mother of the Haitian Revolution and model for female strength and resilience is honored on this day. Both men and women are reminded that the women in our families are the sentinels, seed sowers and gatherers of the community. They are the nurturers, educators, providers, and stabilizing force of society. Women, especially mothers, are the strongest warriors as they will do anything to protect their children and families. This is a time to reflect and give thanks to these pillars of communities and commend women as transmitters of knowledge and a source of security. It is also a time for harvesting the fruits of their labors.

November 1 *Gédè* – All Souls Day or *Remembrance of Ancestors* – As the movement of the sun marks another seasonal change (the end of the cycle of life into the cycle of death, and regrowth) the *Gédè* are associated with those who predeceased us. Those persons who gave their lives, love, protection, and experiences to enable our existence and guide the transactions we make in life daily are joyfully recognized. Because of the lessons acquired and the infinite innovation and creativity the ancestors symbolize, death and the dead are not seen as something morbid and frightening but merely another place of residence. So long as names of are ancestors are remembered they never cease to exist.

Zoroastrianism

Happiness comes to him who brings happiness to all others.

Prepared by:
Maneck N. Bhujwala
Cofounder, Zoroastrian Association of California
Los Angeles, CA
Zoroastrian Association of Northern California
San Jose, CA

Reviewed and approved by:
James R. Russell, PhD
Mashtots Professor of Armenian Studies
Department of Near Eastern Languages and
 Civilizations, Harvard University
Cambridge, MA;
Khojeste P. Mistree
Zoroastrian Scholar and Cofounder, Center for
 Zoroastrian Studies
Mumbai, India

History and Facts

"Zoroastrianism is the oldest of the revealed world-religions, and it has probably had more influence on mankind, directly and indirectly, than any other single faith."[420] The Prophet Zarathushtra, who lived some time around 1500–1000 BCE[421] in ancient Iran, founded a monotheistic religion based on a revelation he received when he was in his early thirties. (Greek philosophers who studied his teachings pronounced his name as Zoroaster.) The religion became well known during the Persian Empire founded by Cyrus the Great of the Achaemenian Dynasty in 539 BCE and was the religion of the majority for over a thousand years. According to western scholars such as Mary Boyce of England, Zoroaster's teachings have influenced later religions including Judaism, Christianity, and Islam.

Zoroaster was the first to teach the doctrines of an individual judgment, heaven and hell, the future resurrection of the body, the general last judgment, and life everlasting for the reunited soul and body. These doctrines were to become familiar articles of faith to much of mankind, through borrowings by Judaism, Christianity and Islam; yet it is in Zoroastrianism itself that they have their fullest logical coherence.[422]

The religion suffered a setback when Alexander the Macedonian (commonly known as Alexander the Great) conquered

---

420 Boyce, M. (1979). *Zoroastrians: Their Religious Beliefs and Practices.* London: Routledge & Kegan Paul, 1.

421 The dates of Zarathushtra's life are uncertain; other sources place the dates for his life as much as 1000 years earlier (2500 BCE); the dates in the text were provided by Professor Russell who, along with Khojeste Mistry, reviewed and approved the content of this chapter.

422 Boyce. *Zoroastrians: Their Religious Beliefs and Practices,* 29.

Persia in 330 BCE, killed many of its priests, destroyed temples, and is alleged to have burned written scriptures stored in the palace complex at Persepolis. Alexander's generals ruled Persia for 80 years before they were overthrown by the Parthian Arsacid Dynasty who reestablished the religion of Zarathushtra and ruled for about 476 years. The Parthian dynasty was followed by the Sassanian dynasty which made the Zarathushti (Zoroastrian) religion the state religion and ruled for over 400 years through 641 CE. After the Arab conquest of the Persian Empire, the religion was replaced by the newly founded Islam, and Zoroastrians were persecuted and driven to remote mountainous and desert areas.

One group of Zoroastrians sought asylum from religious persecution in India, where they were allowed to practice their religion freely. *Parsis*, as Zoroastrians are known in India, prospered through hard work and honesty, both under the local rulers as well as under the British colonial rulers. In consultation with their coreligionists in Iran, they preserved their religious customs and rituals, built temples and established charities. Iranian Zoroastrians, who stayed back in the remote desert and mountainous regions of Iran, suffered massacres and persecutions from various Muslim invaders. In the nineteenth century, the Zoroastrians in Iran were under severe persecution and the Parsis of India sent emissaries to the Iranian rulers to provide relief for their community members; they sent money to build schools and repair destroyed temples.

Not unlike other faith traditions, Zoroastrianism has its own religious texts. *Avesta*, probably meaning "fundamental utterance," is the name given to the sacred scriptures of the Zoroastrians; at its core are the *Gathas* ("Hymns") which form the core of Prophet Spitaman Zarathushtra's divine revelation. Besides the *Gathas*, there are other prayers and commentaries composed by the prophet's followers, based on Zarathushtra's teachings. The text of the most ancient Zoroastrian scriptures is an ancient Iranian language, *Avestan*, akin to the Sanskrit of the Indian Vedas. The manuscripts of the *Avesta* also contain the *Zand*, or interpretive translation, in a more recent form of Iranian called Middle Persian or *Pahlavi*.

The total number of Zoroastrians worldwide is about 130 000 at most, of which about 65 000 live in India and Pakistan; over 15 000 live in North America, about 27 000 in Iran, and the rest scattered elsewhere in the world.

Basic Teachings

The Zoroastrian religion adheres to the principle of *Asha* (righteous living) which is to be achieved by good thoughts, good words, and good deeds. "He serves truth, during his rule, with good word and good action" (*Yasna* 31.22). A large part of the Zoroastrian sacred texts are formed by the 72 chapters of *Yasna*[423] which include 17 chapters of the *Gathas* of Zarathushtra and other texts in the *Avestan* language. The *Yasna* prayer forms the ritual core of the higher inner liturgical ceremonies performed daily by priests in a Fire Temple.

The basic teachings of Zarathushtra are derived from five sacred songs (*Gathas*) composed by him and preserved by his early followers who memorized them and

---

[423] For full text of *Yasna* in English, consult the following website: www.ishwar.com/zoroastrianism/holy_zend_avesta/yasna/ (accessed 23 September 2012).

conveyed them as part of the oral tradition. The following are the main teachings:

- **One God**: There is one God, Ahura Mazda, who creates and maintains the universe through wisdom and a cosmic law of righteousness called *Asha*.

- **Good and Evil**: Twin spirits, opposite in nature, are in an ongoing cosmic struggle that will end as it is promised with the total victory of good at the end of time: the Good Spirit, Spenta Mainya, of Ahura Mazda and its evil opponent, Angra Mainyu, the "Hostile or Evil Spirit." In this respect, Zoroastrianism differs fundamentally and irreconcilably from other great monotheistic traditions by having within it a dualistic doctrine. Christians, Jews,[424] and Muslims assert God is both good and omnipotent and the phenomenon of evil must therefore be a mystery. Zoroastrians, though, believe Ahura Mazda is all good but not all powerful; for if He were, then evil would not have the power it does. Zoroastrians look forward to a victory that good creatures will share with their Creator when the forces of evil have been vanquished and all death and disease, anger and suffering, wickedness and lying, darkness and cold will be no more. For Zoroastrians, evil exists only because the "great war" has not yet been won.

- **Duality**: Zoroastrianism is sometimes understood as a dualistic faith.[425] The

truth is that Zoroastrians do not worship two gods; they only worship the one God, Ahura Mazda. However, prophet Zarathushtra recognized the contrasting, opposing forces in the relative world, implying the concept of ethical duality.

- **God is a Friend and Partner of Man**: Man is a partner of God in the struggle against evil in order to bring about perfection and the defeat of all evil at the end of time. God is a friend who helps men and women. "Take notice of it, Lord, offering the support which a friend should grant to a friend" (*Yasna* 46.2).

- **Equality of Sexes**: Men and women are equal in God's eyes. "May the much desired brotherhood come hither for rejoicing for the men and for the maidens of Zarathushtra, for the fulfillment of the Good Mind" (*Yasna* 54.1).

- **Man has a Free Will**: Men and women are given free will within the physical domain to choose their actions. They are advised to learn and understand the

---

424 Rabbi Harold Kushner, in his best-selling book *When Bad Things Happen to Good People*, suggested that bad things happen because God was not omnipotent. How prevalent that view is in Judaism is unknown.

425 Russell, J. (2008). In a personal response to me on April 3, 2008, after reviewing this chapter, Professor James Russell, a Zoroastrianism scholar from Harvard University, wrote the following.

The misunderstanding of Zoroastrianism as

a religion of dualism does not come from the interpretations of Western scholars, but the Zoroastrian texts themselves (in *Pahlavi*, *dobunishtagih*). What this means is that there are not two Gods, since the evil principle is not a god and neither deserves nor receives worship, but that there are two independent and primordial forces, one good and one bad. Evil is not the absence of good – St. Augustine's *"privatio boni"* – in the Zoroastrian view, but an active and malign force of negation. Since there is manifestly evil in the world, it means the two forces are in conflict, and human beings take a particularly active role in the struggle, endowed as we are with mind and conscience. A consequence of this view is that Zoroastrians cannot placidly regard suffering as an operation of fate, for instance; or death, as a natural event in harmony with God's will. God, being wholly good, may act in mysterious ways at times, but never perverse ones. Instead, these are casualties of war, to be borne with fortitude but never accepted or welcomed; and one hopes and works for a time when infirmity, old age, and death, will be no more.

prophet's teachings before determining what is right and wrong, and making the right choices in their daily lives. "... whereby a person with volition, expresses his preferences" (*Yasna* 31.11).

- **Law of Consequences**: According to the law of *Asha*, choosing the right action will result in good consequences and choosing the wrong action will result in bad consequences. It helps mankind to learn from mistakes in progressing on the right path. "The evil forces who intend to destroy life by means of wicked deeds and power and whom for doing this their own souls and their own consciences are hardened. They will go to Chinvat bridge but their dwelling is forever in the abode of the House of Druj" (i.e., hell) (*Yasna* 46.11).

- **Ethical Choices**: Zarathushtra exhorts his followers to be truthful, industrious, helpful, charitable, kind to all living creations, contented, progressive, peacemakers, moderate in consumption.

Basic Practices

- Life is considered as sacred, and all Zoroastrian practices are intended to promote and celebrate life – materially, psychologically, and spiritually. All elements in nature are considered sacred, so they are symbolically included in rituals, and all basic practices reflect the importance of preserving purity of the elements. Faithful performance and attendance at rituals are considered an important aid to leading a religious life and obtaining a spiritual experience.

- Most Zoroastrians usually worship at home by reciting daily prayers in the presence of a fire in a holder with burning embers, an oil lamp, or some

other source of light; light is symbolic of Ahura Mazda's presence. On special days however, Zoroastrians "charge their spiritual batteries" by visiting a fire temple (an *agiary* or *Atash Behram*) where a consecrated sacred fire is kept burning constantly day and night and is never allowed to be extinguished. An *agiary* is a "fire temple" in which the sacred fire is created by amalgamating four fires taken from the hearth fires of four different professions. The *Atash Behram*, or Fire of Victory, is a fire consecrated by amalgamating sixteen different fires by a group of priests; it has special sanctity as it is a sacred fire of the highest degree.

- Community gatherings, called *Jashans*, take place on certain days like New Year's day, birthdays on the day of initiation and other special days, and/or when a pair or more priests chant the *Avesta* praising Ahura Mazda, His appointed "coworkers," the *Amesha Spentas* (the seven Bounteous Immortals) and the *Yazatas* (the spirits being worthy of worship). The *Jashan* is essentially a thanksgiving ceremony to thank Ahura Mazda for the Creation of the world. These prayers invoke the blessings of Ahura Mazda on the community and also serve as a remembrance ceremony for the souls of the deceased. At these *Jashans*, a fire urn is always present to represent the energy by which Ahura Mazda created the universe. Fruits, flowers, milk, wine, sweet (*halwa*), and dry fruits are kept in metal containers to represent all of Ahura Mazda's principal creations on earth.

- Social ceremonies including those for the occasions of birth, marriage, and death, several types of purification ceremonies, initiation ceremonies for all children, and rituals undergone by those entering the Towers of Silence, rituals for priestly initiation, consecration ceremonies for temples, disposal structures and items used in religious rituals, and liturgical ceremonies, comprise the spectrum of Zoroastrian ceremonies.[426]

○ The initiation ceremony for a child is a religious ritual called the *Navjote* or *Sudreh Pooshi*. During the ceremony, a Zoroastrian priest makes the child ritually wear a white cotton undershirt, which signifies the goodness of the mind and physical and mental purity, and a cord made of lamb's wool which is wound three times around the waist and tied with two knots. The knot in the front represents "deeds of life" performed for Ahura Mazda by the wearer and the knot at the back of the waist represents truth and righteous living. The sacred cord is woven with 72 threads, representing the 72 chapters of the *Yasna*. Prayers are recited during the initiation ceremony when the child is invested with the sacred cord and under shirt in the presence of an audience who bear witness to the initiation.

○ Marriages are solemnized in the presence of a congregation. The ceremony is conducted by two priests reciting prayers and asking certain questions of the Zoroastrian couple and their parents: to ascertain the Zoroastrian Iranian lineage of the bride and groom and asking them to confirm their allegience to Ahura Mazda and the seven *Amesha Spentas*. Both parties are also asked to give their consent to the marriage.

○ Death in Zoroastrianism is not seen as being God ordained. It marks the transition of the soul from the physical to the spiritual existence and ultimately to salvation. As such, excessive mourning is not encouraged; instead relations are urged to recite appropriate prayers to speed the soul's journey to its goal. The body, which starts to decay from the moment of death, is usually disposed of the same day or as quickly as possible in order not to contaminate other living beings. Two priests recite certain portions of the *Avesta* while standing before the corpse and also every month for a minimum period of a year after the body has been disposed. The preferred mode of disposal is in a *dokhma*, a circular structure open to the sky, where birds of prey and the sun's rays eventually dispose of the body. This ensures minimum pollution of the earth and its environment.

• Directed to enjoy life fully but without excesses, Zoroastrians celebrate festival days like New Year's Day, Zarathushtra's birthday, six seasonal festivals called *Gahambars*, birthdays of the fires and waters, and other traditional Persian days with visits to the Fire Temple, good food, new clothes, visiting the theater to see *Parsi/Gujarati* plays, music programs, and other forms of entertainment.

• Traditionally, the Zoroastrian priesthood is hereditary. It is a full-time profession with all the proper priestly customs and practices passed down from father to son as part of the oral tradition, with little distortion. From a very young age, the child is exposed to priestly tradition, and the recitation of prayer by memory comes naturally to him being constantly exposed to the sound of prayer at home. At the

---

426 For a full discussion of religious rituals and customs see www.avesta.org/ritual/rcc.htm for *The Religious Ceremonies and Customs of the Parsees* by Jivanji Jamshedji Modi, PhD.

age of 6, he is put through a religious school or seminary, where he undergoes further training in chanting prayers and also receives general education. At the age of about 10 or 11, he is ordained a *Navar* (first grade). He is expected to recite the whole of the *Yasna* from memory during the *Navar* ceremony which lasts 24 or 30 days within the confines of a Fire Temple. Later, he undergoes the *Martab* ceremony (final grade), lasting 10 days, where he reads the *Vendidad* text beginning at midnight of the last day until sunrise next morning. *Vendidad* or *Videvdat* is an ecclesiastical text that pronounces "the Law against the Demons." It is a prescriptive text dealing with a range of behavior expected from a practicing Zoroastrian and includes, in detail, various purity injunctions. Now, as a fully fledged priest, he assists other senior priests in their duties, while at the same time continuing his religious and secular training until he is ready to perform all the rituals independent of supervision.

- Zoroastrians do not proselytize because of the belief that converting people of other religions implies religious superiority, which is incompatible with the Zoroastrian belief and its innate for respect for other religions.

Principles for Clinical Care
Dietary Issues

- Generally, Zoroastrians do not have rigid restrictions about diet. However, those from the Indian subcontinent traditionally do not eat beef, while those from Iran do not eat pork but do eat other meats.
- Some animals are regarded as noxious in the sacred texts. For example, some Zoroastrians will avoid honey because

it comes from a bee, which is a stinging insect.
- Other animals, such as otters, dogs, and birds (e.g., roosters and eagles), are considered sacred and cannot be killed for any reason.
- There are no kosher requirements.
- Some Zoroastrians may be vegetarians by choice.

General Medical Beliefs

- Whereas the general tendency of Greek medicine was to regard illness as an imbalance of internal humors, the Iranians felt illness arose mainly from external assaults upon the body and soul, which they characterized as demonic. This latter notion approaches the present-day idea of infection. Thus, in Zoroastrianism, it is believed that disorder, disease, and pain are the direct results of the evil spirit which seeks to destroy all that is good in the world. Zoroastrians believe prayers have the power of defeating evil. So, from ancient times, prayers have been used to heal sickness.
- Healing is not understood simply as curing sickness, but also as restoring order and harmony in the world. Healing with the recitation of prayers is mentioned as one of the four types of healing in Zoroastrian scriptures and is considered the best:

> amongst all remedies this one is the healing, one that deals with the Holy Word; this one is that which will best drive away sickness from the body of the faithful; for this one is the best healing of all cures. (*Ardibehesht Yasht* 3.6)

- Zoroastrians generally believe in the positive effects of prayers to aid the healing process. Besides reciting some prayers themselves, ill patients may also ask relatives and friends to pray on their behalf.

- Zoroastrians use *nirangs* (short passages of *Avestan* with invocations and evocations in *Pahlavi*) as holy incantations to cure illness and ward of all sorts of evil.
- Zoroastrians will also hire a priest to recite a hymn, the *Ardibehesht Yasht* (Hymn to the Best Righteousness), which is believed to possess special efficacy in healing.
- Illness is not considered as punishment, but as an affliction of the Evil One.
- Zoroastrian scripture classifies physicians in the following manner:
  - *Asho Baeshazo* (sanitary physician) – one who prevents dissemination of contagious diseases.
  - *Dato Baeshazo* (law physician) – coroner or one who practices forensic medicine.
  - *Karato Baeshazo* (knife physician) – surgeon.
  - *Urvaro Baeshazo* (herbal physician) – one who treats patients with herbal medicines.
  - *Manthro Baeshazo* (holy word physician) – one who cures by use of "holy" words by providing spiritual strength to patients. This specialty occupies a prominent place in the medical community.

O God, do grant us a long life, so that we may achieve our best wishes and desires, the gift that no one but you can grant, that is a full life of service to humanity and actions for progress of the world.[427]

- Zoroastrians are supposed to think rationally, and therefore, they understand

the different causes of illness as discovered by science (physical, mental, genetic, etc.) and believe in following medical treatments prescribed by qualified physicians, psychiatrists, and so forth.

- Rational thinking in making medical treatment decisions is emphasized along with ethical guidelines in determining the right action on a case-by-case basis as long as it does not contravene religious precepts.
- There is no restriction against ingredients in medicine as long as the ingredients are not obtained by taking human life.

Specific Medical Issues

- **Abortion**: Abortion of a normal viable fetus is strictly prohibited as it goes against the general teaching of promoting life.
- **Advance Directives**: In general, the wishes of the person concerned are made known to close friends and relatives. In recent times, particularly in the West, people make living wills which lay down more specific instructions. Zoroastrianism lays great emphasis on the responsibility assumed by the living.
- **Birth Control**: Birth control was indirectly not approved in ancient Persian times, as it was considered important for a person to be married and to have children. However, in modern times, Zoroastrians do use birth control to plan their families. Zoroastrians are taught by their prophet Zarathushtra (Zoroaster) to listen to his teachings and then decide for themselves what is right and what is wrong, so Zoroastrians consider their circumstances (financial and other) to decide the wisdom of bringing a child into their family with the accompanying responsibility of bringing it up properly.
- **Blood Transfusions**: There are no specific

427 *Yasna* 43.2; physician's prayer.

restrictions regarding blood transfusions; it is an individual decision.

- **Circumcision**: Normally, Zoroastrians do not practice circumcision of newborn children.
- **In Vitro Fertilization**: There are no specific restrictions regarding in vitro fertilization; it is an individual decision.
- **Stem Cell Research**: There is no specific restriction or approval regarding stem cell research for therapeutic purposes; it is an individual decision.
- **Vaccinations**: In Zoroastrianism, any action that supports life and increases the well-being and good health of an individual is encouraged. Thus, vaccines are seen as life-enhancing actions and therefore religiously acceptable. More than 95% of Zoroastrians are vaccinated.
- **Withholding/Withdrawing Life Support**: Zoroastrianism actively advocates life-enhancing actions, and any action, including withdrawing life support, which brings one to a quicker death is seen as an action in favor of *Ahriman*, the evil spirit. However, the inevitability of death is a separate issue theologically and, therefore, withholding life support could fit within the modern context of medical futility. In all situations, though, pain relieving medicines are completely endorsed. These are very painful decisions and terminating life can be seen as a merciful act, but this is not so in Zoroastrianism. At the end, in matters such as this, the individual or family members make the decision, as it is they who have to endure the pain and suffering of a loved one.[428]

Note: Zoroastrianism is lax on many of these specific medical issues because there is no central focus of authority such as the pope in Christianity or the Dalai Lama in Buddhism; often decisions are made as a personal choice. However, High Priests do meet periodically and give official opinions on matters of interpretation of religious laws that carry weight in the community.

Gender and Personal Issues

- Personal and public hygiene is important for Zoroastrians as it is important for the prevention of disease and sickness.
- There are no restrictions about gender of caregivers, although most women would feel more comfortable with a female health care provider.

Principles for Spiritual Care through the Cycles of Life
Concepts of Living and Dying for Spiritual Support

- In Zoroastrianism, there is belief in five components of human beings: (1) *Tanu* or physical body; (2) *Ushtana* or Breath of Life; (3) *Urvan* or soul; (4) *Kehrpa*[429] or form or prototype image of the human body; and (5) *Fravashi* or God's guiding spirit and man's guardian spirit. When the physical body dies, the *Urvan* (personal

---

428 "I can only suggest to you what is accurate as per my reading and extrapolation of the texts which does not directly mention such eventualities." The quote here and information provided on withholding/

withdrawing life support was provided by Khojeste Mistree, a reviewer of this chapter.

429 When the *urvan* drops the physical body at death, the *Kehrpa* becomes the vehicle into which the *urvan* finds a resting place. The *kehrpa* is fashioned like the human body in shape and reproduces all the features of a human being .... After death the *urvan*, while making its abode in the *kehrpa* continues to bear the five senses and it bears an exact resemblance to the person of the deceased. By Nurgesh Irani, *A Mystical Explanation of Our Religion*, 46. Available at: http://tenets.zoroastrianism.com/tosee.pdf (accessed 23 September 2012).

soul) and *Fravashi* (guardian spirit) leave the body and continue to exist. The *fravashi* rejoins Ahura Mazda and the soul is under the protection of the spirit being (the *yazata*, *Sraosh*). The soul remains in the earthly realm after death for 3 days and nights. Prayers directed to *Sraosha* are recited by priests (*Sraosha* is the Lord of prayer as one of the celestial assessors who will meet the soul at judgment which takes place on the fourth morning after death). On the early morning of the fourth day after death, the soul is judged for its overall behavior on earth and then proceeds to a future existence depending on the aggregate of good thoughts, words, and deeds done during its lifetime.

- Zoroastrians believe that the soul is immortal and at the time of physical death, it continues to exist. The soul is the spiritual part of a human being. So, a person can take solace in the fact that he/she will continue to exist in the spiritual realm.

- At the end of time, all creation will be restored to a perfect state, so that even though the soul may have to undergo the bad consequences of its actions on earth, it will eventually improve from its experience and become perfectly good.

- The soul of man is judged after death, and the righteous will advance to a heavenly state; whereas those who chose the wrong path will face retribution and suffering in hell, known in Zoroastrianism as the House of Deceit. However, there is no concept of eternal damnation; learning from past mistakes and continuously increasing one's good thoughts, words, and deeds and actively seeking a righteous life is the only path to salvation. Eventually, all souls will progress toward perfection and the entire creation will be restored to a perfect state.

- The promise of a hereafter is an important belief in Zoroastrianism, as man learns to sow the seeds of righteousness in this world, in order to reap the benefits of eternal happiness and immortality in the next world. Thus, the dying person can feel assured that there is hope for a better existence.

During Birth

- According to tradition, when a child is born, a lamp is lighted and it is kept lit for 3 days in the room where the mother is resting. This is especially observed when birth occurs at home.

- The first drink for a child is a sip of sugar water for water represents purity and perfection and sugar for sweetness of life. Furthermore, mothers are supposed to breast-feed the child as long as possible.

- The first name of the child is usually that of an immediate deceased ancestor, one of the spiritual beings, famous Iranian ancestors, and so forth. In Western countries, anglicized versions of traditional names are given for ease of acceptance at schools.

- As stated earlier, Zoroastrians do not normally practice circumcision of newborn children.

- No rituals are generally performed in case of a miscarriage, except that the mother undergoes a purification ceremony once the bleeding ceases. In the case of a stillborn child, the same rituals that apply to adults are performed.

- For spiritual support of patients and families, contact the local Zoroastrian Association through a family member or friend. Usually, the community will come to the aid of the family.

During Illness

- Ideally, a Zoroastrian priest should recite prayers. However, any Zoroastrian who observes a truthful and moral life, knows the correct recitation of prayers, understands the prayers, and who practices physical and spiritual purity can be effective in healing sickness through prayers.
- Besides reciting prayers themselves, patients may also ask relatives and friends to pray on their behalf.
- If an individual is not available to recite prayers, the hospital should allow a cassette recording of prayers to be played.
- Hospitals should allow visitors to bring religious pictures, recite prayers, light an oil lamp, or at the very least have a candle lamp near the patient.
- Visitation of the sick and expressions of moral support are priorities.
- For spiritual support of patients and families, contact the local Zoroastrian Association through a family member or friend. Usually the community will come to the aid of the family.

During End of Life

- Prayers recited by a priest, relative, or friend for the dying person provide a soothing environment due to the vibrations of the *Avestan* chants.
- *See* "A Brief Synopsis of the Death Ritual" in "Scriptures, Inspirational Readings, and Prayers" at the end of this chapter.
- When a person dies in a hospital or at a residence, a member of the Zoroastrian clergy should be contacted to come to the hospital or to the mortuary to recite the *Geh Sarna* (*see* in "Scriptures, Inspirational Readings, and Prayers" at the end of this chapter). Prayers are recited before an oil lamp and a fire in a fire vase (if allowed by the facility) near

the body before it is placed in its final resting place. The *Geh Sarna* is essentially the first *Gatha* (*Ahunavaiti*) which forms part of the revelation of prophet Zarathushtra. It is intended to give courage to family and friends to bear the loss, and as a protection against the spread of evil forces.

- Normally, two priests perform their *Kusti* prayer and with a piece of white cotton cloth connecting them recite the *Geh Sarna* prayer. If only one priest is available, a member of the family can stand with the priest connected to the priest with a piece of cloth. If the deceased person is a pregnant woman in the fifth month of her pregnancy, two pairs of priests perform the *Geh Sarna* ceremony. The reason for having more than one person performing the last rites is to show strength against evil forces said to proliferate the place where the corpse is laid.
- If a priest is not available, any Zoroastrian who can recite the prayer may do so. The priest does not touch the body as it is considered impure.
- If no Zoroastrian is available locally, attempts should be made to call someone (preferably a priest) from out of the area. The North American Mobed (Priest) Council (NAMC) or the Federation of Zoroastrian Associations of North America (FEZANA) (www.fezana.org) can be contacted to help communicate this need. If all else fails, non-Zoroastrian priests have been known to recite prayers for the deceased from their own faith.
- Traditionally, a dog, with two white spots above its eyes, is brought to view the body before, during, and after the *Geh Sarna* ceremony. Various reasons for this ritual include the ability of a dog to determine if there is life in the body. The dog would avoid going close to the body if life was

extinct, but would look at it if life was present. Another reason is the pure nature of the dog is said to keep evil influences away from the body by virtue of its presence and watchful eyes.

Care of the Body

- *See* "A Brief Synopsis of the Death Ritual" in the "Scriptures, Inspirational Readings, and Prayers" section of this chapter.
- The body is treated with respect and when moved from the death bed, it is lifted by two or more persons.
- Prayers are recited continuously by priests, relatives, and friends with a lamp in the room where the body is resting before being moved to a mortuary or final resting place.
- A shroud is placed covering the entire body except the face; the hands are placed cross-wise on the chest, and the big toes are tied together with a strip of cloth to create unity.
- The head of the body should not point in the north direction, as traditionally in ancient Iran it was believed that all kinds of dangers and evils – climatic, physical, mental – came from that direction.
- Immediate relatives wash the body with water, dry it, and then dress it in clean white pajamas and the sacred undervest, including tying the sacred thread (*Kusti*) around the waist while reciting only the *Hormazdae Khodae* prayer.
- All persons, except those involved in cleaning the body and moving the body, are expected to keep a distance from the body, with the purpose of avoiding contact with the evil forces said to afflict the dead body.
- As Zoroastrians are not allowed to pollute the earth, water, or air, the ideal disposal of the body in major cities in India and Pakistan is placement of the body on the floor of an open air circular tower known as the Tower of Silence. The vultures and other birds of prey from nearby trees consume the flesh, and the bones are destroyed over a period of time by the sun's rays. Where the Tower of Silence is not available, the body preferably is to be buried in a concrete or stone coffin. Some Zoroastrians prefer to be cremated with electric heat (for traditional Zoroastrians, fire is a sacred symbol, and only fragrant objects are normally offered to it; thus, using fire for cremation is an irreligious act because a dead body is seen as being polluted).
- There is no specific rule against donation of the body for research, with the exception of one minority group of Zoroastrians (*Ilme Khshnoom*).[430]
- Autopsies and embalming are generally avoided unless required by law.

Organ and Tissue Donation

- There is no specific rule against donation of the organs and/or tissues for research or transplantation. In fact, when bodies are laid to rest in the Towers of Silence, it is considered as a charitable act to donate the bodies for sustenance of the birds of prey.
- A minority group of Zoroastrians following the *Ilme Khshnoom* interpretation of the religion do not allow donation of organs or tissues.

---

430 *Ilme Khshnoom* or *Ilm-e Khshnam*, "Teaching of Joy/Knowledge," is a twentieth-century theosophical offshoot of Zoroastrianism with some relationship to ancient mystical interpretations of Zoroastrianism elaborated in contact with Hindu and Muslim esotericism during the reign of the Mughal emperor Akbar (1556–1605 CE) in India.

Scriptures, Inspirational Readings, and Prayers

- Simple prayers from the *Khordeh Avesta* prayer book as well as the *Geh Sarna* prayers can be recited by any Zoroastrian, although preferably a priest would be involved as he is trained to perform the ceremonies in the proper fashion.
- The prayers recited near the body are the *Kusti* prayers, *Ashem Vohu* prayer and *Geh Sarna* prayer. The text of other prayers can be obtained by accessing the Avesta website (www.avesta.org).

PRAYERS DURING ILLNESS

Prayer for Good Health and Healing

The prayer Airyamana is the greatest of the Holy incantations, the best, fairest most powerful of the Holy spells firm and victorious and healing and the most healing of the Holy spells for the Airyamana (prayer) smites all the legions of the "evil one" for him who worships Truth and righteousness.

—Ardibehesht yasht V.5

Prayer for Removing Disease

O Hom thou art comfort giving the giver of victory for fighting against malice and to bring about healing. O Hom it would be better if thy means of removing diseases spread with brilliance thy healing remedies be used as a means of removing diseases which occur for anyone who praises Hom along with these hymns of the Gathas becomes victorious.

—Hom Yasht V.21

Prayer for Healing

May the Creator the Keeper of the world who is omniscient and nourisher of all, the doer of meritorious deeds … May the Evil one be destroyed may the evil one be far away may the evil one be vanquished and defiled. For the foremost religion is the pure religion of Zarathustr. Ahura Mazda the Exalted, Powerful, Good, Increaser of Good in the world.

—Ardibehesht Yasht Nirang

PRAYERS DURING ILLNESS OR END OF LIFE

Ahunwar

As Ahura Mazda is the chosen lord, so also is He the judge, according to the law of truth. To Him belong the gifts of the Good Mind, of the way of actions of life. To Ahura Mazda is dominion, which He has established for stewardship of the poor in spirit (i.e. the faithful).[431]

Kemna Mazda[432]

Whom hast Thou appointed as guardian for me, O Wise Lord, if the deceitful one shall dare harm me? Whom other that Thy fire and Thy mind through whose actions one has nourished the truth. O Lord? Proclaim that wondrous state to me

---

431 *Ahunwar* or *Ahuna Vairya* is the holiest and most central prayer in Zoroastrianism. Translation into English was provided by Professor James Russell of Harvard University.

432 Mistree, K. (1982). *Zoroastrianism: An Ethnic Perspective.* Mumbai, India: Zoroastrian Studies, 89.

for the sake of the religion. Who shall smash the obstacle (of deceit) in order to protect in accord with thy teachings those pure ones who exist in my house? As a world healer, promise us a judge, and let obedience to him come through the good mind (and) to him whosoever Thou dost wish him to be, O Wise One. Defend us from our foes, O Wise One and O Bounteous Devotion. Begone demonic falsehood, begone the offsprings of the demons, begone the doings and miscreations of the demons, begone O liars; I drive them away northwards in order that they may not do the corporeal world of righteousness any harm. Homage unto Devotion (Ārmāiti).

In the Kēm nā Mazdā prayer we are told that when we are in trouble we should turn to Ahura Mazda for help and guidance.

Ahuramazda Khodae[433]

O Lord Ahura Mazda! May Ahriman be suppressed, removed, held stricken and crushed. May the demons, liars, witches, anti-Zoroastrian rulers, the evil priests, tyrants, evil doers, men of violence, the followers of the Lie and those who cherish the evil mind, be broken. O Ahura Mazda! I repent for all my sins and for all the evil thoughts, words, and deeds which have been thought of by me, and which have proceeded from me; for these sins of thought, word and deed, of body and of soul, and of the corporeal and spiritual worlds, truly do I repent for myself with these three sayings: Glory be unto Ahura

Mazda, May the Hostile Spirit be vanquished, for the most powerful is the will of the truth-doers. I praise the Truth.

Jasa me avanghe Mazda![434]

Come to my aid, O Mazda! Come to my aid, O Mazda! Come to my aid, O Mazda! I am a worshipper of Mazda – I am a Zoroastrian worshipper of Mazda I agree to praise the Zoroastrian religion and to believe in that religion. I praise good thoughts, I praise good words, I praise good deeds, I praise the good Mazda worshipping religion which curtails disputes and quarrels, and which brings about next-of-kin marriages which are righteous; and which of all the religions that have flourished and are likely to flourish, is the greatest, the best, the most excellent, and which is the religion given by Ahura Mazda to Zarathushtra. To Ahura Mazda, I ascribe all good.

This is the profession of the Mazda worshipping religion.

PRAYERS DURING END OF LIFE

Ashem Vohu

Ashem vohu vahishtem asti,
Ushta asti; ushta ahmai
Hyat Ashai vahishtai Ashem
"Truth (is) good, it is the best
It is happiness, happiness (is) unto it the truth,
In accordance for the best truth (itself)."
"Lasting happiness comes to the person who recognizes

---

and affirms the highest truth, for it own."

Kusti Prayer

(I offer this prayer) in the name of the one, worthy of reverence and in the name of the one, who is All-pervasive and in the 1001 names of the one, who is Almighty. (I offer this prayer) in a spirit of good thoughts and good words and good deeds, involving my earthly body and my soul, in earthly and in spiritual experience. In so doing (with these words) I repent, sincerely, for whatever sins I would have committed. (I pray) I will desist from the sins of wicked words and deeds and inclinations and directions, which I hold in enough scorn to repent, sincerely (with these words), for whatever sins I would have committed. Get thee behind me, Aheriman; get thee away from me, Aheriman; get lost, Aheriman. May thy many wicked ways, Ghanamino (i.e. Aheriman) be stricken hard and defeated, restricting thee to the inferno of hell. May it, then, come to pass that thy ultimate annihilation be instituted by Ahura Mazda, in the company of the victorious 33 Yazatas and the Amesha Spentas. May, too, the shining glory of Ahura Mazda keep him forever victorious.[435]

Geh Sarna

In humble adoration, with hands uplifted first of all I pray at this (moment) rejoicing all righteous deeds of the invisible (and) bountiful Ahura Mazda (and) the wisdom of the Good Mind so that I may please the soul of the universe. O Omniscient Lord! I would reach near Thee through the Good Mind. Do Thou grant me benefits of both the worlds, of this the corporeal and (the other) the spiritual, (which may accrue) through truth, joy-giving and happiness.

O Ahura Mazda, Asha (Truth) and Vohu Manah (good mind)! Unto you I shall weave my hymns of praise as never before by whose grace (or from whom) (are obtained) bountiful perfect mentality and the perpetual wealth (i.e., happiness of Heaven) For my rejoicing may you come towards (my) acts of worship!

Being aware of the blessings of deeds of Ahura Mazda (i.e., being aware of the most excellent advantages accrued by performing the deeds approvable to Ahura Mazda) shall I lead my soul to Garothman Heaven through the agency of the Good Mind! As long as I have strength and power, so long will I teach (others) (to abide) by the desire of Truth.

A BRIEF SYNOPSIS OF THE DEATH RITUAL[436,437]

The information provided is based upon the traditions and practices found in Mumbai, India.

---

435 www.avesta.org/ritual/nk_qadimi.htm (accessed 23 September 2012).

436 This section was provided by Khojeste Mistree, a Zoroastrian scholar and reviewer of this chapter.
437 See the following website for a more detailed description: www.avesta.org/ritual/funeral.htm (accessed 23 September 2012). Some of the material

Pre-Death

According to the tradition, a dying person should recite the *Patet* prayer (a prayer of repentance for the mind, body, and soul for the sins which may have been committed) together with as many *Ashem Vohus* (short formularies used regularly often in conjunction with other prayers) as possible; a member of the family may recite some prayers in the ears of the dying person if the patient is unable. (Note: Sins can't be cleansed in Zoroastrianism. Sins can be repented for or overwhelmed by the individual performing greater number of good thoughts, words, and deeds.)

Haoma juice (*Haoma* is the Avestan name for the ephedra plant the sap of which when pounded while reciting a formula of prayers is believed to have divine qualities) may be given to the person in order that the soul may gain strength and immortality, as it is about to embark upon its journey into the spiritual hereafter. An oil lamp (*divo*) should be kept burning close to the head of the person as it is believed that a short while before death, the soul is timid and nervous as it is about to move into a new environment.

Post-Death

Immediately upon death, a prayer vigil should be maintained as the soul is deemed to be frightened and anxious, having been exposed suddenly to another state.

The Sachkar – The Final Ritual Bath

The *sachkar* (ritual bath ceremony which binds and isolates the corpse demons) is done either by a member of the household, or by professional helpers at the *bangli* (a

___

in this section was derived from this article on Parsi rituals.

place where the last rites are performed). Traditionally, the corpse is rubbed with *gaomez* (unconsecrated bull's urine) and washed with lukewarm water.

The body is dressed in clean, old white clothes and the *kusti* (girdle) is tied around the waist of the corpse in the usual manner, with the complete recitation of the *Kusti* prayers. Before the *sachkar*, both the Zoroastrians as well as non-Zoroastrians are allowed to pay their last respects to the dead. But after the *sachkar* has been performed, non-Zoroastrians are not permitted to see the body, traditionally. After the *sachkar* ceremony, the corpse fiends (*nasu*) begin to increase in number in spite of them being ritually contained.

The Sagdid – "Seen By The Dog"

Upon the change of each *gah* (the Zoroastrian day is divided into five watches or time periods called *gahs*; sunrise to 12:40, 12:40 to 3:40, 3:40 to sunset, sunset to midnight, and midnight to sunrise), a *sagdid* (translated literally as "the seeing of the dog") is done, during which a special dog is brought to cast his eyes upon the corpse. The dog is believed to have four eyes (*Vendidad*, 8:16), and its gaze is meant to ward off the evil *nasus*, who, it is said, are frightened away. (*Shayest- la- Shayest*, 2:1).

These dogs are said to have an instinctive ability to detect any form of life, which the body may have.

The Funeral Ceremony (Geh Sarnu)

The funeral ceremony is called the *Geh sarnu* (chanting of the *Gathas*, hymns composed by the Prophet). The *nasisalars* (corpse bearers dressed in white, wearing white caps, gloves, and socks), having done their *padyab-kusti* (ablution and formula for tying the *kusti*) beforehand, enter the room in pairs and in *paiwand* (ritual connection by holding a piece of cloth or cotton tape by two people to show that they are joined). Then having prayed their *Baj of Srosh* (*Srosh* is the spirit being who protects the soul in the afterlife; the *Baj of Srosh* is recited to protect the soul) up to the words "*astavait-ish ashahe*," they intone formula of prayers in accordance with the tradition.

Then, two priests enter in *paiwand*, having done their *padyab-kusti* and having recited various prayers. They stand some distance from the body near the door. At this time, they pray the first part of the *Baj of Srosh*, after which they begin to recite the *Ahunavaiti Gatha* (*Yasna* chapters 28–34) – namely, the words of the prophet himself.

Upon the recitation of the words "yehya vereda vanaema drujim …" "through whose strength we might conquer the Lie …." (*Yasna* 31.4), the priests pause for a short while and turn their faces away (the laity also do the same). During this period, another *sagdid* is done, after which the corpse is transferred to the iron bier by the *nasisalars*. (The priests and laity turn their faces away, for it is believed that there should be no eye contact between the priests/laity and the corpse while it is being transferred from the floor to the iron bier. It is believed that the movement of the body causes a spiritual disturbance enabling the corpse fiends to afflict and harm the living, if they happen to look at the corpse at that time.) The *nasi-salars* either clap or cough to indicate when it is safe to face the corpse, and the priests continue with the recitation of the funeral prayers.

Upon the completion of the chanting of the first *Gatha* by the priests, the *Baj of Srosh* is thereafter concluded, and this brings to an end the main funeral service.

The Sezdo

After the funeral ceremony, the *sezdo* (the paying of respect) takes place. Zoroastrian males, and then the ladies, all pay their homage to the deceased by bowing gently and focusing their eyes around the head of the corpse.

The Final Journey

Upon the completion of the *sezdo*, the corpse-bearers cover the face of the deceased and the body is taken to the Tower of Silence, where the final *sagdid* is done. The mourners pay their very last respects, before the face is once again covered. The body is then carried by the corpse-bearers into the *dakhma* where the body is left for the vultures to devour.

After the Funeral

When a Zoroastrian returns from a funeral, it is mandatory to have a bath in order to remove any ritual contamination of the *nasus* and perform the *kusti* ritual, as the performance of this ritual gives the worshipper a special spiritual protection. It is said that he who wears the *kusti* is "Wise and reminded of the Creator …. thereby the power of the demons is more shattered, the way to sin becomes more obstructed, and the will of the demons greatly lessened" (Dd., Ch. 39, v. 20, 'Persian Rivayat', p. 24).

A *divo* (lamp) should be kept burning for 3 days in the room or house of the deceased.

No meat should be eaten by the family members for the first 3 days, as the *nasus* are said to pollute uncooked meat during that period. On the fourth morning after death, it is obligatory to eat meat when *dhansak* (a Parsi dish) is served.

Grief should be kept to a minimum, as tears for the dead are a hindrance to the progress and well-being of the soul. The *yazata Sraosha* is propitiated continuously for the next 4 days, as he is the protector of the soul of man as well being the Lord of Prayer.

Reason Non-Zoroastrians are Not Allowed to Participate in the Funeral Ceremony

The Zoroastrian point of view about death is quite different from all the other major religions of the world. Death, in Zoroastrianism, is the work of evil and not the doings of Ahura Mazda. Therefore, special precautions, by way of ritual protection, are to be followed, as best as possible, in order to ensure the containment of the corpse fiends.

It is only through the wearing of the *sudreh* (sacred shirt) and the performance of the *kusti* ritual, before and after the actual funeral service, that the living, it is believed, are afforded spiritual protection and are safeguarded from being attacked by the *nasus*. If the sacred shirt (*sudreh*) and girdle (*kusti*) are not worn, then it is not advisable for one to be exposed to the naked aggression of the corpse fiends. It is for this reason that a pregnant Zoroastrian woman is not allowed to participate in the funeral ceremony, as the child in the womb of that woman is ritually unprotected. Similarly, no pre-*navjoted* child (*navjote* is the initiation ceremony of confirmation of a Zoroastrian child into the religion of his birth) is permitted to attend a funeral service, lest the corpse fiends, in some way, afflict the child.

Because non-Zoroastrians cannot wear the *sudreh* and *kusti*, it is for their own spiritual safety and ritual protection that they are forbidden from participating in the funeral service actively, in terms of seeing the face of the corpse.

Special Days: Zoroastrianism

The Zoroastrians have three religious calendars: Fasli (seasonal), Kadmi (old), and Shenshai (royal). The Fasli calendar follows the seasonal timing of the northern hemisphere and is adjusted to account for the leap year. The other two calendars became different from Fasli mainly because the Parsis (Zoroastrians who migrated to India from Iran) forgot to adjust the calendar in India (by adding a month every 120 years), and the Kadmi calendar is 1 month ahead of Shenshai. All three calendars have 30-day months, with 5 extra days, with names of the five Gathas, at year end. The names of the days and months are those of God, Amesha Spentas, and Yazatas. The special days provided in this list are Parsi festivals as per the *Parsi Shenshai* calendar, which is followed by most Parsis all over the world. Most Zoroastrians in Iran (and recent migrants from Iran) follow the Fasli calendar. The English calendar dates are for the year 2010 and will change every leap year.

February 10–14 (month, *Shahrivar*; day, *Ashtad-Aneran*) *Gahambar Paitishahya* (early autumn, bringing in the corn)*

March 12–16 (month, *Mehr*; day, *Ashtad-Aneran*) *Gahambar Ayathrima* (mid-autumn, bringing in the herds)*

March 21 *Jamshedi NoRuz (Irani New Year)* – This festival is celebrated with the advent of spring. According to the tradition, the festival is believed to have been founded by the prophet Zarathushtra himself, whom, it is held, received his first revelation on this day. This day is also associated with the mythical King Jamshed whose golden rule, it is said, lasted for over 600 years. Legend has it that on this day King Jamshed forced the demons to carry him on their shoulders from Mount Demavand to Babylon. It is only in the late nineteenth century that the Parsis of India named this day *"Jamshedi"* NoRuz.

March 26 (day, *Avan*; month, *Avan*) *Avan Ruz nu Parab (Birthday of the Waters)* – This day is celebrated as the birthday of the waters, when Zoroastrians go to the waters and offer thanks to the great nourisher and purifier of the world. Special food and prayers are also offered to the water divinity on this day.

April 24 (day, *Adar*; month, *Adar*) *Adar Ruz nu Parab (Birthday of the Fire)* – This day is celebrated as the birthday of the fire, when Zoroastrians thank the fire for the warmth and light given by it throughout the year. Traditionally on this day, food is not cooked in the house, as the fire is given a rest. Special prayers (including a litany to the fire, the "Atash Niyayesh") are recited in honor of the house fire or before a burning oil lamp (*divo*).

May 11 *Jashn-e Sadeh (Festival of Fire)* – This feast is celebrated in midwinter, 100 days before the advent of spring. It is from this point of time that the day becomes longer than the night, in order that greater light and warmth may permeate the world. The *Jashan* is performed in the fourth watch of the Zoroastrian day after the sun sets. As the Parsi New Year now falls in August, the date of this festival has moved to the month of May, which is not a winter month in the northern hemisphere.

May 26 (day, *Khorshed*; month, *Dae*) *Zarthosht no Diso (Death of Zarathushtra)* – This is the day on which the death anniversary of the prophet falls, symbolically. Special prayers are recited and Zoroastrians traditionally go to the Fire Temple, as a mark of respect and remembrance of their prophet.

May 31–June 4 (month, *Dae*; day, *Mehr-Bahram*) *Gahambar Maidhyairya* (midwinter)*

August 9–18 (month, *Asfandarmad*; day, *Ashtad-Aneran*) *Gahambar Hamaspathmaedya (Fravardegan) (10-day festival of All Souls)** – It is believed that during this 10-day festival the spirits of the dead visit their near and dear ones in the physical world. The priests perform special rituals over cooked food, fruits, and fresh flowers, when the spirits of the departed are invoked in order to seek their protection and blessings, in this world. In the last watch (from midnight to sunrise) of the last day of the year, a special ceremony in honour of the spirits is performed, by way of a gesture to bid the spirits a final farewell from this world.

August 19 (day, *Hormazd*; month, *Farvardin*) *Parsi New Year* – This is the most important day of the year for the Parsi community and is recognized to be the seventh crowning festival, which immediately follows the sixth *Gahambar, Hamaspathmaedya NoRuz* (New Day) is associated with the seventh creation Fire, and is linked to the Bounteous Immortal – the Best Truth. The seventh festival, bridges the old year to the New Year. The resurgence of life takes place during this period with the symbolic victory of the forces of light over those of darkness. It is customary to exchange gifts, wear new clothes, settle disputes, and go to the Fire Temple in order to reaffirm this day to be one of renewal, hope, and joy.

August 24 (day, *Khordad*; month, *Farvardin*) *Khordad Sal (Birthday of Zarathushtra)* – On this day, the Prophet's birthday is celebrated, symbolically.

September 28–October 2 (month, *Ardibehesht*; day, *Khorshed-Daepmehr*) *Gahambar Maidyoizaremaya* (mid-spring)*

November 27–December 1 (month, *Tir*; day, *Mohor-Daepmehr*) *Gahambar Maidyoshema* (mid-summer)*

* There are six *gahambars* in the year that are celebrated in honor of the Sky, the Waters, Earth, Plants, Cattle, and Man. Traditionally, each of these *gahambars* lasted for 5 days and the festivities included much food, merriment, and complex rituals and prayers. For certain intercalation reasons, the sixth *gahambar* was extended to 10 days. The Parsi Zoroastrians popularly know this *gahambar* as *Muktad*, during which period the spirits and souls of the dead are invoked ritually for the living to mingle with the spirits and souls of the spiritual world.

Glossary of Zoroastrian Terms

For a complete glossary of terms for Zoroastrianism, please consult the Avesta website (www.avesta.org/zglos.html).

Concluding Words

"Leave me alone!" "Get out of here!" "You don't know how I feel!" "I really don't want to talk about that." These and similar statements are sometimes voiced by patients in a clinical setting. At the surface, such words seem to convey the message "I want to be alone" or "I am alone in this situation." On the other hand, they may be cries for help or companionship, pleas for someone to join them on the "dark journey" of illness and/or dying.[438]

Communications of this nature, then, could well be reflections of emotional, spiritual, and relational suffering. This type of suffering, though, often cannot be quantified in levels of severity via the ten-point pain scale, nor eradicated by medications. On the contrary, suffering of this nature may only be lessened by transcendental realities such as faith, hope, love, and meaningful relationships with the divine and people.

In situations where suffering exists, patients are looking for someone to be a "bearer of light" to illuminate the current path and the one that lies ahead. They may expect that light bearer to be a physician, nurse, social worker, chaplain, or some other health care provider who will listen to their words of fear, despair, and hopelessness, not only with the ears but also with the eyes, the touch, and the heart. In the listening event, these health care professionals who have been invited into the sacred space should give their undivided attention to the very end of each sentence spoken. The clinician should likewise use all of the senses to "hear" what is not being verbalized. This act of listening should leave patients with the sense that they have been heard and understood.

Listening in this fashion is especially important when there is ambiguity concerning the cause and treatment for some adverse physical and/or mental condition. In these scenarios, interaction with patients as human beings can be equally as important and satisfying as medical procedures to cure the malady.

Finally, patients expect and most often receive excellent physical care by physicians, nurses, and other health care professionals, and yet patient satisfaction scores in hospitals across the country are only mediocre. What is the reason for this? It could well be that patients are looking for an "experience." They want not only their physical problem addressed by competent professionals but also their other needs. They want to be treated as a "whole person" and feel good about and less fearful of their hospitalization. Patients do not want to be treated like patients; they want to be treated like people. When patients are treated in that manner, healing can take place even in the absence of cure.

This book was written to enable health care professionals to sharpen their skills in providing the emotional and spiritual support necessary to facilitate the

---

438 Jeffers, S. (2001). *Finding a Sacred Oasis in Illness.* Overland Park, KS: Leathers Publishing, 121.

"positive experience" that patients expect and deserve.

> To care is to be there physically, emotionally, and spiritually for patients who have entrusted you with the responsibility for their overall sense of well-being.

Sources Cited and Consulted

'Abdu'l-Bahá. (1918). *Divine Philosophy*. Compiled and published by Isabel Chamber Chamberlain. Boston, MA: Tudor Press. Available at: http://bahai-library.com/books/div.phil/ (accessed 23 September 2012).

'Abdu'l-Bahá. (1976, reprint). *Bahá'í World Faith: Selected Writings of Bahá'u'lláh and 'Abdu'l-Bahá*. Wilmette, IL: Bahá'í Publishing Trust.

'Abdu'l-Bahá. (1982). *The Promulgation of Universal Peace*. Wilmette, IL: Bahá'í Publishing Trust.

'Abdu'l-Bahá. (1982, reprint). *'Abdu'l-Bahá in London*. London: Bahá'í Publishing Trust (UK).

Adam, N. (1996). *Kitab Al-Salaat (The Book of Prayer)*. Riyadh: Cooperative Office for Call and Guidance; 2002.

Adams, P., M. Mylander, and S. Oedekerk. (1998). *Patch Adams*. Directed by T. Shadyac. Universal City, CA: Universal Studios.

Adapted from Adventist Health System's SHARE customer service program and *Communication with Compassion*, Adventures in Caring Foundation. Santa Barbara, CA: Win/Win Productions. Available at www.adventuresincaring.org/ (accessed 23 September 2012).

Adler, M. (1986). *Drawing Down the Moon*. New York, NY: Penguin Books.

African Methodist Episcopal Church Book of Worship. (1984). Nashville, TN: AME Sunday School Union.

Albom, M. (1997). *Tuesdays with Morrie*. New York, NY: Doubleday.

Alvord, L. and E. Cohen Van Pelt. (1999). *The Scalpel and the Silver Bear*. New York, NY: Bantam Books.

Amundsen, D. and G. Ferngren. (1995). History of medical ethics. In W. T. Reich, editor in chief. *Encyclopedia of Bioethics*, Vol. 3. New York, NY: Macmillan. p. 1443.

Anandarajah, G. and E. Hight. (2001). Spirituality and medical practice: using the HOPE questions as a practical tool for spiritual assessment. *American Family Physician*, 63(1), 81–88.

Association of Brethren Caregivers. (1998). *Deacon Manual for Caring Ministries*.

Aston, W. trans. (1956). *Nihongi*. London: George Allen & Unwin.

Bach, M. (1982). *The Unity Way*. Unity Village, MO: Unity Books.

Bahá'í Prayers: A Selection of Prayers Revealed by Bahá'u'lláh, The Báb, and 'Abdu'l-Bahá. (1991). Wilmette, IL: Bahá'í Publishing Trust.

Bahá'u'lláh. (1985, reprint). *The Hidden Words of Bahá'u'lláh*. Wilmette, IL: Bahá'í Publishing Trust.

Bahá'u'lláh. (1988). *Gleanings from the Writings of Bahá'u'lláh*. Translated by Shoghi Effendi. Wilmette, IL: Bahá'í Publishing Trust.

Bahá'u'lláh. (1988). *Tablets of Bahá'u'lláh Revealed after the Kitab-i-Aqdas*. Pocket-size ed. Wilmette, IL: Bahá'í Publishing Trust.

Bahá'u'lláh. (1991). *The Compilation of Compilations*. Vols 1 and 2. Ingleside, New South Wales: Bahá'í Publications Australia.

Belavich, T. and K. Pargament. (2002). The role of attachment in predicting spiritual coping with a loved one in surgery. *Journal of Adult Development*, 9(1), 13–29.

Bellah, R. (1970). Beyond Belief. New York, NY: Harper & Row.

Bender, H. *The Anabaptist Vision* [pamphlet, 44 pp]. Scottdale, PA: Herald Press.

Bible, K. ed. (1993). *Sing to the Lord* [hymnal]. Kansas City, MO: Lillenas Publishing.

Book of Discipline of the United Methodist Church, 2004. (2004). Nashville, TN: United Methodist Publishing House.

Book of Resolutions of the United Methodist Church, 2004. (2004). Nashville, TN: United Methodist Publishing House.

Book of Worship: United Church of Christ. (1986). New York, NY: United Church of Christ, Office for Church Life and Leadership.

Booth, B. (2008). More schools teaching spirituality in medicine. *American Medical News*, March 10. Available at: www.ama-assn.org/amednews/2008/03/10/prsc0310.htm (accessed 5 Sept 12).

Boyce, M. (1979). *Zoroastrians: Their Religious Beliefs and Practices.* London: Routledge & Kegan Paul.

Braden, C. (1950). *These Also Believe.* New York, NY: MacMillan.

Brady, M. J., A. H. Peterman, G. Fitchett, et al. (1999). A case for including spirituality in quality of life measurement in oncology. *Psychooncology*, 8(5), 417–428.

Buehrens, J. and F. Church. (1989). *Our Chosen Faith: An Introduction to Unitarian Universalism.* Boston, MA: Beacon Press.

Byock, I. (1997). *Dying Well: The Prospect for Growth at the End of Life.* New York, NY: Riverhead Books.

Cady, H. (2005). *Lessons in Truth: Centennial 1903-2003 Edition.* Unity Village, MO: Unity Books.

Cameron, D. (n.d.). Affirm Life! Online article on Unity School of Christianity website. Available at: http://content.unity.org/prayer/inspirationalArticles/affirmLife.html (accessed 16 Sept 2012).

Canda, Edward. *Kansas City Star*, September 16, 1995, F4.

Canda, E. (2002). Toward spiritually sensitive social work scholarship: insights from classical Confucianism. *Electronic Journal of Social Work*, 1(1), 23 pp.

Carver, R. (1989). What the doctor said. In R. Carver. *A New Path to the Waterfall.* New York, NY: Atlantic Monthly Press. p. 113.

Chapple, C. ed. (2002). *Jainism and Ecology: Nonviolence in the Web of Life.* Cambridge, MA: Center for the Study of World Religion, Harvard Divinity School.

Chen, J. (1990). *Confucius as a Teacher.* Petaling Jaya, Malaysia: Delta Publishing.

Chung, D. (2001). Confucianism. In M. Van Hook, B. Hugen, and M. Aguilar. eds. *Spirituality within Religious Traditions in Social Work Practice.* Pacific Grove, CA: Brooks/Cole. pp. 73–97.

Church of Scientology International staff. (1998). *What is Scientology?* Los Angeles, CA: Bridge Publications.

Cohen, N. Text printed on laminated cards. Reprinted with permission from Mr. Cohen. The text can also be found on the following website: http://naljorprisondharmaservice.org/pdf/FourNobleTruths.htm (accessed 15 Sept 2012).

Coleman, J. (2001). *The New Buddhism: The Western Transformation of an Ancient Tradition.* New York, NY: Oxford University Press.

Collier Complete Works of James Whitcomb Riley. (1916). Vol. 4. New York, NY: Harper and Brothers.

Colville, W. (1906). *Universal Spiritualism.* New York, NY: R. F. Fenno & Company.

Compilations. (1998). Evanston, IL: NSA USA-Developing Distinctive Bahá'í Communities Guidelines For Spiritual Assemblies Office of Assembly Development.

The Concise Oxford Dictionary, 10th edition, London: Oxford University Press; 2001.

Confession of Faith in a Mennonite Perspective. (1995). Scottdale, PA: Herald Press.

Daily Word for Wednesday, February 7, 2007

(Unity Village, MO: *Daily Word* magazine, February 2007), 24.

Darmesteter, J., Dhalla, B. N. Dhabhar, et al. trans. *Holy Zend Avesta – Yasna*. Available at: www.ishwar.com/zoroastrianism/holy_zend_avesta/yasna/ (accessed 23 September 2012).

Dawkins, R. (2006). *The God Delusion*. London: Bantam Press.

De Bary, W., D. Keene, G. Tanabe, et al., eds. (2001). *Sources of Japanese Tradition*. Vol. 1. 2nd ed. New York, NY: Columbia University Press.

Dhammapada. (1993). Boston, MA: Shambhala Publications.

Doctrine and Discipline of the African Methodist Episcopal Church 2004–2008 (2005). Nashville, TN: AMEC Publishing House.

Doege, L. (2000). By what authority? (sermon, First Unitarian Church, South Bend, IN, September 24, 2000).

Dossey, B. and L. Dossey. (1998). Attending to holistic care. *American Journal of Nursing*, 98(8), 35–38.

Droege, T. (1991). *The Faith Factor in Healing*. Philadelphia, PA: Trinity Press.

Dundas, P. (2002). *The Jains*. 2nd ed. London: Routledge.

Dyck, C. (1983). Anabaptism. *The Brethren Encyclopedia*. Philadelphia, PA: Brethren Press.

Earhart, H. (1974). *Religion in the Japanese Experience: Sources and Interpretations*. Encino, CA: Dickenson Publishing Company.

Easwaran, E. (1987). *The Upanishads*. Tomales, CA: Nilgiri Press.

Eddy, M. (1953). *Miscellaneous Writings, 1883–1896*. Boston, MA: Christian Science Publishing Society/Christian Science Board of Directors.

Eddy, M. (1971). *Science and Health with Key to the Scriptures*. Boston, MA: Christian Science Publishing Society/Christian Science Board of Directors.

Effendi, S. trans. (1983). *Gleanings from the Writings of Baha'u'llah*. Wilmette, IL: Bahá'í Publishing Trust.

Effendi, S. trans. (1987). *Prayers and Meditations by Bahá'u'lláh*. Wilmette, IL: Bahá'í Publishing Trust.

Ehman, J. W., B. B. Ott, T. H. Short, et al. (1999). Do patients want physicians to inquire about their spiritual or religious beliefs if they become gravely ill? *Archives of Internal Medicine*, 159(15), 1803–1806.

Faculty of Anderson University School of Theology. (1979). *We Believe: A Statement of Conviction on the Occasion of the Centennial of the Church of God Reformation Movement*. Anderson, IN: Anderson University School of Theology.

Fillmore, C. and C. D. Fillmore. (1941). *Teach Us to Pray*. Unity Village, MO: Unity Books.

Fillmore, M. (1954). *Myrtle Fillmore's Healing Letters*. Unity Village, MO: Unity Books.

Frankl, V. (1959). *Man's Search for Meaning*. New York, NY: Washington Square Press.

Freeman, J. (1987). *The Story of Unity*. Unity Village, MO: Unity Books.

Freer L, editor. *Jara Sutra – Samyuttanikaya Mahavagga*. PTS (the Pali Text Society's English version of the Tipitaka). Volume 5 Oxford: Pali Text Society: 1976.

Freer L, editor. *Tinakatta Sutta – Samyuttanikaya Mahavagga*. PTS (the Pali Text Society's English version of the Tipitaka). Volume 2 Oxford: Pali Text Society: 1976: 179.

Frothingham, R. (1865). *A Tribute to Thomas Starr King*. Boston, MA: Ticknor & Fields.

General Conference of Mennonite Brethren Churches. (2000). *Confession of Faith: Commentary and Pastoral Application*. Winnipeg, MB: Kindred Productions.

Gómez, L. O. trans. (1996). *The Land of Bliss: The Paradise of the Buddha of Measureless Light; Sanskrit and Chinese Versions of the Sukhāvatīvyūha Sutras*. Honolulu: University of Hawaii Press.

Gosho Translation Committee. trans. (1999). *The Writings of Nichiren Daishonin*. Vol. 1. Tokyo, Japan: Soka Gakkai.

Graber, D. and J. Johnson. (2001). Spirituality and healthcare organizations. *Journal of Healthcare Management*, 46(1), 39–50.

Groopman, J. (2004). God at the bedside. *New England Journal of Medicine*, 350(12), 1176–1178.

Gross, R. (1993). *Buddhism After Patriarchy*. Albany: State University of New York.

Guilbert, C. (Custodian of the *Standard Book of Common Prayer*). (1990). *The Book of Common Prayer*. New York, NY: Oxford University Press.

Gunnemann, L. (1977). *The Shaping of the United Church of Christ*. New York, NY: United Church Press.

Habito, R. (2005). *Experiencing Buddhism: Ways of Wisdom and Compassion*. Maryknoll, NY: Orbis Books.

Hall, E. (1959). *The Silent Language*. New York, NY: Doubleday.

Hall, E. (1969). *The Hidden Dimension: Man's Use of Space in Public and Private*. London: Bodley Head.

Harakas, S. (1990). *Health and Medicine in the Eastern Orthodox Tradition*. New York, NY: Crossroad.

Hardacre, H. (1986). *Kurozumikyō and the New Religions of Japan*. Princeton, NJ: Princeton University Press.

Harris, M. *Unitarian Universalist Origins: Our Historic Faith*. Boston, MA: Unitarian Universalist Association.

Hassinger, A. (2007). Eating ethically. *UU World*, 21(1), 28–34.

Healing Affirmations. Available at: http://content.unity.org/prayer/prayers Affirmations/healingPrayerAffirm.html (accessed 16 Sept 2012).

Heart Sutra, The. Buddha Dharma Education Association/BuddhaNet. Available at: www. buddhanet.net/e-learning/heartstr.htm (accessed 5 Sept 12).

Heisey, D. (2004). *Healing Body and Soul: The Life and Times of Dr. W. O. Baker*. Grantham, PA: Brethren in Christ Historical Society.

Hinton, D. trans. (1999). *Mencius*. Washington, DC: Counterpoint.

Hofstede, G. (1994). *Cultures and Organizations: Software of the Mind*. London: Harper Collins.

Holley, H. ed. (1923). *Bahá'í Scriptures: Selections from the Utterances of Bahá'u'lláh and 'Abdu'l-Bahá*. New York, NY: Brentano's Publishers.

Holyoake, G. (1896). *English Secularism*. Chicago, IL: Open Court Publishing Company.

Hopko, T. (1981). *The Orthodox Faith*. Vol. 1, *Doctrine*. New York, NY: Department of Religious Education, Orthodox Church in America.

Hostetter, N. (1997). *Anabaptist-Mennonites Nationwide USA*. Morgantown, PA: Masthof Press.

Hubbard, L. (1965). *The Golden Dawn*. East Grinstead, England: Church of Scientology.

Hubbard, L. (2007). *Scientology: A New Slant on Life*. Los Angeles, CA: Bridge Publications.

Huberman, J. (2007). *The Quotable Atheist*. New York, NY: Nation Books.

Hymnal: A Worship Book. (1992). Elgin, IL: Brethren Press.

Hymns for Praise and Worship. (1984). Nappanee, IN: Evangel Press.

Idler, E. L. and S. V. Kasl. (1997). Religion among disabled and nondisabled persons: I. Cross-sectional patterns in health practices, social activities, and well-being. *Journal of Gerontology: Social Sciences*, 52(6), S294–S305.

Ikeda, D., R. Simard, and G. Bourgeault. (2003). *On Being Human: Where Ethics, Medicine and Spirituality Converge*. Santa Monica, CA: Middleway Press.

Irani, N. *A Mystical Explanation of Our Religion*. Available at: http://tenets. zoroastrianism.com/tosee.pdf (accessed 23 September 2012).

Ironson, G., G. F. Solomon, E. G. Balbin, et al. (2002). The Ironson-Woods Spirituality/ Religiousness Index is associated with long survival, healthy behaviors, less stress, and low cortisol in people with HIV/AIDS.

Annals of Behavioral Medicine, 24(1), 34–48.

Jaini, J. (1916). *The Outlines of Jainism.* Cambridge: Cambridge University Press.

Jaini, P. (1979). *The Jaina Path of Purification.* Berkeley: University of California Press.

Jakobovits, I. (1975). *Jewish Medical Ethics: A Contemporary and Historical Study of the Religious Attitude to Medicine and Its Practice.* New York, NY: Block.

James Dillet Freeman, http://content. unity.org/prayer/prayersAffirmations/ iAmTherePoem.html (accessed 16 Sept 2012).

Jeffers, S. (2001). *Finding a Sacred Oasis in Illness.* Overland Park, KS: Leathers Publishing.

Jeffers, S. L., and D. Kenny. (2008). *Putting Patients First: Best Practices in Patient-Centered Care.* 2nd ed. San Francisco, CA: Jossey-Bass.

Jeffers, S., M. McKenna, and A. Schwartz. (2006). Physicians and clergy in concert. Unpublished manuscript.

Jones, R. M. (1922). *Spiritual Exercises in Daily Life.* New York: Macmillan, vii.

Jowett, B. (1924). Charmides. *The Dialogues of Plato.* Vol. 1. New York, NY: Oxford University Press.

Kalanya Sutra. PTS [Pali Text Society's English version of the *Tipitaka*]. Oxford: Pali Text Society.

Kennedy, L. (1999). *All in the Mind: A Farewell to God.* London: Hodder & Stoughton.

Ketchell, A., L. Pyles, and E. Canda. *World Religious Views of Health and Healing.* Spiritual Diversity and Social Work Resource Center. Available at: www.socwel. ku.edu/candagrant/papers/World.htm (accessed 23 September 2012).

Keum, J. (2000). *Confucianism and Korean Thoughts.* Seoul, Korea: Jimoondang Publishing.

Kirkwood, N. (1988). *A Hospital Handbook on Multiculturalism and Religion.* New York, NY: Morehouse Publishing.

Klitzman, R. (2008). *When Doctors Become Patients.* New York, NY: Oxford University Press.

Koenig, H. (1999). *The Healing Power of Faith.* New York, NY: Simon & Schuster.

Koenig, H. (2001). Religion and medicine IV: religion, physical health, and clinical implications. *International Journal of Psychiatry in Medicine*, 31(3), 321–336.

Koenig, H. (2001). Religion, spirituality, and medicine: how are they related and what does it mean? *Mayo Clinic Proceedings*, 76(12), 1189–1191.

Koenig, H. (2002). *Spirituality in Patient Care.* Philadelphia, PA: Templeton Foundation Press.

Koenig, H. G., H. J. Cohen, L. K. George, et al. (1997). Attendance at religious services, interleukin-6, and other biological parameters of immune function in older adults. *International Journal of Psychiatry in Medicine*, 27(3), 233–250.

Koenig, H., K. I. Pargament, J. Nielsen, et al. (1998). Religious coping and health status in medically ill hospitalized older adults. *Journal of Nervous and Mental Disease*, 186(9), 513–521.

Koenig, H., G. R. Parkerson Jr., and K. G. Meador. (1997). Religion index for psychiatric research. *American Journal of Psychiatry*, 154(6), 885–886.

Koenig, H. G., M. E. McCullough, and D. B. Larson. (2001). *Handbook of Religion and Health.* New York, NY: Oxford University Press.

Kotva, J. (2002). *The Anabaptist Tradition: Religious Beliefs and Healthcare Decisions.* Chicago, IL: Park Ridge Center for the Study of Health, Faith, and Ethics.

Kraybill, D. (1997). Anabaptist Habits. Lecture at Bethel College Mennonite Church, North Newton, KS, October 26, 1997.

Kraybill, D. and C. Hostetter. (1944). *Anabaptist World USA.* Scottdale, PA: Herald Press.

Kuhn, C. (1988). A spiritual inventory of the medically ill patient. *Psychiatric Medicine*, 6(2), 87–100.

Kumar, M. and M. Prakash. Anuvrat Anushasta Saint Tulsi: a glorious life with a purpose. *Anuvibha Reporter.* 2007; 3(1), 42, 71.

Larson, D. and S. Larson. (2003). Spirituality's potential relevance to physical and emotional health: a brief review of quantitative research. *Journal of Psychology and Theology*, 31(1), 37–51.

Legge, J. trans. (1960). *The Chinese Classics in Five Volumes.* Hong Kong: Hong Kong University Press.

Levin, J. S. (1994). Religion and health: is there an association, is it valid and is it causal? *Social Science Medicine*, 38(11), 1375–1382.

Li, D. trans. (1999). *The Analects of Confucius: A New-Millennium Translation.* Bethesda, MD: Premier Publishing.

Lo, B., T. Quill, and J. Talky. (1999). Discussing palliative care with patients. *Annals of Internal Medicine*, 130(9), 744–749.

Lock, M. (2005). Preserving moral order: response to biomedical technologies. In J. Robertson, ed. *A Companion to the Anthropology of Japan.* Malden, MA: Blackwell Press. pp. 483–500.

Lock, M. (1980). *East Asian Medicine in Urban Japan.* Berkeley: University of California Press.

Lukoff, D., F. Lu, and R. Turner. (1992). Toward a more culturally sensitive DSM-IV: pyschoreligious and psychospiritual problems. *Journal of Nervous and Mental Disease*, 180(11), 673–682.

Mansen, T. and S. Haak. (1996). Evaluation of health assessment skills using a computer videodisk interactive program. *Journal of Nursing Education*, 35(8), 382–383.

Mansfield, C., J. Mitchell, and D. E. King. (2002). The doctor as God's mechanic? Beliefs in the southeastern United States. *Social Science and Medicine*, 54(3), 399–409.

Matthews, D. (1998). *The Faith Factor.* New York, NY: Penguin Group.

Maugans, T. A. (1996). The SPIRITual history. *Archives of Family Medicine*, 5(1), 11–16.

Maugans, T. and W. Wadland. (1991). Religion and family medicine: a survey of physicians and patients. *Journal of Family Practice*, 32(2), 210–213.

McCaffrey, A. M., D. M. Eisenberg, A. T. Legedza, et al. (2004). Prayer for health concerns: results of a national survey on prevalence and patterns of use. *Archives of Internal Medicine*, 164(8), 858–862.

McCullough, M. E., W. T. Hoyt, D. B. Larson, et al. (2000). Religious involvement and mortality: a meta-analytic review. *Health Psychology*, 19(3), 211–222.

McSherry, E., S. Salisbury, M. Ciulla, et al. (1987). Spiritual resources in older hospitalized men. *Social Compass*, 34(4), 515–537.

Michiko, M. (2001). Japanese society and religion on the eve of the 21st century. *Nanzan Bulletin*, (21), 43–54. Translated by Robert Kisala.

Mirza, H. (1987). *Outlines of Parsi History.* Mumbai, India: Jak Printers/Amalgamated Industries.

Mistree, K. (1982). *Zoroastrianism: An Ethnic Perspective.* Mumbai, India: Zoroastrian Studies.

Mitroff, I. (1999). *A Spiritual Audit of Corporate America.* San Francisco, CA: Jossey-Bass.

Modi, J. J. (1922) *The Religious Ceremonies and Customs of the Parsees.* Mumbai, India: British India Press. Available at: www.avesta.org/ritual/rcc.htm (accessed 23 September 2012).

Morris, R, editor. *Anguttaranikaya Pancaka-Chankkanipata.* Volume III PTS (the Pali Text Society's English version of the Tipitaka). Oxford: Pali Text Society; 1994, 144.

Morris R, editor. *Thana Sutta. Anguttaranikaya Pancaka-Chankkanipata.* Volume III PTS (the Pali Text Society's English version of the Tipitaka). Oxford: Pali Text Society; 1994, 72.

Mosher, L. (2007). *Faith in the Neighborhood: Understanding America's Rligious Diversity.* Vol. 3, *Loss.* New York, NY: Seabury Books.

Mueller, P. S., D. J. Plevak, and T. A. Rummans. (2001). Religious involvement, spirituality, and medicine: implications for clinical practice. *Mayo Clinic Proceedings,* 76(12), 1225–1235.

National Center for Cultural Competence of Georgetown University. (n.d.). *Planner's Guide.* Washington, DC: Georgetown University Center for Child and Human Development. Available at: http://www11.georgetown.edu/research/gucchd/nccc/documents/Planners_Guide.pdf (accessed 15 Sept 2012).

National Spiritual Assembly of the Bahá'ís of the United States. (1998). *NSA USA – Developing Distinctive Bahá'í Communities: Guidelines for Spiritual Assemblies.* Evanston, IL: Office of Assembly Development.

Nelson, J. (1996). *A Year in the Life of a Shinto Shrine.* Seattle: University of Washington Press.

Newman, K. (1991). *Fashioning Femininity and English Renaissance Drama.* Chicago, IL: University of Chicago Press.

Ni, H. trans. (1979). *The Complete Works of Lao Tzu: Tao Teh Ching and Hua Hu Ching.* Los Angeles, CA: SevenStar Communications.

Ni, H. trans. (1979). *The Taoist Inner View of the Universe and the Immortal Realm.* Los Angeles, CA: SevenStar Communications.

Ni, H. (1984). *Workbook for Spiritual Development of All People.* Los Angeles, CA: SevenStar Communications, 163.

Ni, H. (1990). *Power of Natural Healing.* Los Angeles, CA: SevenStar Communications.

Ni, H. (1991). *The Key to Good Fortune.* Los Angeles, CA: SevenStar Communications.

Nicene Creed [currently used in the celebration of the Divine Liturgy]. (1967). In *The Divine Liturgy of St. John Chrysostom.* Syosset, NY: Russian Orthodox Greek Catholic Church of America.

Nickalls, J. ed. (1975). *The Journal of George Fox.* Philadelphia, PA: Philadelphia Meeting of the Religious Society of Friends.

Nikhilananda, S. (1992). *The Bhagavad Gita.* New York, NY: Ramkrishna-Vivekananda Center.

Ohkuni-Tierney, E. (1984). *Illness and Culture in Contemporary Japan.* Cambridge: University of Oxford Press.

Oman, M. ed. (1997). *Prayers for Healing: 365 Blessings, Poems, and Meditations from Around the World.* Berkley, CA: Conari Press.

Oman, D. and D. Reed. (1998). Religion and mortality among the community-dwelling elderly. *American Journal of Public Health,* 88(10), 1469–1475.

Pargament, K. God help me: spirituality as a resource in self-care. Care for the Caregiver Bioethics Conference, Loma Linda University, Loma Linda, CA. interview by Steven Jeffers, 2001.

Pargament, K., B. Cole, L. Vandecreek, et al. The vigil: religion and the search for control in the hospital waiting room. *Journal of Health Psychology,* 4(3), 327–341.

Pargament, K. I., H. G. Koenig, N. Tarakeshwar, et al. (2001). Religious struggle as a predictor of mortality among medically ill elderly patients: a 2-year longitudinal study. *Archives of Internal Medicine,* 161(15), 1881–1885.

Pattinson, S. (2002). *The Final Journey: Complete Hospice Care for Departing Vaisnavas.* Badger, CA: Torchlight Publishing.

Payutto, P. (2004). *The Pali Canon: What A Buddhist Must Know.* Bangkok, Thailand: Buddhadharma Foundation.

Philippi, D. trans. (1969). *Kojiki.* Princeton, NJ: Princeton University Press.

Philippi, D. trans. (1990). *Norito: A Translation of the Ancient Japanese Prayers.* Princeton, NJ: Princeton University Press.

Pirkei Avot 1:2; a teaching of Shimon ha-Tzaddik. Available at www.myjewishlearning.com/texts/Rabbinics/Talmud/Mishnah/

Seder_Nezikin_Damages_/Pirkei_Avot/Chapter_One.shtml (accessed 2 September 2012).

Prebish, C. and K. Tanaka. (1998). *The Faces of Buddhism in America*. Berkeley: University of California Press.

Puchalski, C. (2000). Physicians and patient spirituality: professional boundaries, competency and ethics. *Annals of Internal Medicine*, 132(7), 578–583.

Puchalski, C. M. (2001). Spirituality and health: the art of compassionate medicine. *Hospital Physician*, 37(3), 30–36.

Puchalski, C. *Institute for Spirituality in Health of Shawnee Mission Medical Center Conference*, information obtained by Steven Jeffers, 2003.

Puchalski, C. and A. Romer. (2000). Taking a spiritual history allows clinicians to understand patients more fully. *Journal of Palliative Medicine*, 3(1), 129–137.

Rahula, W. (1974). *What the Buddha Taught*. New York, NY: Grove Press.

Reader, I. (1991). *Religion in Contemporary Japan*. Honolulu: University of Hawaii Press.

Reader, I. (1991). Letters to the gods: the form and meaning of *ema*. *Japanese Journal of Religious Studies*, 18(1), 23–50.

Royle, E. (1974). *Victorian Infidels*. Manchester: Manchester University Press.

Sadler, A. trans. (1940). *The Ise Daijingu Sankeiki; or, Diary of a Pilgrim to Ise*. Tokyo: Zaidan Hojin Meiji Seitoku Kinen Gakkai. As reprinted in Earhart, H. Byron. (1974). *Religion in the Japanese Experience: Sources and Interpretations*. Encino, CA: Dickenson Publishing.

Salgia, A. (2002). *Pure Freedom: The Jain Way of Self Reliance*. Self-published (can be found at: www.faithresource.org/showcase/Jainism/jainismbooks.htm (accessed 1 Sept 2012) author can be contacted at: asalgia@yahoo.com).

Sanlatta Sutra. PTS [Pali Text Society's English version of the *Tipitaka*]. Oxford: Pali Text Society. 4.

Satprakashananda, S. (1977). *Goal and the Way: The Vedantic Approach to Life's Problems*. St. Louis, MO: Vedanta Society of St. Louis.

Schmidt, R. (1988). *Exploring Religion*. 2nd ed. Belmont, CA: Wadsworth Publishing.

Schulz, W. ed. (1993). *The Unitarian Universalist Pocket Guide*. 2nd ed. Boston, MA: Skinner House Books.

Shinn, R. (1990). *Confessing Our Faith: An Interpretation of the Statement of Faith of the United Church of Christ*. Cleveland, OH: Pilgrim Press.

Sinkford, W. (2005). Real moral values, *UU World*, Volume XIX (2): 7.

Sloan, R. (1999). Religion, spirituality, and medicine [speech]. Twenty-Second Annual Freedom from Religion Foundation Convention, San Antonio, TX, November 6, 1999.

Sloan, R. (2000). Sounding board. *New England Journal of Medicine*, 342(25), 1913.

Sloan, R., E. Bagiella, and T. Powell. (1999). Religion, spirituality, and medicine. *Lancet*, 353(9153), 664–667.

Smith, J. (1980). *The Quest for Holiness and Unity*. Anderson, IN: Warner Press.

Smyers, K. (1999). *The Fox and the Jewel: Shared and Private Meanings in Contemporary Japanese Inari Worship*. Honolulu: University of Hawaii Press.

Snelling, J. (1991). *The Buddhist Handbook*. Rochester, VT: Inner Traditions International.

Spencer-Oatey, H. (2000). *Culturally Speaking: Managing Rapport through Talk Across Cultures*. London: Continuum.

Sperry, L. (2000). Spirituality and psychiatry: incorporating the spiritual dimension into clinical practice. *Psychiatric Annals*, 30(8), 518–523.

Spirituality and Health [information handout]. (June, 2002). Leawood, KS: American Academy of Family Physicians. Available at: http://familydoctor.org/familydoctor/en/prevention-wellness/emotional-wellbeing/mental-health/spirituality-and-health.html (accessed 23 September 2012).

Steinthal P, editor. *Udana*. PTS [Pali Text Society's English version of the *Tipitaka*]. Oxford: Pali Text Society; 1982.

Stoll, R. I. (1979). Guidelines for spiritual assessment. *American Journal of Nursing*, 79(9), 1574–1577.

Strege, M. (1993). *Tell Me Another Tale*. Anderson, IN: Warner Press.

Sulmasy, D. (1997). *The Healer's Calling*. Mahwah, NJ: Paulist Press.

Tanphaichitr, K. (2006). *Buddhism Answers Life*. Bangkok, Thailand: Horatanachai Printing.

Taraporewala, I. (1979). *The Religion of Zarathushtra*. Mumbai, India: Usha Offset Printing Press/Akshar Pratiroop.

Taylor, E. (1998). Spiritual Dimensions of Health Care [course NURS 422], University of Southern California, Department of Nursing. Course information obtained by Steve Jeffers from lecture notes shared by Dr. Taylor with.

Taylor, R. (1990). *The Religious Dimension of Confucianism*. New York: State University of New York Press.

Teeuwen, M. and F. Rambelli. eds. (2003). Introduction to *Buddhas and Kami in Japan*: Honji Suijaku *as a Combinatory Paradigm*. London: Routledge/Curzon. pp. 1–53.

Truog, R. D., M. L. Campbell, J. R. Curtis, et al.; for American College of Critical Care Medicine. (2008). Recommendations for end-of-life care in the intensive care unit: a consensus statement by the American College [corrected] of Critical Care Medicine. *Critical Care Medicine*, 36(3), 953–963.

Tu, W. (1985). *Confucian Thought: Selfhood as Creative Transformation*. Albany, NY: State University of New York Press.

Tucker, M. E. and J. Berthrong. eds. (1998). *Confuianism and Ecology: The Interrelation of Heaven, Earth, and Humans*. Cambridge, MA: Harvard University Center for the Study of World Religions.

Unitarian Universalist Association. Abortion. 1977 General Resolution, August 24, 2011.

Available at: www.uua.org/socialjustice/socialjustice/statements/20250.shtml (accessed 2 September 2012).

Unitarian Universalist Association. Legality of Living Wills. 1978 Resolution, August 24, 2011, www.uua.org/socialjustice/socialjustice/statements/20279.shtml (accessed 2 September 2012.

Unitarian Universalist Association. National Health Plan, 1971 General Resolution. Last updated August 24, 2011. Available at: www.uua.org/socialjustice/socialjustice/statements/19770.shtml (accessed 2 September 2012).

Unitarian Universalist Association of Congregations. Reproductive Choice. 1998 General Resolution. Last updated March 19, 2012. Available at: www.uua.org/socialjustice/issues/reproductive/reproductivehealth/24042.shtml (accessed 2 September 2012).

Unitarian Universalist Association of Congregations. The Right to Die with Dignity. 1998 General Resolution. Last updated March 19, 2012. Available at: www.uua.org/statements/statements/14486.shtml (accessed 15 October 2012).

Unitarian Universalist Association of Congregations. *Singing the Living Tradition*. (1993). Boston, MA: Beacon Press.

United Methodist Book of Worship. (1992). Nashville, TN: United Methodist Publishing House.

United Methodist Hymnal. (1989). Nashville, TN: United Methodist Publishing House.

Vest, J. L. (2006). Panel: Health Disparities and Native Americans. Fifteenth Annual Meeting of the Association for Practical and Professional Ethics, Saturday, March 4.

Vivekananda, S. (1986). *Vedanta: Voice of Freedom*. St. Louis, MO: Vedanta Society of St. Louis.

Von Staden, H. ed. (1989). *The Art of Medicine in Early Alexandria*. London: Cambridge University Press.

Voytovich, S. (1990). The ministry of those who suffer. Unpublished MDiv thesis.

Walsh, K., M. King, L. Jones, et al. (2002).

Spiritual beliefs may affect outcome of bereavement: prospective study. *British Medical Journal*, 324(7353), 1551–1554.

Watson, B. trans. (1993). *The Lotus Sutra*. New York, NY: Oxford University Press.

Watson, B. trans. (1997). *The Vimalakirti Sutra*. New York, NY: Columbia University Press.

Wesley, J. (1733). Circumcision of the heart. In E. Sugden, ed. (1983). *John Wesley's Fifty-Three Sermons*. Nashville, TN: Abingdon Press. pp. 188–189.

Wittlinger, C. (1978). *Quest for Piety and Obedience*. Nappanee, IN: Evangel Press.

Yaconelli, M. (2002). *Messy Spirituality*. Grand Rapids, MI: Zondervan.

Yao, X. (2000). *An Introduction to Confucianism*. New York, NY: Cambridge University Press.

Yeagley, L. Living with dying. Adventist Health System Mission Conference. Information obtained in interview with Larry Yeagley at the conference, February 2004.

Zedek, M., interview by Steven Jeffers, Center for Practical Bioethics' Compassion Sabbath February 4, 2000.

Websites

AFRICAN METHODIST EPISCOPAL CHURCH

African Methodist Episcopal Church Connectional Health Commission: www.AMECHealth.org (accessed 16 Sept 12).

BAHÁ'Í FAITH

Bahá'í Distribution Service: www.bahaibookstore.com (accessed 16 Sept 12).

Bahá'í Faith: www.bahai.us (accessed 16 Sept 12).

The Bahá'í Faith: www.bahai.org (accessed 16 Sept 12).

Bahá'í Topics: www.info.bahai.org (accessed 16 Sept 12).

BUDDHISM

Buddhist Churches of America (Pure Land Buddhism): http://buddhistchurchesofamerica.org (accessed 16 Sept 12).

Hsi Lai Temple: www.hsilai.org/ (accessed 16 Sept 12).

Soka Gakkai International – USA (Nichiren Buddhism): www.sgi-usa.org (accessed 16 Sept 12).

Zen Mountain Monastery (Zen Buddhism): www.mro.org (accessed 16 Sept 12); email zmmtrain@mro.org

CHRISTIAN SCIENCE

Christian Science: www.spirituality.com (accessed 16 Sept 12).

EASTERN RITE CATHOLIC CHURCH

www.east2west.org/doctrine.htm (accessed 16 Sept 12).

HINDUISM

Hinduism: www.hinduism.co.za/ (accessed 16 Sept 12).

ISLAM

http://humanity.com/islamia/psalms_of_islam.htm (accessed 16 Sept 12).

JUDAISM

"Daily Prayer of a Physician": www.jewishvirtuallibrary.org/jsource/Judaism/mdprayer.html (accessed 16 Sept 12).

MENNONITES

www.themennonite.org/public_press_releases/Anabaptist_Center_for_Healthcare_Ethics (accessed 16 Sept 12).

Associated Mennonite Biblical Seminary: www.ambs.edu/ (accessed 16 Sept 12).

Mennonite Church USA: www.mennoniteusa.org/ (accessed 16 Sept 12).

Mennonite Mutual Aid: www.mmasohio.com (accessed 16 Sept 12).

MHS Alliance, Mennonite Health Services: www.mhsonline.org/ (accessed 16 Sept 12).

Third Way Café: www.thirdway.com (accessed 16 Sept 12).

ORTHODOX CHRISTIANITY

Orthodox Church in America: www.oca.org/ (accessed 16 Sept 12).

www.wellsprings.org.uk/rublevs_icon/trinity. htm (accessed 16 Sept 12).

PAGANISM

http://altreligion.about.com/library/glossary/ symbols/bldefswiccasymbols.htm (accessed 9 Sept 2012).

"Charge of the Goddess": www.reclaiming. org/about/witchfaq/charge.html (accessed 9 Sept 2012).

DONA International: www.dona.org/ mothers/index.php (accessed 9 Sept 2012).

Witchvox: www.witchvox.com (accessed 9 Sept 2012).

UNITED CHURCH OF CHRIST

United Church of Christ: www.ucc.org/ (accessed 16 Sept 12).

UNITED METHODIST CHURCH

United Methodist Church: www.umc.org/ (accessed 16 Sept 12).

UNITY

Frequently asked questions about Unity: www.unityonline.org/discover_faq.htm (accessed 23 September 2012).

Unity: www.unityonline.org/ (accessed 16 September 2012).

www.unitychurchofmemphis.com/ UnityBasics.html (accessed 16 Sept 12).

ZOROASTRIANISM

Ahunwar (most sacred manthra of Zoroastrianism): www.avesta.org/ ka/ka_part1.htm#ahunwar (accessed 23 September 2012).

Aogemadaeca: www.avesta.org/fragment/ aogsbe.htm (accessed 23 September 2012).

English translation of Holy Zend Avesta – Yasna: www.ishwar.com/zoroastrianism/ holy_zend_avesta/yasna/ (accessed 23 September 2012).

www.avesta.org/ritual/funeral.htm (accessed 23 September 2012).

Printed and bound by CPI Group (UK) Ltd, Croydon, CR0 4YY

25/10/2024

01779131-0001